Instructor Resources for Success

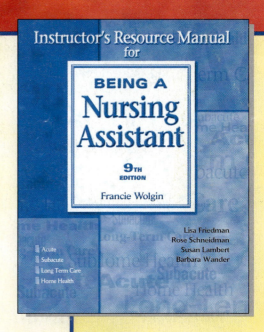

Instructor's Resource Manual for
BEING A Nursing Assistant
9TH EDITION
Francie Wolgin

Lisa Friedman
Rose Schneidman
Susan Lambert
Barbara Wander

Acute
Subacute
Long Term Care
Home Health

INSTRUCTOR'S RESOURCE MANUAL

ISBN: 0-13-177990-7

This **free** manual contains a wealth of material to help faculty plan and manage the nursing assisting course. For each chapter, it includes Learning Objectives, Chapter Overviews, Key Terms, Suggested Teaching Strategies, a Complete Test Bank, and more. For added convenience, The Instructor's Resource Manual also contains an annotated workbook.

INSTRUCTOR'S RESOURCE CD-ROM

ISBN: 0-13-177991-5

This cross-platform CD-ROM includes PowerPoint slides with images and discussion points, an Electronic Test Bank, a printable version of the Instructor's Resource Manual, Videos, and a Transition Guide for a smooth changeover to the new edition. Available to faculty **free** upon adoption of the textbook.

COMPANION WEBSITE SYLLABUS MANAGER

www.prenhall.com/wolgin

Faculty adopting this textbook have **free** access to the online Syllabus Manager feature of the Companion Website, **www.prenhall.com/wolgin**. Syllabus Manager offers a whole host of features that facilitate the students' use of the Companion Website and allow faculty to post syllabi and course information online for their students. For more information or a demonstration of Syllabus Manager, please contact a Prentice Hall Sales Representative.

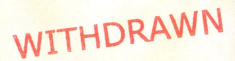

BEING A
Nursing Assistant

9TH EDITION

BEING A
Nursing
Assistant

9TH EDITION

Francie Wolgin, MSN, RN

Community Health Development Program Officer
The Health Foundation of Greater Cincinnati
Cincinnati, Ohio

- Acute
- Subacute
- Long Term Care
- Home Health

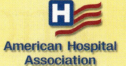

American Hospital Association

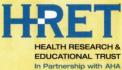

HEALTH RESEARCH &
EDUCATIONAL TRUST
In Partnership with AHA

PEARSON
Prentice Hall

Prentice Hall Health
Upper Saddle River, New Jersey 07458

Library of Congress Cataloging-in-Publication Data

Wolgin, Francie.
    Being a nursing assistant. — 9th ed. / Francie Wolgin.
      p. cm.
    Includes index.
    ISBN 0-13-182873-8
    1. Nurses' aides. 2. Care of the sick.   I. American Hospital
Association.
    [DNLM: 1. Nurses' Aides. 2. Nursing Care—methods.
WY 193 W861b 2000]
RT84.S35 2000
610.73'06'98–DC21
DNLM/DLC
for Library of Congress   99–31931
                                          CIP

Publisher: *Julie Levin Alexander*
Assistant to the Publisher: *Regina Bruno*
Editor-in-Chief: *Maura Connor*
Executive Editor: *Barbara Krawiec*
Managing Development Editor: *Marilyn Meserve*
Development Editor: *Maureen Muncaster*
Editorial Assistant: *Jennifer Dwyer*
Director of Production & Manufacturing: *Bruce Johnson*
Managing Production Editor: *Patrick Walsh*
Production Liason: *Mary C. Treacy*
Production Editor: *John Probst,* The GTS Companies/York, PA
Campus
Manufacturing Manager: *Ilene Sanford*
Manufacturing Buyer: *Pat Brown*
Design Director: *Cheryl Asherman*
Senior Design Coordinator: *Maria Guglielmo Walsh*
Manager of Media Production: *Amy Peltier*
Senior Media Editor: *John J. Jordan*
New Media Product Manager: *Stephen Hartner*
Media Development Editor: *Sheba Jalaluddin*
Senior Marketing Manager: *Nicole Benson*
Marketing Assistant: *Janet Ryerson*
Channel Marketing Manager: *Rachele Strober*
Composition: The GTS Companies/*York, PA Campus*
Illustrator: *Precision Graphics*
Cover Printer: *Lehigh Press*
Printer/Binder: *Von Hoffman Press*

Published for The Hospital Research and Education Trust by Prentice-Hall Inc., Upper Saddle River, New Jersey 07458

Printed in the United States of America
1 2 3 4 5 6 7 8 9 10

ISBN 0-13-182873-8

Pearson Education Ltd.
Pearson Education Australia Pty, Limited
Pearson Education Singapore, Pte. Ltd
Pearson Education North Asia Ltd
Pearson Education Canada Ltd
Pearson Educación de Mexico, S.A. de C.V.
Pearson Education—Japan
Pearson Education Malaysia, Pte, Ltd
Pearson Education, Upper Saddle River, New Jersey

Dedication

I would like to dedicate this book to my daughter, Rebecca, and to my colleagues, committed to empowering and developing others.

NOTICE

The procedures described in this textbook are based on consultation with nursing authorities. The author and publisher have taken care to make certain that these procedures reflect currently accepted clinical practice; however, they cannot be considered absolute recommendations.

The material in this textbook contains the most current information available at the time of publication. However, federal, state and local guidelines concerning clinical practices, including without limitation, those governing infection control and universal precautions, change rapidly. The reader should note, therefore, that new regulations may require changes in some procedures.

It is the responsibility of the reader to familiarize himself or herself with the policies and procedures set by federal, state and local agencies, as well as the institution or agency where the reader is employed. The authors and the publishers of this textbook, and the supplements written to accompany it, disclaim any liability, loss or risk resulting directly or indirectly from the suggested procedures and theory, from any undetected errors, or from the reader's misunderstanding of the text. It is the reader's responsibility to stay informed of any new changes or recommendations made by any federal, state and local agency as well as by his or her employing health care institution or agency.

Note on Gender Usage

The English language has historically given preference to the male gender. Among many words, the pronouns, "he" and "his" are commonly used to describe both genders. The male pronouns still predominate our speech, however, in this text "he" and "she" have been used interchangeably when referring to the Nursing Assistant and/or the patient. The repeated use of "he or she" is not proper in long manuscript, and the use of "he or she" is not correct in all cases. The author has made great effort to treat the two genders equally. Throughout the text, solely for the purpose of brevity, male pronouns and female pronouns are often used to describe both males and females. This is not intended to offend any reader of the female or male gender.

Notice Re "The Nursing Assistant in Action"

The names used in the case studies throughout this text are fictitious.

To the Student

A self-instructional workbook for this text is available through a college bookstore under the title, *Workbook for Being a Nursing Assistant,* 9th edition ISBN # 0-13-117986-9. If not in stock, ask the bookstore manager to order a copy for you. If your course is being offered off-campus, ask your instructor where to obtain a copy. The workbook can help you with course material by acting as a tutorial review and study aid.

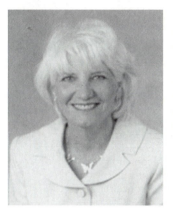

Francie Wolgin, MSN, RN Francie Wolgin serves as Community Health Development Program Officer for THE HEALTH FOUNDATION OF GREATER CINCINNATI. She maintains a relationship with colleagues currently teaching nursing assistants, patient care technicians and nursing students in several states. She serves on the advisory board of Cross Country University and the Medcom Nursing Advisory Board. She was awarded the University of Cincinnati College of Nursing Distinguished Alumni Award in 1999.

Ms. Wolgin's previous positions include System Leader for Education and Employee Development, St. Joseph Mercy Hospital (SJMH), Ann Arbor, Michigan. She served four years as Director of Operations Support and Practice Development at SJMH, and as president of the National Nursing Staff Development Organization. In addition, Ms. Wolgin served as an adjunct faculty member at the University of Michigan School of Nursing. She serves on the advisory board of Cross Country University, and on the editorial board of *Nursing Management.*

Ms. Wolgin has been Director of Nursing Practice Development and Clinical Associate at the School of Nursing, Duke University Medical Center; she has held several management, staff development, and administrative positions at the University of Cincinnati Hospital; and a faculty appointment at the University of Cincinnati College of Nursing and Health. She served on the *Journal of Nursing Staff Development* editorial board for several years. She is the author of *Advanced Skills for Caregivers, Being a Nursing Assistant, 7th and 8th editions,* as well as many articles. She regularly contributes to books on staff development, competency, and training of advanced nursing assistants. Extensive experience as a direct caregiver in a variety of positions gives her both perspective and firsthand knowledge of the challenges and opportunities available throughout the health care continuum.

Guidelines and Procedures

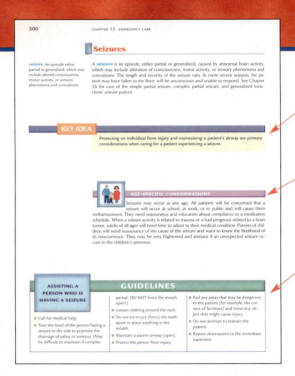

KEY IDEA

Important points are highlighted with a Key Idea icon.

AGE-SPECIFIC CONSIDERATIONS

This feature points out age-specific considerations to take into account when performing a task or skill.

GUIDELINES

Important principles of care are highlighted throughout the text to guide your care of the patient.

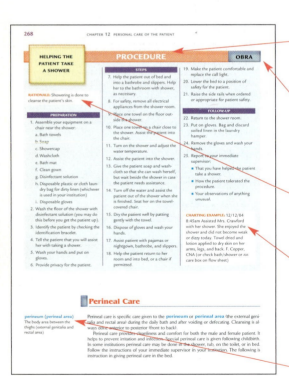

PROCEDURES

Preparation and Follow-up steps are included with procedures when appropriate, so you have everything you need to successfully complete each procedure in one easy-to-find place.

OBRA DESIGNATION

This icon identifies mandatory OBRA content.

RATIONALE

Explains why the procedure is done.

CHARTING

This feature provides an example of what you would document.

MARGIN GLOSSARY

Key Terms are presented in the margin with each term printed in color and followed by the definition.

End-of-Chapter Review

CHAPTER REVIEW

Fill-in-the-blank and multiple choice questions test your understanding of chapter content and help you prepare for the certification exam.

TIME OUT/TIPS FOR TIME MANAGEMENT

Designed to promote your personal and career growth and development, these tips appear at the end of each chapter and help you develop communication, planning and organizational skills, as well as self-discipline.

NURSING ASSISTANT IN ACTION

Provides scenarios based on real-life issues and challenges that you may encounter on the job.

CRITICAL THINKING

These questions will challenge you to apply what you have learned about:

Customer Service

Cultural Care

Cooperation within a Team

EXPLORE MEDIALINK

Calls your attention to activities and resources on the **free** CD-ROM which includes videos and an audio glossary, and website that accompany your textbook.

Click on www.prenhall.com/wolgin for:

Objectives present the learning outcomes

Chapter Outline provides the chapter-specific content outline for student reference

Audio Glossary provides key terms, definitions, and correct pronunciations

Certification Exam-style Review Questions provide practice and immediate feedback for exam-style questions

Case Study provides a brief client scenario followed by critical thinking questions

Study Tip provides helpful suggestions for learning challenging skills and concepts

Toolbox provides additional handy reference material

Web Links present hyperlinks

Faculty Office provides lecture notes for your convenience

Syllabus Manager allows faculty and students the convenience of creating and easily updating an electronic syllabus

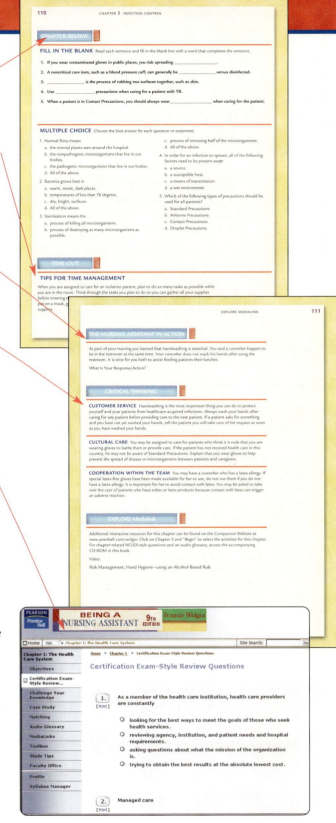

You are entering a challenging and ever-changing health care environment. Being a nursing assistant isn't just another job, but a serious occupation where you are an important part of a team providing health care services. Nursing assistants work in a variety of settings, ranging from within the home, to an office or a clinic, or to an extended care or acute care hospital setting. *Being A Nursing Assistant, 9th Edition* and all the accompanying supplements have been significantly revised, redesigned, and expanded to provide practical core material which makes up the foundation of your practice. As you may know, nursing programs are frequently requiring students to enter the program with nursing assistant certification or training evidence. What you learn as a nursing assistant will become your basic foundation of health care knowledge if you choose to enter a nursing program.

Some of the chapters will be more important to you than others, depending on your practice area or workplace setting. Material that may not seem necessary to know today can become vital if you find yourself being cross-trained to work in a different position, or to accept a job in a different health care setting.

Continuing developments in care technology and increased use of computers to document patient care will necessitate changes or, perhaps, the elimination of certain procedures and tasks. There are, however, core aspects of caring that will be ongoing. Examples include communicating effectively and providing compassionate care that takes into consideration the patient's physical, emotional, and spiritual needs, as well as cultural and age-specific considerations.

This book has been revised and rewritten following an extensive assessment process. The ideas and expressed needs of instructors and students across the country were given serious consideration. Colleagues and educators who have both experience and practical expertise in a variety of practice settings and specialties have contributed as chapter authors and reviewers. Their varied areas of expertise, knowledge, and competency assessment have been skillfully edited and integrated into this book. As a result, *Being a Nursing Assistant, 9th Edition* has been completely updated to prepare you for today's health care environment with new content and technology that includes:

- **Free** Student CD-ROM with certification review, multiple choice questions, nursing skills videos, and an audioglossary.

- **Age-Specific Considerations** are integrated throughout the book.

- **Expanded end-of-chapter exercises** will help you prepare for the certification exam with fill-in-the-blank and multiple-choice questions. Critical thinking components will challenge you to apply what you have learned, while time management tips will help you develop communication, organizational, and planning skills. The Medialink section brings it all together with multimedia activities using our companion Website, CD, and videos.

- **Career-Related Topics** include a section on computer skills as well as information on accepting, keeping, and resigning from a job.

- **Updated Infection Control Chapter** includes hand hygiene, Hepatitis C, revised Contact Precautions, and an introduction to aseptic and sterile technique for nursing assistants who will be working in areas where this information is needed.

- **New Material** has been added to keep you up-to-date with the latest developments and trends in health care, including SARS precautions, new restraints and related policies, care of patients with Alzheimer's disease, noninvasive blood pressure monitoring; restorative care; skin care; communication skills; computer skills; GI system and ostomy care; adults >75 to 100+; care of patient following a total hip or total knee replacement; cancer; AIDS care; sun downing; home health care; mental health care; substance abuse; and depression. Advanced Procedures for practitioners in states that permit NAs to use these skills.

- **New Procedures and Guidelines** cover care of patients with stroke, burns, hemorrhage, shock and seizures, and feeding a patient with dysphagia.

- **Rationales and Charting Examples** for all Procedures make the purpose of the procedure explicit and train the student in documentation.

- **Nursing Assistant in Action feature** provides new scenarios based on actual, real-life issues and challenges which you may encounter on the job. This feature appears for each chapter.

- **Tear-Out Clinical Pocket Translator** provides Spanish translations of commonly encountered words and phrases to help enhance patient care through improved communication.

Your instructor will modify content or steps of procedures when necessary to comply with the standards of your community or state. Because there are significant differences and state variations as to which skills may be performed by nursing assistants, your instructor offers the most current information that applies to your role. You are responsible for knowing what the scope of your role is, as well as the particular policies, protocols and procedures of your employer. Your instructor or employer may provide you with this information, if not, it is important that you ask where you can obtain such information. Only perform those procedures you have been educated or validated to do.

Being a Nursing Assistant, 9th Edition will prepare you to be a successful nursing assistant by providing the core content and procedures you will need to function in a wide variety of practice settings. Welcome to the continuously challenging and learning environment that is health care!

Student and Instructor Resources for Success

Instructors and students who have used previous editions of *Being a Nursing Assistant* will notice that we've created a new interior and exterior design to be more appealing to today's students. While we've changed our look, we didn't change the basics that have helped students successfully master material, such as exceptional readability, clear, easy-to-follow procedures, and a complete supplements package. Our supplements package includes all the traditional components such as an instructor's guide and student workbook and, in addition, has been updated to take advantage of new technology:

- **New Companion Website** (www.prenhall.com/wolgin), tied chapter-by-chapter to the text, gives students an on-line study guide that provides immediate feedback. The Companion Website also enables instructors to create a customized syllabus.

- **Free Student CD-ROM** helps students master key terminology with an audio glossary.

- **Instructor's Resource Manual** makes managing and preparing for class a snap with teaching suggestions, chapter overviews, objectives and key terms, student assignments, answers to end-of-chapter questions, as well as full page reproductions of student workbook pages with answers.

- **Student Workbook** features a variety of activities, including multiple-choice questions, labeling, fill-in-the-blank, and matching. We've also included competency checklists where appropriate for self-assessment.
- **Instructor's Resource CD-ROM** will help you prepare tests with a large bank of test questions. Additional teaching aids include Power Point slides with images and lecture outlines, and videos.

Brief Contents

Detailed Contents

DETAILED CONTENTS

DETAILED CONTENTS

DETAILED CONTENTS

Procedures

■ Indicates mandatory OBRA content. The page number follows the procedure title.

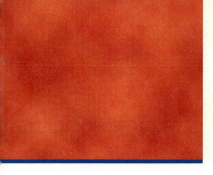

Guidelines

■ Indicates mandatory OBRA content. The page number follows the guideline title.

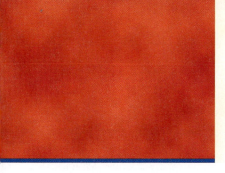

Acknowledgments

This Ninth Edition of *Being a Nursing Assistant* has been prepared by Francie Wolgin, MSN, RN, CNA and her dedicated team of professionals. Individually, they each worked with extraordinary commitment on this revision. Together, they formed a team of highly dedicated professionals who have upheld the highest standards of current instruction for Nursing Assistants.

For their contributions to the Ninth Edition, we gratefully thank:

Jane Campbell, MSN, RN, CS   Gerontology Clinical Nurse Specialist, UNC Memorial Hospital, Chapel Hill, NC

Doris A. Clark, RN, BC, BSN, MSN   PN Faculty, Harrison Center for Career Education, Washington D.C.

Patricia DeiTos, RN, MSN   Program Developer, Continuing Education and Workforce Development, Northern Virginia Community College, Annandale, VA

Lisa Friedman, MS, RN,   Education Specialist, Education and Employee Development, Saint Joseph Mercy Hospital, Ann Arbor, MI

Gail Howard, RN   Clinical Instructor, Staff Development Department, University of Louisville Hospital Louisville, KY

Sofia Moyano-Kleckner, MA, MEd   Training Director, Santa Maria Community Services, Cincinnati, OH

Russell Olmsted, MPH, CIC   Saint Joseph Mercy Hospital, Infection Control, Ann Arbor, MI

Ann Perrin, LISW, CCDC III   Program Officer for Substance Abuse Focus Area for the Health Foundation of Greater Cincinnati, Cincinnati, OH

Deborah L. Stevenson, RN, BSN   Instructor, Hillsborough Community College, Tampa, FL

Gloria Sveller, MSN, RN   Education Coordinator, Education and Employee Development, Saint Joseph Mercy Hospital, Ann Arbor, MI

Thanks to the following Eighth Edition Contributors:

Phylis Brandon-Root, BSN, RN   Infusion Specialist, St. Joseph Mercy Home Care, Ann Arbor, MI

Barb Boylan Lewis, BSN, MA, CETN   Enterostomy Therapy Nurse, St. Joseph Mercy Hospital, Ann Arbor, MI. Member of the Wound, Ostomy, and Continence Nurses' Society (WOCN)

Marti A. Burton, RN, BS   Former Practical Nursing Instructor at Metrotech Technology Center, Oklahoma City, OK

Jane M.Campbell, MSN, RN, CS   Gerontology Clinical Nurse Specialist, UNC Memorial Hospital, Chapel Hill, NC

Ruth Churly-Strohm MSN, RN, PNP   Education Specialist, Education and Employee Development SJMHS, Ann Arbor, MI

Lisa F. Friedman, MS, RN   Education Specialist, Education and Employee Development, SJMHS, Ann Arbor, MI and Coordinator Policies and Procedures

Julee Huss, RN   Supervisor and Nurse Educator, The Shook Home, Chambersburg, PA

Christeen Conlin Holdwick, MA, RN, CNAA System Leader Organization Development, SJMHS, Ann Arbor, MI

Gloria Sveller, MSN, RN Education Coordinator, Education and Employee Development, SJMHS, Ann Arbor, MI. Coordinator of the Patient Care Assistant Education and PCT Program

Kathy Wickman, BSN, MA, CETN Wound, Ostomy and Continence Specialist, St. Joseph Mercy Hospital, Ann Arbor, MI

Jan Treston-Aurand, MS, RN, CIC Infection Control Practitioner, St. Joseph Mercy Health System, Ann Arbor, MI

Thanks to the following Seventh Edition contributors:

Terry Ainsworth, MS, RN, NP Duke University Medical Center

Barb Boylan Lewis, BSN, MA, CETN St. Joseph Mercy Hospital, Ann Arbor, MI

Christeen Conlin Holdwick, MA, RN, CNAA St. Joseph Mercy Hospital, Ann Arbor, MI

Martha Dawson, MSN, RN, VP University of Louisville Hospital

Lou Ebrite, PhD, MS, BS, RN University of Central Oklahoma, Edmond, OK

Cinda Fluke, MEd, RN, CNAA Director of Medical Nursing, Parkland Hospital, Dallas TX

Lisa F. Friedman, MS, RN St. Joseph Mercy Hospital, Ann Arbor, MI

Geraldine Heneghan, MS, RN, CETN, CRN EKA-Division Medical, Capital Heights, MD

Amy F. Larson, MS, RN, CNRN St. Joseph Mercy Hospital, Ann Arbor, MI

Melodee J. Leimnetzer, MSM, RN Lifelink Corporation, Bensenville, IL

Lisa McDowell, MS, RD, CNSD Coordinator of Clinical Nutrition, St. Joseph Mercy Hospital, Ann Arbor, MI

Jerene Maune, MS, RN, CETN, CVN Johns Hopkins Wound Healing Center, Baltimore, MD

Mary Morochnick, BA, RN Nurse Manager Rehabilitation, DUMC

Glenda Pavia, RN, CRRN Rivergate Terrace, Riverview, MI

JoLynn Pulliam, MS, RN, CPHQ St. Joseph Hospital and Supervisor at St. Mary Hospital in Livonia, MI

Caroline Schultz, MS, OTR Work Capacity Services, St. Joseph Mercy Hospital, Ann Arbor, MI

T. Jane Swain, MS, RN, VP St. Elizabeth Medical Center, Covington, KY

Jan Treston-Aurand, MS, RN, CIC St. Joseph Mercy Hospital, Ann Arbor, MI

Kelly M. Warnock, RN Duke University Medical Center, Durham, NC

In addition, the author would like to acknowledge and thank the following organizations and individuals for contributing immeasurably to this edition.

Prentice Hall Health

Julie Alexander, publisher, Prentice Hall Health, for the implementation of her visionary approach and creative ideas.

Maura Connor, editor-in-chief, nursing/health related professions/health occupations, for guidance in making the text user friendly and a pleasure to use.

Barbara Krawiec, acquisitions editor, for her intuition and understanding of the task; for supporting the author in assembling a contributing group of professionals with the expertise and the knowledge needed for this ambitious project.

Marilyn C. Meserve, senior managing editor, development, health related professions, for providing hands-on commitment, zealous energy, and unique coordinating skills from the beginning of the project through its completion.

Jennifer Dwyer, editorial assistant, Prentice Hall Health, for providing critical editorial support and assistance in various stages of the project.

Nicole Benson, marketing manager, Prentice Hall Health, for the development and the implementation of the marketing strategies, the outreach, and the promotions for all components of the program.

Pat Walsh, managing editor, production, Prentice Hall Health, for providing production leadership and guidance to meet the needs of the project, including the text, the multimedia components, and the additional supplemental parts of the program.

Mary Treacy, project manager, production, for her management, coordination of materials, cross-checking all phases of production, the control and mastery of technical details, and communication with all involved on the project.

Ilene Sanford, senior manufacturing manager, for her planning and management of the many details and schedules behind the printing and binding process.

Maria Guglielmo, senior design coordinator, Prentice Hall Health, for her patience and creative contributions in bringing together the design of the book, including both the interior and the cover.

Organizations

Special thanks to Garry Faja, President and CEO, Saint Joseph Mercy Health System, and Julie MacDonald, Senior VP, St. Joseph Mercy Hospital, Ann Arbor, MI, for their support throughout the project and for granting permission to reprint or adapt, within this book and its supplements, materials and forms from Saint Joseph Mercy Health System, St. Joseph Mercy Hospital and Home Care. Appreciation is also extended to Kathleen Rhine, VP, Human Resources, SJMHS.

Technical Advisors

The publisher wishes to acknowledge the cooperation of organizations and individuals who assisted in the photography program. For their invaluable contribution to the accuracy of these photographs, the technical advisors who supervised the procedures portrayed in these photographs were:

Lisa Friedman, MS, RN	Education Specialist
David Micham, BS, RRT	RT Education Coordinator
Gloria Sveller, MSN, RN	Education Coordinator
Dolores McAdoo, RN	Instructor
Susan Reddel, RN	Instructor

For assistance in the photography shoots by providing space, technical assistance, materials, and a pool of extremely competent CNAs to model in our photographs, or very special thanks to:

Mary Lou Proch, Director of Education
Sara Anthony, Education Department
Nurses and Staff of Eight Tower East
Sarasota Memorial Hospital
Sarasota, FL

Victoria Haines, Staff Services Assistant
Sarasota Memorial Hospital Staff Services
Sarasota, FL

Paul Farineau, Education Director
Home Health Services of Sarasota
Sarasota, FL

Elizabeth Bess, Director
Cindi Aun, RN, Director of Nursing
Joyce Stobbs, BS Director of Social Services
Heartland Health Care and Rehabilitation Center
Sarasota, FL

Deborah Metheny, RN, MS, Assistant Director SCTI
Pamela Bull LaGasse, RN, EdD, Department Chairperson, Allied Health
Sarasota County Technical Institute
Sarasota, FL

David Bobish, Director of Nursing
Physicians Dialysis Center
Sarasota, FL

Photography Models: For their gracious assistance in finding models to portray the patients
in our photographs:
Cynthia Clements, Jan Wright and members of the following organizations:
The New Sarasotans Club
Sarasota, FL

First Congregational United Church of Christ
Sarasota, FL

St. Andrew United Church of Christ
Sarasota, FL

Broadway Theatre Academy
Susan Swanson, Director
Sarasota, FL

Credits

ACE is the registered trademark of Peg Bandage, Inc.
Acetest is the registered trademark of Miles, Inc., Diagnostics Div.
Band-Aid is the registered trademark of Johnson & Johnson Medical, Inc. and Johnson
   & Johnson Consumer Products, Inc.
Clinitest is the registered trademark of Miles, Inc., Diagnostics Div.
K-Pad is the registered trademark of Katecho, Inc.
T.E.D. is the registered trademark of The Kendall Co.
Velcro is the registered trademark of Velcro USA, Inc.

Reviewers

The following reviewers provided invaluable feedback and suggestions. We wish to thank
each of these professionals for their contributions.

Reviewers for the Ninth Edition

Gloria Bizjak MEd, EMT

Instructor Trainer, Curriculum Developer
Maryland Fire and Rescue Institute, University of Maryland
College Park, MD

Patricia Deitos, RN, MSN
Program Developer, Continuing Education and Workforce Development
Northern Virginia Community College
Annandale, VA

Sandra Gustafson, MA, RN
Nursing Faculty
Hibbing Community College
Hibbing, MN

Patty Leary, MSEd
Instructor
Mecosta Osceola Career Center
Big Rapids, MI

Russell N. Olmsted, MPH, CIC
Epidemiologist, Infection Control Services
Saint Joseph Mercy Health System
Ann Arbor, MI

Vickie T. Poole, RN
Instructor, Health and Medical Sciences
Halifax County High School
South Boston, VA

Ann E. Sims, RN, BSN
Nursing Assistant Programs Director
Albuquerque Technical Vocational Institute
Albuquerque, NM

Victoria Skiles, RN, BSN
Staff Development/Infection Control Coordinator
Tel Hai Nursing Center
Honeybrook, PA

Tammy J. Taylor, RN
Assistant Professor of Nursing, CNA Program Coordinator
Heartland Community College
Normal, IL

Reviewers for the Eighth Edition

Patti Biro
Director of Healthcare Programs
Del Mar College
Corpus Christi, TX

Marie Boucher RN
Director
Helping Hands Trade School
Waterville, ME

Judith T. Kautz MS, RN
Education Director
Pima Medical Institute
Tucson, AZ

Catherine Mainville RN, BS
Rhode Island Central Directory for Nurses
Providence, RI

ACKNOWLEDGMENTS

Nancy Pimentel RN
Life-Stream/Cognosco
New Bedford, MA

Diane Weeks RN
Onondaga Cortland Madison Boces
Cortland, NY

Kathy Williford RN, MSN
Department Chair - Nursing
Edgecomb Community College
Tarboro, NC

Reviewers for the Seventh Edition

Judith Ann Avie, RN, BSN, MEd IT
Vice President
United Training Services
Professional Services Department
Southfield, MI
Also: Instructor
              Instructional Design and Development
              Wayne State University
Also: Instructor
              College of Health Science
              University of Detroit Mercy

John Bennett, RN, BSN, MSN
Instructor
Education and Training
South Hills Home Health Agency
Homestead, PA

Introduction

Welcome to the diverse and challenging field of health care. You are, or will be, working in the health care system where the delivery of patient care services is the focus of employer and employee alike. Whether you work in a large metropolitan hospital, a suburban nursing home, an inner-city or rural outpatient clinic, or the patient's home, *the patient* is the most important person. All personnel are there to provide care or to treat the sick and injured.

Being a Nursing Assistant offers you an extensive resource to help you as you study—learn and train—and as you are on the job. Your instructor will guide your learning/training during class, lectures, practice sessions, and clinical experiences, and will teach you the procedures and policies that are required in your state and in the institution, agency, or delivery site where you will be working because **methods and policies vary from state to state and from one health care setting to another.**

Health care delivery systems are continually changing to meet the ever-growing demands for health care services. Institutions, agencies, and their personnel must respond rapidly to make use of new research findings, insights, techniques, or equipment changes. If this text, or any other source, takes one approach to a situation and your instructor takes a different approach, follow your instructor. Your instructor is an expert in health care delivery and is the authority for your course.

On the job, you will be supervised by the nurse manager, supervisor, or team leader. They may not necessarily be the same person, although they might be. We use the term immediate supervisor throughout this book to refer to the person who supervises you and keeps a record of your performance. During your training, if you do not understand a procedure, ask your instructor for help. On the job, ask your nurse manager or team leader. It is far better to get help if you are not sure, than to do something wrong.

The more you know about how *Being a Nursing Assistant, 9th Edition* is organized the more help you will gain from using it. Take the time now to read the next few pages to find out what's in *Being a Nursing Assistant, 9th Edition*—where it is and how to find it.

Contents

All chapters and main headings, as well as procedures and guidelines, that appear in the chapters are listed in the Contents.

Introduction

A paragraph at the beginning of each chapter highlights the content, issues, or concepts presented in the chapter. You may find it helpful to consider what you already know about the chapter content and to develop a list of questions you hope to answer as you read the chapter. Such efforts at focusing on the content are very helpful. Other techniques for studying are provided in *Using This Textbook* which follows the Glossary description.

Objectives

Each chapter begins with a list of objectives that tells you what you should be able to do by the end of the chapter. The objectives describe measurable or reachable goals—procedures or tasks to be performed, guidelines to be followed, information to be recalled and used. Use the Chapter Review at the end of the chapter to help you review the content and assess how well you have understood the content and met the objectives.

Always be sure to:

- Take notes (write words or phrases, or perhaps make drawings or sketches).
- Make connections with what you already know about the topic.
- Make a list of questions (no more than three or four) about what you want to learn.

Read the chapter carefully, paying particular attention to the Objectives, Key Terms, Key Ideas, and Age-Specific Considerations. They will help you identify key concepts, ideas, and issues in the chapter. Follow your instructor's directions, and note information about policies and practices that relate to your institution.

Always be sure to:

- Keep in mind the Objectives for the chapter.
- Note words or phrases that are **bold** or seem important to you.
- Take a closer look at tables, charts, photographs, and illustrations.
- Jot down information that answers your preview questions.
- Use the Chapter Review to help you recall and meet the objectives.
- Ask your instructor for help with concepts, procedures, or guidelines you find difficult.
- Re-read sections related to questions you are unable to answer.

CD-ROM Start Up

- From the START menu select RUN
- Type your CD-ROM drive letter, then type :\setup.exe (CLICK OK)
- Follow the on screen instructions
- See read me file for additional information

For support call 1-800-677-6337; 8-5; M-F CST or email: media.support@pearsoned.com

Employment Opportunities

The health care field, like any other, offers options to the Nursing Assistant who is pursuing that "first job" as well as the one who is seeking "opportunities for advancement." Chapter 35 provides information about where to look for work, how to interview, accepting a job, and making career moves along the employment continuum. Continuing education that supports cross-training and career path planning that encourages multi-skilling are also presented. Take the opportunity to discuss your short-term and long-term goals with your instructor or supervisor.

Medical Terms and Abbreviations

The Appendix provides an extensive list of medical terms, abbreviations, and specialties. You should learn as many medical terms and abbreviations as you can. Understanding terminology and abbreviations used in the health care field will make you more confident, help you understand instructions you are given, and assist you in reporting accurately. Knowledge of the "words" used will greatly improve your ability to communicate effectively.

Glossary

The end-of-book Glossary provides a complete alphabetical listing of all the Key Terms used in the text. Following the definition of each term, the number(s) of the chapter(s) in which the term is used appears in parentheses. For example, "**seizure** An episode, either partial or generalized, which may include altered consciousness, motor activity, or sensory phenomena and convulsions (13, 26)."

Using This Textbook

After you purchase *Being a Nursing Assistant, 9th Edition,* or when your instructor gives you your first assignment, take a little time to get to know this textbook. Make a quick survey of the text. Look at the *Detailed Contents* and find out what's listed there. As you read the chapter titles, you will get a sense of how the content is organized.

Chapter 1 introduces the "big picture" of the health care system. In Chapter 2 you learn about the role of the nursing assistant. The importance of good communication skills in caring for patients is presented in Chapter 3. Chapter 4 discusses patients, residents, and clients and you learn that individuals in need of care are referred to differently in different settings. Continue going through the entire *Detailed Contents* on your own, noting what's in each chapter. You may want to star or highlight chapter content that is of special interest or importance to you. There is more material in this book than needed for many nurse assisting NA courses. As you begin your career, you will find having this book as a reference will help when you need extra information or are caring for patients with different problems or diseases.

Be sure to find the Appendices: Medical Terms, Abbreviations, and Specialties and What's New in Patient Restraints. Also, don't forget the Glossary and Index listed at the end.

Preview Before You Read

As you read or study each chapter in this book, you will find it helpful to preview the chapter first. Whenever you are reading and learning new material you wish to remember, take the time to focus your energies and to set up the proper internal environment for learning. Preview first.

Preview the chapter by reading the Introduction, Objectives, Key Terms, Main Headings, and Summary. Notice that you have not read the chapter itself, just the skeleton or bare bones. Examine photographs, illustrations, drawings, charts, and tables.

Chapter Review

Each chapter presents a *Chapter Review* in the form of fill-in-the-blank and multiple choice questions. These questions will help you review the chapter's main ideas. The questions also will remind you of the things you have learned and the objectives you have met. The questions are not intended to be a test or quiz. You may wish to discuss the answers to the questions with classmates and/or your instructor. This type of discussion will help you to remember what you have learned. Reread and study any parts of the chapter that deal with a question you could not answer.

 ## Time Out

In this section you will find *Tips for Time Management*. These tips will help you develop communication, planning, and organizational skills.

 ## The Nursing Assistant in Action

These scenarios are based on actual, real-life issues and challenges you may encounter on the job. The statement of each situation is followed by a probing question. Use these situations and the questions accompanying them to explore your moral, ethical, or legal obligations in the situation described. Also, take advantage of actual situations as they present themselves to develop questions of your own to assist you as you seek solutions or appropriate responses.

Applying Critical Thinking

You will be able to expand your understanding by applying your critical-thinking skills to the scenarios presented in this section. For each of the scenarios presented, you are asked to think of what you might do to solve the problem.

CUSTOMER SERVICE Customer Service is a vital part of health care. Most patients or residents have choices as to where they seek health care. Very small things make the interactions with healthcare providers either positive or negative. Think about customer service in terms of the patient or family's needs and expectations. In your training or orientation to a new position you will observe many examples of patient interactions with staff. Frequently it takes no more time to show the consideration expected by your patients. Once patients or family members are dissatisfied or unhappy with the way they were treated, it is very difficult and time consuming to regain their trust or respect.

CULTURAL CARE The patients and staff in most health care settings are very diverse and difference. Some practices may seem wrong or strange if you have had little experience with a particular culture. This is a new addition to help identify situations you may encounter. The more you can learn about the culture of individuals you provide care for or come in contact with, the easier your job will be.

COOPERATION WITHIN A TEAM The best patient outcomes occur when all members of the health care team work together and cooperate with each other to get all the necessary work done. Employees, patients and families all benefit when there is cooperation. This feature provides an example in each chapter. In a new job you may not know how to begin team cooperation. Offering to help others and treating everyone with respect are the best places to start. The ideas presented in each chapter will provide discussion points for students and help you recognize when team members are working together.

Explore MediaLink

In this section you will find suggestions and help through the use of multimedia extension activities.

Preparing for the Competency Evaluation Exam

Expanded end-of-chapter exercises will help you prepare for the certification exam with fill-in-the-blank and multiple-choice questions. In addition, in Chapter 35 you will find a sample test with an answer key containing questions similar to those that appear on the Nurse Assistant Competency test. General information you will need to know to help you prepare/qualify for the Competency Evaluation Exam is also provided. For example, there is information about OBRA regulations regarding course requirements, explanations of the clinical skills exam and written/oral exam, test fees and time requirements. Be sure to ask your instructor about specific state requirements that apply to you.

1 The Health Care System

OBJECTIVES

When you have completed this chapter, you will be able to:

- Explain the purpose and organization of the health care delivery system.
- Explain how managed care influences the health care delivery system.
- Describe the effects of DRGs on the American health care system.
- Describe five ways of organizing the patient care services/nursing health care team.
- Identify the members of the patient care services/nursing health care team.
- Explain the purpose and function of a multidisciplinary team approach to patient care.
- Explain the difference between the qualifications of the registered nurse and the licensed practical nurse, and between the jobs of the patient/nursing assistant and the unit clerk/secretary.

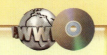

MediaLink

www.prenhall.com/wolgin

Use the address above to access the free, interactive Companion Website created for this textbook. Get hints, instant feedback, and textbook references to chapter-related NCLEX-style questions. Link to other interesting sites.

AUDIO GLOSSARY:

Use the Companion Website, or the CD-ROM disk enclosed with your textbook, to hear the pronunciation of key terms in the chapter.

KEY TERMS

diagnosis
diagnosis-related groups (DRGs)
functional nursing
health care institution (facility)
Health Insurance Portability and Accountability Act (HIPAA)
hospice
hospital
immediate supervisor
multidisciplinary team
nurse
nurse manager
nursing assistant
patient-focused care
preferred provider organization (PPO)
primary nursing
task oriented
team leader
team nursing

INTRODUCTION

This chapter introduces you to the health care system. It is a challenging, ever changing environment that embraces the delivery of health care services to individuals in need of care, the facilities in which these services are provided, and the health care providers who deliver these services. Some factors affecting the health care environment include an aging population, advances in medicine, new possibilities for delivering care, governmental legislation and regulations, managed care plans, and insurance companies. Patient care is delivered in a variety of ways on an inpatient and outpatient basis in a variety of long-term and short-term care settings, including the patient's home. In all situations, health care providers are expected to provide quality compassionate care in a cost-effective manner.

Different types of facilities and services are presented along with several nursing models. One of the newest models, patient-focused care, is a multidisciplinary team approach that places the patient and the patient's needs first—at the center, prompting and directing the delivery of services. It is important for you as a nursing assistant to understand the environment of the health care system, the organizational structure of your particular setting or facility, and the nursing model, or structure, on which your health care team is based.

The Health Care Environment

The health care environment is a continually changing and challenging place to work. Health care organizations and the people who work in them strive to improve their roles and work. Even as they provide compassionate, quality patient care and contribute to society at large, **health care institutions (facilities)** and their care providers study to improve their knowledge and develop in their roles as caregivers. These efforts to learn new skills are important because change in the health care system is happening faster than ever.

The health care delivery system is designed to meet the health care needs of all individuals. The five basic functions of a *health care delivery system* are to:

1. Provide care for ill and/or injured people
2. Prevent disease
3. Promote individual and community health
4. Provide facilities for the education of health workers
5. Promote research in the sciences of medicine and nursing

To give more people access to health care, to get the best possible results, and to keep costs down, health providers are constantly reviewing agency, institution, and patient needs and hospitalization requirements. Health providers continually ask questions like these:

- What do they do or what is their mission?
- Where do they do it?
- Who can do the work?
- How can they get the best results at the lowest cost?
- What does the individual patient or family desire from the health care providers?
- Is this treatment needed, necessary, or in the patient's best interests?

health care institution (facility) Hospital, hospice, nursing home, convalescent home, or clinic where health care services are provided both on an inpatient and outpatient basis

Efforts to answer these questions make providers:

- Think about or focus on the bigger issues of disease prevention and the health status of entire communities, not just about medical care for the sick and injured who come to an institution for help.
- Rethink the roles of hospitals and the ways different institutions and providers can cooperate. For example, people might go to walk-in or same-day surgery clinics rather than to hospitals, and many services might be provided in people's homes.
- Rethink what must be handled by a doctor or nurse and what can be done by others, including helping patients and their families assume active roles in self-care.
- Look for the best ways to meet the goals of those who seek health services.
- Listen to what patients and their families say they want in addition to the actual services and treatments people seek.
- Discuss with patients various treatments, goals, costs, and/or alternatives to treatment in order to provide the best care for the patient.

Health Care Reimbursement

Trying to reduce or control the ever increasing costs of health care has been a big challenge. Most health care administrators struggle to reduce their expenses yet provide the quality of care expected by patients, families, and accreditation bodies. Managed care or managed lives contracts are negotiated with major employers. **Preferred provider organizations (PPOs)** may contract with an employer to offer health care and physician services for a discounted group rate. Employees who use any providers outside the plan usually will not be reimbursed and must pay out of their own pockets for any health care services received. Price, access, outcomes, satisfaction, and quality all influence the choice of a health care provider. Often when individuals change jobs or employers, they are required to change physicians and use the services of a specific hospital or health care system.

preferred provider organization (PPO) Organization that contracts with an employer to provide health care and physicians' services to employees at a discounted rate

Medicare and Medicaid

Medicare and Medicaid are two different government programs that greatly influence health care. Medicare is a federal U.S. government program funded by Social Security and available to all individuals over age 65, regardless of income. It also covers the health care of some persons with disabilities or handicaps, regardless of age.

Medicaid is a separate program, funded by each state to help meet the medical and health care needs of low-income individuals or families. Medicaid programs and eligibility vary from state to state. Children of single mothers who have minimal income or who are unemployed receive medical coverage through Medicaid. Some individuals may qualify for coverage under both Medicare and Medicaid, for example, an 80-year-old woman who has very limited income. The largest portion of state Medicaid dollars goes to pay for nursing home care for elderly or blind persons or those with disabilities.

Many of the questions providers ask relate to insurance companies, managed care plans, and government legislation. For example, the federal Medicare program and other insurers look at services used by patients who fall into **diagnosis-related groups (DRGs)**. A **diagnosis** is a physician's determination of a patient's disease or condition. Researchers look at groups of patients with related or similar diagnoses (a DRG) and develop statistics on the average length of hospital stay and average cost.

diagnosis-related groups (DRGs) Diagnostically related groups of patients; a DRG includes patients whose diagnoses are related, usually by body system or broad disease type, such as heart disease

diagnosis Finding out what kind of disease or medical condition a patient has; a diagnosis is always made by a physician

HIPAA

Through federal regulation, the **Health Insurance Portability and Accountability Act (HIPAA)** governs and protects individuals' privacy and the security of health information. It also standardizes electronic transactions and the use of unique indentifiers (for example, the

Health Insurance Portability and Accountability Act (HIPAA) Federal regulation governing the privacy of medical records and encouraging electronic transactions

employers' tax identification number). In August 2000, the U.S. Department of Health and Human Services (HHS), in accordance with HIPAA of 1996, issued final electronic transaction standards to streamline the processing of health care claims, reduce the volume of paperwork, and provide better service for providers, insurers, and patients. The new standards establish standard data content, codes, and formats for submitting electronic claims and other administrative health care transactions. By promoting the greater use of electronic transactions and the elimination of inefficient paper forms, these standards are expected to provide a net savings to the health care industry of $29.9 billion over 10 years. All health care providers will be able to use the electronic format to bill for their services, and all health plans will be required to accept these standard electronic claims, referral authorizations, and other transactions.

In December 2001, Congress adopted legislation that allowed most covered entities to obtain a 1-year extension to comply with the standards, from October 16, 2002, to October 16, 2003. To qualify for the extension, the covered entity had to submit a plan for achieving compliance by the new deadline.

Privacy Standards

HIPAA also deals with the privacy of medical records. In December 2000, HHS issued a final rule under HIPAA to protect the confidentiality of medical records and other personal health information. The rule limits the use and release of individually identifiable health information; gives patients the right to access their medical records; restricts most disclosure of health information to the minimum needed for the intended purpose; and establishes safeguards and restrictions regarding disclosure of records for certain public responsibilities, such as public health, research, and law enforcement. Improper uses or disclosures under the rule are subject to criminal and civil sanctions prescribed in HIPAA. Most covered entities had until April 14, 2003, to comply with the patient privacy rule.

Diagnosis-Related Groups

DRGs were developed at Yale University and in 1983 they became a basis for payment for Medicare patients as well as a method for doctors to assess patients for the provision of quality care. There are over 400 DRGs. Age, comorbidities (more than one disease or chronic illness; for example, a person with diabetes and hypertension), and complications will influence the assigned DRG coding number. Payments are set fees based on the DRG assigned.

Current Procedural Terminology (CPT-4)

CPTs are currently in their 4th edition. These are groups of five numbers used to classify procedures or medical services performed for billing purposes.

Managed Care

Managed care is a term used to describe a wide variety of prepayment agreements, negotiated contracts and discounts, agreements for prior service authorization or approval, and performance audits. In managed care there is a standard benefit package, open enrollment, information or data on quality of care, and payments or contributions paid to a benchmark plan. A benchmark is a comparison or reference point, for example, the comparison of an organization's costs to the regional or national averages of similar providers. Physicians are encouraged to—and are rewarded for—practicing efficiently through fixed payments. In essence, managed care is a business strategy whereby health care financing and delivery are combined into one organization for the purposes of balancing costs, quality of care, and access. No evidence is seen of a long-term cost savings or decline in quality of care in patients covered by managed care, although patients have been dissatisfied with delays in seeing specialists and by their inability to see a preferred specialist.

Health Care Delivery Sites

Health care delivery sites and professional and nonprofessional workers depend on the revenue received in exchange for services provided to patients based on standard, contracted, or negotiated prices. The amount of money received by providers is frequently predetermined by national standards or based on statistics such as the average length of hospital stay and average cost. Health care professionals also use DRGs to group patients and determine the best answers to the questions outlined earlier in this chapter. These answers will change with advances in patient care techniques and technology.

Health care is delivered in an ever expanding variety of settings, facilities, and sites. Examples include:

- Acute care facility
- Adult day care
- Adult group living center
- Assisted living
- Birthing center
- Community care home
- Free-standing surgical center
- Home health agency (home care)
- **Hospice** inpatient center
- Long-term care nursing facility
- Mental health facility or partial treatment unit
- Outpatient clinic
- Physician offices
- Rehabilitation facility
- Residential care home
- Respite care
- Skilled nursing facility
- Subacute care facilities

hospice An extended, or long-term, care facility that provides health care services to terminally ill patients and their families

Each facility or health care delivery site requires an organizational structure that supports the purpose and functions of the delivery site. Figure 1–1◆ provides an organizational plan for a **hospital** organizational chart identifying the various departments required in such a facility. It highlights the nursing branch and indicates the line of communication and responsibility—chain of command—within the facility. A flatter management style is used in a skilled nursing facility (Figure 1–2◆).

As prevention becomes increasingly important, health care screening and assessment sites will be found at shopping malls, fairs, senior citizen centers, schools, churches, or other places where people gather. Patients are staying fewer days in the hospital and in many cases are receiving the majority of their health care, including surgical procedures, in outpatient or ambulatory settings. This means there are sicker, more critically ill patients in the hospital settings and a higher demand for health care workers in the variety of sites and places where health care is given to people.

hospital A short-term, or emergency, care facility that provides health care services to patients

KEY IDEA

You will learn new terms and see many changes as you work in the health care field. Remember: The goal of all health care professionals is to improve patient care and the health of the community. If you stay focused on that important aim, you'll accept change as a necessary step to achieve that goal.

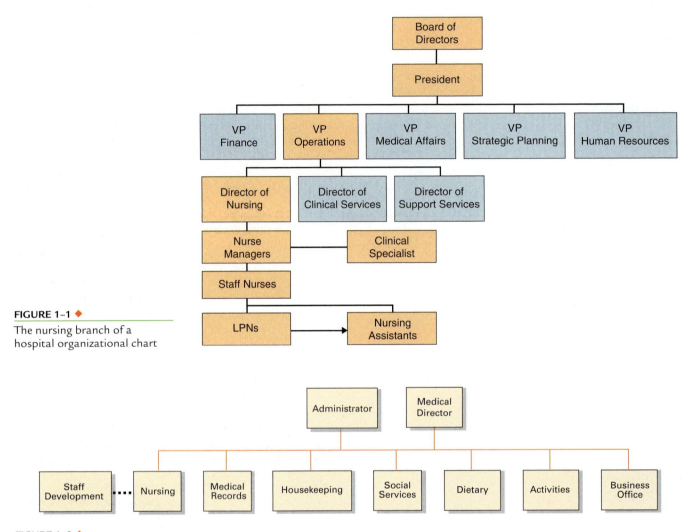

FIGURE 1–1 ◆

The nursing branch of a hospital organizational chart

FIGURE 1–2 ◆

Organization of a long-term care facility

The Patient/Health Care Team

The structure, or organization, of each health care team is unique. The size, complexity, and scope of services will determine the need for administration and/or layers of management. The current trend is to flatten the levels of administration and have decision making as close to the patient or at the lowest level as it can reasonably occur within the organization. The health care team model fits within the larger organizational structure of the facility. Refer to Figure 1–1 to identify the nursing branch of a health care facility.

Organization of the Health Care Team

Some models will work better in some settings than others. The nature of the patient care required, function, size, and location of a patient care facility affect staffing needs. What works best in a major metropolitan area is not necessarily the best option for a rural location. Also, the needs of the patients or residents in a hospice, nursing home, hospital, or home care setting differ greatly. Several models of patient/health care teams are described here. Each model indicates the relationship of the members of the nursing staff to each other and directs the interaction of staff with patients. Become familiar with the health care team models discussed here and realize that wherever you work the organization of the team may vary. Each one's role is important to the patient's care.

- **Functional nursing:** The **nurse manager** or charge nurse assigns and directs all patient care responsibilities for the nursing staff. This system is sometimes called *direct assignment*. In this organization, one nurse would be responsible for all medications; another for taking all vital signs.

- **Team nursing:** The nurse manager is sometimes called the *resource nurse*. She or he divides the staff into teams. Each team has a leader. The nurse manager assigns a group of patients to each team. The team leader then makes out the patient care assignments for all the members of the team. Team members may be registered nurses (RNs), licensed practical nurses (LPNs), **nursing assistants** (NAs) or patient care assistants (PCAs) (Figure 1–3◆). The **team leader** is teacher, adviser, and helper to all the team members. This system is **task oriented**. This means that nursing care is arranged according to what must be done for a group of patients.

- **Primary nursing:** Primary nursing is a method of patient care delivery in which the professional **nurse** is responsible and accountable for the entire nursing care of the patient 24 hours a day. The nurse is responsible for assessing the patient's needs and for planning, implementing, and evaluating the patient's nursing care. The purpose is to ensure that the professional nurse works directly with the patient. In addition, responsibilities include family teaching, patient education, discharge planning, and coordinating discharge plans with community agencies to assist the patient after discharge. This system is patient oriented. This means that the nursing care is arranged according to the total needs of the individual patient; it is

functional nursing A method of organizing the health care team in which the head nurse assigns and directs all patient care responsibilities for the nursing staff; this is sometimes called *direct assignment*

nurse manager The RN leader responsible for the care delivery, personnel supervision, and operating budget of a unit, area, or facility

team nursing A task-oriented method of organizing the health care team in which the team leader gives patient care assignments to each team member

FIGURE 1–3 ◆

The nursing care health team

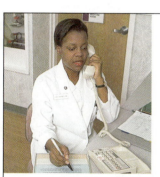

PROFESSIONAL REGISTERED NURSE (RN)
Four-year university education with a bachelor's degree
or
Two-year junior or community college education with an associate degree
or
Three-year diploma from a hospital nursing school
and
Passed state board examinations

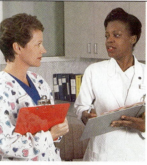

LICENSED PRACTICAL NURSE (LPN)
or
LICENSED VOCATIONAL NURSE (LVN)
One-year training program
Passed state board examinations
PLPN/MLPN–Pharmaceutical Licensed Practical Nurse is one who administers drugs or medications after taking a special course and passing a special examination

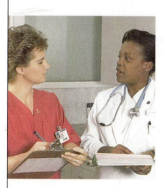

PATIENT CARE TECHNICIAN
PERSONAL CARE ATTENDANT
PERSONAL CARE ASSISTANT
HOMEMAKER
NURSING ASSISTANT
NURSING AIDE
NURSE'S AIDE
NURSE'S ASSISTANT
HOME HEALTH AIDE
HOME HEALTH ASSISTANT
GERIATRIC AIDE
GERIATRIC ASSISTANT
ORDERLY
NURSING ATTENDANT
All are names used for the nonprofessional worker who, under the direction and supervision of registered nurses, carries out basic bedside nursing functions

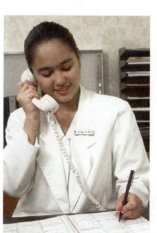

HEALTH UNIT SECRETARY
HEALTH UNIT CLERK
HEALTH UNIT COORDINATOR
Works at the desk of the nurses' station
—Does clerical work
—Answers the telephone at the nurses' station
—Helps to direct traffic on the floor
—Fills out requisition slips
—Transcribes physicians' orders

nursing assistant A person who helps the registered nurse to care for patients; nursing assistants work in hospitals, long-term care or other health care facilities, or in the patient's home

team leader The nurse responsible for one area of a nursing unit, including patient care assignments

task oriented Nursing care that is arranged according to what must be done

primary nursing A patient-oriented method of organizing the health care team in which the professional registered nurses are responsible for the total nursing care of the patient

nurse A person educated and trained to provide health care for people and to help physicians and surgeons; nurses are licensed as registered nurses (RNs) and licensed practical nurses (LPNs)

patient-focused care A care delivery model in which multidisciplinary teams plan, make decisions, and deliver care with the patient's needs being the focus rather than the needs or convenience of various departments or caregivers

multidisciplinary team A team of professionals and nonprofessionals from different disciplines that plans, makes decisions, and implements the delivery of patient care that is focused, or centered, on the patient's needs rather than any particular discipline's (department's) needs

sometimes called *patient-oriented* or total nursing care. The primary nurse will be assisted by associate nurses who provide care when the primary nurse is not scheduled on duty.

- ■ **Partners in practice:** Patient care is delivered with a combination of a nurse or primary care nurse working in partnership with a patient care assistant as a team. An assigned patient group is shared between these two partners who work closely to meet the care needs of their patients. In some settings, this model schedules both the nurse and NA to work the same schedule as much as possible to enable them to deliver care more effectively. Depending on the needs of the unit, other partner examples could include nurse and LPN or RN and respiratory therapist.

Patient-Focused Care

Along with the nursing models just described, one increasing trend in health care is to use a **patient-focused care** delivery model. This model may involve a small team of cross-trained caregivers assigned to deliver patient care in a specific unit or area. In this case, the members are cross-trained to draw blood samples, run EKG strips, and provide other skilled care as needed. The patient receives more personalized care because there are fewer personnel in direct contact with each patient.

Figure 1–4◆ represents a patient-focused care delivery model involving a **multidisciplinary team** used in a health care facility. The team plans, makes decisions, and delivers care with the patient as the central point of focus, rather than the needs of various departments and services. This design intends to provide seamless care across the continuum or episode of health care. The managers are more like coaches in this model, and the health care team workers are all working toward the common goal of delivering personalized, cost-effective care focused or centered on patient needs. A multidisciplinary team involves as many or as few departments (members) as the patient's needs require.

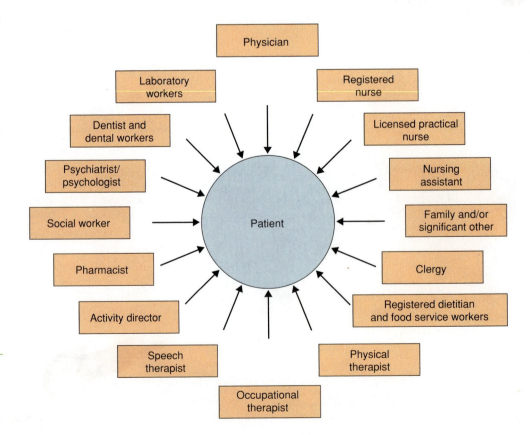

FIGURE 1–4 ◆

A multidisciplinary team provides patient-focused/patient-centered care; when possible the team includes the patient and the patient's family

Health care institutions not only provide care based on different models, but also according to the age of the patient. This is called *age-specific care.* This means that health care institutions recognize that patients are not all the same and need to be treated and cared for in ways that are appropriate for the stage of life in which they are. While the goals of care may be the same for all patients, how the caregivers interact with the patient, how the patient is taught, the equipment used for various ages, and safety measures needed for different age groups may vary widely. Age-specific care recognizes that as patients grow, mature, and age, they need different approaches to care in order to best meet their care needs.

The Nursing Assistant: Part of the Team

As a nursing assistant, you are a member of a health care team (Figure 1–3). Everyone on the team must understand teamwork and know what they are supposed to do and then do it to the best of their abilities with a spirit of cooperation. You will be working under the supervision of a professional nurse and cooperatively with other members of the nursing service staff. The figure provides a list of the many names used when referring to a health care worker who carries out the basic bedside nursing functions. Remember that the nurse recognizes the nursing assistant as a valuable worker and team member. Look to your nurse manager, team leader, or **immediate supervisor** as someone who will help you to learn and understand your job.

It is not uncommon to see a variety of care delivery models even within the same facility. Some models work more effectively in a given unit or area. As different ideas evolve, and the realities of decreasing reimbursement or payment for health care services continue, you can count on being exposed to different delivery models in your career. There will also be significant differences in the role expectations of nursing assistants. Figure 2–1 in Chapter 2 provides an example of the different duties and roles of the PA/NA, the advanced NA, and the patient care technician.

immediate supervisor An individual responsible for providing direction, critiquing performance, and giving feedback related to that performance

Relationship of Nurse and NA/PCA

You are an important member of the health care team. Your assignments and expectations will vary in different facilities and on different units. A key to your success in your role is to discuss your assignment, duties, and any questions you may have with your supervisor or the nurse with whom you are working. Review the photos and information in Figure 1–3 for specific information about the credentials and responsibilities of the nursing health care team. This figure identifies the health care team members and describes some of the training they receive to function or be licensed in the role of RN, LPN, and clerk/secretary.

As a result of the Omnibus Budget Reconciliation Act (OBRA) of 1987, nursing assistants working in skilled and nursing care facilities are required to complete an approved training program. Then they must pass a competency evaluation program consisting of a written test and a skills test. Refer to Chapter 35 for more information about competency requirements and evaluation for nursing assistants.

SUMMARY

The health care environment is continually changing. Members of the health care team work in a variety of inpatient and outpatient settings or in the home. These health care workers are expected to provide quality, compassionate care using a variety of patient care models, but always in a cost-effective manner. Medicare, managed care companies, PPOs, networks, insurers, and others set their payments to, or negotiate contracts with, health care institutions in exchange for the services provided to patients. In addition, HIPAA regulations and compliance standards uniformly protect the privacy and security of individuals' health information and medical records from improper use or disclosure. Your employer will explain your responsibilities for patient care charges as they relate to your particular setting. Examples are charting or accounting for supplies used. Patient-focused or patient-centered care, wherein multidisciplinary teams plan, make decisions, and place the patient at the center of their care delivery, is a current trend. Understanding the organizational structure of your particular setting or facility will help you to understand how and where your nursing team fits in the overall structure of your facility or agency and to appreciate the specific function your team and you in particular serve in the delivery of patient services.

NOTES

CHAPTER REVIEW

FILL IN THE BLANK Read each sentence and fill in the blank line with a word that completes the sentence.

1. The _____ is the nurse responsible for one area of a nursing unit.

2. An _____ is a chart that shows the chain of command within an institution.

3. An extended care facility that takes care of terminal patients is called a _____.

4. _____ is a type of insurance that is based on prepayments, negotiated contracts, and agreements for prior service authorization.

5. Patient-focused care is a _____ model for assigning care to patients.

MULTIPLE CHOICE Choose the best answer for each question or statement.

1. Which of the following is not a function of a health care delivery system?
   a. Provide care for the ill and injured
   b. Prevent disease
   c. Provide free care to the indigent
   d. Provide facilities for the education of health care workers

2. A physician's determination of a patient's condition or disease is called a
   a. hospice.
   b. referral.
   c. diagnosis.
   d. HIPAA code.

3. Which of the following is not a health care delivery site?
   a. Birthing center
   b. Fitness center
   c. Skilled nursing facility
   d. Community care home

4. Which of the following is not a care delivery model?
   a. Primary nursing
   b. Quad care
   c. Team nursing
   d. Partners in practice

5. HIPAA's primary concern is
   a. Financing health care
   b. Fighting obesity
   c. Regulating hip replacements.
   d. Protecting patient privacy and treatment information

6. Nursing assistants who work in nursing homes must complete
   a. competency evaluation programs.
   b. college.
   c. training programs.
   d. written tests.

TIME-OUT

TIPS FOR TIME MANAGEMENT

You will be required to attend in-services and unit meetings occasionally during your shift. Watch for notices of these mandatory meetings. Plan to come to work a bit early on that day to organize your care around the meeting.

NURSING ASSISTANT IN ACTION

You will be working with a group of people you do not know. You report to the unit and a team member approaches you saying, "Oh you must be the new guy. I was told to show you around."

What Is Your Response/Action?

CRITICAL THINKING

CUSTOMER SERVICE Patients and their families are your customers. They are coming to your place of employment for their health care needs. Think of two experiences you had when you needed to see a doctor or when you or a family member were in a hospital. What actions taken by health care providers come to mind? Often, a bad experience or insensitive staff encounter comes to mind. Consider what could have been done differently to avoid the unpleasant situation.

CULTURAL CARE As a nursing assistant you will encounter patients and families from various cultures. You will hear many thoughts, attitudes, beliefs, or opinions that are different from your own. If you are not sure what the particular differences are, be sure to ask first if there are any particular things the patient can tell you that would help you to provide his or her care.

COOPERATION WITHIN THE TEAM Members of the health care team bring their own contributions and skills to the team. The patient and family needs are important. Learning what each member needs will help promote understanding and cooperation within the team. When individuals focus only on what their particular jobs are and do not pay attention to how others are affected, cooperation and teamwork cannot result.

EXPLORE MediaLink

Additional interactive resources for this chapter can be found on the Companion Website at www.prenhall.com/wolgin. Click on Chapter 1 and "Begin" to select activities for this chapter. For chapter-related NCLEX-style questions and an audio glossary, access the accompanying CD-ROM in this book.

2 Your Role as a Nursing Assistant

When you have completed this chapter, you will be able to:

- Display qualities that are desirable in a good patient/nursing assistant.
- Identify duties and role functions of nursing assistants.
- Practice good personal hygiene.
- Organize your work efficiently.
- Behave ethically.
- Keep confidences to yourself.
- Work accurately.
- Be dependable.
- Follow rules and instructions.
- Develop cooperative staff relationships.
- Show respect for patients' rights.
- Explain how laws affect you and the patients you care for.
- Report incidents.

MediaLink
www.prenhall.com/wolgin

Use the address above to access the free, interactive Companion Website created for this textbook. Get hints, instant feedback, and textbook references to chapter-related NCLEX-style questions. Link to other interesting sites.

AUDIO GLOSSARY:

Use the Companion Website, or the CD-ROM disk enclosed with your textbook, to hear the pronunciation of key terms in the chapter.

KEY TERMS

accountable
accuracy
competency
cooperation
dependability
ethical behavior
hazard
hygiene
incident
informed consent
interpersonal skills
malpractice
negligence
stress

The nursing assistant is an important member of the health care team. Depending on where you work and the role you play on the team, your duties may include a range of direct and indirect patient care tasks. Job descriptions identify specific expectations, roles, and duties. Job descriptions will vary among institutions and agencies, but they reflect the institution's mission, patient care service philosophy, objectives, and/or policies. In addition to performing the required job duties, each caregiver is expected to demonstrate good interpersonal skills in interacting with other members of the health care team and with patients. Good organizational skills—time management and goal setting—and the ability to relieve personal stress are real assets in nursing assistants. A personal code of ethics and an awareness of the legal aspects of being a nursing assistant are essential in order to function as a caregiver.

The Nursing Assistant: An Important Caregiver

accountable To be answerable for one's behavior; legally or ethically responsible for the care of another

competency A demonstrable skill or ability

Being a nursing assistant is not just another job—it is a serious occupation. There are many new things to learn and so many things to do as a caregiver. The fundamental patient care tasks and procedures for which you will be **accountable** can be found on the health care institution's or agency's job description. Your instructor can review any state licensing or certification **competency** requirements that apply to you.

KEY IDEA

Remain sensitive to what you would want if you or one of your loved ones were the patient. *Empathy* and *understanding* from those caring for a patient are part of the treatment. Frequently, they are as important as medicine or therapy in helping the patient to get well.

Role of the Nursing Assistant

You will find a variety of job titles are used for nursing assistant positions. Whether you are called nursing assistant, patient care assistant, patient care associate, certified nurse assistant, or some other title to reflect these roles, you will be working under the supervision of the nurse manager or team leader. We will use the terms *nursing assistant* and *immediate supervisor* to refer to you and the person who supervises you. Your immediate supervisor usually makes your assignments, provides feedback on how well you are doing, and keeps track of your overall performance. Ask your immediate supervisor for help when you do not know how to do an assigned procedure or when you are unsure of yourself. It is better to get help than to do something wrong.

If you think you are being asked to do more than you were taught to do, remember that everything you do as a nursing assistant will be supervised by a registered professional nurse. That professional nurse can either provide any additional instruction you may need or will direct you to the proper person or department for such education. Everyone in health care is expected to be continually learning new and updated information on how to best care for patients and their loved ones.

Duties and Functions of the Nursing Assistant

A general summary of a job description will state that the nursing assistant works under the direct or general supervision of a registered nurse, contributing to the delivery of patient care through performance of selected day-to-day activities; maintenance of a functional and aesthetic environment conducive to patient well-being; demonstration of unit/area designated competencies; and interaction with patients considering their developmental, age-specific, cultural, and spiritual preferences. Refer to Table 2–1◆ to review an example of the specific duties and functions expected of three different levels of nonlicensed caregivers. Special education is provided for each level. Note that the job duties of a nursing assistant vary from state to state. Your instructor or employer should be familiar with the acceptable practice duties and functions for your particular situation and should instruct you as to the specifics.

> **KEY IDEA**
>
> Caregivers are expected to have good interpersonal skills that enable them to get along well with others, approach and resolve conflicts constructively, problem solve, and maintain confidentiality of information acquired in their role as caregivers.

 ## Personal Qualities

You have decided that you want to be the best nursing assistant you can be and do the best possible job. What kind of person makes a good nursing assistant? Certain traits, attitudes, and habits are often observed in people who are successful in their work in health care institutions, especially on the nursing team. **Interpersonal skills**, such as courtesy and **cooperation**, enable people to interact or work together in a productive and satisfying manner. Some of these traits are built into your personality—you have had them all along. Others can be learned through practice. Refer to Chapter 3 for more information about interpersonal skills and communicating with patients and coworkers.

Use the Traits and Attitudes Checklist to see where you stand. Put a check mark in the "Yes" column to indicate qualities you already have or in the "Can Learn" column next to those you think you can work on to make them a part of your personality.

interpersonal skills Skills used in interacting with other persons, such as courtesy; good interpersonal skills enable people to interact or work together in a productive and satisfying manner

cooperation Working or acting together; uniting to produce an effect or to share an activity for mutual benefit

Traits and Attitudes Checklist

	Yes	Can Learn
1. I am trustworthy, dependable, and honest.	_____	_____
2. I relate easily to new people.	_____	_____
3. I make friends quickly.	_____	_____
4. I enjoy working with people.	_____	_____
5. I get along well with others.	_____	_____
6. I am sensitive to the feelings of others.	_____	_____
7. I am considerate and tactful.	_____	_____
8. I want to help people.	_____	_____
9. I try to be gracious and polite at all times.	_____	_____
10. I get satisfaction when serving others.	_____	_____
11. I show sympathy and patience with others.	_____	_____
12. I try to control my temper.	_____	_____
13. I believe the work I do is important.	_____	_____

Traits and Attitudes Checklist

	Yes	Can Learn
14. I want to improve my performance.	_____	_____
15. I like to learn new things.	_____	_____
16. I rarely let my private life interfere with my work.	_____	_____
17. When the work is heavy and everyone is tense, I try a little harder.	_____	_____
18. I have a sense of humor.	_____	_____
19. I exercise regularly and/or have a way to reduce stress in my life.	_____	_____
20. I feel comfortable helping those who are less able to help themselves.	_____	_____

Personal Hygiene and Appearance

hygiene The science that deals with the preservation of health; when used to describe an object or a person, it means clean and sanitary

All members of the nursing team are teachers by the example they set. They influence each other to become better in their jobs. The practice of good personal **hygiene**, as used in a health care environment, becomes a teaching tool. Here are things to remember about personal cleanliness and your appearance:

- Dress properly and neatly. Follow the dress code of the health care institution where you work.
- Use good personal hygiene, bathing or showering daily.
- Keep your mouth and teeth clean and in good condition.
- Keep your hair clean and neatly combed. Long hair should be braided, pulled back, or pinned up.
- Keep your nails short and clean. Wear only clear nail polish, if any.
- Wear no or very little makeup.
- Try to be completely free of odor. Do not use heavy perfume, scented sprays, or heavy shaving lotion. Use an unscented deodorant.
- Have a physical checkup every year.
- Eat a well-balanced diet every day.
- Get plenty of sleep. Be alert when you come to work.
- Keep your body fit; do daily exercises.
- Wear clean clothes every day.
- Wear comfortable, low-heeled, enclosed shoes with nonskid soles and heels.
- Keep your shoes polished and the laces clean.
- Repair rips and hems and replace missing buttons on your clothing.
- Never wear jewelry, such as large, dangling earrings, bracelets, or pendants.
- Wear a white sweater if you are cold.
- Always wear your name pin and institutional badge.
- Always wear a wristwatch with a second hand.
- Always carry a pen and a pad of paper.

Patients believe a health care environment is, or should be, one of the cleanest places in the world. You will want, therefore, to be especially clean and fresh looking yourself.

TABLE 2–1 ◆

Patient Care Team—Nonlicensed Caregivers' Duties/Functions

PATIENT CARE TECHNICIAN	PATIENT CARE ASSOCIATE II	PATIENT CARE ASSOCIATE I
TREATMENT/PROCEDURES AS FOLLOWS:	BASIC HYGIENE/ADLS:	PREPARE AND MAINTAIN CLEAN ENVIRONMENT FOR PATIENTS:
■ Venipuncture ■ Blood cultures ■ Start or discontinue IV (not to include regulating rate) ■ Suctioning–tracheal, oral ■ Routine nebulizer mist Tx ■ Routine oxygen therapy ■ Pulse oximetry ■ Intermittent clean caths ■ Insert/d/c of urinary cath ■ Sterile/clean dressing changes (may use thirds solution chlorpactin, normal saline, bacitracin), no blind packing ■ PCIS documentation ■ Peripheral vascular checks ■ ROM/splints ■ Emergency equipment check ■ Assist patient with cough and deep breathing ■ Flush heplocks with normal saline ■ Trach care ■ Blood glucose monitoring ■ Remove nasogastric tubes ■ Respond to call lights UNIT SPECIFIC TASKS: ■ Obtain blood specimens (arterial lines, heplock, CVC) ■ Flush A-lines, heplocks, and CVCs (as a function of blood drawing) ■ Hold pressure post PTCA sheath removal and/or intra-aortic balloon pump cath	■ Bathing/showering patients ■ Vital signs ■ Blood glucose monitoring ■ Obtain body weights ■ Strip/make beds ■ Oral hygiene, skin care ■ Shampooing, shaving ■ Foley care ■ Toileting ■ Transfer, turn, ambulate patients ■ Set up for meals or deliver trays ■ Pass trays and nourishment ■ Document calorie counts ■ Record I&Os (oral intake) ■ H. S. care ■ Transport functions ■ Body fluid cleaning ■ Respond to call lights ■ PCIS documentation ■ Assist w/menu selecting ■ Prepare body postmortem ■ Orient patient/family to room ■ Collect/dispose of soiled linen ■ Order late trays ■ Collect meal trays ■ Deliver soiled tray cart to soiled sending room ■ Drain IV bags; d/c IVs ■ D/C foley catheters ■ Assist with minor treatments/procedures ■ ROM ■ Unit tests per unit policy (i.e., guaiac stool, obtain sterile urine specimen from indwelling catheter) ■ Assist patient with C & DB ■ Use of equipment such as K-pad, Hoyer lift, bed scale, cardiac chair safely ■ Enemas ■ Simple clean dressing change	■ Mop floors in rooms/halls/spot mop ■ Clean toilets/sinks in patient rooms ■ Clean nursing stations ■ Clean soiled utility room ■ Clean med room ■ Clean supply room ■ Dusting furniture, ceiling, and windows ■ Discharge cleaning of patient rooms ■ Empty trash in patient rooms* ■ Strip beds* ■ Make beds–unoccupied/occupied w/assistance ■ Prepare room for patient arrival ■ Replenish soaps, toilet papers, towels, etc., in patient rooms* ■ Disinfect showers/tub between use/daily general clean* ■ Body fluid cleaning* ■ Needlebox exchanges* ■ Stock/clean pantry area ■ Stocking of other supplies ■ Minor maintenance duties ■ Monitor level of linen ■ Assist w/stocking and replenishing of unit supply carts/medication carts ■ Check/restock emergency equipment/supplies housed in patient rooms ■ Answer phones and communicate messages* ■ Assure working condition of selected equipment UNDER THE DIRECTION OF THE **RN**: ■ Respond to call lights ■ Assist other nursing associates with making occupied beds and assisting with patient ADLs ■ Assist with meal setup, delivery of trays, and return of food cart ■ Escort patients in a wheelchair for procedures or discharge
All basic hygiene/ADLs as listed under PCA II Prepare and maintain clean environment for patients (responsible for * items under PCA I) Note: **Not all-inclusive lists.** PCIS = patient care information system.	Prepare and maintain clean environment for patients (responsible for * items under PCA I)	

SOURCE: Chart courtesy of St. Joseph Mercy Hospital, Ann Arbor, Michigan.

Organizing Your Work

Most people working in health care today find the demands of their jobs very hard to meet. Along with your patient assignment, you will be given a list of other duties to complete. Some information you need will be given in a report or written on the patient's care plan or care map. It is helpful to plan how you will complete your assignment and begin immediately. Avoid putting off or delaying completion of your work.

Time Management

Time management is planning, prioritizing, and organizing your work or tasks to be completed in a given period of time, usually measured in hours and minutes. You will need to *prioritize* your work, meaning you do the most important things first. You decide which things are most important by reviewing your assignment, noting what needs attention first, second, and so on. Decisions you make will be influenced by doctors' orders, nurses' instructions, scheduled tests or appointments, and immediate physical, safety, or welfare needs of your patients.

Patient needs take priority over housekeeping or cleaning needs. Your supervisor will help you determine when you need to change your priorities. Frequently, new needs and unexpected situations arise in the workplace that require you to adjust your priorities, for example, requests to assist with other patients' needs or unforeseen emergencies. If you use your time to complete assigned tasks, including cleaning and returning equipment and supplies and charting sooner than the last part of your scheduled shift, you will be less hurried and feel more satisfied in your work. It is helpful to make and carry a written list to remind you of your assignments. This list can be checked as you complete assigned duties and provide patient care, and it serves as a reminder of what you need to do.

Goal Setting

Goal setting means identifying a target or desired end and developing an action plan to move toward it. You set a goal when you decided to become a nursing assistant. For example, you identified the educational program and applied for acceptance, or you secured a position where the education was provided as part of your orientation. Attending classes, studying, practicing your new skills, and preparing for your final tests and/or examination are the action steps to accomplish this goal.

Stress Reduction

stress A physical, mental, or emotional tension or strain triggered by a stimulus that requires some response or type of adjustment

Stress is a physical, mental, or emotional tension triggered by a stimulus that requires some response or type of adjustment. Everyday sources of stress are loss, fear, threat, frustration, uncertainty, and conflict. The demands you experience in your personal life and in your role as a nursing assistant can cause you to feel an uncomfortable level of stress or anxiety.

KEY IDEA

When there is too little *stress*, nothing much happens or gets done. Too much stress can leave one feeling overwhelmed, even immobilized.

Stress can come from inside or outside. Internal (inside) stresses are self-imposed by what a person thinks or does. External (outside) stresses are caused by demands posed by other people, things, circumstances, or events.

There are many things you can do to relieve stress. It is best to try several ways to see what works for you. The means one person uses to relieve stress may not relieve stress for another person. It may even cause additional stress.

WAYS TO REDUCE STRESS	GUIDELINES	
■ Exercise physically at least three times a week for 20 to 30 minutes. The activity can be the same each time or any combination of the following: running, walking briskly, swimming, dancing, playing bas-	ketball or soccer, or aerobic exercises—activities that increase your heart rate. ■ Do gardening, yard work, house cleaning, or hobbies. ■ Listen to music that is soothing and relaxing to you.	■ Talk with understanding friends or family members who can help you put things in perspective. ■ Use humor, watch comedies, or listen to funny people. ■ Read, meditate, or pray. ■ Soak in a hot bath.

Avoid people, situations, or things that can increase your stress. Some people drink alcohol to excess, use street or recreational drugs, or gamble to have fun or "relax." For many, these activities lead to serious addiction and/or dependency, become serious personal or money problems, and interfere with the ability to work, causing attendance problems. If you or your loved ones are having problems, numerous confidential community resources are available for individuals desiring help or support to change.

Ethical Behavior

Ethical behavior means doing what you ought to do because it is right and consistent with good and moral conduct. As a member of the nursing team, a patient/nursing assistant will be expected to subscribe to the same high standard that professional nurses and health care providers do. Nursing has a Code for Nurses that outlines the values, norms, and ideals of the profession. It provides guidance for ethical conduct and a framework within which to look at and evaluate nursing actions. As a nursing assistant, you should observe this code for ethical behavior.

Patients derive their images of the nursing service primarily from the behavior of the individuals with whom they come in contact. All members of the nursing team must adhere to standards of personal ethics that reflect credit on the nursing profession. Members of the nursing team are responsible for their individual conduct in accord with the professional

ethical behavior To keep promises and do what you should do; to act in accordance with the rules or standards for right conduct or practice

CODE OF ETHICS	GUIDELINES	OBRA
■ Be conscientious in the performance of your duties. This means do the best you can. ■ Be generous and sensitive in helping your patients and your fellow workers. ■ Carry out faithfully the instructions you are given by your immediate supervisor. ■ Perform *only* procedures that you have been educated to do or that	are on (or below) the level of duties/responsibilities listed in your job description. ■ Respect the right of all patients to beliefs and opinions that might be different from yours. ■ Let the patient know that it is your pleasure, not just your job, to assist him or her. ■ Try to demonstrate that you are sincere in your involvement in the care of a human being. Always	show that the patient's well-being is of the utmost importance to you. ■ Do not accept tips from patients. You are expected to do a good job for the salary paid by your employer. Graciously decline any tips offered and reassure patients they do not need to offer tips to receive or reward good care.

standards of care. Each member of the health care team has the ability to positively or negatively influence the individuals with whom they come in contact.

KEY IDEA

Ethical behavior means doing what you ought to do because it is right and consistent with good and moral conduct.

Practicing high ethical behavior does more than reflect well on the patient's opinion of the nursing profession. It will help you personally improve the status of the nursing assistant. A patient or visitor who observes a conscientious, willing, and honest nursing assistant will think well of that person and the entire nursing staff. All members of the nursing team must adhere to standards of personal ethics that will reflect credit on the nursing profession.

- **Ethics of confidentiality:** Figure 2–1◆ outlines patient confidentiality considerations.

accuracy The quality of being exact or correct; exact conformity to truth and rules; free from errors or defects

- **Ethics of accuracy: Accuracy** is a part of being dependable (Figure 2–2◆). In a health care institution, you are concerned with human lives. What might appear to you to be a tiny mistake or oversight could delay the recovery of a patient. It is vitally important for you to follow your nurse's or team leader's instructions exactly. Be accurate when you are recording a temperature. Be alert when you answer the patient's call light. Should a mistake occur, report it to your immediate supervisor at once. If you do not understand something, ask again. Always remember: There is a reason for every step in the policies of the health care institution.

- **Ethics of dependability:** Your health care institution is organized to function efficiently when a certain number of people are on the job. If you are not there, patients could be deprived of the care they need. Also, your absence may cause your fellow workers to be overloaded with work. It is essential that you arrive promptly every day unless you are ill. If you are sick, call the nursing office at the appropriate time. **Dependability** means more than coming to work on time every day. It means that the immediate supervisor who asks you to do something can rely on you to do it at the proper time and in the proper way (Figure 2–3◆).

dependability A quality shown by coming to work every day on time and doing what is asked at the proper time and in the proper way

Everybody follows instructions and goes by rules. Otherwise, the job would never get done. Even the top people in the health care institution have to follow rules. Below are some useful guidelines to remember in your work. They can help to make you a better nursing assistant.

WORK RULES AND INSTRUCTIONS   **GUIDELINES**   **OBRA**

- In your written or verbal communication, be *accurate* to the best of your ability.
- Follow carefully the instructions of your immediate supervisor.
- If you do not understand something, ask your immediate supervisor for more information or to explain the reason why.

- There are good reasons for every work rule and every procedure in the health care institution. Be aware of them all or at least know where you can look them up.
- Report accidents or errors immediately to the immediate supervisor.
- Keep confidences to yourself, except when it might be dangerous to a patient. For example, a

patient tells you she is not taking her medicine. Report this to your immediate supervisor.
- Do not waste or destroy supplies or equipment.
- Be ready to adjust quickly to new situations.
- Try to get things done on time. Use a systematic work schedule.
- Work to be a good team member.

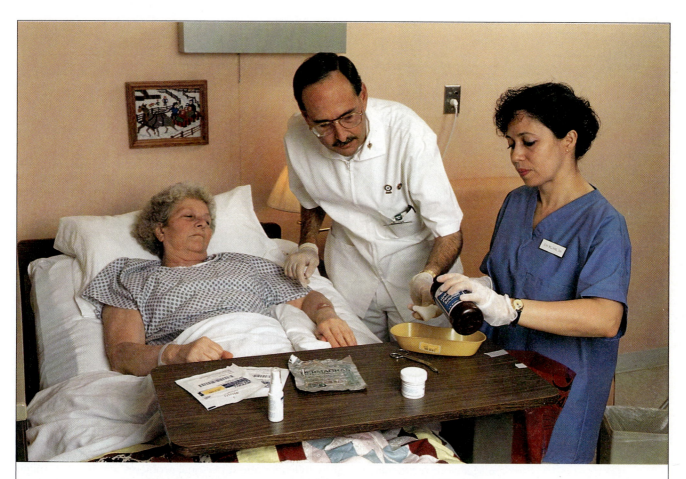

Discuss patient information only with the doctor, the RN, your team leader, or your supervisor. Patient information should be discussed in areas where you will be able to maintain confidentiality and not be overheard by others.

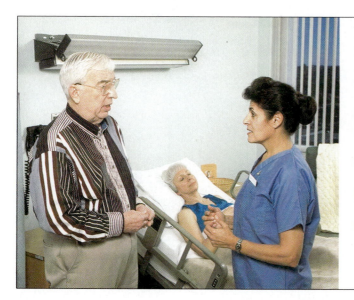

Do not discuss patient information with:

- Another patient
- Relatives and friends of the patient
- Visitors to the hospital
- Representatives of the news media
- Fellow workers, except when in conference
- Your own relatives and friends
- Individuals calling the unit requesting confidential information

FIGURE 2–1 ◆

The ethics of confidentiality

FIGURE 2-2 ◆

Be accurate; for example, check the patient's ID bracelet for accuracy

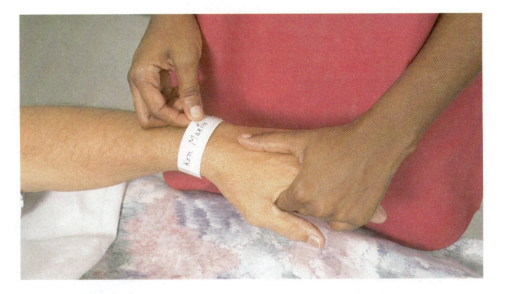

Staff Relationships

You will find your fellow workers and other health care personnel more agreeable and helpful if you treat them properly (Figure 2–4◆). Some good practices are:

- Report to the immediate supervisor whenever you leave the unit for any purpose and at the end of your shift. Report to the supervisor again when you return.
- Volunteer to assist coworkers as time allows or when you recognize your help is needed.
- Direct all questions you may have about patients and their care to your immediate supervisor.
- Tell your nurse manager or team leader about personal problems that you feel might be interfering with your work. There may be confidential employee assistance programs to help you.

FIGURE 2-3 ◆

Be dependable

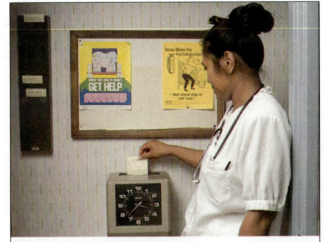

■ Report to work on time.
■ Keep absences to a minimum.
■ Keep promises.
■ Do an assigned task as well as you can; finish it quickly, quietly, and efficiently.
■ Perform a task you know should be done, without having to be told.

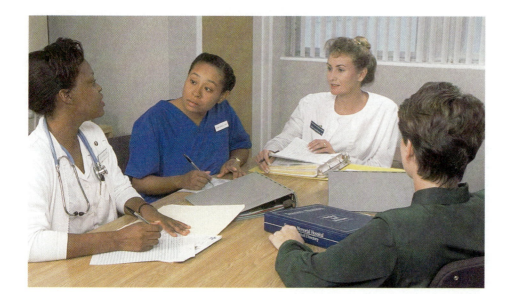

FIGURE 2–4 ◆
Staff conference

- Avoid talking about your personal problems with other staff members; never discuss your personal problems with patients.

- Follow all instructions given to you by your immediate supervisor. If you are unsure or confused about any of your assignments, discuss them with your immediate supervisor.

- Report all complaints from patients and visitors to the immediate supervisor. Never ignore complaints, no matter how silly or unreasonable they may seem to you.

- Perform all your duties in a spirit of cooperation and follow orders willingly (Figure 2–5◆).

FIGURE 2–5 ◆
Cooperate with your fellow workers

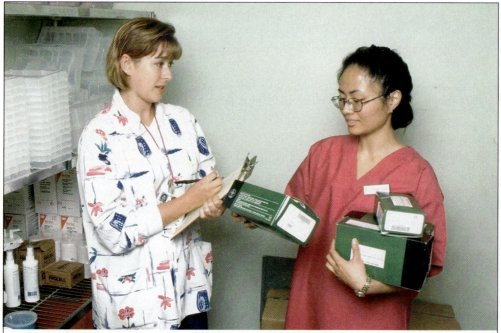

"I'll do my best to get the job done right."
- ■ Accept jobs assigned to you without complaint.
- ■ Follow the advice of your supervisors.
- ■ Show a willingness to learn.

■ Be courteous and express your appreciation when interacting with team members. Of course, always remember to say *please* and *thank you.*

Legal Aspects of Patient Care

Laws concerning patients and workers in health care institutions are written to protect both the patients and the workers. As nursing assistants, you need to understand how the law affects you and the patients you care for. One important legal aspect you will learn about is incident or occurrence reporting. This plays an important role in responsible patient care and the safety program of your institution. It is advisable that you know the laws of your particular state.

The Patient Care Partnership

The American Hospital Association has written a *The Patient Care Partnership* to be used as a guide by doctors, health care providers, employees in hospitals, and patients. This document describes the basic rights to which the patient is entitled. Figure 2–6◆ lists the complete 12 provisions. Patients are responsible for knowing and exercising their rights in accordance with the laws of their state.

negligence The commission of an act or failure to perform an act, where the respective performance or nonperformance deviates from the act that should have been done by a reasonably prudent person under the same or similar conditions

malpractice Negligence when applied to the performance of a professional

The words *negligence* and *malpractice* are often used interchangeably, as if they were the same thing. Officially, **negligence** is the commission of an act or failure to perform an act where the respective performance or nonperformance *deviates* from the act that should have been done by a reasonably prudent person under the same or similar conditions. **Malpractice** is negligence when applied to the performance of a professional. When a nursing assistant does not follow the directions of an immediate supervisor, and such failure causes or results in injury to the patient, then the nursing assistant has committed a negligent act. Examples of negligent acts nursing assistants might commit follow:

■ Failure to raise the side rails on a patient's bed and the patient falls

■ Failure to open the bottom of the mechanical lift to its widest position before use and the patient falls

■ Failure to follow instructions to turn the patient every 2 hours, and to document same, and the patient develops decubitus ulcers

■ Failure to place the patient's feet on the provided footrests of the wheelchair and as a result the wheels of the wheelchair run over and injure the patient's feet

Standards of care are based on laws, administrative policy, and guidelines published for nursing assistants. The professional standards of care are usually defined with respect to community, state, or national standards. These standards of care permit you to be judged based on what is expected of someone with your education and experience. All health care institutions and home health agencies have their standards of care, which you must follow.

Good Samaritan laws have been developed to protect individuals trying to give assistance to people requiring emergency care outside the health care institution. In the states that have Good Samaritan laws, you will be granted immunity if you act in good faith to provide care to the level of your education, to the best of your ability, as a reasonable and prudent person.

Consent is given by an adult who is conscious and clear of mind and results in acceptance of your care. Along the same lines, adults have the right to *withhold consent*, that is, refuse your care. Whatever their reasons, adults have this right. A parent or legal guardian can refuse to let you care for her child. You, the nursing assistant, must report to your immediate supervisor if any adult refuses to permit you to care for him or a significant other.

THE PATIENT CARE PARTNERSHIP

UNDERSTANDING EXPECTATIONS, RIGHTS AND RESPONSIBILITIES

When you need hospital care, your doctor and the nurses and other professionals at our hospital are committed to working with you and your family to meet your health care needs. Our dedicated doctors and staff serve the community in all its ethnic, religious and economic diversity. Our goal is for you and your family to have the same care and attention we would want for our families and ourselves.

The sections below explain some of the basics about how you can expect to be treated during your hospital stay. They also cover what we will need from you to care for you better. If you have questions at any time, please ask them. Unasked or unanswered questions can add to the stress of being in the hospital. Your comfort and confidence in your care are very important to us.

WHAT TO EXPECT DURING YOUR HOSPITAL STAY

HIGH QUALITY HOSPITAL CARE

Our first priority is to provide you the care you need, when you need it, with skill, compassion, and respect. Tell your caregivers if you have concerns about your care or if you have pain. You have the right to know the identity of doctors, nurses and others involved in your care, and you have the right to know when they are students, residents or other trainees.

A CLEAN AND SAFE ENVIRONMENT

Our hospital works hard to keep you safe. We use special policies and procedures to avoid mistakes in your care and keep you free from abuse or neglect. If anything unexpected and significant happens during your hospital stay, you will be told what happened, and any resulting changes in your care will be discussed with you.

INVOLVEMENT IN YOUR CARE

You and your doctor often make decisions about your care before you go to the hospital. Other times, especially in emergencies, those decisions are made during your hospital stay. When decision-making takes place, it should include:

■ *Discussing your medical condition and information about medically appropriate treatment choices.* To make informed decisions with your doctor, you need to understand:

— The benefits and risks of each treatment.

— Whether your treatment is experimental or part of a research study.

— What you can reasonably expect from your treatment and any long-term effects it might have on your quality of life.

— What you and your family will need to do after you leave the hospital.

— The financial consequences of using uncovered services or out-of-network providers.

Please tell your caregivers if you need more information about treatment choices.

■ *Discussing your treatment plan.* When you enter the hospital, you sign a general consent to treatment. In some cases, such as surgery or experimental treatment, you may be asked to confirm in writing that you understand what is planned and agree to it. This process protects your right to consent to or refuse a treatment. Your doctor will explain the medical consequences of refusing recommended treatment. It also protects your

right to decide if you want to participate in a research study.

■ *Getting information from you.* Your caregivers need complete and correct information about your health and coverage so that they can make good decisions about your care. That includes:

— Past illnesses, surgeries or hospital stays.

— Past allergic reactions.

— Any medicines or dietary supplements (such as vitamins and herbs) that you are taking.

— Any network or admission requirements under your health plan.

■ *Understanding your health care goals and values.* You may have health care goals and values or spiritual beliefs that are important to your well-being. They will be taken into account as much as possible throughout your hospital stay. Make sure your doctor, your family and your care team know your wishes.

■ *Understanding who should make decisions when you cannot.* If you have signed a health care power of attorney stating who should speak for you if you become unable to make health care decisions for yourself, or a "living will" or "advance directive" that states your wishes about end-of-life care; give copies to your doctor, your family and your care team. If you or your family need help making difficult decisions, counselors, chaplains and others are available to help.

PROTECTION OF YOUR PRIVACY

We respect the confidentiality of your relationship with your doctor and

(continued)

FIGURE 2–6 ◆

The Patient Care Partnership (Reprinted with permission from the American Hospital Association, Copyright 2003.)

other caregivers, and the sensitive information about your health and health care that are part of that relationship. State and federal laws and hospital operating policies protect the privacy of your medical information. You will receive a Notice of Privacy Practices that describes the ways that we use, disclose and safeguard patient information and that explains how you can obtain a copy of information from our records about your care.

PREPARING YOU AND YOUR FAMILY FOR WHEN YOU LEAVE THE HOSPITAL

Your doctor works with hospital staff and professionals in your community. You and your family also play an important role in your care. The success of your treatment often depends on your efforts to follow medication, diet and therapy plans. Your family may need to help care for you at home.

You can expect us to help you identify sources of follow-up care and to let you know if our hospital has a financial interest in any referrals. As long as you agree that we can share information about your care with them, we will coordinate our activities with your caregivers outside the hospital. You can also expect to receive information and, where possible, training about the self-care you will need when you go home.

HELP WITH YOUR BILL AND FILING INSURANCE CLAIMS

Our staff will file claims for you with health care insurers or other programs such as Medicare and Medicaid. They also will help your doctor with needed documentation. Hospital bills and insurance coverage are often confusing. If you have questions about your bill, contact our business office. If you need help understanding your insurance coverage or health plan, start with your insurance company or health benefits manager. If you do not have health coverage, we will try to help you and your family find financial help or make other arrangements. We need your help with collecting needed information and other requirements to obtain coverage or assistance.

While you are here, you will receive more detailed notices about some of the rights you have as a hospital patient and how to exercise them. We are always interested in improving. If you have questions, comments, or concerns, please contact _____.

© 2003 American Hospital Association. All rights reserved.

FIGURE 2–6 (continued)
The Patient Care Partnership

---

informed consent A voluntary act by which a conscious and mentally competent person gives permission for someone else to do something for him

Informed consent is a voluntary act by which a conscious and mentally competent person gives permission for someone else to do something for him.

Civil rights must be guaranteed to all citizens. This includes freedom from discrimination because of *religion, ethnic origin, sex, race, physical handicap,* and *age.*

For example:

- An employer cannot discriminate in hiring practices.
- A nursing assistant cannot discriminate in care for patients.

Defamation of character refers to making false or damaging statements or misrepresentations about another person that defame or injure her reputation. There are two types of defamation of character:

Slander: A spoken statement (gossip)

Libel: A written statement

Abandonment is the act of leaving, walking off the premises, deserting, or neglecting a patient. If the nursing assistant is unable to care for his patient, suitable and qualified substitutes must be made with consent of the patient; otherwise, a breach of duty could occur. An example would be leaving a patient care unit/area at the end of your shift when there was no one else there to care for the patients.

Criminal law applies to felonies against society. The elements of crime and punishment are usually part of each state's legislation and judicial opinions.

False imprisonment refers to a situation in which a person is restrained or detained without proper consent. Restraints cannot be applied to any patient without a written order from the physician. It is important to review your facility's restraint policy and procedures and follow them as outlined.

For additional legal terms, see Table 2–2♦.

TABLE 2–2 ◆

Additional Legal Terms and Definitions

TERM	DEFINITION
Accident/incident	An unforeseen event that occurs without intent.
Accountability	The act of being liable or legally responsible.
Advanced directive (living will)	Instructions given in advance that life-support systems shall not be used in the event that the patient's death will occur soon and a physician has determined that there can be no recovery and the application of life-support systems would only artificially prolong the dying process.
Assault	An unsuccessful attempt or threat to commit bodily harm.
Battery	An assault that is actually carried out where the person is injured.
Civil law	Concerned with the legal rights and duties of private persons.
Crime	A violation against a citizen or society.
Invasion of privacy	Invasion of the right to live in seclusion without being subjected to undesired publicity.
Liability	An obligation incurred or that might be incurred through any act or failure to act.
Wills	A statement for the distribution of personal belongings and property following death.

Incidents

An **incident**, or occurrence, is an event that is outside or does not fit the routine operation of the health care institution or the routine care of the patients. It may be an accident or something that might cause one. For example, a staff person stumbles into a patient in a wheelchair because someone spilled liquid and failed to wipe it up. Such incidents can affect the patients, visitors, and members of the institution's staff. Prevent accidents. Report **hazards**. Be alert for potential dangers, such as spilled liquids and trash.

incident An unforeseen event that occurs without intent

hazard A source of danger; a possible cause of an accident

Types of incidents are:

- Patient, visitor, or employee accidents
- Thefts from patients, visitors, or employees
- Thefts of facility property
- Accidents occurring on outlying hospital property, such as sidewalks, parking lots, or entrances

KEY IDEA

Prevent accidents. Report hazards. Be alert for potential dangers, such as spilled liquids and trash.

Whenever an incident occurs, a report must be made. Each agency will have a special form to use. Your supervisor or instructor will review the specific accident/incident form with you (Figure 2–7◆). Report any incident you observe immediately. Also report any unsafe conditions you think might lead to an incident. Reporting is very important to the safety program of the health care institution and for the protection of all health care

FIGURE 2–7 ◆

Accident/incident report

MEMORIAL HOSPITAL
ACCIDENT/INCIDENT REPORT

Medical Record # _____

1. Patient ☒   Visitor ☐   Employee ☐   Other ☐
2. Date of this report 12/25 20 xx   Date of incident _____ 12/25/xx

3. Name ____ Johnson, Henry A. ____   Age 43   Sex Male Marital Status _____
   Department _____   Position _____

4. Location incident occurred at ____ Room 407 ____   Time 1:00 a.m.
                                                                                                p.m.

5. Reported to _____   Patient seen by Dr. ___ Ralph A. Jones ___
   _____ Time ____ a.m.   _____ Time 1:05 a.m.
                                          p.m.   p.m.

6. Statement of doctor or resident (diagnosis, parts of body affected and treatment)
   ____ Patient examined—no injuries sustained—left elbow slightly ____
   ____ abraded. ____

   _____ Attending Physician _____ M.D.

7. Describe incident and how accident occurred. (Statement of nurse or person in charge.)
   ____ Patient found on floor—stated he attempted to get out of bed, slipped off and fell to floor. ____
   ____ Slight abrasion of left elbow. No hospital property damaged. ____
   Signed _____   Title _____
8. Witness name ___ Fred R. Smith ___   Address ___ 33 Yale St., New Brunswick, N.J. ___
   Witness name _____   Address _____
9. Name of machine involved _____
10. Kind of work performed by machine _____
11. Part of machine causing injury _____
12. Any protective device on machine _____
13. Action taken to prevent recurrence _____

   _____ Signed _____ Title _____
                                                                    mo   day   yr
14. Did employee lose time?   Yes ☐ No ☐   If yes, give last day worked ☐   ☐   ☐
    If unable to resume work, give probable date of return mo day yr   if already returned mo day yr
                                                             ☐   ☐   ☐   ☐   ☐   ☐
15. If patient accident, signed _____ Date _____
    Ass't. Adm. Nursing Service
                                               a.m
    Reported to administration on ____ at ____ p.m. Signed _____ Adm.

Department director must complete necessary information in duplicate. Duplicate must be forwarded immediately to chairman of the safety committee.

Reviewed by safety committee on _____ Signed _____ Chairman.
                                    (FILL OUT IN DUPLICATE)

workers. For the institution to have adequate records and be prepared for possible liability suits or damage claims, all the facts related to the incidents must be known. Incident reports are filed with the hospital's administration and are not part of the patient's chart. Employee failure to report an incident, particularly one in which a patient is injured or harmed, can result in disciplinary action or termination.

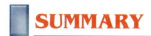

SUMMARY

The nursing assistant is an important member of the health care team. In your role as caregiver, you will be ensuring that patients do not suffer any extra pain and will be making a patient's stay in the health care institution easier. Good interpersonal skills and hygiene are expected in a nursing assistant. Good organizational skills can help make the many duties and responsibilities of the job more manageable and less stressful. As a member of the nursing team, a nursing assistant will be expected to subscribe to the high standard that professional nurses and health care providers set for themselves. Always remember that patients are entitled to respect for their human rights. They must be kept safe and properly cared for at all times. Laws concerning patients and workers in health care institutions protect both the patients and the workers. Be aware of the legal aspects of your job and understand the importance of reporting incidents in your institution's overall safety program.

NOTES

CHAPTER REVIEW

FILL IN THE BLANK Read each sentence and fill in the blank line with a word that completes the sentence.

1. When you are legally or ethically responsible for the care of another, you are said to be _____.

2. Working or acting together for mutual benefit is called _____.

3. Good _____ includes good personal cleanliness and appearance.

4. You demonstrate good _____ when you plan, prioritize, and organize your work in order to get it done in a given time period.

5. _____ behavior includes keeping promises, doing what you should do, and acting in accordance with the rules and standards for right conduct and practice.

MULTIPLE CHOICE Choose the best answer for each question or statement.

1. Positive traits in a nursing assistant are all of the following except
   a. being trustworthy.
   b. enjoying working with others.
   c. liking things only a certain way.
   d. liking to learn new things.

2. The code of ethics includes which of the following standards?
   a. Carrying out faithfully the instructions you are given
   b. Respecting the right of all patients to beliefs that are different from yours
   c. Letting the patient know it is your pleasure to do your job
   d. All of the above

3. Do not discuss patient information with
   a. other patients.
   b. relatives and friends of the patient.
   c. your family.
   d. All of the above.

4. Doing something or not doing something when a reasonably prudent nursing assistant would have done it under the same conditions is called
   a. negligence.
   b. invasion of privacy.
   c. accountability.
   d. battery.

5. An incident is an unforeseen event that occurs without intent
   a. it does not need to be reported.
   b. only serious patient injuries are reported.
   c. failure to report it could lead to losing your job.
   d. there is no liability for it.

TIME-OUT

TIPS FOR TAKING CARE OF YOURSELF

You may be treated unfairly by a supervisor at work. This can cause you to feel hurt or angry. Take time to cool down before you react to the situation. Think through the causes of the supervisor's behavior. Avoid wasting time by discussing the unfairness with other staff members. Approach the supervisor at a later time and ask to calmly discuss what occurred. Clear the air by hearing both sides of the situation.

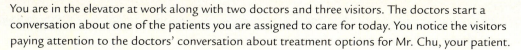

NURSING ASSISTANT IN ACTION

You are in the elevator at work along with two doctors and three visitors. The doctors start a conversation about one of the patients you are assigned to care for today. You notice the visitors paying attention to the doctors' conversation about treatment options for Mr. Chu, your patient.

What Is Your Response/Action?

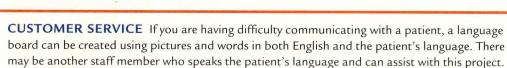

CRITICAL THINKING

CUSTOMER SERVICE If you are having difficulty communicating with a patient, a language board can be created using pictures and words in both English and the patient's language. There may be another staff member who speaks the patient's language and can assist with this project. If not, arrangements can be made to call a family member or interpreter when it is necessary to communicate important information or ease anxiety.

   The communication board should have a space where you can write your name so she will be able to more easily recall her caregiver's name.

CULTURAL CARE As a nursing assistant you will encounter many cultural differences among coworkers and patients. It may not be easy to understand and appreciate the large or small differences you notice or experience. Some relationships will develop quickly, whereas others will develop over time. Be pleasant and patient with coworkers who are quiet or reserved.

COOPERATION WITHIN THE TEAM Dependability is one of the most important personal qualities you can bring to a team. Coworkers and supervisors need to know they can count on you to do your Job and be on time when you are scheduled to work or are expected back from a break. Coworkers will appreciate your consideration and be more likely to value team members who are dependable and considerate of each other.

EXPLORE MediaLink

Additional interactive resources for this chapter can be found on the Companion Website at www.prenhall.com/wolgin. Click on Chapter 2 and "Begin" to select activities for this chapter.

For chapter-related NCLEX-style questions and an audio glossary, access the accompanying CD-ROM in this book.

KEY TERMS

body language
boot up
central processing unit (CPU)
communication
courtesy
cursor
cyanosis
data
edema
empathy
feedback
hardware
keyboard
light pen
log on
memory
monitor
mouse
network
objective observations
objective reporting
observation
password
pediatric patient
personal identification number
   (PIN)
printer
prompt
retrieval
screen
secretions
software
subjective observations
subjective reporting
tact
terminal

OBJECTIVES

When you have completed this chapter, you will be able to:

■ Demonstrate a courteous and professional manner toward patients, families, visitors, and coworkers.

■ Keep your emotions under control while on the job.

■ Deal with patients and visitors in an empathetic and tactful manner.

■ Show interest and concern about the patient's welfare.

■ Communicate effectively with pediatric patients and their parents.

■ Use communication skills effectively when relating to patients and their visitors.

■ List seven barriers to effective communication.

■ Answer the patient's call light signal promptly.

■ Meet the patient's physical and psychological needs.

■ Teach a patient with a visual or hearing impairment how to use the call light.

■ Take complete and accurate telephone messages.

■ Use your senses of sight, touch, hearing, and smell to observe your patients.

■ List the behaviors to observe in a patient.

■ List the behaviors to report when they are observed in infants or children.

■ Differentiate between objective and subjective reporting.

■ Report observations promptly, accurately, and objectively.

■ Identify the basic parts and functions of a computer used to document and communicate patient information.

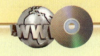

MediaLink

www.prenhall.com/wolgin

Use the address above to access the free, interactive Companion Website created for this textbook. Get hints, instant feedback, and textbook references to chapter-related NCLEX-style questions. Link to other interesting sites.

AUDIO GLOSSARY:

Use the Companion Website, or the CD-ROM disk enclosed with your textbook, to hear the pronunciation of key terms in the chapter.

This chapter describes how communication occurs through words and actions. As a nursing assistant, you will communicate with patients, their families or significant others, and other health care staff. It is important that you be positive and effective as a communicator. Personal qualities that promote positive communication and that you will use in communicating with patients, their families, and other health care staff are discussed. Some barriers to effective communication are also presented. Special consideration will be needed when communicating with individuals who have visual or hearing impairments as well as the pediatric patient. Information on how to communicate and document objectively or report your observations of patients is also presented.

INTRODUCTION

Communication Skills

Communication refers to the exchange of information with others. This information can be about facts, feelings, opinions, or ideas. Communication may be verbal or nonverbal. Verbal communication may be spoken or written. Greetings like "Hello" and "Good morning," phone conversations, and letters and greeting cards are examples of verbal communication. Nonverbal communication involves body language. It may be as simple as a wave of the hand or a wink, or it may involve the entire body. All communication, whether verbal or nonverbal, involves these three important elements:

- a sender: the one sending the message
- a receiver: the one receiving the message
- a message: the information shared or emotion expressed

Even if all three elements are present, the communication may not be understood, or it may be misinterpreted. For example, the sender may speak too quickly, the receiver may be busy or preoccupied and not listening, or the message may include difficult or unknown terms. Any one of these factors may affect the communication. Certain responsibilities or criteria are attached to each element in the communication. Only when these criteria are met will the communication be understood and less subject to misinterpretation.

- The sender must obtain the receiver's attention, be organized, speak clearly, and make sure the message is understood.
- The receiver must listen carefully, respond appropriately, and ask for clarification, if needed.
- The message must be organized, simple, and clear.

Verbal Communication (Communicating through Words)

Verbal communication occurs through the exchange of spoken words. Ideas, facts, or information is transferred from the sender to the receiver. For example, when you arrive at your workplace and greet a coworker, you are communicating verbally. You are the sender, your coworker is the receiver, and your greeting is the message. Likewise, your coworker who receives your message then responds to your greeting. This response to the message, which actually may repeat the message, is called **feedback**. The exchange of greetings between you and a coworker can express very different meanings, depending on the tone of your voice, the speed or quickness of your spoken words, your inflection, and the actual words you use. If your greeting is warm and lighthearted, you convey the idea

communication The exchange of thoughts, messages, or ideas by speech, signals, gestures, or writing between two or more people

feedback Response of the receiver to the sender's message; the response, or feedback, lets the sender know if the message is acknowledged and clearly understood

that you are having a good day and are pleased to be there. Such a greeting may (but not necessarily) draw a similar positive response from your coworker even if he or she is not having an equally pleasant day.

Written Communication

Written communication occurs when you use handwritten or printed words, photographs, or drawings to communicate. The patient's record or chart is a form of written communication. Your assignment, too, may be written on a sheet of paper or posted on the unit bulletin board. Other examples of written communication are the patient's ID bracelet, NPO and OXYGEN IN USE signs, and the different color stripes and arrows the hospital may utilize in main corridors to help you get from place to place within the facility.

Nonverbal Communication and Body Language

Spoken and written words are used for most communications. But other ways are sometimes more effective to get a message across. Hand movements (gestures), expressions on your face, and body movements may tell the story better than words. Although no words are spoken, a powerful message can be sent. Often, one can look at a person and see that the person is happy, sad, angry, willing, or unwilling to perform a requested task. For example, if someone is slamming charts or refusing to answer a question by turning his or her body away from you, the nonverbal message is negative, but you do get a message. A very different message is communicated when you see someone hugging another, smiling, or making eye contact with another person.

KEY IDEA

The three key elements in all communication are the sender, the receiver, and the message. The same message can have different meanings depending on how quickly or slowly you speak, your tone of voice, your facial expression, or gestures you make.

Barriers to Effective Communication

Good or effective communication is communication in which the "sender" conveys (sends) the intended message and draws an appropriate response (feedback) from the "receiver." Communication is good or effective when it is respectful, honest, clear, and appropriate. Bad, negative, or ineffective communication fails to convey the intended message or draws an inappropriate response. Communication can fail or break down for many reasons. It will be helpful to learn what ways of speaking, topics, issues, or situations may be barriers to communications. Some barriers to effective communication are:

1. Clichés, familiar, or overused phrases said with little or no thought, such as "Don't worry" or "It was meant to be"
2. Questions that can be answered with "yes" or "no" responses
3. Language misunderstandings or misinterpretations of meaning
4. Cultural differences, including beliefs and practices
5. Sensitive topics
6. Judgmental attitudes on the part of the sender or receiver
7. Failure to listen to feedback (response to your message) or giving the receiver only partial attention

Aids to Effective Communication and Relating to People

Relating to people means making a connection between yourself and another person. The relations between yourself and patients, visitors, parents, and fellow workers depend on your approach and response to them. If you have a kind, courteous, sensitive, tactful, empathetic, and open manner, you will find it easier to form positive connections (Figure 3–1◆). Relationships depend on receiving as well as giving information, so listening attentively is as important as what you say. Communication skills are necessary to be successful as a nursing assistant.

Taking care to be nonjudgmental when you listen and observe others will help to improve your communication with them. Maintaining emotional control by not allowing others to easily upset you with their words and actions is an essential skill for health care providers. When people are worried, anxious, or sick, their ability to control their fear and stress is reduced. Patients, coworkers, or your supervisor may share that they do not like the way you are doing a particular task or assisting them. Try to focus on the suggestion or constructive criticism being offered, rather than becoming angry or upset with the person sending the message to you.

Remember that courtesy, empathy, tact, and emotional control do much to enhance positive communication. Consider them here and think of ways to make them part of your personality.

- **Courtesy:** consideration and respect shown for another person's needs. It means cooperating, sharing, and giving. Being polite and considerate of others shows that you care about them. Think how you would feel if you were in their place, and you will understand how far a cheerful word and a smile can go.

- **Empathy:** feelings, thoughts, and motives of one person are understood and/or felt by another person without pity. A nursing assistant should use empathy or empathize with the patient, visitor, and coworkers.

courtesy Being polite and considerate

empathy The ability to put yourself in another's place and to see things as they see them

FIGURE 3–1◆

Helpful personal qualities include courtesy, emotional control, empathy, and tact

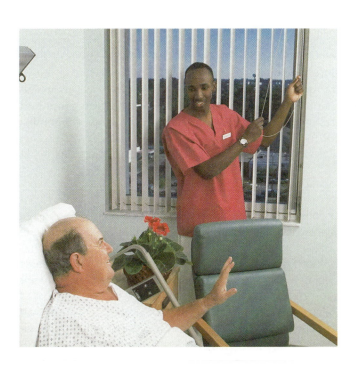

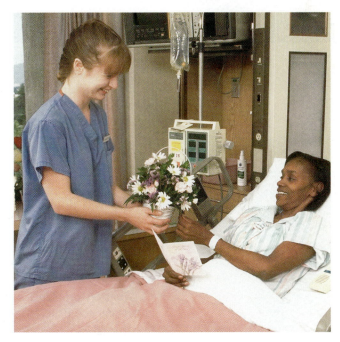

tact Doing or saying the right things at the right time

- **Tact:** doing and saying the right things at the right time. Tact also includes knowing when it is best to say nothing. Avoid asking questions that could embarrass the patient who has visitors.

- ***Emotional control:*** calm and self-control in the presence of a patient, another staff member, or a visitor who may upset or anger you. You may feel like making a rude or nasty remark or reply. Don't do it. Stop and realize that the patient may be worried, nervous, or tense. This may also be the case for family and friends who visit the patient. Fellow workers may be under stress because of a problem at home or on the job. Try to be understanding and learn to control anger and cope with all situations.

Learning to accept constructive criticism and suggestions without feeling you are being personally attacked is an essential part of your job. Try to avoid becoming defensive. If your supervisor criticizes you or tells you to do something, you may feel like saying, "That is not my job" or "Why do you pick on me?" Stop and examine your attitude. Calm down and then perform the right or correct action. It can be helpful to discuss the situation at a later time after you and your supervisor/coworker are better able to hear each other and consider a different point of view. Try to focus on the work or skill being discussed. It is easy to personalize criticisms or suggestions. Consider that your supervisor may be wanting to help you modify or improve your skills or interactions, while still valuing you as a person.

Relationships with Patients

Many things make a difference in a patient's behavior and attitude during an illness. The patient may become frightened, angry, or sad. Some factors or influences are the diagnosis, seriousness of the illness, age, previous illnesses, past experience in hospitals, and mental condition. Other things that might make a difference are the patient's personality, disposition, and financial condition.

Each patient's reaction to pain, treatment, annoyances, and even kindness is different. Always treat each patient as an individual, a person who needs your help. Respect confidences the patient shares with you, recognizing that giving the patient the opportunity to speak about physical problems or other concerns is a real kindness. Refer to Chapter 2 for more information regarding confidentiality and a code of ethics for health care staff.

KEY IDEA

> Keep confidences. Never talk to anyone except your immediate supervisor about a patient's condition. Take care to see that you are out of earshot from others when you are discussing a patient's problem. Discussing one patient's medical condition with another patient is an invasion of privacy. Never discuss your patients with family members or friends.

Always try to give the patient confidence in the hospital, the doctors, and the nursing staff. Never discuss or criticize any of your fellow staff members in front of a patient.

Remember that the patient's behavior is the result of things that worry or bother him (Figure 3–2◆). The patient may be hostile, mean, and nasty. You may simply be the nearest person to talk to or to lash out against. Try not to take what is said to you personally and respond in kind.

Whatever problems a patient has, you can be sure one person considers them very important—the patient. Try to be understanding. Be a good listener, even when you would rather leave.

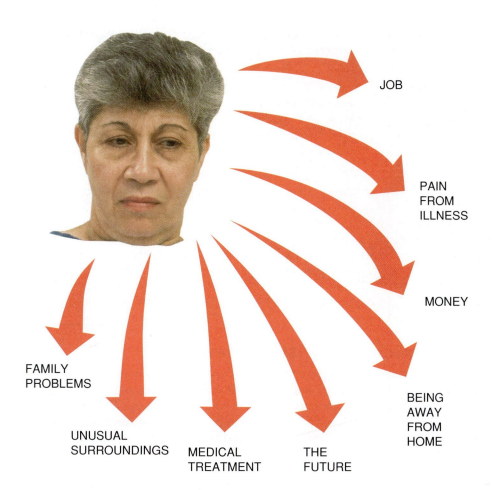

JOB

PAIN FROM ILLNESS

MONEY

BEING AWAY FROM HOME

THE FUTURE

MEDICAL TREATMENT

UNUSUAL SURROUNDINGS

FAMILY PROBLEMS

FIGURE 3–2◆

A patient worries about many things

Patients and visitors often relieve their feelings of helplessness and hopelessness through words and behavior. It may sometimes appear that they are trying to take it out on you. Be patient with them as much as possible. Remember that the patient may be suffering emotionally as well as physically; talking may relieve the emotional suffering.

Try to be as tactful as you can. When a patient begins to recover, give praise and encouragement. Do not hold a patient's behavior against them. Remember some behaviors are difficult but the individual is not a bad person because they are unkind or focused on themselves.

Always listen when a patient makes a complaint or brings up a problem. Patients' questions about the doctor or the time and plans for discharge should be referred to your immediate supervisor.

While these considerations apply to adult and pediatric patients alike, the following is particularly important to remember as you relate to children, or pediatric patients.

Sometimes a child cries when his parents are getting ready to leave the hospital. You can show empathy to both the child and parents by making the separation easier for them. Pick up the child (if permitted) and pat and soothe him. Turn the child's attention to something other than the anxiety, fear, and pain of being separated from the parents.

Crying is the normal, natural way for children to express their feelings and fears. Try to understand why a child is crying excessively. Do not let it irritate you.

Never tell a child that you are going to take his temperature or blood pressure. The child may think you are going to take something away. Say you are going to measure his temperature or blood pressure instead. Explain the procedure; let the child examine the stethoscope or such to gain confidence and trust.

FIGURE 3-3◆

Explaining and clarifying information is part of the nursing assistant's job

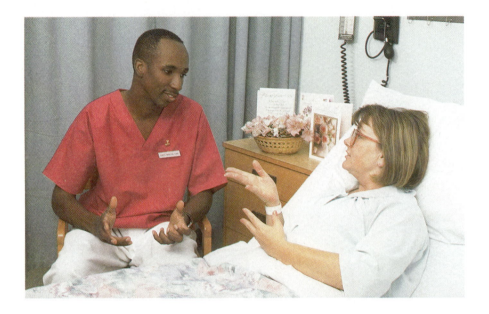

Communicating with Patients

As a nursing assistant, you are close to patients during their stay in the hospital. Often they tell you about their needs, pains, and worries. As you listen, you are both in close communication. Every time you touch a person's body, whether you speak any words or not, you are communicating something. How you assist a person in any action that involves touching the body says something. If you are careful, firm, and gentle, it tells the person something far different than if you are rough.

Pay attention to your posture. The way you move when you enter a patient's room or how you stand by the bed are ways of communicating through **body language**. Try to make these movements communicate energy, a sense of interest, and a willingness to help. A frown, an impatient body movement, or a shrug may give the patient the message "Do not bother me." Also, a certain way of standing or walking may send the message "I am lazy" or "I don't want to be bothered."

When you feel rushed, take a moment to collect yourself and focus on the patient. Look at the patient when you speak to her (Figure 3–3◆). This tells the patient that she has your attention. If you are looking away when talking, the patient gets the impression that your attention is elsewhere. Speak clearly and distinctly in a normal tone of voice. Talk with the patient, not just to or at her. Ask the patient what she likes or dislikes, thinks, or wants. Wait for the response and listen to the responses in an interested manner. If you are particularly busy, let a patient know when you will have some time to be able to sit and talk with her. If you think there will be a delay in your return with something the patient requested, be sure to let her know.

Vulgar words or slang are not appropriate or necessary. Also, do not use medical terms or abbreviations when talking to patients and their visitors. If you use medical language and the patient does not understand, you might give the wrong idea about what is happening to the patient (Figure 3–4◆).

body language

Communication through hand movements (gestures), facial expressions, body movements, and touch

KEY IDEA

Keep your voice pleasant, not too loud or too high pitched. Speak clearly and slowly enough to be easily understood. Never whisper or mumble, even when you think the patient is asleep or cannot hear you. This is annoying to the patient.

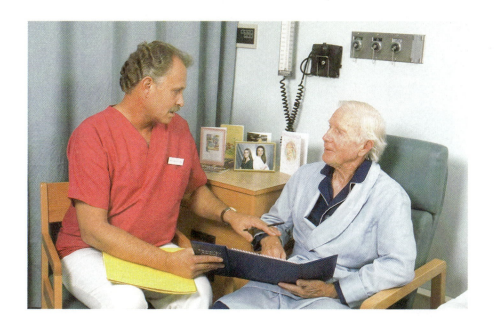

FIGURE 3-4◆
Communicating with patients is an important part of the nursing assistant's job

Remember that, although some patients seem to be semicomatose, comatose, or unconscious, they may be fully aware of what is happening around them and can often hear what is happening. Therefore, always speak and behave as if the patient can hear every word. They may hear more than you think. Patients frequently report conversations that occurred when they were seemingly comatose or unconscious.

Be sensitive to those times when the patient does not want to talk. Respect changes in the patient's mood or behavior. Saying nothing may have more meaning than any words or facial expressions. Sometimes a pat on the shoulder or holding a hand means more to a patient than anything you might say. Simply being near the stretcher or bed at the moment of trouble may be the most comforting message of all. It may help to silently sit near the patient for a few minutes when you know the patient is upset, afraid, or lonely. Use these guidelines when interacting with your patients (Figure 3-5◆).

Acknowledge the Need for Privacy and Avoid Being Overheard

All patients have the right to personal privacy. Information about their condition or diagnosis should not be displayed in a place where visitors or health care workers not immediately

COMMUNICATING WITH PATIENTS	GUIDELINES	OBRA
■ Address adults using Mr., Ms., or Mrs. and their last name unless they request otherwise. ■ Show an interest in what the patient is saying. ■ Let your facial expressions show that you are interested (Figure 3–4). ■ Use good manners.	■ Speak clearly, distinctly, and slowly. Speak in a normal, pleasant tone. ■ Use language that the patient can understand. ■ Respect the patient's moods. Sometimes silence can help. ■ Make your body movements look pleasing and energetic.	■ When someone in need asks you for assistance, whether to bathe or turn her or to get something that is out of reach, you should give your assistance willingly and graciously, no matter whose assigned patient it is. Avoid communicating a rushed or unhelpful response.

FIGURE 3–5◆

Show empathy with patients and their families

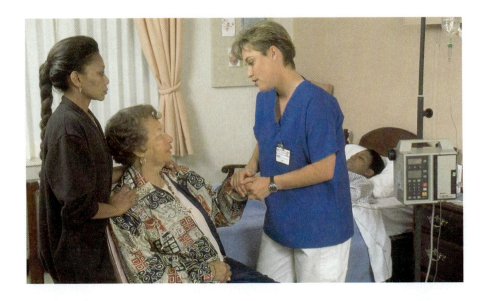

involved in their care can see it. Additionally, patients' confidentiality is respected by not discussing their case or situation in places where your conversation can be overheard by the patient, visitors, or coworkers.

Guidelines include the following:

- Curtains should be pulled or doors closed before providing personal care to any patient or exposing his or her body. Expose only the required or necessary area of the body.

- Do not stand outside a patient's room and discuss his or her case with visitors or coworkers in public areas such as the elevators or cafeteria.

- Avoid commenting about the patient to coworkers in front of the patient.

- Do not ask patients for personal information in a waiting area when others are present. If there is no private place, try to obtain this information in writing from the patient or ask in a quiet voice, standing close to the patient.

- Cover patients with sheets, towels, or gowns when possible to provide privacy.

SITUATION	INAPPROPRIATE COMMUNICATION	APPROPRIATE COMMUNICATION
Two caregivers standing outside a patient's room	"I cannot wait—tomorrow we will have one less cranky patient!"	"Can you meet me for a break in the staff lounge?"
Caregiver at the registration area of a urology ambulatory care office	"So, Mr. Smith, any luck with your Viagra?"	"Mr. Smith, your doctor will see you in five minutes."
Two caregivers talking in an elevator with visitors present	"That family in 304—are they weird or what? Can you believe she puts up with him beating her?"	"Remind me to call the social worker after lunch" or "I wonder what the cafeteria is serving today?"
Caregiver passing an elderly patient's room where the door is open and he is dressing	Caregiver says "How are you coming along?" and keeps on walking.	"Mr. Alvarez, let me close this door for you. I'll check back in a couple minutes."

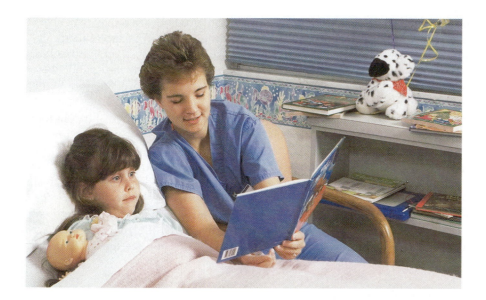

FIGURE 3–6 ◆
Pediatric patients have special needs

Communicating with the Pediatric Patient

In most hospitals, anyone under age 16 is called a **pediatric patient** (Figure 3–6◆). These patients may be grouped in several ways. For example, pediatric patients are sometimes grouped according to age because children of different ages need different kinds and amounts of care. Children also may be grouped according to their medical or surgical condition. Refer to Chapter 15 for information on chronological-age considerations and nursing assistant behaviors in communicating with the pediatric patient. Also, see Chapter 31 for information about communicating with pediatric patients and medical and surgical conditions that necessitate hospitalizing pediatric patients.

Call a child by his first name or nickname. Using his name tells the child that you know who he is. It shows respect for the child as a person and is a mark of courtesy.

Do not use commands (Figure 3–7◆). Do not call any child "stupid" or "dumb." Using such words can be very harmful to a child, because if they are repeated often enough

pediatric patient Any patient under the age of 16 years

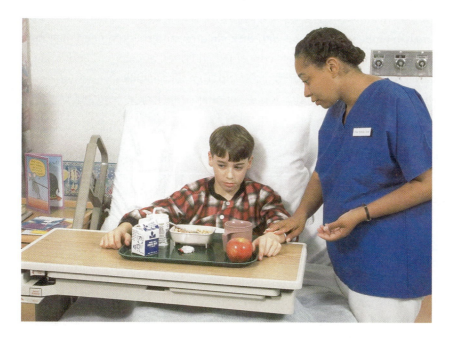

FIGURE 3–7◆
Do not say "Don't play with your food"; you could say "Aren't you hungry?"

children may begin to think of themselves as stupid or dumb. Then they may begin to behave as if they were stupid, because they think this is what is expected of them.

Very small children simply cannot tell you in words what they want. It is hard for them to communicate with you. Children will try to tell you things by the sounds they make, through the use of gestures or pointing, and by the way they move. You should try to understand what their sounds and movements mean.

Try to learn the reason for their crying and then try to comfort them. Reasons for crying, of course, depend on how old the child is and perhaps on what happened before they started crying.

When you are giving children personal care, use every chance you have to show your interest in them and your affection for them. This is done in different ways with children of different ages. Although children may not complain or seem to feel sorry for themselves, they may be uncomfortable or unhappy. They need your kindness and empathy. Your smile, a tender touch, or affectionate words can tell the child that you are interested in and care about him or her. Refer to Chapter 15 for age-specific considerations and recommendations.

Importance of the Child's Family

A child is still a member of a family, even when in the hospital. The person or persons who care for the child at home represent the family. Many hospitals and pediatric patient care units have a policy of allowing a family member to stay with the child and even encourage them to do so.

KEY IDEA

This may be the first time the child has been away from home. The child may be frightened or may view hospitalization as punishment. Such a patient needs to be held, touched, and talked to in order to be comforted and reassured.

Several important things need to be considered and remembered with the pediatric patient:

- Family members need to be with their children, and children need their families.
- Family members are normally concerned and often are worried and frightened.
- Most children first learn about the world from their families.
- The younger the child, the more important the family is in helping to ease the child's fears.

Things you can do to help are:

- Do the best possible job of caring for the child. This is usually reassuring to the family members.
- Show interest and concern about the family members' welfare. Ask, "Is there something we can do?"
- Do not make judgments about the family members' attitudes or behavior, even if they seem strange to you.
- Encourage and allow family members to help take part in the child's care when possible and if permitted.
- Sometimes family members seem to be worried about something concerning their child's stay in the hospital and are afraid to talk about it. If you suspect this, tell your immediate supervisor.

Communicating with Older Adults

Most older adults are able to easily communicate. Changes in vision or reduced hearing occur with many elderly persons. However, communicating with patients who have Alzheimer's disease can be challenging because they are confused and disoriented. Refer to Chapter 32 for guidelines and more detailed information.

Communicating with Family and Visitors

Visiting hours are often the highlight of the day for patients. Knowing that family and friends are interested and concerned can do a lot to relax a patient's tensions, ease feelings of loneliness or isolation, relieve fears, and cheer the spirit.

Visitors may be worried and upset over the illness of a member of the family. They need your kindness and patience. Pleasant comments about flowers or gifts brought by visitors for the patient may be helpful (Figure 3–8◆).

If it appears that visitors are upsetting or tiring the patient, notify your immediate supervisor, who can caution the visitors or ask them to leave.

In some situations, visiting hours may be longer or shorter. Sometimes special circumstances require exceptions to be made to meet the needs of particular families or visitors. Usually a note is put in the patient's chart or plan of care to alert staff that a particular exception has been made. Your instructor will tell you about the visiting hours and any rules for visitors in your health care institution. These rules, of course, must be followed. Two main rules usually apply to visitors in any health care institution:

- Visitors are not allowed to take institutional property away with them.
- Visitors cannot bring food or drink to the patient unless permission has been given by the nurse or doctor.

Certain actions are helpful in your contacts with visitors. Follow these guidelines when interacting and communicating with visitors.

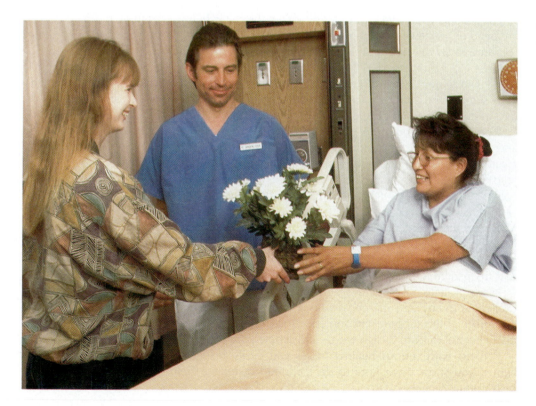

FIGURE 3–8◆

The nursing assistant should make visitors feel welcome

<table>
<tr><td>

COMMUNICATING WITH VISITORS

</td><td>

GUIDELINES

</td><td>

OBRA

</td></tr>
</table>

- Listen to the visitor. Whether it is a suggestion, a complaint, or "passing the time of day," listen to the person. Some suggestions by visitors can be very helpful. Some complaints may be valid. When a complaint is presented, tell the person, "Thank you for bringing this matter to my attention. I will tell my supervisor about this," and then report it to your immediate supervisor.

- Do not get involved in the family's private affairs and feelings. Never take sides in family quarrels. Never give information or opinions to someone about other family members.

- Be prepared to give information regarding the hospital to visitors. Tell them what facilities are available for coffee, snacks, or meals, and the hours of operation. Tell them where to find a public telephone. Direct them to other places in the institution, for example, the business office or the gift shop.

Communicating with Sensory-Impaired, Blind, or Deaf Patients

Patients with sensory loss present special challenges. Your patients who are visually impaired, or blind, will have the same personal care needs as your other patients. Providing care will be much easier if you explain what you wish to do and encourage the patient's cooperation. Your patient has probably accepted his visual disability and learned to do things for himself quite well. Assume your patient has normal intelligence and treat him with the respect and courtesy you would any other patient. The patient's care plan should identify how the patient can best see or hear. If this information is not available to you, then ask your patient if he has any vision at all and determine if the patient sees light, dark, shadows, and so on. Discuss things that might be helpful to the patient. For example, where his cane should be placed if the patient has one or describing the size and shape of the room, the location of the bathroom, the bedside chair, overbed table, and nightstand.

For patients who have serious vision losses, the call light is used differently. Patients who are blind or visually impaired must be shown and taught how to use the signal. Have them feel around for the cord and practice using it while you are there.

If the call light is the kind that you push to turn on, you can call it a "push" button. If it works like a light switch, you can compare it to that. When working with patients who have serious visual losses, you should not expect them to turn off the signal. You can do that routinely when you respond to the signal call.

Communicating with the patient who is deaf or hearing impaired and is able to read and write will be easier if you remember to carry a small pad and a pen. You can communicate with your patient in writing. Print short questions that are easy for the patient to read. The patient can respond by writing the answers. Use questions that can have either "yes" or "no" answers, if possible. Pictures or drawings can be used with patients who cannot read.

Also, if the patient wears a hearing aid, be sure it is operating and assist the patient if he has difficulty manipulating it. Refer to Chapter 26 for care of hearing aids.

Some patients can read lips. If this is true for your patient, always position yourself so that the patient is able to see your lips. Speak slowly and distinctly. Don't shout!

Many facilities have staff available to communicate with patients who present particular challenges to any staff members who do not have the training to sign, for example. Take advantage of this support staff and encourage your patient to do so. You may find it particularly helpful to learn to sign words and simple phrases.

Patients with serious hearing losses can easily learn how to pull or push the call light if you show them how to do it instead of telling them. Remember, they cannot hear you.

Communicating with Non-English-Speaking Patients

Sometimes patients come to the hospital who do not speak English or for whom English is a second language. It would be ideal if your facility employed workers who speak languages other than English or if you could learn certain medical terms or phrases in several languages to assist you in communicating with your patients. There may be a list of personnel or volunteers who can be called to translate when it is necessary to communicate with non-English-speaking patients. Some hospitals have contracts established with AT&T to provide translators via telephone when needed in urgent or emergency situations. Also, communication boards with pictures or drawings of equipment, such as a bedpan, TV, phone, water pitcher, and so on, are helpful tools to use in communicating with patients. In the absence of these options, a family member or friend can be very helpful.

Communicating with Other Staff Members

Communication is essential in providing patients with the coordinated care they need. Staff communicate through the patient record, in report or team meetings, in conversations or consultations about particular patient needs or problems, and verbally.

Answering the Patient Call Signal

Every patient has a way of sending a signal to the nursing staff when something is needed. It is important to answer the patient's call for service or help without delay (Figure 3–9◆).

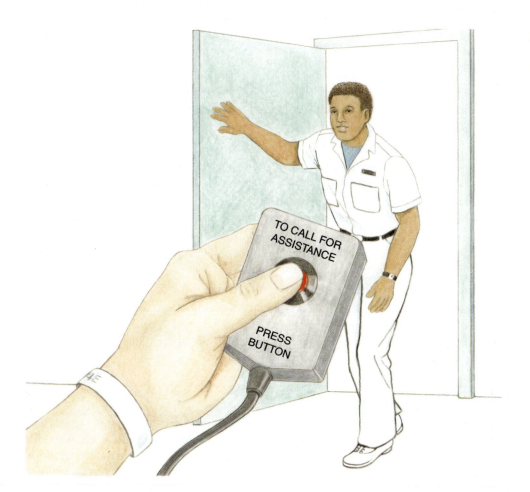

FIGURE 3–9◆

Answer the patient's call as quickly as possible

FIGURE 3–10◆

Take patients' family concerns seriously

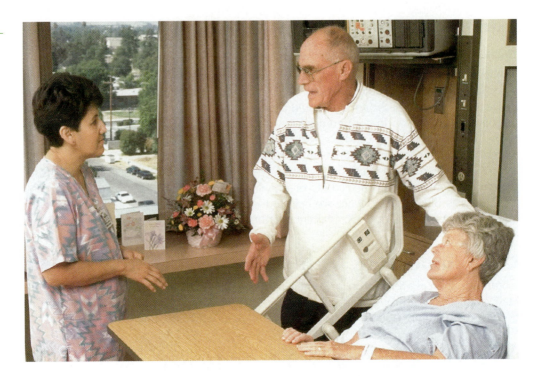

FIGURE 3–10◆ Take patients' family concerns seriously

All patients have a call light or signaling device. It is important to show the patient and family how to use the call light system at the time of admission. When the patient presses the button on the end of the cord, a light flashes near the nurses' station and over the patient's door. This device may be called a *call light* or *call bell*. A hand bell system can be used if no electronic system is available. You should always keep alert for such signals. Answer the signal as soon as it flashes. Every minute seems forever to the patient who is waiting. When the patient signals:

- Go to the patient at once, quietly and in a friendly way.
- Turn off the call signal and address the patient by name.
- Say, "Mr. Jones, what can I do for you?"
- Do whatever the patient asks, but be sure it is correct and safe for this patient. If you are in doubt, ask your immediate supervisor. Relate what the patient wants and then follow your supervisor's directions.
- Take patient and visitor concerns seriously (Figure 3–10◆). If you are unable to do something to correct the situation, refer the matter or problem to your supervisor.
- When necessary, use the emergency signal to get qualified personnel to assist you. Emergency signals are usually in one or more convenient locations: at the bedside, in the bathroom, shower, or tub room.
- Place the call light where the patient can reach it easily.
- *Caution:* A young child or an incapacitated adult may not be able to use the call light. Listen for calls for help from these patients and go quickly to see what they need. Check these patients often to see if they need something. Often, special call lights are available for patients with handicaps.

Using the Telephone

When you use the telephone or an intercommunication system (intercom), speak clearly and slowly. When you answer the telephone, for example, say, "Third floor, west. Mrs. Brown, nursing assistant, speaking." When you take a message for someone else, write it down immediately. Then repeat it to the person calling to make sure it is correct. Verify the spelling of the caller's name so you are sure you have it right. Record the following:

- The person being called
- The date and time the call was received
- The caller's name and phone number
- The message
- Your name and title

Reporting Incidents

Incidents can occur at any time, and no incident should be viewed as too insignificant to report. When you are unsure if a situation warrants an incident report, discuss the matter with your supervisor. A simple notation on the patient's chart may be adequate. Always ask for help when you are unsure. Your concern indicates that you care and that you are responsible. Remember: The patient's safety and well-being are your first responsibility. Refer to Chapter 2 for more detailed information on reporting incidents.

Complaints and Grievance Procedures

There are times when employees, patients, or families have concerns or issues that they want to bring to the attention of supervisors or administration. This communication occurs in the form of a verbal or written letter of complaint. Some facilities have formal grievance procedures for employees to use when they have been unable to resolve an issue with their coworkers or supervisor. If there is such a procedure in your facility, it will be mentioned during your orientation. The human resources staff or individual can review this process with you should you need more information.

Observing the Patient

Get into the habit of observing the patient during all your contacts. These contacts include the bed bath, bed making, mealtimes, visiting hours, and any other time you are with the patient. **Observation** of the patient is a continuous process. Observing begins the first time you see a patient and ends when he is discharged from the hospital.

observation Gathering information about the patient by noticing any change

Observation means more than just careful watching. It includes listening and talking to the patient and asking questions (Figure 3–11◆). It means being aware of a situation and

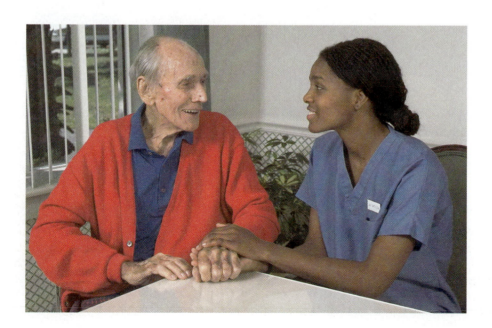

FIGURE 3–11◆

Observation of the patient includes listening and talking

interpreting it. Be alert to changes in a patient's condition or anything unusual that occurs whenever you are with a patient. Report any changes in the patient's condition or appearance. Also watch for changes in the patient's attitude, moods, and emotional condition. Pay attention to any complaints. For example, report to your immediate supervisor if:

- A patient who had an abdominal operation 2 or 3 days ago says, "The calf of my leg is sore."
- A patient who is being given a blood transfusion says, "I feel itchy."

Methods of Observation

Learning how to make useful observations is one of the most important things you will do in your work and will give you satisfaction and a feeling of achievement (Figure 3–12◆). The process of observation never ends, and you learn by doing. Because observations are so important in the total care of all patients, doctors, nurses, and all health care givers never stop learning.

Objective Observations: Signs

objective observations Signs that can be observed and reported exactly as they are seen

edema Abnormal swelling of a part of the body caused by fluid collecting in that area; usually the swelling is in the ankles, legs, hands, or abdomen

Use all your senses (looking, listening, touching, smelling) when making **objective observations**:

- You can see some signs of change in a patient's condition. By using your eyes, you can observe a skin rash, reddened areas, or swelling (**edema**).
- You can feel some signs with your fingers: a change in the patient's pulse rate, puffiness in the skin, dampness (perspiration).
- You can hear some signs, such as a cough or wheezing sounds, when the patient breathes.
- You can smell some signs, such as an odor on a patient's breath.
- Listen to the patient talking for other changes in his condition.

FIGURE 3–12◆

Be alert when making observations. Touching, listening, and looking help you gather information about the patient

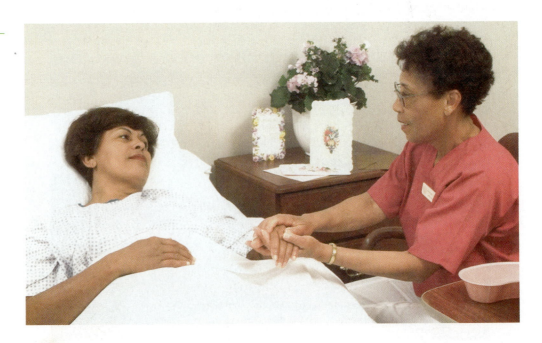

Subjective Observations: Symptoms

Subjective observations are symptoms that can be felt and described only by the patient. Examples are pain, nausea, dizziness, ringing in the ears, or headache. Table 3–1◆ provides a list of things to observe in the patient.

Observation of an Infant or Child

Observing an infant or a child means looking at her appearance and physical condition, bodily functions and **secretions**, and movements and behavior. When you observe changes in any of these, it is very important that you report them to your immediate supervisor right away. Report things that can be measured, such as a high temperature. Also report the things you see in a pattern of change, such as the child's behavior. Your careful observation and quick reporting could save a baby's life. The following are things to report when you observe them in infants or children:

Appearance and Physical Condition

- The child's temperature is high or very low.
- The pulse is unusually fast, slow, or irregular.
- The child is breathing rapidly or is having trouble breathing.
- The abdomen seems to be swollen.
- The child's skin does not look normal; it may be yellow, show purplish patches, appear unusually pale, or have a blue cast.
- There may be blueness (**cyanosis**) in the fingernails or lips.
- Secretions, bleeding, or odor is coming from the baby's navel (umbilicus).

Bodily Functions and Secretions

- The child has not urinated during your hours of work or has voided very little.
- The child has diarrhea.
- A large amount of mucus is being secreted from the mouth or nose.
- The child is producing a large amount of saliva.
- The child is having trouble swallowing.
- The child is coughing or choking.
- The child is vomiting.

Movement and Behavior

- The child is lying in an abnormal position.
- The muscles are twitching.
- There is no movement in the legs or arms.
- The child is lying very quietly or seems unusually still.
- The child is crying or is excessively irritable.

Reporting and Recording Observations

Reporting and recording observations involves care and accuracy. You will have to sort out and report appropriately objective and subjective information. Forms you will use and charting techniques will vary from facility to facility. Some records will be handwritten; others will be computerized. You will be taught whatever system is in use in your facility or agency.

---

subjective observations Symptoms that can be felt and described only by the patient himself, such as pain, nausea, dizziness, ringing in the ears, and headache

secretions The substances that flow out of or are produced by glandular organs; the process of producing this substance; for example: sweat, bile, lymph, saliva, or urine

cyanosis When the skin looks blue or gray, especially on the lips, nailbeds, and under the fingernails; in a black patient, it may appear as a darkening of color: This occurs when there is not enough oxygen in the blood

TABLE 3–1◆

Things to Observe in a Patient

WHAT TO OBSERVE	QUESTIONS TO ASK YOURSELF
General Appearance	Has this changed? If so, in what way? Is there a noticeable odor (smell)?
Mental Condition or Mood	Does the patient talk a lot? Very little? Does he talk about the future or the past? Does he talk about where he hurts? Is the patient anxious and worried? Is he calm? Or is he very excited? Is he talking sensibly? Or not making sense? Is he confused or disoriented? Is he speaking rapidly? Slowly? Is he cooperative? Uncooperative? Is he belligerent or aggravated?
Position	Does the patient lie still, or does he toss around? Does he like to lie in one position better than others? Does he prefer being on his back? On his side? Is he able to move easily?
Eating and Drinking Habits	Does the patient complain that he has no appetite? Does he dislike his diet? How much does he eat? Does he eat some of each kind of food? Is he always thirsty, or does he very seldom drink water? Does he eat all the food on his tray? Does he eat half the food on his tray? Does he refuse to eat?
Sleeping Habits	Is the patient able to sleep? Is she restless? Does she complain about not being able to sleep? Do these complaints agree with your observations? Does she sleep more than is normal? Is she constantly asleep?
Skin	Is the patient's skin unusually pale (pallor)? Is it flushed (red)? Is the skin dry or moist? Are his lips and fingernails turning blue (cyanotic)? Is any swelling (edema) noticeable? Are there reddened areas? Are these at the end of the spine, or on the heels, or at other pressure points? Is the skin shiny? Is there any puffiness? Is there puffiness in the legs and feet? Is his skin cold and clammy? Is it hot? Are there bruises or unusual markings?
Eyes, Ears, Nose, and Mouth	Does the patient complain that she sees spots or flashes before her eyes? Does bright light bother her? Are her eyes red (inflamed)? Is it hard for her to breathe through her nose? Does she seem to have large amounts of mucous discharge from the nose? Does she complain that she has a bad taste in her mouth? Is there an odor on her breath? Is the patient able to hear you?
Breathing	Does the patient wheeze? Does she make other noises when she breathes? Does she cough? Does she cough up sputum and how much? What is the color? Is it bloody? Does she have difficulty breathing (dyspnea) or shortness of breath?
Abdomen, Bowels, and Bladder	Does the patient's stomach appear to be distended (puffed up)? Does he complain of gas, belching, or nausea? Is he vomiting (having emesis)? What is the appearance of the vomitus? Does it contain red blood? Does it look like coffee grounds? Is the patient constipated? How often does he have a bowel movement? What is the color and consistency (hard or soft) of feces (stool)? Is there any blood, or clumps of mucus, or pieces of white material in the feces? How often does the patient void (urinate)? How much does he void each time? Does he say that he has pain during urination or that it is difficult to start to urinate? Is there sediment (cloudiness) or blood in the urine? Is it concentrated? Does the urine have a peculiar odor or color? Is the patient unable to control his bowels or urine (incontinent)?
Pain	Where is the pain? How long does the patient say she has had it? How does she describe the pain? Is it constant? Does it come and go? Does she say that it is sharp, dull, aching, or knifelike? Has she had medicine for the pain? Does the patient say that the medicine relieved the pain?
Daily Activities	Does the patient dress himself? Does he walk without help? Does he walk with help? Does he avoid walking altogether?
Personal Care	Without help, does the patient brush his teeth? Comb his hair? Go to the bathroom? Wash his face? Does he ask for assistance?
Movements	Is the patient shaking (having tremors or spasms)? Is she limp? Are her movements uncontrollable?

Subjective and Objective Reporting

It is very important for you to understand the difference between **objective reporting** and **subjective reporting**. Reporting subjective information must be done accurately by repeating what the patient tells you regarding herself. Remember, only the patient can describe or make a judgment about what she feels. Examples are pain, nausea, dizziness, ringing in the ears, and headaches.

Objective reporting means reporting exactly what you measure or observe, that is, what you see, hear, feel, or smell. Examples of measurements include temperatures, vital signs, blood pressures, weights, size, or actual amounts. The nursing assistant must always use objective reporting (see Figure 3–13◆).

Here are some examples of objective reporting:

- Mrs. Barbary in Room 110, window bed, is perspiring profusely.
- Mr. Ellis in Room 432, door bed, had a bowel movement that was white; a specimen was collected.
- Mrs. Delcara, Room 510, A bed, has an area on her left heel that is hard, red, and it measures the size of a quarter.
- Mrs. Walker in Room 330, A bed, lips are dark blue.
- Mrs. Carlin in Room 101, window bed, right ankle is much larger than her left ankle.
- Mr. Joseph in Room 404 is clenching his teeth together and is talking very differently than he was talking at breakfast.
- When Mr. Roberts in Room 581, B bed, breathes he makes loud wheezing sounds, which he was not doing when I made his bed an hour ago.
- Mrs. Smith, Room 8031, is breathing rapidly, and the breaths appear to be shallow.
- Mr. Williams, Room 204, B bed, urine looks red tinged; a urine specimen was collected.

objective reporting
Reporting exactly what you observe

subjective reporting
Giving your opinion about what you have observed; the nursing assistant should never use subjective reporting

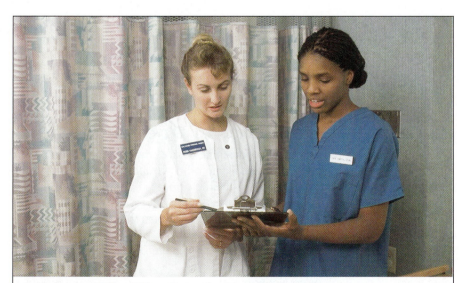

FIGURE 3–13◆
Guidelines to follow when reporting observations

Guidelines to Follow When Reporting Your Observations
- Write down the patient's name, room number, and bed number.
- Write or report your observations to the nurse or team leader as soon as possible.
- Report the time you made the observation.
- Report the location of the observation.
- Report exactly, but report only what you observe, that is, report objectively.

FIGURE 3–14◆
Subjective versus objective
reporting

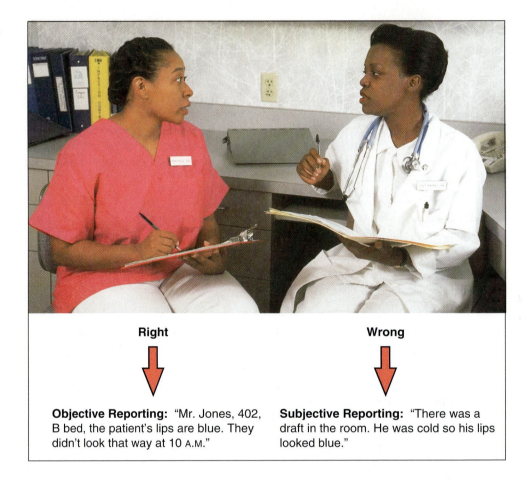

Right

Wrong

Objective Reporting: "Mr. Jones, 402, B bed, the patient's lips are blue. They didn't look that way at 10 A.M."

Subjective Reporting: "There was a draft in the room. He was cold so his lips looked blue."

- Cindy Jones, Room 107, A bed, has a red area the size of a dollar bill on her upper right back.
- Mr. Jones, Room 101, A bed, urine was bright red; left in urinal in his bathroom for you to see.

Figure 3–14◆ gives examples of the right way and the wrong way of reporting.

Forms and Records Used in Documentation

Every facility has its own forms and record keeping or documentation system. Some facilities' records are written down in long hand while other facilities have computerized their documentation system (Figure 3–15◆). Your instructor or staff development educator will explain the particular way you are expected to chart the care you have given to patients. Refer to Figure 12–2 in Chapter 12 for an example of a form you may be asked to use to chart daily care of patients.

Recording the date and time of your observations accurately is a very important part of documentation. Some facilities/agencies use a 24-hour "clock," or military time, for recording rather than the standard, or conventional, 12-hour clock with A.M. and P.M. Table 3–2◆ is a conversion table that gives the 12-hour clock for the A.M. and P.M. hours (conventional time) on the left and the corresponding 24-hour clock hours (military time) on the right. If you are using military time, the hours from midnight to noon are referred to as "___ hundred hours." For example, 2:00 A.M. is "0200" (two hundred hours). The P.M. hours (after noon to midnight) on the 12-hour clock can easily be converted to military time by adding the time on the 12-hour clock to 12. Therefore, if it is 4:00 P.M., military time would be 12 + 4 or 1600 hours.

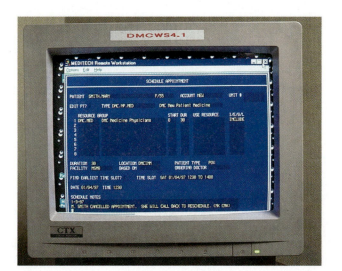

FIGURE 3–15◆
Computerized charting

Computerization of Medical Records

Health care facilities are increasingly computerizing their records. It is necessary for all health care givers to be trained to document on the computerized record (Figure 3–15). This training usually lasts for several days, especially if the caregiver has had little or no computer training or **keyboard** (typing) experience. Even those employees or students who do have some computer experience will need to learn how to use the system—computer equipment and **software** programs—in use in their particular facility. A **password** is given or chosen by each person to give them access to the system. A particular advantage of a computerized record-keeping or charting system is that a particular patient's chart or record can be pulled up in multiple places. For example, a physician can chart, check lab results, or write orders from another location in the facility or from an office outside the facility.

Advantages of computerized records are:

- Various caregivers can access the records with ease.
- The problem with reading handwriting is avoided because the record is clearly printed.
- Eventually record storage will be kept on disks rather than on volumes of paper.

keyboard An input device similar to a typewriter keyboard; has additional keys that allow the user to make selections to direct computer activity

software Set or sets of instructions that direct computer operations; computer programs

password A word or phrase that identifies a person and allows access to or entry to a program or record

TABLE 3–2◆

24-Hour Clock Conversion

12-HOUR CLOCK (CONVENTIONAL TIME)	24-HOUR CLOCK (MILITARY TIME)	12-HOUR CLOCK (CONVENTIONAL TIME)	24-HOUR CLOCK (MILITARY TIME)
1:00 A.M.	0100	1:00 P.M.	1300
2:00 A.M.	0200	2:00 P.M.	1400
3:00 A.M.	0300	3:00 P.M.	1500
4:00 A.M.	0400	4:00 P.M.	1600
5:00 A.M.	0500	5:00 P.M.	1700
6:00 A.M.	0600	6:00 P.M.	1800
7:00 A.M.	0700	7:00 P.M.	1900
8:00 A.M.	0800	8:00 P.M.	2000
9:00 A.M.	0900	9:00 P.M.	2100
10:00 A.M.	1000	10:00 P.M.	2200
11:00 A.M.	1100	11:00 P.M.	2300
12:00 (Noon)	1200	12:00 (Midnight)	2400 (0000)

- Patients can be issued cards with computer chips that contain pertinent medical history. These cards can be presented to emergency departments, health care providers, and/or clinics, as needed. The possibility of errors and delays in treatment can be reduced.

- Fewer questions will arise about services provided and payments can be processed sooner.

Computer Documentation

The use of computers has become commonplace in health care during the past decade. Many organizations have expanded the technology used in ordering, reporting, and documenting patient care to include electronic or computer as well as handwritten systems. Computers are used for many different reasons—from ordering laboratory tests and food service to recording information about the patient's progress and activities of daily living. Health care workers are expected to have basic familiarity with computers and how computers function. For some, the thought of using a computer is unnerving while others consider it a fact of life. The basic function of a computer is to break knowledge down into a simple form, store it, then rapidly move it from one place to another in a very efficient and rapid fashion. Computers are tools to assist in communicating information and getting work done.

Basic Parts, or Components, of a Computer

Computers are made up of two key components: a **central processing unit (CPU)**, or "brain," and a data storage device, or **memory**. The central processing unit performs several functions and moves pieces of data, one at a time, to and from data storage or memory. Several other pieces of equipment or hardware are necessary to know about in order to become comfortable using a computer. We discuss this equipment next.

Hardware

Hardware includes all of the parts that physically make up the computer, the electronic and mechanical parts of the computer that can be touched or manipulated. Hardware includes the keyboard, **mouse**, **monitor**, or terminal, and the **printer**. The hardware is used to enter **data** into the central processing unit, the brain of the computer, where it is processed for storage or for output and printing. The central processing unit and memory are contained in a box or tower that can be found near the computer monitor, which is also called a **terminal** (Figure 3–16◆).

Similar to a television, the terminal or computer monitor displays data or information on a **screen**, usually in color. The **cursor** is a blinking or flashing line or box that indicates the user's location on the computer screen. A message that appears on the computer screen is called a **prompt**. A prompt is a signal that the user needs to either make a selection on the screen or to enter data in order for the computer program to continue.

Data can be entered by way of a keyboard or by making selections with a mouse or light pen. The computer keyboard is similar to a typewriter, with additional keys that allow the user to make selections to direct computer activities. The arrow keys on the keyboard allow a user to move the cursor up or down and to the right or left on the computer monitor. There are also special *function keys* on a computer keyboard. The function keys are spare keys, which operate differently depending on the *software*, or *program*, being used. On the right of the keyboard, there is a number pad, similar to a calculator, which is used for entering numerical data for calculations. As a computer user, you will need to be familiar with the placement of letters, numbers, and function keys on the keyboard so you can record data or execute other computer functions. In addition, you will need to know how to use a mouse or light pen (Figure 3–17◆).

---

central processing unit (CPU) Central processing unit, the "computer brain" where information is stored or directed to appropriate pathways

memory The capacity of the computer to store data

hardware The actual physical equipment that is used by a computer to process data

mouse A pointing and selecting device to input data; a small tabletop electronic pointing device used to make selections on a computer screen

monitor A screen, similar to a television screen, that allows the user to see input and output

printer An output device for creating a hard copy

data Information that a user enters into a computer

terminal A computer monitor that allows the computer operator to see input and output on a screen

screen A portion of data that is displayed at one time within the confined area of the computer monitor

cursor Flashing bar, or symbol, that indicates where the next character is to be placed or location on the computer screen

prompt A reminder that the user must take some action so further processing of the data can continue

FIGURE 3–16◆

Computer system components

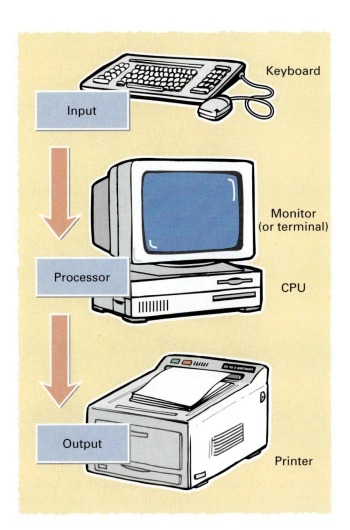

A mouse is one type of electronic pointing device used to make selections on a computer monitor. To become comfortable using a mouse requires eye–hand coordination and a bit of practice. The user lightly rests his/her hand on the mouse and gently moves it on a desk or tabletop. When the mouse is moved on the top of the table or desk, the cursor moves on the monitor. Once the cursor is in the desired position on the screen, the user presses or "clicks" the left button to make a selection. The right button is used less frequently and is similar to the spare keys on the keyboard; it offers options for additional functions with specific software.

Another electronic pointing device is the **light pen**, which looks exactly like its name implies, an oversized pen. A wire connects the light pen to the CPU on one end and emits a small light signal to which the computer can respond at the other end. Sometimes there is a button on the side of the light pen that the user pushes to make the selection on the screen. The light pen can be held as a pen when designed to make selections by scanning the data, such as bar codes. Otherwise, the light pen can be held across the palm of the hand, like a knife handle, using the index finger to push the button for making selections. The latter method for making selections is the "point-and-click" method. With either method, the user requires practice to refine the skill. Portable wireless pen-based computers, or laptop computers, are increasingly used in office settings, outpatient clinics, and home care (Figure 3–18◆).

A printer is used to transfer data from memory into information on paper. Different types of printers are available. A laser printer burns the ink into the paper while an ink-jet printer sprays tiny dots of ink onto the page. Both laser and ink-jet printers feed paper

light pen A hand-held device shaped like a pen that has an electronic sensor for making selections on a computer screen

FIGURE 3–17◆

Caregiver enters data using
a keyboard

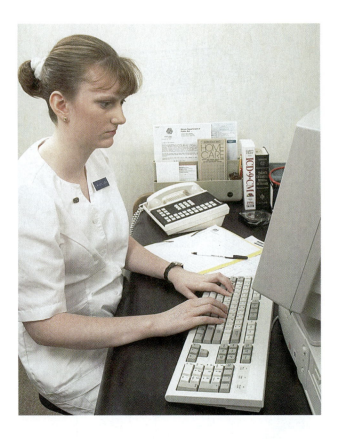

through the rollers one page at a time. A dot matrix printer has small metal pins that press ink from a ribbon on the page and feeds perforated paper on tractor pins through the printer. With the continuous-feed paper, users sometimes experience problems with paper jams or inappropriately torn paper resulting in misalignment of the next page. It is important to tear the paper only at the perforated end of the page or to feed the paper through to the end of the page. A printer may be found next to the other hardware at an individual workstation or in a central location where several workstations have access to it.

Hardware is connected to the CPU by cables. Occasionally, the cables become loose and create problems with the hardware. Simple problem solving can be done by tracing wires to their ports and checking the connections. Hardware varies from one manufacturer

FIGURE 3–18◆

Portable wireless pen-based
computer

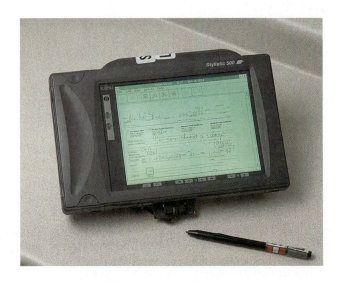

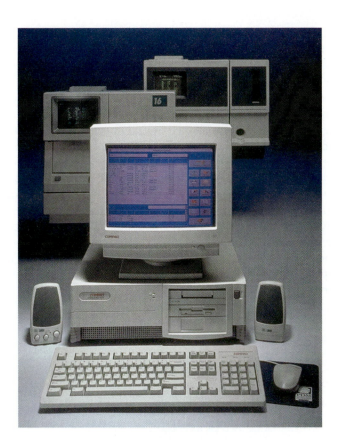

FIGURE 3–19◆
Windows software on a patient management system

to another. Once you are comfortable with one type of hardware, you often can figure out what to do with a similar piece of hardware from a different manufacturer.

Software

Software is a term used to describe the programs or set of instructions that make the computer work. Software, or the computer program, contains instructions that direct computer activity. Without software the computer would not function. Software is loaded, or installed, on the computer by computer analysts or programmers who are familiar with information systems (IS) (Figure 3–19◆).

Computer programs exist for a number of activities. The most common types of software seen in patient care areas are used for:

1. Ordering patient care activities
2. Recording patient care information
3. Interfacing with other departments to obtain information or reports

Organizations usually provide training to prepare employees to use new software. The training is often done directly on the computer and is known as *computer-based training* (CBT). Learning to use new software takes time, practice, and patience.

Network

When working in a large organization, several computers may be connected to each other by cables or telephone lines or via wireless means to create a **network**. If a workstation is connected to a network, the user can have access to any of the software or hardware that is part of the network. In fact, a user could go to any workstation in the organization, *log on* to the network, and use that computer to enter data.

network Several computers that are connected together, having access to central computer programs; can interface to obtain information; located at different workstations

log on To sign on to the computer using a password or personal identification number

personal identification number (PIN) password

boot up To start up the computer

Computers that are part of a network are often left on and ready to use. The monitor may be blank or have a *screen saver* of some nature. The user simply needs to touch any key to get to the log-in screen. A user will **log on** when he enters his user identification (ID) and password, which is a confidential code allowing network access. The user ID and password are listed in the computer for security purposes. This is the same concept as a **personal identification number (PIN)** used at an electronic bank teller machine. If the ID is in the list of people identified as valid and legitimate users and the password matches the ID, then the user will have access to the network. If the ID or password does not match those on the list, access will be denied. Security is important to eliminate inappropriate users.

Individual, or stand-alone, workstations may need to be turned on and off daily. Turning a computer on is called **booting up**. When a user wants to turn off the computer, he must exit the programs that are running and log out. The user must always log off the computer appropriately or the ID and password will continue to be in operation. This means that another person wanting to use the computer may actually be doing so under the previous user's name rather than her own. Be sure to log off or sign off each time you complete recording patient information so your electronic signature and the patient data are removed from the screen. The terminal will then be ready for the next user. Table 3–3◆ contains additional definitions for frequently used computer terms.

TABLE 3–3◆

Frequently Used Computer Terms

TERMS	DEFINITIONS
Boot	To start up the computer.
Downtime	Time a computer cannot be used because of maintenance or mechanical failure.
Drive	Pathway that sends signals to the right place at the right time.
Hard copy	A printed copy of data in a file; printout; output.
Information systems	Refers to managing data through the use of computers; a unit or department in an organization deals with computers.
Input	Entering data into the computer system.
Interface	Technology that allows two or more computers to exchange programs and data. Also referred to as a *network*.
Log on	To sign on to use the computer.
Main memory	The part of the central processing unit that stores data and program instructions. It does not perform any of the logical operations, for example, computations or sorting.
Memory	The capacity of the computer to store data.
Output	Processed data translated into final form information.
Program	A set or sets of instructions that tell the computer hardware what to do in order to complete the required data processing. Also called software.
Report	Structured information provided upon request or at selected intervals.
Retrieve	Recall data from computer memory.
Security code	A group of characters that allows an authorized computer user access to certain programs or features. Password.
Screen	A portion of data that is displayed at one time within the confined area of the computer monitor.
Sign-on code	Secure password to prevent unauthorized persons from using the system.
Workstation	A location that contains a CPU, computer monitor, keyboard, and mouse or light pen; may be an individual unit or part of a network.

Confidentiality

All patient-centered computer information is considered confidential because it deals with the private and personal information about patients and their conditions. Most computer systems have a method of protecting patient confidentiality, such as tracking the number of entries or excursions made into the patient's database. If anyone other than the designated caregiver is looking at the patient data in the computer, there is a breach of patient confidentiality. Only those delivering care to the patient at a given time are permitted access to patient data.

Most computer systems have the capacity to track the number of entries or excursions into the system. If a person not actually involved with patient care explores data, the system manager will be able to detect it. Staff members who breach patient confidentiality may be subject to disciplinary action, including termination of employment.

Computers are expensive and a large investment for organizations. Many organizations have limited numbers of computers in given patient care areas. In some areas, such as intensive care, a computer may be at each patient's bedside, whereas in other areas there may be one workstation for every four patients. Computers make it efficient to record and store information for **retrieval** or recall. The patient medical record can be available for others to access when necessary. It is especially useful for large hospital systems to have a computerized patient record so information from across the patient's continuum of care can be retrieved. Although data are stored in the computer, a hard, or printed, copy of the patient's record is also available. In the future, employers will expect most caregivers to be computer literate.

retrieval To recall data stored in computer memory

Medical Terminology

Refer to the Appendix for a listing of medical terms and abbreviations commonly used in health care facilities. The Appendix also provides an extensive listing of medical specialties, with title of the physician delivering each specialty and a brief description of the specialty itself. Learn where the general medical reference materials are kept in your facility and in the unit(s) or area(s) to which you are assigned.

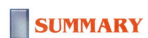

SUMMARY

Communication occurs through the exchange of gestures and words and the observation of actions. This chapter has identified ways to communicate effectively with patients, their families, and other health care providers using your actions, words, and observation skills. Both your verbal and written communication skills are important. Subjective reporting includes what you learn directly from a patient. Objective reporting refers to what you are able to hear, see, feel, or smell. In your work, you will be educated (taught/trained) and expected to chart or document on a variety of forms and systems.

CHAPTER REVIEW

FILL IN THE BLANK Read each sentence and fill in the blank line with a word that completes the sentence.

1. Signs that can be observed and reported exactly as they are seen are called _____ _____.

2. _____ _____ is a type of communication through movements (gestures), facial expressions, body movements, and touch.

3. For the pediatric patient, _____ is extremely important in helping calm the fears of the patient.

4. It is very important to answer the _____ _____ when the patient signals so that she can receive help without delay.

5. _____ are an electronic medical record that makes it easy for institutions to record and store information for retrieval or recall.

MULTIPLE CHOICE Choose the best answer for each question or statement.

1. Communication
   a. may be written.
   b. may be spoken.
   c. is an exchange of information with others.
   d. All of the above.

2. Which of the following is not a key element of communication?
   a. The sender must obtain the receiver's attention and make sure the message is understood.
   b. The sender must speak loudly.
   c. The receiver must listen carefully and respond appropriately.
   d. The message must be organized, simple, and clear.

3. The patient's medical record is an example of
   a. verbal communication.
   b. written communication.
   c. nonverbal communication.
   d. body language.

4. To maintain patient confidentiality, you should do all of the following *except*
   a. discuss one patient's problems with another patient.
   b. keep confidences.
   c. keep out of earshot of others when discussing a patient's concerns.
   d. only discuss the patient's problems with your supervisor.

5. Which of the following guidelines does not promote good communication?
   a. Showing an interest in the patient
   b. Speaking loudly at all times
   c. Using good manners
   d. Using language the patient can understand

TIME-OUT

TIPS FOR TAKING CARE OF YOURSELF

Write information on a pocket note pad for reporting or recording later. Do not depend on your memory. You will deal with a great many numbers, and you will confuse one patient's vital signs and another patient's intake if you do not write it down. If you don't write out the information, you will waste time repeating the task to get the correct numbers. Writing information down will also help you reduce the number of terrors or mistakes you make.

THE NURSING ASSISTANT IN ACTION

You are working as a CNA in a long-term care facility assisting a group of residents during their dinner. You overhear a confused resident, Ms. Loud, rebuffing a newly admitted tablemate, Mrs. Brauns, who just introduced herself. Mrs. Loud says, "I have told you a thousand times what my name is so do not ask me again! I will not tell you again what my name is!" Mrs. Brauns now is in tears.

What Is Your Response/Action?

CRITICAL THINKING

CUSTOMER SERVICE If you know that a patient asked you to do something, but you cannot remember what it was, be honest and tell her: "I'm sorry I know you asked for something or requested one other item. Please remind me again so I can get it for you right away."

   Address patients using the name they prefer. If you cannot remember how a patient wants to be addressed, ask him. Introduce yourself when you first care for a new patient. Remind a patient who you are if it has been a few days since you last cared for him: "Mr. Cox, I am Alberta Kwansa, the nursing assistant who will be caring for you today."

CULTURAL CARE There is a wide variation in personal space and how much distance is acceptable or comfortable for communication. Your personal space comfort level will differ from that of individuals from other cultures. In some cultures comfortable personal space is 1½ ft. while in others, it extends to 4 ft. Social distance varies from 4 to 12 ft. Adjust to accommodate the comfort level of the patient.

COOPERATION WITHIN THE TEAM Charting is the way patient care is communicated and legally documented. You will encounter coworkers who have different levels of computer skills. You can assist your coworker by showing what steps are necessary to get the software operating. It is not appropriate to share your log-in password, chart procedures you did not perform, or to sign your coworker's name. If a coworker asks you to chart for her ask what else you can do to help her out instead.

EXPLORE MediaLink

Additional interactive resources for this chapter can be found on the Companion Website at www.prenhall.com/wolgin. Click on Chapter 3 and "Begin" to select the activities for this chapter.

For chapter-related NCLEX-style questions and an audio glossary, access the accompanying CD-ROM in this book.

4 Patients, Residents, and Clients

KEY TERMS

client
culture
customer-focused care
ethnic diversity
need
patient
physical crisis management
resident
service

OBJECTIVES

When you have completed this chapter, you will be able to:

- Describe seven goals of customer focused care.
- Demonstrate an understanding of cultural differences among patients, residents, and clients.
- Provide service that meets the basic human needs of those who are in your care.
- Identify actions you can take to promote rest and sleep for your patients.
- Describe how unmet needs can influence patient behavior.
- Use methods to deal with disruptive behavior.

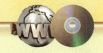

MediaLink

www.prenhall.com/wolgin

Use the address above to access the free, interactive Companion Website created for this textbook. Get hints, instant feedback, and textbook references to chapter-related NCLEX-style questions. Link to other interesting sites.

AUDIO GLOSSARY:

Use the Companion Website, or the CD-ROM disk enclosed with your textbook, to hear the pronunciation of key terms in the chapter.

All individuals are influenced by the values and beliefs of their cultures. Cultures share similarities as well as differences when it comes to dealing with pain, the causes and treatment of illness, and death. This chapter offers an overview of cultural diversity and suggests some strategies to enable you to provide customer-focused service and to meet the physical and psychological needs of your patients, residents, or clients. The importance of rest is presented along with approaches or actions you can take to promote sleep. The chapter also reviews approaches to dealing with difficult behaviors.

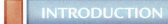 **INTRODUCTION**

Understanding and Relating to Patients, Residents, and Clients

In various health care settings or facilities, you will hear the individuals to whom you are providing care referred to as patients, clients, or residents. **Patients** usually refers to those admitted to inpatient or outpatient hospitals, physician offices, or clinics. Individuals in nursing homes, long-term care, or extended care facilities are frequently referred to as **residents**. (Residents usually live at a facility for an extended period of time.) Individuals cared for by home health agencies or providers are generally referred to as **clients**. While your place of employment may refer differently to those you provide care for, the most important thing to remember is to treat all individuals within your care with respect and courtesy, keeping in mind any cultural differences.

Customer-Focused Care

Chapter 1 reviewed the various ways care is delivered or provided to individuals. See Chapter 1 for more information about customer-focused care.

> **ALERT**
>
> For all patient contact, adhere to Standard Precautions (Chapter 5, pages 83–85). Wear protective equipment as indicated.

patient An individual admitted to an inpatient or outpatient hospital, physician office, or clinic

resident An individual cared for in a nursing home or other long-term/extended care facility

> **KEY IDEA**
>
> The common aspect of all care is that it should be directed to meet the needs of the individual and his family. You are providing care for, and service to, those who are unable to care for themselves.

Service is an important part of patient care. Patients, families, and visitors will judge the care given to their loved ones based on attentiveness, quality of food, cleanliness of the environment, and employee behavior. Most important are personal interactions, attention, and perceived helpfulness of the staff. Many studies have been done to determine the degree of customer satisfaction with health care. Leebov (1990)[1] found that employee behavior toward customers is the most powerful marketing and customer satisfaction tool available to an organization or facility. It is important to know that dissatisfied customers or patients usually do not complain. Instead, 9 out of 10 will go to another health care provider rather than return. They will also tell an average of 20 other relatives, friends, or acquaintances about their experience. A negative experience hurts the overall reputation of the facility.

client An individual cared for by a home health agency or provider

service Factors such as attentiveness, quality of food, and cleanliness of environment, which affect the care and comfort of the individual receiving health care

---

[1] Leebov, W. *Customer Service in Healthcare,* Chicago: American Hospital Publishing, 1990, p. 3.

FIGURE 4–1◆

Treat individuals who are in your care, as well as their families, the way you would like to be treated

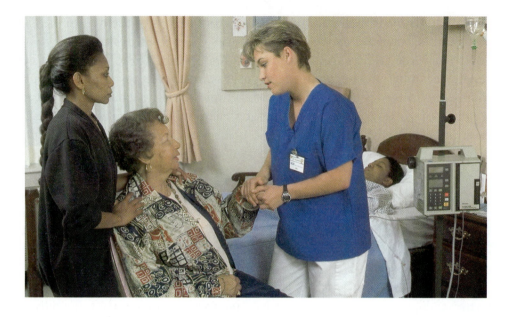

When you care for others, treat them and their families the way you would like to be treated (Figure 4–1◆). Provide the service and care you would expect if they were your loved ones.

Seven Goals of Customer-Focused Care

customer-focused care Care designed to meet the needs of patients, residents, and clients (customers)

There are seven goals of **customer-focused care**, which is designed to meet the needs of patients, residents, and clients (customers). While all of them are important, the care needs of your patients should be your primary concern.

1. Care provided reflects respect for the individual.
2. Caregivers are working together in a planned way, so that care is coordinated.
3. Information is communicated.
4. The patient's physical comfort and care needs are met.
5. The patient is relieved of fear when possible.
6. Family and/or friends are involved.
7. Care is considered over the continuum, rather than a discrete episode or time period. Many conditions or illnesses, such as pregnancy, cancer, AIDS, and diabetes, will require medical care and services from a variety of providers.

Cultural Differences and Diversity

ethnic diversity The variety of races, religions, and cultures in the world

culture The thoughts, beliefs, and values of a social group

Ethnic diversity refers to the variety of races, religions, and cultures in the world. A **culture** is the thoughts, beliefs, and values of a social group. Ethnic diversity is increasing in the United States. Currently, one in every four Americans is Hispanic, African American, or Asian. Latin Americans comprise the largest ethnic minority group in the United States, and one-third of children attending schools are nonwhite.

Thus, as part of a nursing care team, it will be very important to increase your knowledge of the various cultural differences and similarities and how they affect viewpoints about pain, the causes of illness, treatment, and death. Your supervisor can provide more specific information regarding cultural differences and similarities.

KEY IDEA

The more you can learn about an individual's cultural beliefs and differences, the more able you will be to provide sensitive care and services to your patients, residents, or clients.

APPRECIATING CULTURAL DIVERSITY

GUIDELINES

- Learn as much as you can about other cultures, especially those cultures of patients in your care or those of your coworkers.
- Treat everyone with respect.

- Develop an understanding for differences.
- Appreciate the talents and contributions of others.
- Be open, flexible, and adaptable.
- Practice effective communication skills.

- Be quick to apologize if you see you have offended someone.
- Thank others who help you better understand or teach you more about their culture.

Transcultural Nursing

Since you have chosen to be a nursing assistant, we assume that you enjoy working with and helping people. For sick people to feel well again, they must first be helped to feel relaxed, comfortable, accepted, and safe, regardless of their ethnic background (Table 4–1◆).

As part of the nursing care team, you will assist with the delivery of nursing care to people from many different countries and backgrounds (Figure 4–2◆). People may adhere to religious beliefs, values, traditions, practices, or rituals that are very different from your own. They may have very different food habits, manners, lifestyles, social roles, family

TABLE 4–1◆

Cross-Cultural Communication Guidelines

- Establishing and building relationships is the core and aim of all effective communication in a cross-cultural setting.
- Recognize your own cultural filters, including the values (and stereotypes) that shaped them. Work at understanding your own cultural preferences.
- Speak at a comfortable pace for your foreign associates. Repeat what was said. Summarize often; confirm and clarify.
- Be respectful of (cultural) differences. Listen, observe, and describe, rather than evaluate.
- Don't settle for surface meaning. Patiently search for what is really being communicated.
- Respect the appropriate level of formality in other cultures.
- Avoid taboos; pay particular attention to your nonverbal behavior.
- Beware of jokes; they cannot readily be translated into another language, culture, or value system.
- Check yourself constantly for cultural assumptions.
- Be very conscious of the context in which the communication takes place.

SOURCE: Reprinted with permission from Gottfried Oosterwal, Ph.D., *Community in Diversity: A Participant Workbook*, 1995, p. iii–21.

FIGURE 4–2◆

As a nursing assistant, you will help deliver care to people from different countries and backgrounds

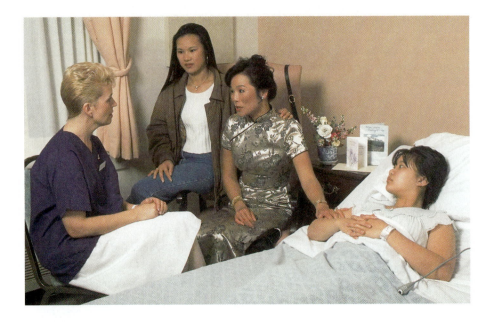

systems, birth and death practices, or perceptions of privacy, territoriality, and touch. They may use languages, customs, or behavior patterns completely foreign to you. You must learn to be tolerant, accepting, and understanding of these differences. Behave in ways that show respect for the patient's customs and beliefs.

Different does not mean better or worse, merely another way of doing or seeing things. Because your own ways are familiar to you, they seem like the right ways, and other languages, values, lifestyles, traditions, or diets may seem strange. Your customs may seem just as strange to the patient as her customs seem to you. This can lead to misunderstandings. Remember, there is no right or wrong in these matters.

KEY IDEA

Many patients are frightened by illness and the hospital or health care setting. Part of your job is to show the patient that the health care institution is a friendly place and that your major concern is for her well-being.

Patients born in other countries may be fearful because of problems in understanding our language and culture. Be sure to discuss these problems with your immediate supervisor, who can suggest ways of dealing with these patients effectively, for example:

- If the patient speaks and understands little or no English, your nurse manager or team leader may suggest the use of flash cards, pictures, nonverbal communication, a translator, or materials written in the patient's language to communicate with the patient and thereby reduce stress and anxiety (Figure 4–3◆).

- There are no universal gestures. For example, the American "thumbs up" or "OK" sign may be a terrible insult to Turkish, Greek, or Brazilian individuals. Unless you know and understand the meanings of gestures in another culture, avoid using them.

- Space has different meanings to different people. It is better to ask before approaching or touching someone. Each culture has its own comfort zone in which communication takes place. It may be 18 inches or arm's length in the United States or Canada, but the range in other countries can be 5 inches to 50 inches. Caregivers may have patients or visitors who unknowingly intrude on each other's space or comfort zones.

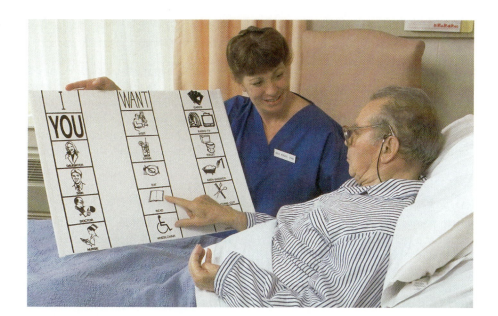

FIGURE 4–3◆

Try using different methods to help communicate with patients who do not speak your language

■ A patient from another culture may answer "yes" to all questions asked because in his culture it is rude to say no. Your nurse manager or team leader may suggest that you phrase your questions so that a "yes" or "no" answer is not required. For example, instead of asking, "Do you want the lights out now?" you could say, "What time would you like me to turn off the lights?"

■ A patient may refuse to eat hospital food because of religious or cultural dietary laws or beliefs. In many Latin American cultures, for instance, the concept of keeping the body in balance involves the use of foods identified as "hot" foods or "cold" foods. Depending on the illness, which is also considered "hot" or "cold," a patient may prefer to eat a particular food in order to bring the body into balance. An example of a "hot" food among Puerto Ricans might be corn meal or peas, while a "cold" food would be bananas or lima beans. There are also hot and cold medicines and herbs. Similar beliefs are found among Asian cultures, which believe in the philosophy of Tao. According to Taoism, harmony is maintained through a balance of yin and yang. Yin represents cold, darkness, and female, while yang represents hot, light, and male. Certain conditions or illnesses are considered either yin or yang and require the opposite types of food or herbs for treatment. A yin food would include mostly fruits and vegetables, while yang foods include meat, chicken, and most, but not all, kinds of fish.

   Some groups avoid certain types of food altogether. A patient may be a strict vegetarian, avoiding not only meat, fish, and poultry, but also all dairy products. Other patients may avoid certain foods on certain religious occasions. Some may fast on religious holidays. Patients have the right to decide what they will eat and when they will eat it. Your nurse manager or team leader may be able to make special arrangements for this patient's food. If the facility cannot provide the requested foods, arrangements can be made for the family or friends to bring food.

■ People from many cultures place more importance on modesty than Americans. They may want to keep certain parts of the body, such as the head, the face, arms, or legs, covered at all times. Your nurse manager or team leader may suggest ways of draping the patient so necessary care can be given without violating the patient's sense of modesty, dignity, and privacy.

■ People have different ideas about death and the hereafter. Adherents of some religions believe that the body should not be touched or moved after death until the proper religious authority arrives. Your nurse manager or team leader may suggest that you straighten the patient's limbs before death occurs.

Basic Human Needs

need A requirement for survival

Every person has basic physical and psychological needs that must be met. A **need** is a requirement for survival. Most people can satisfy their own needs; however, sometimes they need help. As a nursing assistant, you will help your patients meet some of their most basic needs until they no longer need your assistance. Your knowledge of these needs and your objective observations, when reported promptly, will help your supervisor, nurse manager, or team leader to determine if all the patient's needs are being met by the plan of care.

Basic Physical and Psychological Needs

All human beings have basic physical needs that must be met in order to live. These needs do not all have to be met completely every day. But the more each person's needs are fulfilled, the better the quality of life.

Psychological needs must be satisfied to have a healthy emotional and social outlook. These, also, do not have to be met completely every day. However, the more completely each need is met, the better the emotional state of the individual.

Some psychologists divide human needs into five categories, arranged into a hierarchy, or order of priority, developed by Abraham Maslow (Figure 4–4◆). Maslow's idea is that human beings work on meeting lower level, physical needs (food, water, shelter) first, then move on toward meeting higher level needs (security, belonging, and so on).

Rest and Sleep

Your body requires rest and sleep. One must first be in a state of rest to fall asleep. Rest is a state wherein one feels comfortable, calm, and free of stress and anxiety. Certain activities may be restful to one individual, but not so for others. Examples are listening to music, reading, watching TV, swimming, walking, sewing, golfing, drawing, or gardening.

FIGURE 4–4 ◆

Maslow's hierarchy of needs

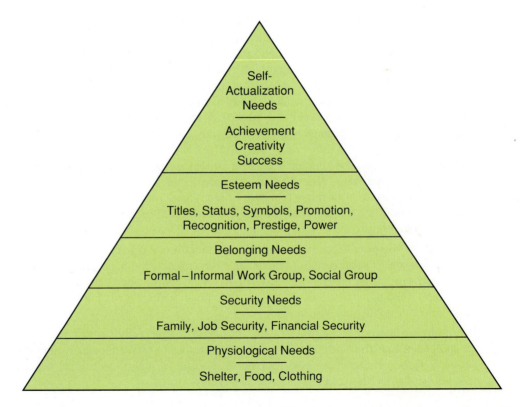

Determining those activities that are restful for each individual is important because it will help you to promote rest. Basic needs for water, food, and comfort must be met for a person to rest (Table 4–2◆).

Sleep is a natural periodic suspension of consciousness during which the natural restorative powers of the body occur. In this state of unconsciousness, there is reduced voluntary muscle activity and lowered metabolism because the body requires less energy during sleep. In sleep, the body is at rest. The blood pressure, temperature, pulse, and respirations are lower than when awake. While there is a general unawareness of the environment and people around you while asleep, most individuals are easily awakened by noise, alarms, the sound of a baby crying, etc.

Sleep is an essential and distinctive aspect of human behavior. Each person's body has individual requirements regarding their basic needs for sleep and rest. Nearly one-third of the average adult life span is spent sleeping. Sleep requirements decrease with age. Newborns average 20 hours of sleep per day, while elderly persons require 5 to 6 hours per day. Infants and children sleep more soundly and have a harder time awakening than older adults.

It is during sleep that tissues heal and the body is restored or refreshed. One's mental alertness and energy levels are restored during sleep. Stress, tension, and anxiety are reduced. Following sleep, one can usually think more clearly and function more effectively.

Individuals have different sleep/wake patterns or rhythms during a 24-hour period. You are probably aware of your preferred biological clock or pattern. Some individuals require only a few hours of sleep while others need 8 to 10 hours to feel refreshed. Your body may or may not require brief nap periods. You may be alert in the early morning, awaking before your alarm rings, but ready to go to sleep early in the evening. Yet others prefer to sleep in the early morning, but have no trouble staying up late at night. Health care facilities routinely interfere with the sleep cycles of both the health care providers and the

TABLE 4–2◆

Rest and Sleep

FACTORS AFFECTING SLEEP	APPROACHES/ACTIONS
Age	Be aware that older persons awaken easily and children tend to sleep more soundly.
Anxiety/Stress/Emotional Problems	Listen and offer emotional support. Encourage the patient to talk about what is bothering him. Resource persons may be available for consultation/support or medications ordered to reduce anxiety. Check with your supervisor.
Environment/Strange Sounds/Noise	Keep the door closed at night to reduce noise. A child may want a toy or blanket from home to comfort him. Reduce noise: Try not to use the intercom system at night, speak in low voices to prevent awakening patients unnecessarily.
Light	Keep bathroom light on or off, per patient's preference.
Strange Bed/Pillow	Patient may be allowed to have her preferred pillow brought in from home.
Exercise	Avoid exerting patients less than 2 hours prior to sleeping time.
Caffeine/Nutrition	Cheese and milk can promote rest and sleep. Offer decaffeinated drinks, water, or juices rather than tea, coffee, or cola drinks at bedtime or in the evening.
Illness Symptoms: Pain	Need for sleep is increased. Try repositioning or pain medication as ordered. Report if it does not help. Distractions such as TV, reading, and humor may promote rest.
Vomiting, Diarrhea, Other	Medications usually are ordered to treat the symptoms; offer skin care and mouth care as needed.
Lifestyle Changes	The patient may not be comfortable with his roommate—a change may be needed. The recent death of a close relative or friend may be causing depression. Encourage the patient to talk about her grief/loss.

TABLE 4–3◆

The Sleep Cycle

Presleep	NonREM Stage 4
NonREM Stage 1	Deepest stage of sleep
Lightest sleep state	Hard to awaken
Easily aroused	Body rests and restores
NonREM Stage 2	Lower vital signs
Sound sleep	Lasts 15–30 minutes
Increased relaxation	REM Sleep
Lasts 10–20 minutes	Vivid dreaming
NonREM Stage 3	Mental restoration occurs
Begin deep sleep	Review problems and events of the prior
Muscles completely relax	day
Slow and regular respiratory and	Hard to arouse
heart rates	Starts 50–90 minutes after sleep begins
Lasts 15–30 minutes	

SOURCE: Material adapted from J. Fry, "Sleep Disorders," *Merritt's Textbook of Neurology*, Baltimore, MD: Williams & Wilkins, 1995.

patients. Caregivers are needed around the clock, and various aspects of patient care occur at times that are unwelcome to the patients. Whenever possible, it is important to consider each individual's preferences and needs when you plan their care needs. For example, you may have a patient who prefers to sleep in the morning and have their bath in the early afternoon. It is possible to plan your assignment to accommodate their preferences.

There are two phases of sleep, REM (rapid-eye movement) and NonREM (nonrapid-eye movement). REM sleep accounts for 25 percent of the time spent sleeping, while NREM sleep makes up 75 percent of the time.

The sleep cycle lasts about 85 to 100 minutes and repeats itself three to five times over a 6- to 8-hour period of sleep (see Table 4–3◆ on the sleep cycle). An adult will usually fall asleep within 10 to 15 minutes, and go through a sequence of stages 1, 2, 3, and 4, followed by the reverse (stages 4, 3, and 2). Next, the first REM sleep period occurs. The cycles of sleep will continue three to five times. Deep sleep occurs more often during the first half of the total time spent in sleep. Vivid dreaming in the REM sleep episodes increases in intensity and duration during the second half of sleep. When people are ill or hospitalized, they frequently do not experience prolonged blocks of sleep time and thus experience less time in REM sleep, leaving them feeling less restored or rested.[2]

Influences on Patient Behavior: Unmet Needs

When basic needs are not met, most people show some reaction or change in behavior. If a physical need is not met, the person might become irritable or weak. When an emotional need is not met, the person's reactions may include anxiety, depression, aggression, anger, or a physical ailment without apparent cause. An unwanted diagnosis, a serious illness, age, and previous experience, along with personality, financial situation, and family relationships can all be the source of unmet needs, thus affecting a patient's behavior.

Report these reactions to your immediate supervisor. By reviewing a patient's actions, your supervisor will be able to determine if a need is unmet and evaluate the plan of care to attempt to fulfill the need and thus change the patient's behavior.

---

[2] Material adapted from J. Fry, "Sleep Disorders," *Merritt's Textbook of Neurology*, Baltimore, MD: Williams & Wilkins, 1995.

Remember, too, that each person has a different reaction to pain, treatment, and even attempted kindness, so when you try to make adjustments to fulfill needs, you should consider him to be an individual. If you observe the patient's behavior carefully, you will be better able to report it and make changes to fulfill needs.

 ## Dealing With Difficult Behavior

Patients, their families, and friends are usually experiencing varying amounts of stress and anxiety. An illness can be very frightening and can reduce a person's ability to cope with a stressful situation. Some patients or their significant others may have a particularly hard time dealing with or accepting an illness or injury. An individual may be overcome by stress, grief, or guilt. An individual may be suffering from a mental problem or other illness and may not be able to understand or recognize her own behavior. Some medications can also cause side effects that leave a person disoriented, combative, or hallucinating (Figure 4–5◆).

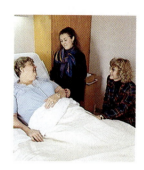

FIGURE 4–5◆
Some patients, finding themselves in the role of a sick person, realize that they now get more attention from everyone, including visitors. Secondary gains such as this extra attention might promote helplessness and difficult behavior

KEY IDEA

Your challenge as a nursing assistant is to deal with a patient's disruptive behavior in such a way that keeps you, the patient, and others in the environment safe from harm.

Below are some causes of disruptive behavior, along with appropriate actions.

Causes or Reasons	Appropriate Actions
1. Illness or injury (insulin shock, head injury, respiratory problems)	Keep safe from injury. Reassure. Make minimal attempts to reason with the individual.
2. Mental illness/emotional problems	Reduce stimuli. Give short, concrete directions. Do not ask "why" questions. Do not argue or correct grandiose delusions. Ignore strange behaviors, focus on safety. Acknowledge the person's difficulty.
3. Medication reactions; confused/disoriented, "feel bugs crawling on them"	Focus on safety. Report to your supervisor.
4. Stress	Be supportive. Acknowledge the stressor, if you know it.
5. Anger	Remain calm.
6. Misbehavior	Don't focus on negative behavior. Be clear about limits.

 ## Physical Crisis Management

Physical crisis management refers to how you deal with a dangerous situation. Many facilities have training programs or courses for employees who work in high-risk areas, such as psychiatry or the emergency department. There is a high probability that you will encounter

physical crisis management
Methods for dealing with a dangerous situation involving a patient, resident, or client

DEALING WITH THE DISRUPTIVE INDIVIDUAL

GUIDELINES   OBRA

- Be objective.
- Remain calm, but firm and controlled.
- Act appropriately and do not raise your voice or yell back.
- Do not display your own anger or threaten the person.

- Respect personal space, stay at least an arm's length away from the person.
- Be alert.
- Take time to determine the facts, whenever possible.
- Watch body positioning and non-verbal body language.

- Do not stare or avoid eye contact.
- Remember many people want their "say," not their "way."
- Call for help or assistance if you cannot defuse the situation.

GENERAL TECHNIQUES TO TRY

GUIDELINES

- Be honest about your fear of violence.
- Listen and reflect back what you hear.
- Do not minimize a person's feelings.

- Point out reality.
- Offer hope.
- Offer alternatives quickly; be sure these are choices, not threats.
- Avoid sharing personal information about yourself.

- Do not turn your back toward the person.
- Be aware of how to get help in case of emergencies.

someone who is unable to control his behavior or emotions because he has a physical or mental illness or is under the influence of drugs or alcohol. When patients or visitors are very stressed, they may not be in control of their feelings or emotions. Sometimes they yell and become insulting or verbally abusive to health care givers in any setting. It is helpful to anticipate this and review some basic guidelines to assist you in coping with these kinds of problems.

SUMMARY

Seven goals of customer-focused care, which is designed to meet the needs of patients, residents, and clients, help you provide service to those who are in your care. It is important to keep cultural variations in the way people view illness and treatment in mind when you communicate with and provide care for patients whose ethnic backgrounds differ from your own. When you encounter a patient whose behavior is disruptive, you can use a number of techniques to try to defuse the situation.

NOTES

_____

_____

_____

_____

CHAPTER REVIEW

FILL IN THE BLANK Read each sentence and fill in the blank line with a word that completes the sentence.

1. A _____ is an individual cared for by a home health agency or provider.

2. A _____ is an individual cared for in a long-term/extended care facility.

3. The more you learn about an individual's _____ and differences, the better you can provide sensitive care and services to your patients, residents, or clients.

4. A _____ is a requirement for survival.

5. Every person has basic _____ and _____ needs.

MULTIPLE CHOICE Choose the best answer for each question or statement.

1. Which of the following actions do not promote sleep and rest?
   a. Being aware of the noise around you
   b. Always turning off all the lights
   c. If possible, allowing the patient to use his own pillow
   d. Offering skin and mouth care as needed

2. Which of the following is not a good technique to try when dealing with a disruptive patient?
   a. Yell back at the patient.
   b. Be objective.
   c. Be alert.
   d. Remain calm, but firm.

3. Which of the following is considered a physiological need?
   a. Social groups
   b. Status, titles
   c. Shelter
   d. Family

4. Which of the following is *not* a guideline for appreciating cultural diversity?
   a. Treat everyone with respect.
   b. Take what the patient says literally.
   c. Be open, flexible, and adaptable.
   d. Thank others who help you to better understand about their culture.

5. Which of the following is true?
   a. Use flash cards and pictures with patients who do not speak English helps to reduce stress and anxiety.
   b. Use the universal "OK" sign to communicate with people of all cultures.
   c. Hold the patient's hand and look directly in her eyes when talking with women of all cultures.
   d. All of the above.

TIME-OUT

TIPS FOR TIME MANAGEMENT

Avoid the temptation to do more talking than working. Save social talk for break time. Make your conversations patient-centered, not self-centered. Keep your conversations with coworkers professional and positive.

THE NURSING ASSISTANT IN ACTION

You are caring for Mr. George, a seriously ill 32-year-old man. Following a head injury, he is being treated for an infection. When you come to assist him with lunch, he yells at you, "Get that slop out of here or I will throw the tray on the floor!"

What Is Your Response/Action?

CRITICAL THINKING

CUSTOMER SERVICE Many patients have a difficult time getting enough rest or sleep. Do not awaken patients when you are assigned to provide care procedures that can wait. Usually the bed can be changed or the patient bathed at a later time in your shift.

CULTURAL CARE Some patients and families will have very different ways of communicating. They may use many gestures, argue with each other, and talk loudly. This behavior is normal for them and may not be a problem for the patient. It may be seen as frightening to a roommate from a more reserved culture. If you notice a problem and are uncomfortable handling it alone, talk the situation over with your supervisor.

COOPERATION WITHIN THE TEAM You may be better able to communicate with some patients than other members of the team, especially if you are more familiar with the patient's culture or language. If you see this is the case, offer to help other team members communicate with the patient or family or share important cultural considerations they may not know about.

EXPLORE MediaLink

Additional interactive resources for this chapter can be found on the Companion Website at www.prenhall.com/wolgin. Click on Chapter 4 and "Begin" to select activities for this chapter.

For chapter-related NCLEX-style questions and an audio glossary, access the accompanying CD-ROM in this book.

5 Infection Control

OBJECTIVES

When you have completed this chapter, you will be able to:

- Differentiate between helpful and harmful microorganisms.
- List four conditions affecting the growth of bacteria.
- Summarize the history of infection control.
- List five ways microorganisms are spread.
- Explain how microorganisms are destroyed.
- Describe the three main purposes of asepsis.
- Identify what precautions are used for all patients.
- List the three elements necessary for transmission of infection.
- Demonstrate the procedures for handwashing and hand hygiene.
- Demonstrate the procedures for donning gloves, mask, and gown.
- Identify OSHA standards for occupational exposure to bloodborne pathogens.
- Identify recommendations for prevention and control of hepatitis C.
- Demonstrate sterile techniques.

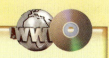

MediaLink
www.prenhall.com/wolgin

Use the address above to access the free, interactive Companion Website created for this textbook. Get hints, instant feedback, and textbook references to chapter-related NCLEX-style questions. Link to other interesting sites.

AUDIO GLOSSARY:
Use the Companion Website, or the CD-ROM disk enclosed with your textbook, to hear the pronunciation of key terms in the chapter.

KEY TERMS

asepsis
aseptic
autoclave
bacteria
disinfection
friction
hand hygiene
health care-associated infection (HAI)
hepatitis B
hepatitis C
infection
infection control
isolation
microorganism
normal flora
nosocomial infection
pathogen
Rickettsiae
severe acute respiratory syndrome (SARS)
spores
sterile field
sterilization
transmission
virus

INTRODUCTION

The health care environment is an area that requires the people who work there to have a basic knowledge and understanding of disease and disease transmission. This chapter introduces the nursing assistant to the history of germ theory and its evolution into today's practice. Health care workers and patients alike have benefited from knowledge about disease transmission. An example of this is the recently updated guideline from the Centers for Disease Control and Prevention (CDC) for the protection of health care workers in health care institutions. CDC's expanded guideline consists of two tiers of precautions: Standard Precautions and Transmission-based Precautions. In this chapter, the relationship between Universal Precautions and the new CDC guideline, particularly Standard Precautions, is presented. With the information and examples provided on infection control, nursing assistants will be able to protect themselves more fully, as well as their patients, from acquiring one of the most serious and dreaded complications of hospitalization—a *nosocomial* infection or health care-associated infection. The importance of asepsis and sterile technique is introduced. Guidelines for maintaining a sterile field and procedures to put on sterile gloves and open sterile packages are included.

History of Infection Control

People once believed that sickness was caused by evil spirits. About 500 years ago, scientists began to suspect that some diseases were caused by very small living things they called *germs*. The germ theory of disease was not actually *proven* until about 100 years ago. A French scientist named Louis Pasteur made two important discoveries about bacteria. First, he discovered that many diseases are caused by **bacteria**. Second, he discovered that bacteria could be killed by excess heat.

bacteria Unicellular microorganism

Pasteur's name has been used to refer to the heat method of killing germs. For example, *pasteurization* is the process of heating milk to 140°F (60°C) and keeping it at that temperature for one-half hour. Pasteurization kills harmful bacteria and makes milk safe for us to drink.

A few years after Pasteur's discoveries, a British surgeon, Joseph Lister, found that germs could also be killed by carbolic acid. Lister recognized that many deaths in hospitals seemed to be connected with unclean conditions. He was the first to *demand* that surgical wounds be kept clean and the air in the operating room pure. His success was demonstrated by a reduction in deaths in people undergoing amputation, which decreased from 45 to 15 percent.

aseptic Germ free, without disease-producing organisms

Lister's theories led to changes in hospitals by introducing the principles and methods of aseptic surgery. **Aseptic** means germ free, or without disease-producing organisms. Lister developed a technique to keep germs out of open wounds and also identified a method to destroy germs. His method was to spray the skin around the wound with carbolic acid. Also, surgical instruments were made aseptic by being dipped in a carbolic acid solution. This technique was a major advance in the battle against disease.

Nosocomial or Health Care-Associated Infections

People working in hospitals began to realize that some disease-producing germs were everywhere. Scientists learned that germs multiply very rapidly—every 12 minutes. They also found that if germs are not controlled, they may spread infection and disease from one person to another. Therefore, it was necessary to apply the principles of asepsis to the health care practice in order to prevent **nosocomial infections** (infections acquired while a person/patient is in the hospital).

More recently, a broader understanding has been reached that infections can be caused by health care given by caregivers or by exposure to caregivers or other individuals who have a contagious disease in a variety of health care settings outside a hospital, including homes, long-term care facilities, or physician offices. The term **health care–associated infection (HAI)** is used to describe these more broadly acquired infections and is rapidly replacing *nosocomial*. In addition, some infections such as a surgical site infection most often develop after the patient has been discharged. **Severe acute respiratory syndrome (SARS)** virus is an example of a virus spread by infected health care workers and individuals who were unaware they were infecting others with whom they came in contact.

Nosocomial infections range from simple and uncomplicated to major and life threatening. Patients often have weakened immune systems and are prone to exposure from the people, equipment, and environment within a health care facility. Additionally, patients are at risk for iatrogenic infection, which can occur following surgery, medication, or a treatment. *Iatrogenic* means *caused by medical treatment*. Bacteria causes two common nosocomial infections: methicillin-resistant *Staphylococcus aureus* (MRSA) and *Psuedomonas aeruginosa*. They are both resistant to antibiotic treatment and difficult to control. Vancomycin-resistant enterococci (VRE) is another difficult-to-control germ that has been seen in both hospitals and long-term care facilities.

The success of modern medicine in controlling and preventing infection is due to the focus, or emphasis, on the individual health care worker as the primary source, or means, of spreading infection and thus the means of preventing infection.

Nature of Microorganisms

A germ is a microorganism. *Micro* means very small. *Organism* means living thing. So a **microorganism** is a living thing that is so small it cannot be seen with the naked eye, only through a microscope. Different kinds of microorganisms (also called *microbes*) are bacteria (**Rickettsiae**), fungi, protozoa, and viruses. Microorganisms occur nearly everywhere in nature. They occur most abundantly where they find food, moisture, and a temperature suitable for their growth and multiplication. Since conditions that are favorable for microorganisms are those under which people normally live, it is inevitable that we live among numerous microbes.

Microorganisms are best known to the average person by the diseases they cause in human beings. The disease-producing microorganisms or *germs* are called **pathogens**. Figure 5–1◆ demonstrates the role different pathogens can play in disease causation. They grow best at body temperature, 98.6°F; 37°C. Pathogens destroy human tissue by using it as food. They may also give off waste products called toxins that are absorbed into and poison the body.

Some microorganisms, particularly bacteria and fungi, are helpful and necessary for healthy functioning of a person and are referred to as normal flora. **Normal flora** in the human digestive system breaks down the foods not used by the body and turns them into waste products. Also, certain microbes cause a chemical change in food called *fermentation*. Fermentation is the change that produces cottage cheese from milk, beer from grains, and cider from apples.

Microbes each have their own normal environment, or home, called their natural habitat. When organisms gain access to areas of the body in which they do not belong (Figure 5–2◆), they become pathogens. For example, *Escherichia coli* belongs in the colon where it helps to digest food. When it gets into the bladder or into the bloodstream, it can cause a urinary infection, or a *bloodstream* infection.

---

nosocomial infection
Hospital-acquired infection

health care–associated infection (HAI) An infection acquired in a health care setting.

severe acute respiratory syndrome (SARS) A viral respiratory illness spread by close person-to-person contact.

microorganism A living thing that is so small it cannot be seen with the naked eye but only through a microscope

rickettsiae An example of bacteria found in the tissues of fleas, lice, ticks, and other insects; Rickettsiae are transmitted to humans by insect bites

pathogen Disease-producing microorganism

normal flora Microorganisms that are necessary for health, and usually live and grow in specific locations; they are nonpathogenic when in or on a natural reservoir

FIGURE 5–1 ◆

Pathogens cause disease in the human body

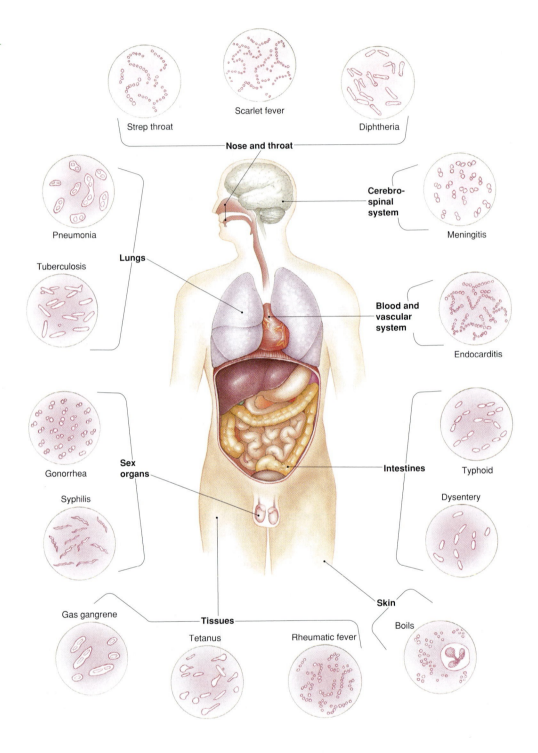

Bacteria grow well in moist, warm, dark areas. For example, meat must be stored at extremely cold temperatures and then cooked to extremely high temperatures in order to eliminate the risk of potential bacterial contamination that has occurred through improper handling or cooking. Some bacterial microbes require oxygen to live. Figure 5–3◆ describes four conditions that affect the growth of bacteria.

In the hospital you will often hear the words *staph*, or *staphylococcus*, and *strep*, or *streptococcus*. Staphylococcus and streptococcus are examples of two types of bacteria that may become pathogens if given the right opportunity. They are commonly found on the human skin and may enter the body through a portal of entry. A portal of entry is an area

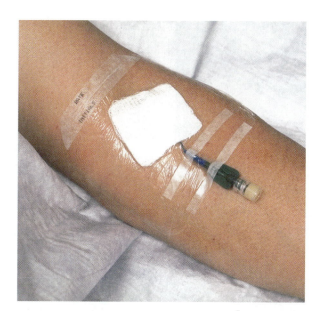

FIGURE 5–2 ◆
Bacteria may enter the body through invasive points of entry such as IV sites, indwelling catheters, and surgical sites. Bacteria may also enter the body through cuts or through the nose and mouth

where the primary defense to an organism is violated and results in direct access to the inside of the body. Our primary defense is the skin, and it is violated every time the skin is cut, such as when a surgical incision is made or when a tube/drain is placed. When staphylococci get inside the skin, they may produce a local infection. Soreness, tenderness, redness, and/or pus (infection) may result. Sometimes staphylococcus infections can affect the whole body.

A **virus** is another type of microorganism. Viruses are much smaller than bacteria and cause many of our diseases. Examples are measles, AIDS (acquired immunodeficiency syndrome), and influenza. Viruses can survive only in other living cells.

virus A type of microorganism; much smaller than bacteria and can survive only in other living cells

FIGURE 5–3 ◆
Four conditions affecting the growth of bacteria

1 Moisture

- Bacteria grow well in moist places

2 Temperature

- 170°F. – High temperature kills most bacteria
- 50°F. to 110°F. – Most disease-causing bacteria grow rapidly
- 98.6°F. – Normal human body temperature. Bacteria thrive easily on and in the human body
- 32°F.– Low temperatures do not kill bacteria, but retard their activity and growth rate

170°
110°
98.6°
50°
32°

3 Oxygen

- Aerobic bacteria require oxygen to live

- Anaerobic bacteria can survive without oxygen

4 Light

- Light is bacteria's worst enemy. When exposed to direct sunlight, they become sluggish and die rapidly

LIGHT

- Darkness favors the development of bacteria. They become very active and multiply rapidly

DARKNESS

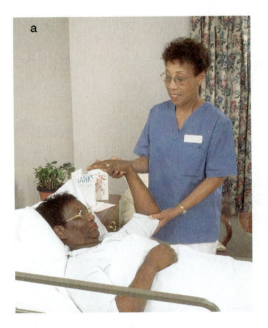

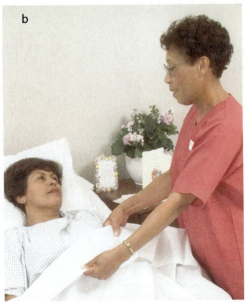

Figures 5–4a◆ and 5–4b◆ show ways that microorganisms are NOT spread. Touching a patient does not require use of gloves or other protective equipment, provided the patient's skin is intact and not draining or weeping. Visiting with a patient and adjusting the bed sheets also does not require protective equipment unless the linen is soiled. Examples of situations with the potential for spreading microorganisms and for which protective equipment such as gowns, gloves, and masks may be indicated are the emptying of a urinary bag, starting an IV, and doing a dressing change.

Preventing the Spread of Infection

infection control The effort to prevent the spread of pathogens

It is a major goal of health care institutions to prevent the spread of pathogens. This battle is called **infection control**. In spite of the best efforts of health care personnel, there are always some harmful microorganisms around us. We can reduce the number of organisms, however, by maintaining simple cleanliness procedures. We can keep ourselves clean by bathing and frequent handwashing. We can keep the institution and its equipment clean with soap, water, and special solutions that assist in the removal of bacteria and also inhibit bacterial growth.

Disinfection and Sterilization

Two very important methods for killing microorganisms or keeping them under control are:

disinfection The process of destroying as many harmful organisms as possible

sterilization The process of killing all microorganisms, including spores

spores Bacteria that have formed hard shells around themselves as a defense

autoclave Device used to achieve sterility of an item through heat, pressure, and steam

1. **Disinfection:** the process of destroying as many harmful organisms as possible. It also means slowing down the growth and activity of the organisms that cannot be destroyed.

2. **Sterilization:** the process of killing all microorganisms, including spores, in a certain area.

Spores are bacteria that have formed hard shells around themselves as a defense. These shells are like a protective suit of armor. Spores are very difficult to kill; some can even live in boiling water. Spores can be destroyed by being exposed to pressurized steam at a high temperature. Machines called **autoclaves** can produce this high-temperature, pressurized steam (Figure 5–5◆). Autoclaves are used to kill spores and other disease producing bacteria. Another method of sterilization uses a chemical gas instead of heat to destroy microorganisms. This method can be used to sterilize equipment made of plastics without melting it. When an object is free of all microorganisms, it is called *sterile*. These are both effective ways of sterilizing objects used in a health care institution.

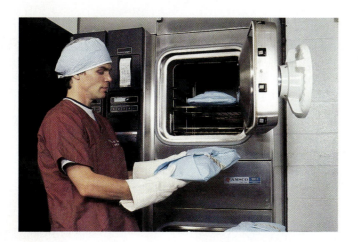

FIGURE 5–5 ◆

Autoclaves are used to kill spores and other disease-producing bacteria

Sterilization is necessary if the article or device will be inserted into the bloodstream or will come into direct contact with a sterile area. Examples include IV catheters or scalpel blades used in the operating room to cut into tissue or an open wound. Such a needle or blade is referred to as a surgical instrument. Surgical instruments are considered to be *critical* items and must be sterilized. Other devices, including endoscopes, only have contact with mucous membranes (inside the mouth). Therefore, sterilization is not necessary, but a high level of disinfection is required between each patient use. Disinfection of these reusable devices kills all germs except low levels of spores. These devices are classified as *semicritical.* Noncritical items are supplies and equipment that are used in the care of patients, but do not come in contact with an open or draining area, for example, a blood pressure cuff. Therefore, noncritical items can be cleaned with a hospital-approved disinfectant, between patient use, to prevent the spread of disease or **infection** (Figure 5–6◆).

infection Results from a pathogen producing a reaction that may cause soreness, tenderness, redness, and/or pus, fever, change in drainage, and so on

FIGURE 5–6 ◆

The IV pole is cleaned with approved disinfectant

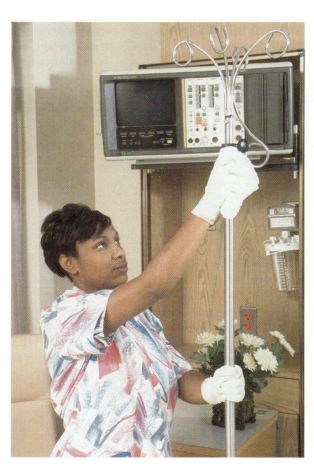

Asepsis

asepsis The absence of microorganisms (germs)

Asepsis means the absence of microorganisms. Asepsis can be achieved by preventing the conditions that allow pathogens to live, multiply, and spread. As a nursing assistant, you will share the responsibility for preventing the spread of disease and infection by using aseptic techniques. The main purposes for asepsis in caring for patients are as follows:

- Protecting the patient against becoming infected a second time by the same microorganism. This is called *reinfection*.
- Protecting the patient against becoming infected by a new or different type of microorganism from equipment, another patient, or a member of the hospital staff. This is called *cross-contamination*.
- Protecting the patient from becoming infected with the patient's own organisms.

When the patient acquires an infection that was not present prior to or at the time of admission to the hospital, it is called a nosocomial, or hospital, acquired infection. For the transmission of any infection within a hospital, three things are necessary:

- A source of the infecting microorganisms
- A patient or susceptible host
- A means of transmission for the microorganism

The presence of these three factors, or components, is also referred to as the *chain of infection*. Infection control strategies are aimed at interrupting this chain of infection.

The source of the microorganisms may be the patient, the health care worker, or basically anyone, as well as the inanimate environment, for example, equipment. The patient becomes a susceptible host (one who can catch the disease or become infected) because the ability to resist an infection varies with different people. Certain criteria, such as age, underlying disease, current medication, or treatments, can greatly affect an individual's ability to "resist" infection. The final component that is necessary for an infection to develop is a route of transmission. You must understand the concept of **transmission**, or how the disease is spread, in order to protect yourself as well as your patient. Three main routes of transmission need to be focused on within a hospital: contact, droplet, and airborne.

transmission The spread of microorganisms

KEY IDEA

Most diseases are spread through body fluids. Some diseases are spread through the air. Hospitals have isolation policies designed to protect health care workers from exposure to infectious diseases.

Isolation To separate or set apart

Isolation Precautions

The Centers for Disease Control and Prevention (CDC) have updated their guideline for protecting health care workers (HCW) and patients from exposure to infectious diseases. The guideline consists of two tiers of precautions.

The first and most important tier contains those precautions designed to decrease the risk of transmission of disease to the HCW and patients through exposure to body fluids. This tier is called *Standard Precautions* and is used when caring for all patients, regardless of the patient's diagnosis and whether or not the patient is known to have an infectious disease.

The second tier of the CDC guideline is designed for patients documented or suspected to be carrying or infected with pathogens that require extra precautions in addition to the Standard Precautions. This second tier of precautions, known as *Transmission-based Precautions,* includes (1) Airborne Precautions, (2) Droplet Precautions, and (3) Contact Precautions.

The CDC's expanded guideline is presented in order to provide an example of safe practice and precautions. It is your responsibility to learn and to follow the isolation policies used at your health care institution.

Not all hospitals will choose to follow the CDC guidelines exactly. Most hospitals will have isolation policies that are similar in underlying principle but may be different in detail. All hospitals that comply with regulatory rules, for example, OSHA, will have at least the following:

1. A barrier-based isolation policy that applies to all patients and is designed to reduce the risk of transmission of microorganisms from blood or other blood-containing body fluids. These policies may be referred to as *Universal Precautions*.

   Many health care institutions have chosen to expand on these required precautions to include not only blood and blood-containing body fluids, but any moist body substance. These expanded precautions are often called *Body Substance Isolation* or *Body Substance Precautions*.

2. An isolation policy to prevent the transmission of infectious diseases that are spread on air currents. These policies are often called *Airborne Precautions* (like the CDC's) or *Respiratory Isolation*.

3. Policy standards for the safe handling of "sharps" to prevent injuries and deep exposure to body fluids. In some cases, standards for sharps handling are included in the institution's barrier-based policies (see item 1).

Most institutions follow basic precautions like those just outlined; others will have expanded and adopted more detailed practices they felt were warranted. Since health care institutions choose to adopt and implement guidelines differently, it is important that you be familiar with the isolation policies used at your institution.

Many institutions will choose to use the new terminology and implement the precautions as they are described in this chapter. In those health care facilities where CDC guidelines are not followed, staff training will provide information regarding changes in policy and practice. Your immediate supervisor will provide direction and clarification, as needed.

Standard Precautions

All health care institutions have isolation precautions that are designed to reduce the risk of exposure to microorganisms and prevent the spread of infectious diseases. Typically, the main system of precautions used by health care institutions applies to all patients, since many diseases, such as **hepatitis B** virus (HBV), **hepatitis C** virus (HCV), and human immunodeficiency virus (HIV), the virus that causes AIDS, can be spread before the patient even develops symptoms of the disease. Therefore, Standard Precautions must be used when caring for all patients.

Both HBV and HIV are spread through several routes:

1. Parenteral (direct inoculation of blood on a needle through the skin)
2. Mucous membranes (blood contamination of the eye or mouth)
3. Sexual
4. Perinatal (from infected mother to newborn infant)

Standard precautions, precautions to be used for all patient care as recommended by the CDC, are designed to provide safety to health care workers and patients and to assist in controlling the transmission of HAIs.

hepatitis B Bloodborne disease that affects the liver and is easily transmitted within the health care setting following parenteral exposure

hepatitis C Prior to 1988 known as nonA-nonB hepatitis. Transmitted best through needle sticks and may result in chronic liver disease

KEY IDEA

Remember: The CDC's Standard Precautions are similar to Universal Precautions in that both are directed at body fluids that are blood or blood serum derived or fluids that contain blood, but Standard Precautions are broader in that they also include precautions for any moist body substance. Examples are tears, eye drainage, saliva, ear drainage, vaginal secretions, semen, urine, stool, sputum, nasal drainage, and drainage from open wounds or incisions

Standard Precautions apply to:

1. Blood
2. All body fluids secretions and excretions, except sweat, regardless of whether or not they contain visible blood
3. Nonintact skin
4. Mucous membranes

To comply with these precautions the practices listed on page 85 must be followed.

Nursing assistants will adhere to the precautions in Table 5–1◆ when delivering care to all patients. Table 5–1 lists selected procedures or patient interactions for which Standard Precautions are necessary and indicates the specific precautions (equipment) to be used.

TABLE 5–1◆

Selected Procedures and Standard Precautions Required

PROCEDURES	HANDWASHING	GLOVES	GOWN	MASK	EYEWEAR
Talking to patient					
Obtaining patient's blood pressure	X				
Hands become soiled with blood/ body fluids	X				
Examining patient *without* touching blood, body fluids, or mucous membranes	X				
Touching blood, body fluids, mucous membranes, broken skin, lesions, or contaminated equipment	X	X			
Drawing blood	X	X			
Doing heel stick	X	X			
Inserting an intravenous catheter	X	X			
Between patient contact	X				
Suctioning a patient's respiratory tract **Note:** Use gown, mask, and eyewear if blood/body fluid exposure is likely.	X	X			
Handling soiled waste, linen, and other materials **Note:** Use gown if waste or linen is saturated and may soil employee's clothing.	X	X			
Operative and other procedures that produce splattering/spraying of blood or body fluids	X	X	X	X	X

Note: Use of waterless alcohol hand antiseptic is an acceptable alternative to handwashing for obtaining blood pressure, exam without touching blood/body fluids, inserting a catheter, and between patient contacts.

STANDARD PRECAUTIONS

- *Hand Hygiene*: Must wash hands after all patient care. Wash hands with soap and water when hands are visibly dirty or contaminated with body substances or are visibly soiled with blood or other body fluids or after touching blood, body fluids, secretions, excretions, and contaminated items, regardless of whether gloves are worn.

- *Waterless Alcohol Hand Antiseptics*: If hands are not visibly soiled, use an alcohol-based hand antiseptic (e.g., gel, foam, or rinse) for routinely decontaminating hands prior to performing patient care, such as inserting IVs or urinary catheters, or after removing gloves. Note, if there is any dirt or body substances on hands it must be removed with soap and water. Waterless alcohol hand antiseptics are not effective if hands are visibly dirty.

- *Gloves*: Must be worn when in contact with blood, all body fluids, secretions, and excretions (except sweat) regardless of whether or not they contain visible blood, nonintact skin, and mucous membranes. (See procedures for applying and removing gloves later in this chapter.) Nursing assistants who have open cuts, sores, or dermatitis on their hands must wear gloves for all patient contact or be removed from patient contact until hands are healed.

- *Gowns or Aprons*: Must be worn during procedures or situations when exposure to body fluids, blood, draining wounds, or mucous membranes may occur. (See procedures for applying and removing gowns later in this chapter.)

- *Mask and Protective Eyewear*: Wear a mask and protective eyewear or face shield to protect eyes, mouth, or nose during patient care activities that are likely to generate splashes or sprays of blood, body fluids, secretions, or excretions (Figure 5–7◆).

- *Transportation*: When transporting any patient, ensure that precautions are maintained to minimize the risk of transmission of microorganisms to other patients and contamination of environmental surfaces or equipment.

- *Multiple-Use Patient Care Equipment*: When using common equipment or items, for example, a stethoscope or blood pressure cuff, it must be adequately cleaned and disinfected after use or whenever it becomes soiled with blood or other body fluids. (See procedure for care and cleaning of noncritical items later in this chapter.)

hand hygiene General term that applies to either handwashing, antiseptic handwash, antiseptic hand rub, or surgical hand antisepsis

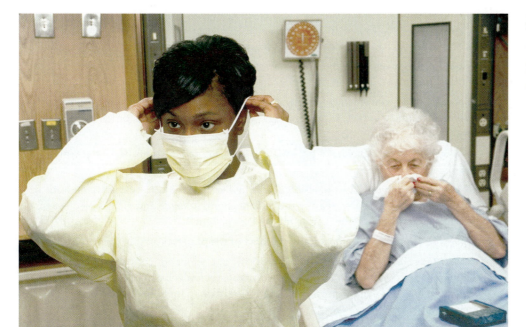

FIGURE 5–7 ◆

The face mask that covers both mouth and nose is worn to prevent exposure to blood, body fluids, or when the patient is coughing excessively

Transmission-based Precautions

Transmission-based Precautions, or the second tier of isolation, are designed for patients documented or suspected to be infected or colonized with highly transmissible or epidemiologically important pathogens for which precautions beyond Standard Precautions are needed to interrupt disease transmission in health care settings. (This is determined by the facility. For example, a facility might decide that frequency of a multi-antibiotic-resistant germ requires additional precautions on top of Standard Precautions; similarly, a pediatric facility is concerned about preventing transmission of respiratory syncytial virus (RSV) and therefore uses Contact Precautions on top of Standard Precautions.)

There are three types of Transmission-based Precautions: Contact Precautions, Droplet Precautions, and Airborne Precautions. Figures 5–8a♦, 5–8b♦, and 5–8c♦ give specific instructions regarding visitors and required procedures or protective equipment for Contact, Droplet, and Airborne Precautions. These precautions may be combined for diseases that have multiple routes of transmission and are to be used in addition to Standard Precautions. Table 5–2♦ lists numerous infections or conditions and identifies the precautions—type and duration—to be used in caring for patients with these infections or conditions.

Contact Precautions

Contact Precautions are to be used for the specific patient who is known to be infected with a microorganism that is not easily treated with antibiotics and can be transmitted easily by direct contact between the patient and health care worker or patient to patient

FIGURE 5–8a ♦

Contact Precautions

CONTACT PRECAUTIONS

Visitors report to nursing station before entering room.

- *Indications:* For patients infected with a microorganism that is not easily treated with antibiotics or that can be transmitted by direct contact. Examples of germs included in this category are *Clostridium difficile*, *Shigella*, respiratory syncytial virus, herpes, and impetigo.

- *Patient Placement:* Private room (if not available, place patient with another patient with similar microorganism, but with no other infection).

- *Gloves:* Wear gloves when entering the room and for all contact of patient and patient items, equipment, and body fluids.

- *Gown:* Wear a gown when entering the room if it is anticipated that your clothing will have substantial contact with the patient, environmental surfaces, or items in the patient's room.

- *Masks and Eyewear:* Indicated if potential for exposure to infectious body material exists.

- *Hand Hygiene:* If hands are not visibly soiled, use waterless alcohol-based hand antiseptic prior to or just after leaving the patient room. If hands are visibly soiled, wash with soap and water before caring for another patient.

- *Transport:* Limit the movement and transport of the patient.

- *Patient Care Equipment:* When possible, dedicate the use of noncritical patient care equipment to the patient. When using common equipment or items, they must be adequately cleaned or disinfected upon removal from patient's room or between patient uses.

Always use Standard Precautions.

DROPLET PRECAUTIONS

FIGURE 5–8b ◆
Droplet precautions

Visitors report to nursing station before entering the room.

■ *Indications:* For patients infected with microorganisms that are transmitted by droplets and can be generated by the patient during coughing, such as invasive *Haemophilus influenzae, Neisseria meningitidis,* influenza, and diphtheria.

■ *Patient Placement:* Private room (if not available, place patient in a room with a patient who has active infection with the same microorganism).

■ *Gloves:* Must be worn when in contact with blood and body fluids.

■ *Gowns:* Must be worn during procedures or situations where there will be exposure to body fluids, blood, draining wounds, or mucous membranes.

■ *Masks and Eyewear:* In addition to Standard Precautions, wear mask when working within three feet of patient (or when entering patient's room).

■ *Hand Hygiene:* If hands are not visibly soiled, use waterless alcohol-based hand antiseptic prior to or just after leaving the patient room. If hands are visibly soiled, wash with soap and water before caring for another patient.

■ *Transport:* Limit the movement and transport of the patient from the room to essential purposes only. If necessary to move the patient, minimize patient dispersal of droplets by masking the patient, if possible.

■ *Patient Care Equipment:* When using common equipment or items, they must be adequately cleaned or disinfected after each use.

Always use Standard Precautions.

AIRBORNE PRECAUTIONS

FIGURE 5–8c ◆
Airborne precautions

Visitors report to nursing station before entering room.

■ *Indications:* For patients known or suspected to be infected with microorganisms transmitted by airborne droplet nuclei that remain suspended in the air, such as tuberculosis, chicken pox, and measles.

■ *Patient Placement:* Private room. Negative air pressure in relation to the surrounding areas. Keep doors closed at all times.

■ *Gloves:* Same as Standard Precautions.

■ *Gown or Apron:* Same as Standard Precautions.

■ *Respiratory Protection and Eyewear:* For known or suspected active pulmonary tuberculosis, put on an N-95 mask or more protective respirator prior to entering room. For known or suspected airborne viral disease (for example, chicken pox or measles), standard mask should be worn by any person entering the room unless the person is not susceptible to the disease. When possible, persons who are susceptible should not enter the room.

■ *Hand Hygiene:* If hands are not visibly soiled, use waterless alcohol-based hand antiseptic prior to or just after leaving the patient room. If hands are visibly soiled, wash with soap and water before caring for another patient.

■ *Patient Transport:* Limit the transport of the patient to essential purposes only. If transport is necessary, place a mask on the patient if possible.

■ *Patient Care Equipment:* When using equipment or items (stethoscope, thermometer), they must be adequately cleaned and disinfected before use by another patient.

Always use Standard Precautions.

(hand or skin to skin) or with indirect contact with environmental surfaces or patient-care items. Examples of such illnesses include:

1. Gastrointestinal, respiratory, skin or wound infections, or colonization with multidrug-resistant bacteria
2. Enteric (intestinal) infections with a low infectious dose or prolonged environmental survival, including:
   a. *Clostridium difficile*
   b. For diapered or incontinent patients: enterohemorrhagic *Escherichia coli* 0157:H7, *Shigella*, hepatitis A, or rotavirus
3. Respiratory syncytial virus, parainfluenza virus, or enteroviral infections in infants and young children
4. Skin infections that are highly contagious or that may occur on dry skin, including:
   a. Diphtheria (cutaneous)
   b. Herpes simplex virus
   c. Impetigo
   d. Major (noncontained) abscesses, cellulitis, or decubiti
   e. Pediculosis
   f. Scabies
   g. Staphylococcal furunculosis in infants and young children
   h. Zoster (disseminated or in the immunocompromised host)
5. Viral/hemorrhagic conjunctivitis
6. Viral hemorrhagic infections (Ebola, Lassa, or Marburg)

Droplet Precautions

In addition to Standard Precautions, use Droplet Precautions for patients known or suspected to be infected with microorganisms transmitted by droplets that can be generated by the patient during coughing, sneezing, talking, or the performance of procedures that induce coughing. Examples of such illnesses include:

1. Invasive *Haemophilus influenzae* type b disease, including meningitis, pneumonia
2. Invasive *Neisseria meningitidis* disease, including meningitis, pneumonia, and sepsis
3. Bacterial respiratory infections spread by droplet including:
   a. Diphtheria
   b. Mycoplasma pneumonia
   c. Pertussis
   d. Pneumonic plague
   e. Streptococcal pharyngitis, pneumonia, or scarlet fever in infants and young children
4. Serious viral infections spread by droplet transmission, including:
   a. Adenovirus
   b. Influenza
   c. Mumps
   d. Parvovirus B19

TABLE 5–2◆

Type and Duration of Precautions Needed for Selected Infections and Conditions

INFECTION/CONDITION	PRECAUTIONS	
	TYPE*	DURATION†
Acquired immunodeficiency syndrome (AIDS)	S	
Chicken pox (varicella)[1]	A, C	F1
Conjunctivitis		
Acute bacterial	S	
Chlamydia	S	
Gonococcal	S	
Acute viral (acute hemorrhagic)	C	DI
Diphtheria		
Cutaneous	C	CN[2]
Pharyngeal	D	CN[2]
Hepatitis, viral		
Type A	S	
Diapered or incontinent patients	C	F[3]
Type B-HBsAG positive	S	
Type C and other unspecified non-A, non-B	S	
Type E	S	
Impetigo	C	U24 HRS
Influenza	D	DI
Lice (pediculosis)	C	U24 HRS
Measles (rubeola), all presentations	A	DI
Meningitis		
Aseptic (nonbacterial or viral meningitis)		
(also see enteroviral infections)	S	
Bacterial, gram-negative enteric, in neonates	S	
Fungal	S	
Haemophilus influenzae, known or suspected	D	U24 HRS
Listeria monocytogenes	S	
Neisseria meningitidis (meningococcal), known or suspected	D	U24 HRS
Pneumococcal	S	
Tuberculosis[9]	S	
Other diagnosed bacterial	S	
Multidrug-resistant organisms, infection or colonization[4]		
Gastrointestinal	C	CN
Respiratory	C	CN
Pneumococcal	S	
Skin, wound, or burn	C	CN
Pertussis (whooping cough)	D	F[5]
Respiratory infectious disease, acute (if not covered elsewhere)		
Adults	S	
Infants and young children	C	DI
Roseola infantum (exanthem subitum)	C	
Scabies	C	U24 HRS
Severe acute respiratory syndrome (SARS)	A, C, S	
Staphylococcal disease (*S. aureus*)		
Skin, wound, or burn		
Major[6]	C	DI
Minor or limited[7]	S	
Enterocolitis	S[8]	
Multidrug-resistant (see multidrug-resistant organisms)		
Pneumonia	S	
Scalded skin syndrome	S	
Toxic shock syndrome	S	

(continued)

TABLE 5–2◆

Type and Duration of Precautions Needed for Selected Infections and Conditions (*continued*)

Streptococcal disease (group A *Streptococcus*)		
Skin, wound, or burn		
Major[6]	C	U[24 HRS]
Minor or limited[7]	S	
Endometritis (puerperal sepsis)	S	
Pharyngitis in infants and young children	D	U[24 HRS]
Pneumonia in infants and young children	D	U[24 HRS]
Scarlet fever in infants and young children	D	U[24 HRS]
Tuberculosis		
Extrapulmonary, draining lesion (including scrofula)	S	
Extrapulmonary, meningitis[9]	S	
Pulmonary, confirmed or suspected, or laryngeal disease	A	F[10]
Skin-test positive with no evidence of current pulmonary disease	S	
Zoster (varicella-zoster)		
Localized in immunocompromised patient, disseminated	A, C	DI[11]
Localized in normal patient	S[11]	
Microorganisms that might be used in bioterrorism situations		
Anthrax	S	
Pneumonic plague	D,S	
Smallpox	A, C, S	
Botulism	S	

*TYPE OF PRECAUTIONS	†DURATION OF PRECAUTIONS
A - Airborne	CN - Until off antibiotics and culture negative
C - Contact	DH - Duration of hospitalization
D - Droplet	DI - Duration of illness (with wound lesions, DI means
S - Standard	until they stop draining)
When A, C, and D	U - Until time specified in hours (HRS) after initiation of
are specified, also use S	effective therapy
	F - See footnote number

Reference:
1. Maintain precautions until all lesions are crusted. The average incubation period for varicella is 10 to 16 days, with a range of 10 to 21 days. After exposure, use varicella zoster immune globulin (VZIG) when appropriate, and discharge susceptible patients if possible. Place exposed susceptible patients on Airborne Precautions beginning 10 days after exposure and continue until 21 days after last exposure (up to 28 days if VZIG has been given). Susceptible persons should not enter the room of patients on precautions if other immune caregivers are available.
2. Until two cultures taken at least 24 hours apart are negative.
3. Maintain precautions in infants and children <3 years of age for duration of hospitalization; in children 3–14 years of age, until 2 weeks after onset of symptoms; and in others, until 1 week after onset of symptoms.
4. Resistant bacteria judged by the infection control program, based on current state, regional, or national recommendations, to be of special clinical and epidemiologic significance.
5. Maintain precautions until 5 days after patient is placed on effective therapy.
6. No dressing or dressing does not adequately contain drainage.
7. Dressing covers and adequately contains drainage.
8. Use Contact Precautions for diapered or incontinent children <6 years of age for duration of illness.
9. Patient should be examined for evidence of current (active) pulmonary tuberculosis. If evidence exists, additional precautions are necessary (see tuberculosis).
10. Discontinue precautions only when TB patient is on effective therapy, is improving clinically, and has 3 consecutive negative sputum smears collected on different days, or TB is ruled out. Also see CDC Guidelines for Preventing the Transmission of Tuberculosis in Health Care Facilities.
11. Persons susceptible to varicella are also at risk for developing varicella when exposed to patients with herpes zoster lesions; therefore, people who are susceptible should not enter the room if other immune caregivers are available.

e. Rubella

f. SARS

Airborne Precautions

In addition to Standard Precautions, use Airborne Precautions for patients known or suspected to be infected with microorganisms transmitted by airborne droplet nuclei that remain suspended in the air and can be widely dispersed by air currents within a room or over a long distance. Examples of such illnesses include:

1. Tuberculosis

2. Varicella (including disseminated zoster)

3. Measles

Care of the patient in isolation takes extra time and extra effort. It's important to be as efficient as possible, therefore you should combine nursing duties when in the patient's room. Don't forget the patient needs your support and explanation of procedures as much as ever. Being in isolation carries its own set of worries, fears, and stigmas for the patient. You can minimize these obstacles and help your patient overcome them by showing your patient you are not afraid of talking with him nor of spending some time with him. Being in isolation has been identified as being the worst experience for many patients due to their fear of being identified as infectious (Figure 5–9◆). It is important to maintain confidentiality as well as professionalism with this group of patients.

FIGURE 5–9 ◆

Isolation is very difficult for most patients

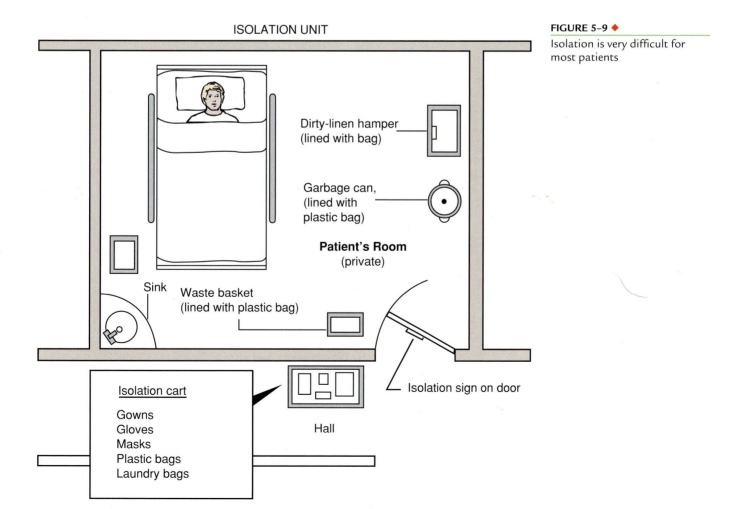

ISOLATION UNIT

A New Disease Called SARS

Severe acute respiratory syndrome (SARS) is a respiratory illness that has recently been reported in Asia, North America, and Europe. This section provides basic information about the disease and what is being done to combat its spread. To access the most current information about SARS, go to www.cdc.gov/ncidod/sars/ and www.who.int/csr/sars/en/.

For all contact with suspect SARS patients, careful hand hygiene is urged, including handwashing with soap and water; if hands are not visibly soiled, alcohol-based handrubs may be used as an alternative to handwashing.

In general, SARS begins with a fever greater than 100.4°F (>38.0°C). Other symptoms may include headache, an overall feeling of discomfort, and body aches. Some people also experience mild respiratory symptoms. After 2 to 7 days, SARS patients may develop a dry cough and have trouble breathing.

The primary way that SARS appears to spread is by close person-to-person contact. Most cases of SARS have involved people who cared for or lived with someone with SARS or who had direct contact with infectious material (for example, respiratory secretions) from a person who had SARS. Potential ways in which SARS can be spread include touching the skin of other people or objects that are contaminated with infectious droplets and then touching your eye(s), nose, or mouth. This can happen when someone who is sick with SARS coughs or sneezes droplets onto themselves, other people, or nearby surfaces. It also is possible that SARS can be spread more broadly through the air or by other ways that are currently not known.

Most of the U.S. cases of SARS have occurred among travelers returning to the United States from other parts of the world with SARS. There have been very few cases as a result of spread to close contacts such as family members and health care workers. Currently, SARS is not spreading more widely in the community in the United States.

Possible Cause of SARS

Scientists at CDC and other laboratories have detected a previously unrecognized coronavirus in patients with SARS. This novel coronavirus, for which CDC recently completed genome sequencing, is believed to be responsible for the global epidemic of SARS. Some close contacts of infected patients, including health care workers, have developed similar illnesses. In response to these developments, CDC has issued revised interim guidance concerning infection control precautions in the health care and community settings. To minimize the potential for transmission, these precautions are recommended as feasible, given available resources, until the epidemiology of disease transmission is better understood.

Care of Patients with SARS

If a suspect SARS patient is admitted to the hospital, infection control personnel should be notified immediately. Infection control measures for inpatients should include:

- Standard Precautions (e.g., hand hygiene); in addition to routine standard precautions, health care personnel should wear eye protection during all patient contact
- Contact Precautions (e.g., use of gown and gloves for contact with the patient or his or her environment)
- Airborne Precautions (e.g., an isolation room with negative pressure relative to the surrounding area and use of an N-95 filtering disposable respirator for persons entering the room)

If Airborne Precautions cannot be fully implemented, patients should be placed in a private room, and all persons entering the room should wear N-95 respirators. Where possible, a qualitative fit test should be conducted for N-95 respirators. If N-95 respirators are not available for health care personnel, then surgical masks should be worn. Regardless of the availability of facilities for Airborne Precautions, Standard and Contact Precautions should be implemented for all suspected SARS patients.

Infection control measures for outpatients include the following:

- Persons seeking medical care for an acute respiratory infection should be asked about possible exposure to someone with SARS or recent travel to an area with SARS. If SARS is suspected, provide and place a surgical mask over the patient's nose and mouth. If masking the patient is not feasible, the patient should be asked to cover his mouth with a disposable tissue when coughing, talking, or sneezing. Separate the patient from others in the reception area as soon as possible, preferably in a private room with negative pressure relative to the surrounding area.

- All health care personnel should wear N-95 respirators while taking care of patients with suspected SARS. In addition, health care personnel should follow Standard Precautions (e.g., hand hygiene) and Contact Precautions (e.g., use of gown and gloves for contact with the patient or his or her environment) and should wear eye protection for all patient contact.

In the home or residential setting, SARS patients should wear a surgical mask during contact with others. If the patient is unable to wear a surgical mask, it may be prudent for household members to wear surgical masks when in close contact with the patient. Household members in contact with the patient should be reminded of the need for careful hand hygiene including handwashing with soap and water; if hands are not visibly soiled, alcohol-based handrubs may be used as an alternative to handwashing.

Protective Equipment and Procedures

The following guidelines, procedures, and illustrations are provided to give a more detailed description of some of the practices previously described.

Hand Hygiene

If hands are not visibly soiled, use an alcohol-based hand antiseptic (e.g., gel, foam, or rinse) for routinely decontaminating hands prior to performing patient care, such as inserting IVs or urinary catheters, or after removing gloves. Note, if there is any dirt or body substances on hands it must be removed with soap and water. Waterless alcohol hand antiseptics are not effective if hands are visibly dirty.

In your work you will be using your hands constantly, therefore it is your responsibility to keep your hands in as good a condition as possible. Try to avoid cuts and chaffing of your hands by wearing gloves when it's cold outside, using a good moisturizing lotion, and generally trying to protect your hands. Fingernails should be kept short, and fake fingernails of any kind should be discouraged. Fake nails and chipped, or cracked nail polish can harbor or entrap microorganisms.

Excessive jewelry, for example, rings or bracelets, should not be worn because they can entrap bacteria. Due to the nature of your job, you will handle supplies and equipment used in the treatment and care of patients. Microorganisms will get on your hands (Figure 5–10◆). They will come from the patient or from the things the patient has touched. Your hands could carry these germs to other persons and places or to your own face and mouth. Washing your hands frequently will help to prevent this transfer of germs.

KEY IDEA

Hand hygiene (handwashing) is the cornerstone of infection control activities and is not to be replaced by the use of gloves. You must use hand hygiene before and after contact with each patient. Hand hygiene is the single most important way to prevent the spread of infection and disease.

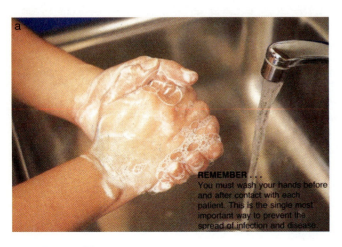

FIGURE 5–10a ◆

Washing your hands is important in preventing the spread of infection

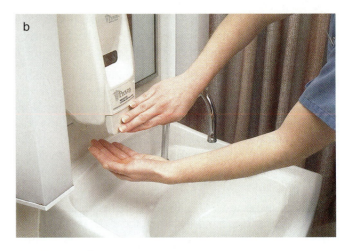

FIGURE 5–10b ◆

Use a soap dispenser

Waterless Hand Hygiene

Most people do not wash their hands as often as they should. To improve or promote hand hygiene among health care personnel, many employers now place an alcohol-based waterless antiseptic gel dispenser near the entrance to the patient's room or at the bedside or in other convenient locations. Some supply individual pocket-sized containers to be carried by health care workers with high workloads and high numbers of patient care contacts. Waterless hand hygiene products are sold in most stores that sell soap products.

friction The process of rubbing two surfaces together, such as skin

---

HANDWASHING   GUIDELINES   OBRA

- Handwashing must be done before and after each nursing task, before and after direct patient contact, and after handling any of a patient's belongings. Also, wash hands before going to work, after work, before and after eating, and before and after going to the bathroom.

- The water faucet is always considered contaminated. This means there are microorganisms on it. If necessary, use paper towels to turn the faucet off. Never touch the faucet.

- If your hands accidentally touch the inside of the sink, start over.

- Take soap from a dispenser; do not use bar soap. Bar soap sits in a pool of soapy water in the soap dish, which is considered contaminated.

- Handwashing is effective only when:
  1. You use enough soap to produce lots of lather.
  2. You rub skin against skin to create **friction,** which helps to eliminate microorganisms. Remember your fingers have four sides.
  3. You rinse with tepid or lukewarm running water. Rinsing is very important to remove the pathogens. *The solution to pollu-*

tion is dilution. Adequate soap, lots of water, lots of friction!

- Hold your hands lower than your elbows while washing. This is to prevent germs from contaminating your arms. Holding your hands down prevents backflow over unwashed skin. Add water to the soap while washing. This keeps the soap from becoming too dry.

- Never use the patient's bar of soap for yourself.

- Rinse well. Soap left on the skin causes drying and can cause skin irritation. The primary reason that skin chaps is because hands are not thoroughly rinsed and dried after handwashing!

PROCEDURE

HANDWASHING

RATIONALE

Handwashing is the most important way you can prevent the spread of infection and disease.

PREPARATION

1. Assemble your equipment. The equipment used for handwashing is found at all times at every sink in all health care institutions.
   a. Soap
   b. Paper towels
   c. Warm running water
   d. Wastepaper basket

STEPS

2. Completely wet your hands and wrists under the running water. Keep your fingertips pointed downward.

3. Apply soap.

4. Hold your hands lower than your elbows while washing.

5. Work up a good lather. Spread it over the entire area of your hands and wrists. Get soap under your nails and between your fingers (Figure 5–11◆).

6. Clean under your nails by rubbing your nails across the palms of your hand.

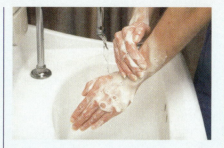

FIGURE 5–11 ◆
Wash up to 2 inches above each wrist

7. Use a rotating and rubbing (frictional) motion for 15 seconds.
   a. Rub vigorously.
   b. Rub one hand against the other hand and wrist.

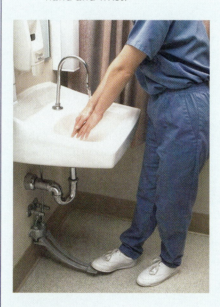

FIGURE 5–12a ◆
Rinse well and, when available, control water using the foot pedal

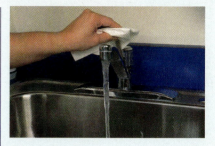

FIGURE 5–12b ◆
Use a towel to turn off a faucet

   c. Rub between your fingers by interlacing them.
   d. Rub up and down to reach all skin surfaces on your hands, between your fingers, and 2 inches above your wrists.
   e. Rub the tips of your fingers against your palms to clean with friction around the nail beds.

8. Rinse well. Rinse from 2 inches above your wrists to the hands. Hold your hands and fingertips down under running water (Figure 5–12a◆).

9. Dry thoroughly with paper towels.

10. Turn off the faucet, using a paper towel. Never touch the faucet with your hands after washing (Figure Figure 5–12b◆).

FOLLOW-UP

11. Discard the paper towel into the wastepaper basket. Do not touch the basket.

Studies show that waterless rinses are quick to use, more effective against many germs than handwashing, and improve skin condition.

Waterless antiseptic gels should be used:

- Before performing invasive procedures (such as inserting a thermometer or urinary catheter) or between direct patient care procedures or contacts
- When caring for patients using Contact Precautions for antibiotic-resistant organisms, especially when leaving the room after contact with patient, equipment, or surfaces

<table>
<tr><td>**WATERLESS HAND HYGIENE**</td><td>**PROCEDURE**</td><td>**OBRA**</td></tr>
</table>

PROCEDURE   **OBRA**

STEPS

1. Locate wall-mounted dispenser and push release lever with one hand while holding the other, open hand underneath the nozzle of the dispenser.

2. One squirt of gel is delivered onto the open hand. Obtain another 1 to 2 mL if needed to have enough to cover the skin of both hands.

3. Rub the gel into the skin of both hands.

4. Allow hands to dry, usually about 30 seconds.

Charting example: Charting unnecessary.

RATIONALE

Waterless antiseptic agents are used when regular handwashing sinks are not within easy reach or when a quick way to perform hand hygiene is needed.

- After patient contact, e.g., obtaining a blood pressure or temperature, when hands are visibly clean
- After removing gloves, as long as hands are not visibly soiled

KEY IDEA

Waterless antiseptic gels do not remove soil or body fluids from the hands. Therefore, if hands are visibly soiled, wash them with soap and running water.

Gloves

The skin, as the primary defense, protects the body against infection. Medical exam gloves, if properly used, provide additional protection for your hands and help protect you and your patients from infection and disease. The utilization of gloves has become essential for all health care workers when touching moist body fluids, when making direct contact with nonintact skin, or when inserting your fingers inside a patient's mouth (Figure 5–13◆).

FIGURE 5–13 ◆

Always put on disposable gloves whenever you may come in contact with the body fluids (except sweat) of patients

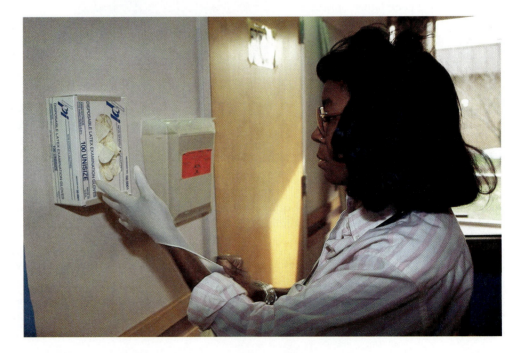

| PUTTING ON DISPOSABLE GLOVES | **PROCEDURE** | **OBRA** |

STEPS

2. Slip your hand into the gloves, one hand at a time.

3. Work the gloves down to the base of the fingers to make sure they fit comfortably.

4. Gloves should neither be too tight nor too loose at the fingertips or wrists.

5. Upon application, inspect gloves for integrity.

Charting Example: Charting unnecessary. Handwashing is assumed and not charted.

RATIONALE

Wearing gloves provides a barrier between your hands and potential contaminants or body fluids.

PREPARATION

1. Remove jewelry and wash hands. Remove two gloves from box or package.

KEY IDEA

If you wear contaminated gloves in public areas and touch things such as telephones, doors, or elevator buttons, you put everyone at risk for infection!

Gloves do not provide total protection because defects, such as holes, do occur in these (latex, vinyl) materials. Gloves do provide a barrier between your skin and a potential contaminant or body fluid but you cannot rely on them for complete protection. The combination of gloves, followed by good hand hygiene upon removal, offers the most complete protection. (Note: Gloves/supplies are available that are made of alternate materials for those with a documented latex allergy.)

KEY IDEA

Gloves must be changed:
- Between each patient contact.
- When integrity of glove is violated (hole or tear).
- Upon completion of each task where contamination with body fluids may have occurred.

The Mask

The mask is intended for protection of the health care worker and/or patient from droplets containing microorganisms expelled from the oropharynx and nasopharynx. Using a mask correctly and for the appropriate indications is essential. The mask is a filter intended to prevent the spread of diseases that are spread via an airborne route, such as chicken pox or measles. Some germs transmitted through the air are small enough to get deep inside the lungs. A more protective device called a *respirator* is recommended for health care workers. Respirators are used to protect against tuberculosis (TB) germs, the SARS virus, or other highly contagious germs that can be inhaled. An N-95 respirator is a type that is

REMOVING GLOVES

PROCEDURE

OBRA

RATIONALE

Removing and correctly disposing of gloves protects your hands from contact with potential contaminants or body fluids.

STEPS

1. With both hands gloved, with the gloved fingers of one hand grasp the glove of the other hand just below the cuff (Figure 5–14a◆).

2. Turn or peel one glove inside out, starting at the cuff. Hold it in the gloved hand, making sure to avoid contact with inside of other hand (Figure 5–14b◆).

3. Place your ungloved index and middle fingers inside the cuff of the remaining glove (Figure 5–14c◆).

4. With the ungloved hand, peel the second glove from the inside, tucking the first glove inside the second as you remove your hand (Figure 5–14d◆).

FOLLOW-UP

5. Upon removal of gloves, be sure to discard used gloves directly into the trash. Wash your hands.

Charting example: Charting unnecessary.

a
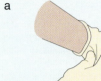

b
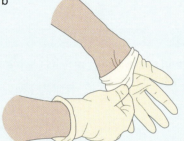

C
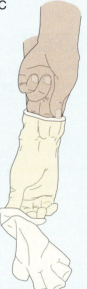

d
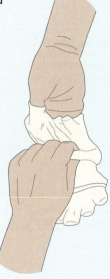

FIGURE 5–14 ◆
Removing gloves

PUTTING ON A MASK

PROCEDURE

OBRA

RATIONALE

Masks worn correctly prevent inhalation of microorganisms and reduce exposure to body fluids or secretions.

PREPARATION

1. Wash hands.
2. Obtain mask.

STEPS

3. Place mask on face and adjust pliable nose piece until it fits securely.

4. Tie strings securely at crown of head.

5. Grasp bottom portion of mask, spread mask to cover below chin.

6. Tie lower strings behind neck.

Masks are designed for a close fit but improper application can negate their efficiency.

Charting example: charting unnecessary.

| WEARING MASKS TO PREVENT CROSS-INFECTION | PROCEDURE | OBRA |

RATIONALE

The mask serves as a filter to protect caregivers and/or patients from exposure to droplets expelled from the oropharynx or nasopharynx.

1. Mask should be handled only by the strings, thereby keeping the hands uncontaminated by a soiled mask. (Figure 5–15◆)

   - Never lower mask to hang loosely around the neck or place it in a pocket.

   - Promptly discard mask into the proper receptacle upon removal.

   - Change mask if it becomes wet or moist.

   - Change mask between procedures or cases in operating rooms or ambulatory surgery settings.

2. An N-95 respirator may be used for a shift when used by the same caregiver providing care to a patient on Airborne Precautions. Should the N-95 respirator become contaminated, it should be changed.

3. If the mask is worn by a health care worker to provide an uncontaminated air environment for patient, and the health care worker has excessive facial hair, a hood must be worn to cover the neck area.

4. Wash hands following discard.

Charting example: charting unnecessary.

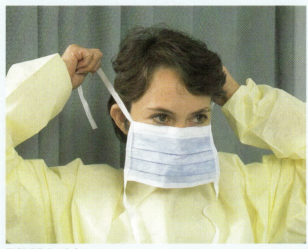

FIGURE 5–15 ◆
Masks should be handled only by the strings to avoid contamination.

commonly used. The *N* stands for non-oil-containing particles and the *95* means it filters 95 percent of the TB germ. The procedure above is utilized when a mask is to be used.

KEY IDEA

The Centers for Disease Control and Prevention mandates that workers who care for clients with suspected/active tuberculosis be provided with a particulate respirator (NIOSH approved). To ensure a good fit, the mask must be "fit tested." Your health care facility will have guidelines on how to achieve this.

Care and Cleaning of Noncritical Items

A noncritical item is one that comes in contact with intact skin but not mucous membranes. Examples of noncritical items include bedpans, blood pressure cuffs, stethoscopes, pulse oximeters, bedside tables, and patient furniture. The risk of transmitting disease from direct contact with inanimate surfaces (noncritical item) is minimized through proper cleaning and maintenance of noncritical items. Intact skin acts as an effective barrier to most microorganisms, and sterility is not critical.

GUIDELINES

CARE AND CLEANING OF NONCRITICAL ITEMS

- Following use of a noncritical item, check for visible contamination, such as blood or other body substances.

  a. If the item is not visibly soiled, carefully wipe the item clean with alcohol or the cleaning solution recommended by the manufacturer and /or the current hospital cleaner.

  b. If the item is visibly soiled with blood or body fluids, the item should first be wiped, cleaned, and then disinfected.

- Recommended cleaning, or disinfecting, solutions and methods must be effective against microbes while not harming the device in any way, for example, corroding the metal or cracking the plastic. The solution may include:

  a. 70 to 90 percent ethyl or isopropyl alcohol

  b. Sodium hypochlorite (household bleach) 1 part bleach to 10 parts water

  c. Phenolic germicidal detergent

  d. Iodophor germicidal detergent

  e. Quaternary ammonium germicidal detergent

PROCEDURE   OBRA

APPLICATION OF A GOWN

RATIONALE

Gowns provide a barrier to reduce exposure to microorganisms, body fluids, or secretions.

STEPS

1. Wash your hands. If you are wearing a long-sleeve uniform, roll your sleeves above your elbows (Figure 5–16a◆).

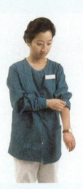

FIGURE 5–16a ◆
Roll up sleeves

2. Unfold the isolation gown so the opening is at the back (Figure 5–16b◆).

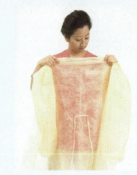

FIGURE 5–16b ◆
Unfold gown so the opening faces you

3. Put your arms into the sleeves of the isolation gown (Figure 5–16c◆).

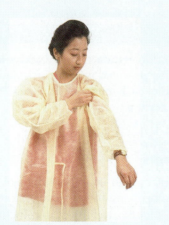

FIGURE 5–16c ◆
Put your arms into the sleeves

4. Fit the gown at the neck, making sure your uniform is covered (Figure 5–16d◆).

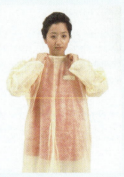

FIGURE 5–16d ◆
Fit gown at your neck

5. Reach behind and tie the neck back with a simple shoelace bow or fasten an adhesive strip (Figure 5–16e◆).

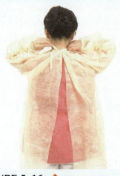

FIGURE 5–16e ◆
Tie neck back with simple bow

PROCEDURE *(continued)*

6. Grasp the edges of the gown and pull to the back (Figure 5–16f◆).

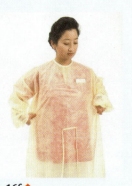

FIGURE 5–16f ◆
Grasp gown edges and pull them back

7. Overlap the edges of the gown, completely closing the opening and covering your uniform completely (Figure 5–16g◆).

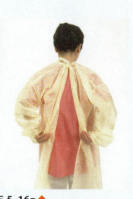

FIGURE 5–16g ◆
Completely cover back of your uniform

8. Tie the waist ties in a bow or fasten the adhesive strip (Figure 5–16h◆).

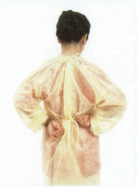

FIGURE 5–16h ◆
Tie waist ties in a bow
Charting example: charting unnecessary

REMOVING A GOWN

PROCEDURE

OBRA

RATIONALE

Careful removal of a gown will prevent exposure or direct contact with potential contaminants, blood, or body fluids.

STEPS

1. Keep gloves on, then untie the waist belt or ties (Figure 5–17a◆).[1]

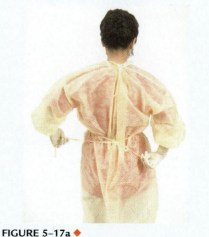

FIGURE 5–17a ◆
Untie waist ties

2. Untie the neck ties, being cautious not to come in contact with neck, or have someone else untie the gown for you (Figure 5–17b◆).

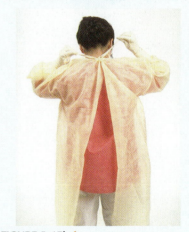

FIGURE 5–17b ◆
Carefully untie neck ties

---

[1]This procedure is based on AORN standards. In practice there are two acceptable approaches regarding removing gloves and gown. The most important point is to avoid contamination or contact exposure to blood and body fluids. In the case where there is blood on your gown and gloves, it is most important to remove your gloves last after you have touched the contaminated gown. Follow your instructor's direction and always wash your hands after removing and discarding gowns, masks, and/or gloves.

PROCEDURE *(continued)*

3. Pull the sleeve off by grasping each shoulder at the neck line (Figure 5–17c◆).

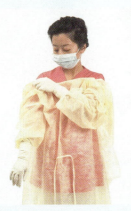

FIGURE 5–17c ◆
Grasp gown at shoulder to pull sleeve off

4. Turn the sleeves inside out as you remove them from your arms (Figure 5–17d◆).

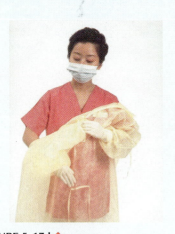

FIGURE 5–17d ◆
Turn sleeves inside out as you remove them

5. Holding the gown away from your body by the inside of the shoulder seams, fold it inside out, bringing the shoulders together (Figure 5–17e◆).

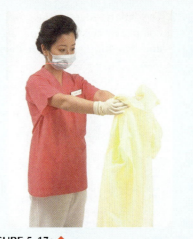

FIGURE 5–17e ◆
Hold gown away from you as you fold it inside out

6. Roll the gown up with the inside out and discard (Figure 5–17f◆).

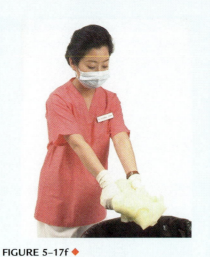

FIGURE 5–17f ◆
Roll gown inside out and discard

7. Remove gloves, being, careful to not contaminate yourself (Figure 5–17g◆). (See description in glove removal.) Be sure to discard used gloves directly into the trash. Wash your hands.

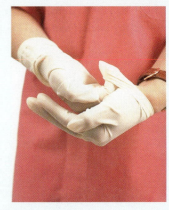

FIGURE 5–17g ◆
Remove gloves

8. Remove mask touching only the strings and discard (Figure 5–17h◆).

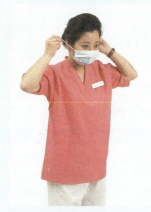

FIGURE 5–17h ◆
Remove mask

FOLLOW-UP

9. Wash hands (Figure 5–17i◆).

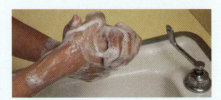

FIGURE 5–17i ◆
Wash hands

PROCEDURE *(continued)*

10. Alternative way to correctly remove gown and mask (Figure 5–17j◆).

Charting example: charting unnecessary.

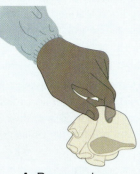

A Remove gloves.

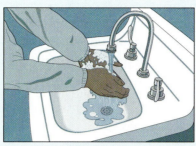

B Wash hands.

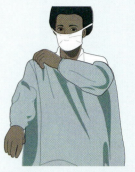

C Grasp each shoulder of gown near neck to remove sleeves.

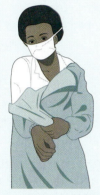

D As you remove sleeves turn them inside out.

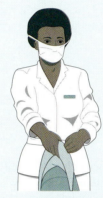

E Fold the gown inside out, holding it away from you.

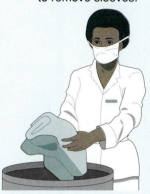

F Roll up the gown and discard it.

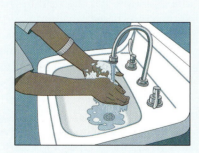

G Wash your hands.

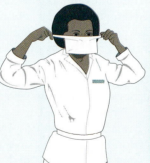

H Remove your mask.

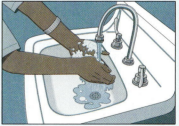

I Wash your hands.

FIGURE 5–17j ◆

Changes in Isolation Strategies

As information on disease transmission becomes more available and more scientific, certain isolation strategies of the past are being eliminated. The practices that have no longer been found necessary consist of the following: double bagging of linen, meltaway bags, special precautions for cleaning dishware and utensils used by patients in isolation, and protective or reverse isolation. The rationale for the change in each isolation strategy follows:

1. Double bagging of linen is unnecessary since all linen is considered infectious and therefore needs to be handled in such a manner as to avoid dispersal of microorganisms. This includes using a plastic bag if the linen is soiled or wet in order to prevent contamination of floors, linen chutes, or bins. The practice of double bagging is not necessary, however.

2. Meltaway bags are unnecessary since all linen is handled as infectious.

3. No additional special precautions are needed for dishes, glasses, cups, or eating utensils for the patient in isolation. Dishes should be handled according to standard hospital procedure or in the home setting may be washed with hot, soapy water or in the dishwasher. Disposable dishes and utensils are not necessary for patients in isolation precautions.

4. Protective or reverse isolation was shown to be ineffective in preventing infection in immunosuppressed patients, as the patient's own flora was primarily responsible for his or her infection. Good handwashing, limiting visitors, and not allowing fresh fruits, vegetables, or flowers is the most effective prevention method for this population. Some hospitals have more specific precautions for immunocompromised patients.

OSHA Standards for Occupational Exposure to Bloodborne Pathogens

Who is at risk? All facilities will identify all job classifications that have occupational exposure to blood and other potentially dangerous body fluids and materials. Since July 6, 1992, OSHA (Occupational Safety and Health Administration, U.S. Department of Labor) standards have mandated that training and immunization must be provided to all employees within 10 days of initial assignment to a job that puts the employee at occupational risk. This training must be updated annually. All employees must be given the choice to elect or refuse immunization. If refused, the employee has the right to change his or her mind at a later date and receive immunization at no charge.

Employers are required to provide a means of protecting their employees from potential exposure to hepatitis B. Employees must use Standard Precautions, protective clothing, protective eye wear or face shields, and equipment to prevent exposure to potentially infectious materials. However, the best defense against infection by hepatitis B is vaccination.

Hepatitis B vaccine (grown on yeast) became available in 1987 and is now the only type produced in this country. Adverse reactions are minimal and there is no possibility of infection from this vaccine. The hepatitis B vaccine is contraindicated for individuals who are hypersensitive to yeast or any component of the vaccine. Employees with a history of cardiopulmonary disease should consult their physician prior to accepting this vaccination.

Immunization is accomplished in a three-injection series. Any employee with a potential for occupational exposure qualifies to receive the vaccine. All costs associated with this immunization must be provided by the employer.

Hepatitis C virus (HCV) is now the most common chronic bloodborne infection in the United States. Most people with HCV are chronically infected and might not be aware of their infection because they do not have any clinical symptoms. Infected persons serve as a source of transmission to others and are at risk of developing chronic liver disease. HCV is transmitted primarily through large or repeated percutaneous exposures to blood. Prior to 10 years ago, HCV was transmitted in blood transfusions; however, today, blood is screened for this virus. Injecting drug use consistently has accounted for a substantial proportion of HCV infections.

Another bloodborne pathogen that puts health care workers at potential risk is human immunodeficiency virus (HIV). The acquired immunodeficiency syndrome (AIDS) caused by HIV is a severe viral disease that affects the immune system and is characterized by opportunistic infections. The risk is due to exposure by semen, vaginal secretions, cerebrospinal fluid, synovial fluid, pleural fluid, pericardial fluid, peritoneal fluid, amniotic fluid, saliva, blood, blood products, and other body fluids and waste. Annual reeducation and the enforced use of standard precautions is the best means of preventing exposure. (AIDS is discussed in Chapter 30.)

AGE-SPECIFIC CONSIDERATIONS

Immunization

Infants less than 3 months of age have an immature immune system. They rely on passive immunity from their mothers. This makes them more prone to infections. The elderly also are more prone to infections. As the body ages, changes in the pulmonary system, such as decreased muscle strength, decreased vital capacity, and decreased cough, make the elderly more prone to infection.

KEY IDEA

At times you may be asked to assist a nurse performing a procedure using aseptic or sterile technique. Do not perform sterile procedures independently unless you have been instructed to do so. Your instructor will be familiar with any practice rules or restrictions

Asepsis and Sterile Technique

When working in a health care environment, it is important to assist patients to maintain their best possible physical state. To do so, caregivers might be required to practice the principles of asepsis (aseptic technique). When practiced correctly, these standards protect the patient from exposure to germs and help prevent infections.

Asepsis means the absence of microorganisms. Asepsis can be achieved by preventing the conditions that allow pathogens to live, multiply, and spread. As a caregiver, you share the responsibility to prevent the spread of infection by using aseptic, or sterile, technique. (*Aseptic technique* and *sterile technique* are terms that can be used interchangeably. For the rest of this chapter, we will use the term *sterile technique*.)

Sterile technique encompasses the steps followed to prevent contamination by germs. By following these steps very carefully, you will be able to maintain a sterile, or aseptic (germ-free), environment in which to do certain tasks.

When practicing sterile technique, keep the following guidelines in mind.

GUIDELINES

MAINTAINING A STERILE FIELD

■ A **sterile field** is an area that you can create to work from when you are doing a sterile procedure. This area must remain dry in order to remain sterile. You can use a sterile wrap from a package to create this field, or you can use sterile towels supplied as part of a supply kit.

■ Only sterile items can be on a sterile field. Sterile items have gone through the process of sterilization, which can destroy all living microorganisms. If an unsterile item is placed on the field, the field becomes unsterile. If an unsterile item touches a sterile item, the sterile item becomes unsterile.

■ Only the top of a table or counter of a sterile field is considered to

be sterile. Anything hanging over the edge of a sterile field is unsterile. The edges of a sterile field itself (approximately 1 inch into the field) are considered unsterile, so be careful that you do not touch these areas with sterile items.

■ Do not cross over your sterile field—that is, unless you are wearing sterile gown and gloves, do not reach over a sterile field. Microbes may drop from your arms or hands onto the sterile field, making it unsterile.

■ Do not turn your back on your sterile field. You do not know what is happening when you cannot see your field. Place the sterile field in a location that will allow you to keep it in sight and do your work efficiently.

■ You may not touch the sterile field unless you have sterile gloves on.

■ When you have sterile gloves on, your hands must be kept above your waist, in front of your body, and in your sight at all times. You may not touch anything that is not sterile. If you touch an unsterile item, your gloves become contaminated and must be replaced.

■ You may drop sterile items onto a sterile field, but if they touch any unsterile items or the unsterile edge of the field, the sterile item becomes contaminated.

■ Anything on your sterile field that absorbs moisture from an unsterile item becomes unsterile. For example, if there is wetness on the table on which you open your sterile package and this wetness soaks into your sterile field, the field becomes contaminated.

---

sterile field An area created to work from when you are doing a sterile procedure

Surgical conscience is a term used to describe the way you must act and think when you are working with sterile technique. It is your responsibility to be aware of and maintain your own sterile technique. For example, if no one is around and you contaminate your sterile field, you must be aware of this and start over. This protects the patient from microorganisms and germs that could cause an infection.

It is important to know the difference between clean technique and sterile technique. Some procedures are performed with clean technique. For example, clean technique might be used to change a dressing over a closed surgical wound or to reinforce a dressing. Clean technique involves using clean gloves and clean supplies (they do not need to be sterile, but they may be). You do not need to use sterile technique when doing something "cleanly," but you must still avoid contaminating your clean supplies and clean gloves. Clean items become contaminated if you drop them on the floor; clean gloves become contaminated if you use them to touch something dirty. The RN will tell you what type of technique (clean or sterile) to use during a procedure.

PUTTING ON STERILE GLOVES

PROCEDURE

Sterile gloves must be carefully applied to avoid contamination.

STEPS

1. Wash hands or apply waterless hand antiseptic.

2. Select a pair of wrapped gloves in a size that will fit your hands snugly.

3. Check to be certain that the gloves are sterile.

   a. Package intact with no signs of dampness?

   b. Seal of sterility?

4. Place package on a clean, dry, flat surface.

5. Open the wrapper, handling only the outside (Figure 5–18a◆ and 5–18b◆).

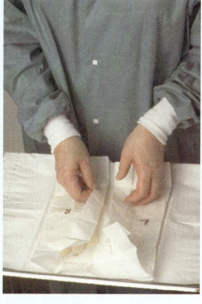

FIGURE 5–18b ◆
Handle only outside of wrapper

folded cuff (Figure 5–19◆) *Do not touch the outside of the glove!*

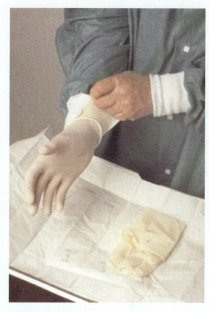

FIGURE 5–20 ◆
Put glove on your right hand

8. Use your gloved right hand to pick up the left glove:

   a. Place the finger of your gloved right hand under the cuff of the left glove (Figure 5–21◆).

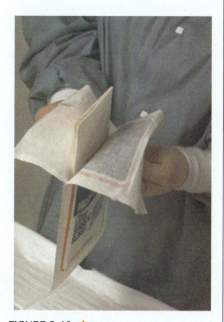

FIGURE 5–18a ◆
Open wrapper

6. Use your left hand to pick up the right glove. Touch only the inside

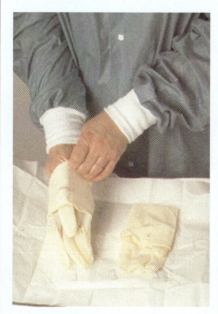

FIGURE 5–19 ◆
Touch only the inside of glove

7. Put the glove on your right hand (Figure 5–20◆).

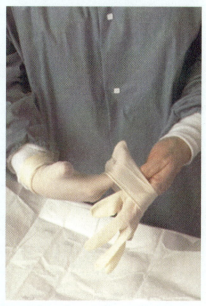

FIGURE 5–21 ◆
Place fingers of gloved hand inside left-hand glove cuff

PROCEDURE *(continued)*

b. Lift the glove up and away from the wrapper, and pull it onto your left hand.

c. Continue pulling left glove up to wrist. Be certain that the gloved right thumb does not touch your skin or clothing (Figure 5–22◆).

9. With your gloved left hand, place fingers under the cuff of the right glove and pull it up over your right wrist.

10. Adjust the fingers of the glove as necessary.

11. If either glove tears, remove them both and begin the procedure again with another pair.

Charting example: charting unnecessary

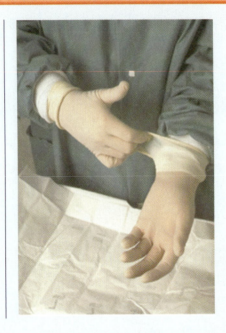

FIGURE 5–22 ◆

Pull glove on hand up to wrist

OPENING A STERILE PACKAGE

PROCEDURE

RATIONALE

Sterile packages must be carefully opened to avoid contamination.

STEPS

1. Wash hands.

2. Assemble the equipment and supplies
   a. Sterile gloves
   b. Sterile package

3. Check to be certain all supplies are sterile:
   a. Package intact, with no signs of dampness?
   b. Seal of sterility?

4. Place the package on dry, flat, clean work surface (an over-bed table, for example). Position the package so that the first edge to be unfolded will be pulled away from you. (By opening the package away from you with the first motion, you will not have to reach across your sterile area again.) The outer wrap of the package will serve as a sterile field to work on (Figure 5–23a◆).

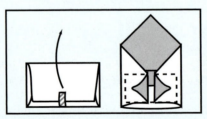

FIGURE 5–23a ◆

Open first edge of package away from you

5. Slowly pull the corners at the right and left of the package (Figure 5–23b◆). This exposes the inside of the package.

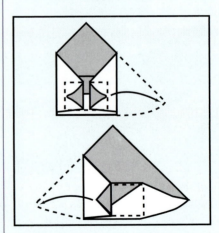

FIGURE 5–23b ◆

Pull right and left corners of package to expose inside

PROCEDURE *(continued)*

6. Carefully pull back the corner pointing toward you (Figure 5–23c◆).

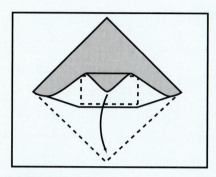

FIGURE 5–23c ◆
Pull the last edge of package toward you

7. If you are going to add sterile items to your field, do so now. Remember that the edge (1 inch around) of your sterile field, and anything hanging over the edge of your work area, is contaminated (Figure 5–24a◆).

8. Do not touch anything inside your sterile package or sterile field until you have put your sterile gloves on.

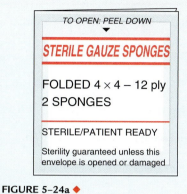

TO OPEN: PEEL DOWN
▼

STERILE GAUZE SPONGES

FOLDED 4 × 4 – 12 ply
2 SPONGES

STERILE/PATIENT READY

Sterility guaranteed unless this
envelope is opened or damaged

FIGURE 5–24a ◆
Check that sterile package is clean and dry

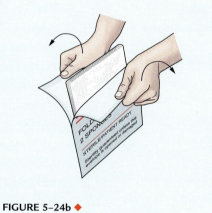

FIGURE 5–24b ◆
Grasp each side of package at the top

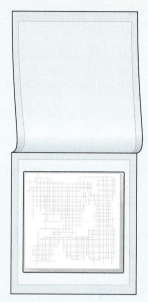

FIGURE 5–24c ◆
Peel down the sides of package and lay flat. The sterile gauze may be dropped onto a sterile field. Aseptic and sterile technique are particularly important in any area where surgical procedures are performed or in an operating environment. An instructor will review objectives and performance expectations specific to the procedures that are performed.

SUMMARY

The work of being a nursing assistant is not without risk. However, these risks are greatly minimized or eliminated by following the recommendations in this chapter, such as when to wear protective items, handwashing, and having the hepatitis B vaccine. Handwashing is the most important measure you can take to prevent the spread of microorganisms. Knowing how disease or infection is transmitted is the first step, but you then must utilize the Standard and Transmission-based Precautions necessary to interrupt the chain of transmission effectively. It is your responsibility to do all you can to prevent infections in your patients and yourself by following the described practices.

CHAPTER REVIEW

FILL IN THE BLANK Read each sentence and fill in the blank line with a word that completes the sentence.

1. If you wear contaminated gloves in public places, you risk spreading _____.

2. A noncritical care item, such as a blood pressure cuff, can generally be _____ versus disinfected.

3. _____ is the process of rubbing two surfaces together, such as skin.

4. Use _____ precautions when caring for a patient with TB.

5. When a patient is in Contact Precautions, you should always wear_____ when caring for the patient.

MULTIPLE CHOICE Choose the best answer for each question or statement.

1. Normal flora means
   a. the normal plants seen around the hospital.
   b. the nonpathogenic microorganisms that live in our bodies.
   c. the pathogenic microorganisms that live in our bodies.
   d. All of the above.

2. Bacteria grows best in
   a. warm, moist, dark places.
   b. temperatures of less than 76 degrees.
   c. dry, bright, surfaces.
   d. All of the above.

3. Sterilization means the
   a. process of killing all microorganisms.
   b. process of destroying as many microorganisms as possible.

   c. process of removing half of the microorganisms.
   d. All of the above.

4. In order for an infection to spread, all of the following factors need to be present *except*
   a. a source.
   b. a susceptible host.
   c. a means of transmission.
   d. a wet environment.

5. Which of the following types of precautions should be used for all patients?
   a. Standard Precautions
   b. Airborne Precautions
   c. Contact Precautions
   d. Droplet Precautions

TIME-OUT

TIPS FOR TIME MANAGEMENT

When you are assigned to care for an isolation patient, plan to do as many tasks as possible while you are in the room. Think through the tasks you plan to do so you can gather all your supplies before entering the isolation room. You can save the time and supplies you would use if you had to put on a mask, gown, and gloves several times to perform different tasks or to go get additional supplies.

THE NURSING ASSISTANT IN ACTION

As part of your training you learned that handwashing is essential. You and a coworker happen to be in the restroom at the same time. Your coworker does not wash his hands after using the restroom. It is time for you both to assist feeding patients their lunches.

What Is Your Response/Action?

CRITICAL THINKING

CUSTOMER SERVICE Handwashing is the most important thing you can do to protect yourself and your patients from healthcare-acquired infections. Always wash your hands after caring for any patient before providing care to the next patient. If a patient asks for something and you have not yet washed your hands, tell the patient you will take care of her request as soon as you have washed your hands.

CULTURAL CARE You may be assigned to care for patients who think it is rude that you are wearing gloves to bathe them or provide care. If the patient has not received health care in this country, he may not be aware of Standard Precautions. Explain that you wear gloves to help prevent the spread of disease or microorganisms between patients and caregivers.

COOPERATION WITHIN THE TEAM You may have a coworker who has a latex allergy. If special latex-free gloves have been made available for her to use, do not use them if you do not have a latex allergy. It is important for her to avoid contact with latex. You may be asked to take over the care of patients who have tubes or latex products because contact with latex can trigger an adverse reaction.

EXPLORE Medialink

Additional interactive resources for this chapter can be found on the Companion Website at www.prenhall.com/wolgin. Click on Chapter 5 and "Begin" to select the activities for this chapter. For chapter-related NCLEX-style questions and an audio glossary, access the accompanying CD-ROM in this book.

Video:

Risk Management; Hand Hygiene—using an Alcohol-Based Rub

6 Safety

KEY TERMS

ambulate
ambulation
bed alarm
cannula
chair alarm
clove hitch
cognition
confusion
delirium
dementia
flowmeter
gait training
nasal
OBRA regulations
oxygen
pressure-sensitive mat
protective devices
restraint alternative
restraints

OBJECTIVES

When you have completed this chapter, you will be able to:

- List the general rules of safety in a health care setting.
- List safety precautions in caring for older adults and children.
- Describe the special safety precautions necessary when oxygen is being used.
- Explain what you can do to prevent fires and what to do in case of a fire.
- Practice restraint application.
- Discuss restraint alternatives.
- Discuss and document care of patients in restraints.
- Identify OBRA regulations regarding the use of restraints.
- List the safety rules for patient ambulation.

MediaLink
www.prenhall.com/wolgin

Use the address above to access the free, interactive Companion Website created for this textbook. Get hints, instant feedback, and textbook references to chapter-related NCLEX-style questions. Link to other interesting sites.

AUDIO GLOSSARY:
Use the Companion Website, or the CD-ROM disk enclosed with your textbook, to hear the pronunciation of key terms in the chapter.

The safety measures presented in this chapter will assist you in creating and maintaining a safe environment for your patient. You will learn about general safety, oxygen safety, fire safety, and patient safety. To ensure the patients' and the health care workers' safety, all health care facilities have fire and evacuation plans. Home health workers are always alert to possible fire hazards in the patient's home. In addition to the fire and safety measures described here, you will need to know and follow the specific evacuation plan for your facility. The most important thing you will learn about safety is prevention. Prevent the accident or fire. You play a key role in creating and maintaining a safe environment for your patient, your coworkers, and yourself.

The proper use of protective devices, alternatives, and restraints is an important component of safety. Seclusion and restraint may be necessary in clinically appropriate and adequately justified situations. It is essential to review and comply with current policy and procedures. Compliance with individual state patient bills of rights, the public health codes, and the standards of the Joint Commission on Accreditation of Healthcare Organizations (JCAHO) and/or OBRA (Omnibus Budget Reconciliation Act of 1987) regulations influence and when revised, require changes in current practice. Patient's rights, dignity, and well-being are supported, maintained, and thoroughly documented.

> ### INTRODUCTION

General Safety Measures

People with health care needs are challenged by illness, disability, concerns, and medications. Many of them cannot care for themselves in an emergency and rely on health care personnel for protection. As a member of the care team you must make every effort to guard against accidents, prevent fires and other kinds of emergencies, and know what to do in case of emergency. Follow the guidelines given below for safety measures. Prevention of accidents or injuries saves the patient pain and suffering. It also avoids expense and staff time required to document and follow up.

In some settings, bed rails are less commonly used and may be considered a form of unnecessary restraint. Be sure you know the policy of your employer with regard to side rails.

> ### ALERT
> For all patient contact, adhere to Standard Precautions (∞ Chapter 5, pages 83–85). Wear protective equipment as indicated.

AGE-SPECIFIC CONSIDERATIONS

For all restraint procedures: Patients of all ages must be treated with respect. Children and the elderly might feel as though they are being punished for doing something wrong. If the patient is confused, being restrained often increases anxiety and attempts to "escape." Talk frequently and reassuringly to all patients in restraints. Explain that the devices are being used to prevent them from accidentally pulling on lines, tubes, or drains or from falling. Check on the patient frequently and advocate for the removal of the restraint as soon as the patient's mental capacity has improved or when the medical device is no longer needed.

In addition to the safety measures followed for adult patients, the care of young children in the hospital or home setting requires additional safeguards to prevent accidents and ensure a safe environment. The following Safety Measures for Young Children guidelines are based on the chronological-age characteristics and needs of young children. Refer to Chapter 15 for information on chronological-age development.

- Use handrails on stairways (Figure 6–1♦). In hallways and stairs, keep to the right and avoid collisions. Take special care at intersections (Figure 6–2♦).
- Use care when opening doors that open into busy areas (Figure 6–3♦).
- Be sure to lock the brakes and any wheels on beds, stretchers, examining tables, wheelchairs, bedside commodes, and shower chairs. Use care in transferring patients to or from them.
- Be very careful of the position of the patient's feet during wheelchair transport. Keep hands and feet in view while transporting by stretcher.
- When you see something on the floor that doesn't belong there, pick it up. Spilled liquids can be very dangerous (Figure 6–4♦). Remember that the housekeeping or environmental department may clean a room or area only once a day. Incidental spills in patient areas are the responsibility of all health care workers.

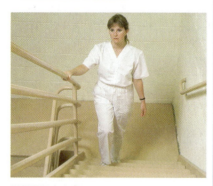

FIGURE 6–1 ♦
Be safety conscious at all times

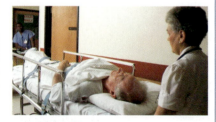

FIGURE 6–2 ♦
Use caution at intersections

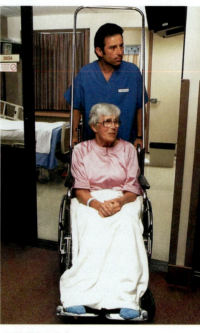

FIGURE 6–3 ♦
Be careful going through doorways

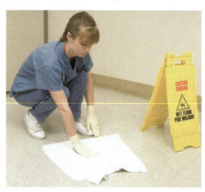

FIGURE 6–4 ♦
Clean up spills immediately

- Follow the instructions of your supervisor while giving care and be aware of special instructions for a patient, such as:
  - No weight bearing.
  - Keep head (or foot) of bed elevated at all times.
  - Do not position patient on right side.
  - May be out of bed with assistance only.
  - Do not use left arm to take blood pressure.

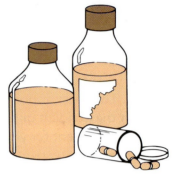

FIGURE 6–5 ♦
Never use the contents of an unlabeled container; take the container to your supervisor immediately

- Never use the contents of an unlabeled container; take it to your supervisor at once (Figure 6–5♦). Store cleaning fluids only in assigned areas, which should be locked.
- Check meal trays for dentures and check soiled linen for overlooked items such as misplaced instruments, needles, or other articles, and dispose of them properly.
- Place used disposable razors in approved containers, never in a waste basket.
- Use disposable gloves when the possibility of coming in contact with blood or body fluids is present.
- If ordered, keep bed side rails up and in the locked position (Figure 6–6♦).

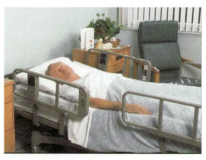

FIGURE 6–6 ♦
Keep the side rails up and in the locked position for patients who are confused, restless, or coming out of anesthesia

<table>
<tr><td colspan="3">

SAFETY MEASURES FOR YOUNG CHILDREN

GUIDELINES
</td></tr>
</table>

Children are not responsible for their own actions and are dependent on adults to protect them.

- Keep all patient care items out of the child's reach.
- Be certain a child cannot reach any regulation valves on IV tubing, oxygen flowmeters, or any other tubes or equipment.
- Cover electrical outlets not in use.
- Do not stock any extra needles or syringes in the child's room.

- Use care to remove items that could be harmful to young children.
- Children must be watched closely to prevent injuries.
- Never leave small children unattended unless they are in a protective crib.
- Frequently check a child in a protective device.
- Keep out of the child's reach all articles used in the child's care.
- Keep crib railings up and locked. Bed rails for toddlers and older children should be used according to physician's order.

- Keep exit doors, stairway doors, and linen chutes closed when not in use and locked if possible.
- Keep drapery and window blind cords out of child's reach.
- Examine all toys for small or loose parts that can cause choking.
- Remove from the bed or floor large objects the child can stand on, increasing the risk of falls.
- Be sure windows are closed and locked.
- Lock the wheels on beds and cribs.

Oxygen Safety

A special device called a regulator or **flowmeter** is needed when **oxygen** is used (Figure 6–7◆). It controls and regulates the rate or flow of oxygen that is being administered to the patient. If your patient is being given oxygen be sure that you know the policies of your employer regarding its use and care of the equipment. The amount of oxygen given to a patient is expressed in liters and is given according to the order of a physician or respiratory specialist. As the nursing assistant, you may be instructed to set up and monitor liter flow in some institutions. *The physician's or respiratory therapist's order must be followed exactly.*

Respiratory therapy departments or technicians take care of administration of oxygen and of the equipment used in most hospitals. In some settings, the nursing assistant may be expected to transport oxygen tanks and must know the facility's policies regarding safety in handling and storage of the tanks.

Room air is 21 percent oxygen. Oxygen, by itself, does not burn. However, it is one of the elements needed to cause fire, along with heat and fuel. Special precautions must be taken when more than the normal amount of oxygen is present, such as in a patient's room where oxygen is being administered. Extra oxygen supports combustion and can make things catch fire and burn more rapidly than in normal room air. Since patients may also be given oxygen therapy in the home, it is important that you advise the patient and/or the patient's caregiver of the caution they must take when oxygen is in use. Observing the following safety rules for oxygen use can help to prevent fires.

flowmeter A device used to control and regulate the flow of oxygen

oxygen A colorless, odorless, tasteless gaseous element that is essential for respiration; air is 21 percent oxygen

Oxygen Therapy

Use of an oxygen mask or **nasal cannula** is determined by the physician or respiratory therapist, depending on the needs of the patient. Both devices are made of plastic and come in direct contact with the patient's skin during use. Any area—behind the ears, on the cheeks, and at the nostrils—where there is contact combined with perspiration and moisture must be checked frequently for breakdown and protected if necessary.

nasal Pertaining to the nose and nasal cavity

cannula A flexible tube that can be inserted into a body cavity and used to draw fluids out or give oxygen or fluids

FIGURE 6–7 ◆

Although some oxygen delivery systems look different, they all have the same parts and function

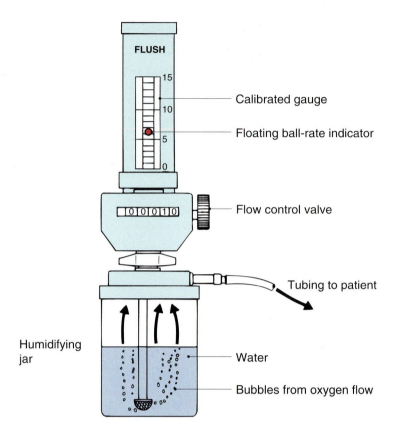

FLUSH

15

10

5

0

Calibrated gauge

Floating ball-rate indicator

Flow control valve

Tubing to patient

Humidifying jar

Water

Bubbles from oxygen flow

GUIDELINES   **OBRA**

OXYGEN SAFETY

■ Place a NO SMOKING–OXYGEN IN USE sign on the door of the room and over the patient's bed (Figure 6–8◆).

■ Keep the oxygen tubing free of kinks (see Figure 6–7).

■ Monitor any electrical appliance or device in the patient's room that could potentially create a spark, including items such as electric razors, hairdryers, and heating pads.

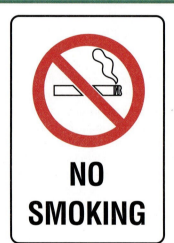

NO SMOKING

FIGURE 6–8 ◆

No Smoking sign should be used when oxygen is in use

■ Be observant for any lighters, matches, or smoking materials the patient or visitors may have and report them to your supervisor at once.

■ If a humidifying jar is used, the correct level of distilled water must be maintained in the jar and the water in the jar should "bubble" as the oxygen passes through it (see Figure 6–7).

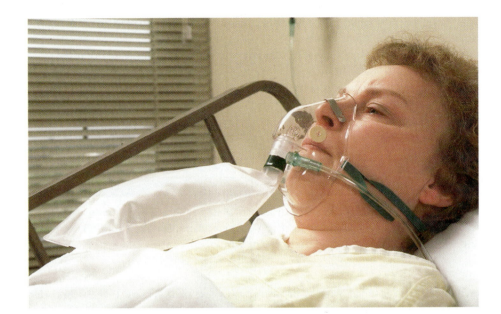

FIGURE 6–9 ◆
Oxygen is administered by an oxygen mask

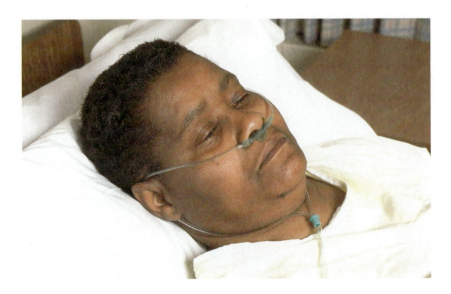

FIGURE 6–10 ◆
The tubing of cannulas is flexible

The oxygen mask, used most often for a patient who cannot be relied on to consistently breathe through his nose, covers the mouth and nose (Figure 6–9◆). Keep the mask in place and the inside of the mask clean at all times.

The oxygen cannula is placed inside the patient's nostrils, extending upward about 1/2 inch. Two small holes in the tubing provide the patient with oxygen. The tubing of cannulas is flexible (Figure 6–10◆). In one type, the tubing wraps around the patient's ears and is secured under the chin; in another, the tubing extends from the nostrils across the cheeks and wraps around the patient's head. Nasal cannulas move easily, so their placement should be checked frequently (Figure 6–11◆).

 ## Fire Safety and Prevention

Fire can start at any time in any setting. It may come as the aftermath of a disaster or a single incident. All health facilities have fire and disaster plans to provide safe transport and evacuation of patients and health care workers to a safe environment within the facility or

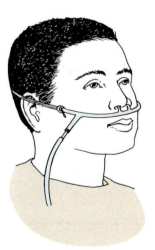

FIGURE 6–11 ◆
Nasal cannulas move easily, so check their placement frequently

outside the facility. If you work in a home setting you will develop an evacuation plan with your client and/or the client's caregiver. The best plan, however, is prevention, and preventing fires is everyone's job—be sure you know and observe all fire safety rules.

If a fire breaks out, you must:

1. Know what to do.
2. Remain calm.
3. Carry out what you have learned.

KEY IDEA

Elevators are not to be used without approval of the Fire Department. An electrical failure could cause the elevator to stop between floors. Smoke could fill the elevator and the individuals trapped in the elevator would suffocate.

Be sure you are familiar with your institution's fire plan (Figure 6–12◆) and disaster plan. Know where your facility's fire extinguishers are located and what type of rating they have. Fire extinguishers may be rated A, B, or C according to the type of fire on which they can be used.

FIGURE 6–12 ◆

Fire safety planning

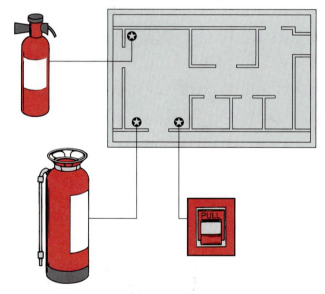

- Know the floor plan of your department and the hospital as a whole

- Pay particular attention to exit routes

- Know the exact location of fire alarms and fire extinguishing devices

- Know how to report a fire

- Know the emergency and disaster plan of your hospital and what you should do

- Know how to use fire extinguishers

Types of Fire Extinguishers and Their Use

A for paper, wood, and trash

B for burnable liquids such as oil or grease

C for electrical fires

ABC for use on any type of fire

K for kitchen fires; used in restaurants or large kitchens

If a situation does require the actual use and discharge of a fire extinguisher, remember the word **PASS:**

P Pull the safety Pin on the upper handle (Figure 6–13a◆).

A Aim low. Point the nozzle at the base of the fire (Figure 6–13b◆).

S Squeeze the handles releasing the extinguisher's agent.

S Sweep from side to side aiming at the base of the fire until the fire goes out or is extinguished (Figure 6–13c◆).

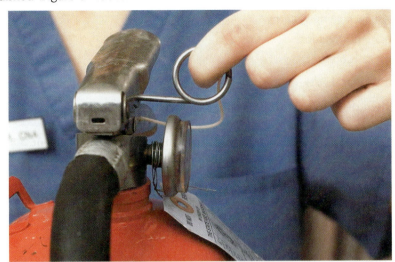

FIGURE 6–13a ◆

Pull the pin on the upper handle of the fire extinguisher

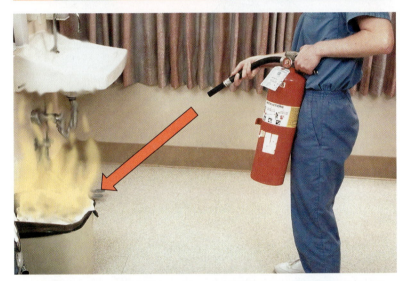

FIGURE 6–13b ◆

Aim low toward the base of the fire

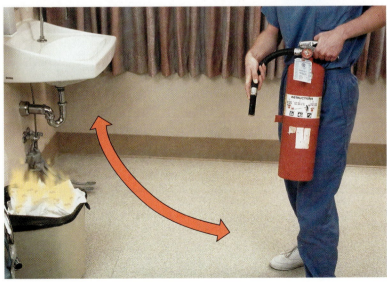

FIGURE 6–13c ◆

Sweep the area from side to side

Major Causes of Fire

- Smoking and matches
- Misuse of electricity
- Defects in heating systems
- Spontaneous ignition
- Improper rubbish disposal

Remember that it takes three things to start a fire (Figure 6–14◆):

- HEAT, in the form of sparks or flame
- FUEL, any burnable material
- OXYGEN, present in the air we breathe

FIGURE 6–14 ◆

Three things are needed to start a fire: heat, fuel, and oxygen

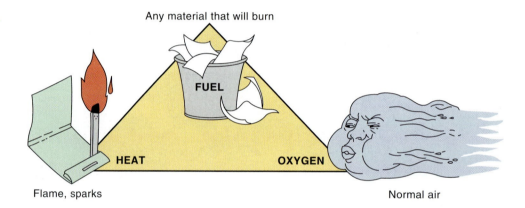

FIGURE 6–15 ◆

Smoking and nonsmoking areas are clearly identified

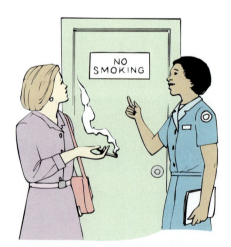

Smoking

Smoking is the number one cause of fires in health care institutions. Many facilities have adopted a nonsmoking policy (Figure 6–15◆). Some have identified areas where smoking is permitted. It is important that employees, visitors, and patients smoke only in approved areas and observe the following rules:

- Provide ashtrays for those who smoke. Never use or allow anyone else to use disposable cups or dishes as ashtrays.

- Be sure that ashtrays are not emptied into trash containers until all smoking materials are safely extinguished.

- Provide supervision for any patient who wishes to smoke if the patient is confused or weak. Sedated patients should not smoke.

- Report any violation of your employer's smoking policy to your supervisor at once.

Misuses of Electricity

- Use care to be sure electrical equipment does not come in contact with water.

- Limit use of extension cords; if used, make sure they are in accordance with your faculty's policies.

- Many electrical devices are equipped with three-pronged grounding plugs. Do not use any such device if the rounded middle pin on the plug has been broken or cut off.

- Check cords and plugs for fraying or cracking prior to use. Report all electrical hazards at once (Figure 6–16◆).

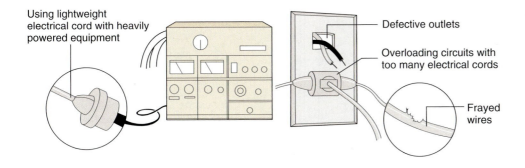

Using lightweight electrical cord with heavily powered equipment

Defective outlets

Overloading circuits with too many electrical cords

Frayed wires

FIGURE 6–16 ◆

Misuses of electricity

In Case of a Fire

If a fire occurs, remain calm and remember that many lives can depend on your actions. Keeping in mind the word **R A C E** can assist you in remembering what to do (Figure 6–17◆):

- **R**emove the patient from the immediate vicinity of the fire.

- **A**ctivate the alarm and alert other staff members that a fire exists, following the policy of your employer.

- **C**ontain or confine the fire by closing all the doors in the area.

- **E**xtinguish the fire if it is safe to do so.

Know and follow your employer's evacuation plan. Your institution will hold scheduled fire "drills" to assist staff in knowing exactly what to do in case of fire, including specific rescue techniques. Be sure that you dispose of all rubbish in the manner and place designated by your facility.

If you are working in a home setting, have fire drills regularly. In case of a fire, be sure to follow the evacuation plan that you developed earlier with the patient and/or the caregiver or other family members if they are present. Having an evacuation plan in advance of such a situation will help you to remain calm and facilitate the removal of your client to a safe environment.

FIGURE 6–17 ◆

In case of a fire, remember the word **R A C E**

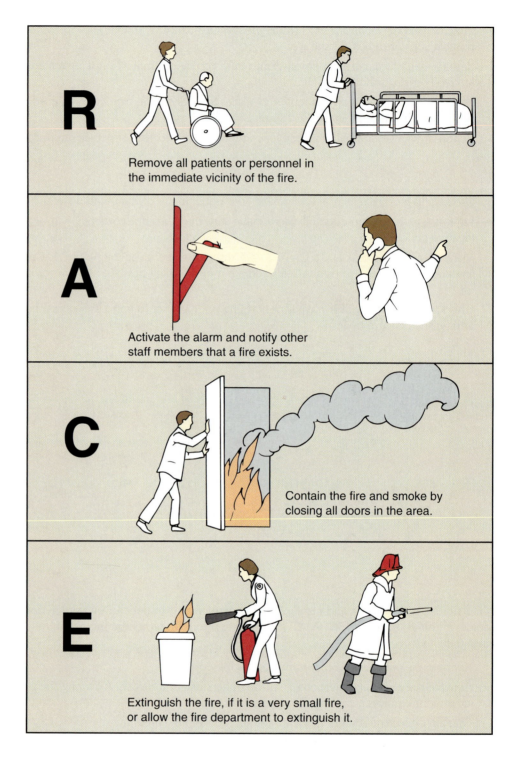

R Remove all patients or personnel in the immediate vicinity of the fire.

A Activate the alarm and notify other staff members that a fire exists.

C Contain the fire and smoke by closing all doors in the area.

E Extinguish the fire, if it is a very small fire, or allow the fire department to extinguish it.

Most areas of the country have enhanced 911 in effect. If you are calling from a landline phone, your call and location are easily traced. If you are calling from a cell phone, be prepared to tell the 911 operator the address and floor or apartment number where you need the fire department to respond.

Fight the fire only in these situations:

■ Everyone has left or is leaving the building.

■ After 911 or the Fire Department has been called.

■ The fire is small and in a contained area (trash basket, pillow, small appliance, etc.).

- You can fight the fire with your back to your escape route.
- You have access to the correct extinguisher and it operates.
- You have been trained to use the fire extinguisher and know how it operates.

If you have any doubts or encounter a problem, do not attempt to fight the fire. Close the door behind you and leave immediately.

DO NOT fight a fire with a portable extinguisher in these situations:

- It is a large fire or is already spreading beyond the area where it started.
- Your escape route could be blocked by the fire.
- You are unsure how to use the fire extinguisher.
- You are unsure what type of fire extinguisher to use on the fire at hand.

Disasters

A disaster is an extraordinary event that causes great damage, destruction, many injuries and loss of lives or property, and extensive damage to the environment. Disasters can be natural or caused by people.

Natural disasters cannot be prevented or controlled. Disaster plans are developed to respond to the event or to protect people by setting off warnings, alarms, or sirens to take cover or evacuate the area before a hurricane strikes or flood waters rise. Examples include:

- Snow or ice storms
- Hurricanes or tornados
- Floods
- Earthquakes

Disasters caused by people include:

- Transport vehicle (airplane, train, bus, truck, car, etc.) crashes or bombings
- Nuclear power plant accidents
- Gas or chemical leaks
- Fires or explosions
- Riots and wars
- Terrorism or bioterrorism

Some man-made disasters can sometimes be averted or controlled, and are preventable in many cases. Other disasters such as bioterrorism or the September 2001 terrorist attacks on the World Trade Center are intentional.

When a disaster occurs or is pending, you are responsible for knowing your community's or facility's disaster plan. These plans are reviewed annually by employers and practiced in drills. Disaster drills prepare you to:

- Review the written plan for evacuation and discharge plan to safely remove patients.
- Notify police, fire, or other agencies or organizations that assist in disaster situations.
- Take action in various types of disasters.
- Work as a team with others to provide as safe an environment as possible for every one involved.
- Notify needed personnel and review roles of all involved.
- Practice gearing up to provide emergency care to injured persons.
- Identify where there are gaps or problems in the plan and make needed changes.

Patient Safety

Falls in health care facilities account for a large percentage of patient-related accidents. You can help prevent falls by:

- Anticipating the patients' needs
- Placing call light and personal items within easy reach
- Correctly positioning patients in beds and chairs
- Practicing safe patient lifts and transfers
- Maintaining a clutter-free environment
- Answering call lights promptly
- Cleaning up spills at once
- Knowing and following your employer's fire emergency plan

Falls and Restraints

Prevention of falls is the most common reason for use of physical restraints in the acute care setting. Older patients are far more likely to be restrained than younger patients. The literature reports that the application of a restraint to prevent injury may actually increase the risk. There is no evidence that the use of restraints prevents patient accidents and, in fact, there are reports that patients are in more danger when restrained (Table 6–1 ◆).

Modifying Risk Factors for a Fall

- Emphasize proper gait and stress the need to turn around slowly. Encourage patients to pick their feet up with each step.
- Ensure that patients have shoes or slippers that fit well.
- Evaluate the need for a walking aid in collaboration with physical therapy if needed.

TABLE 6–1 ◆

Factors That Put Older Patients at High Risk

GAIT/POSTURE	OTHER PHYSIOLOGICAL CHANGES
■ Older men and women don't pick up their feet as high. ■ Increased postural sway is due to slowed proprioception leading to loss of balance. ■ Ability of body to right itself from unexpected trip or step is lessened with age due to impaired muscular control.	■ Increased muscle weakness ■ Tendency toward orthostatic hypotension ■ Autonomic reactivity and decrease in vascular compliance
SENSORY/VISION	**PATHOLOGY FACTORS**
■ Impaired night vision ■ Decreased depth perception ■ Increased susceptibility to glare ■ Decreased ability to discriminate colors and see near objects	■ Decreased cognitive function results in falls primarily due to poor judgment. ■ Alcohol and drug side effects may result in falls. ■ Cerebrovascular disease may precipitate falls. ■ Parkinson's disease causes gait disturbance.
ENVIRONMENTAL FACTORS	**EQUIPMENT/TUBES/LINES**
■ Improper or poorly fitting shoes increase the risk of falls. ■ Floor obstacles lead to increased tripping and falls. ■ Poor lighting. ■ Bed and chair wheels unlocked.	■ Foley catheter tubes/bags can be tripped over. ■ IV lines and poles can be obstacles. ■ Oxygen tubing can cause tripping.

- Encourage patients to avoid rising quickly from sitting or lying positions.
- Encourage physical activity such as walking to improve balance and motor control and muscle strength.

The more deconditioned a patient becomes from lack of mobility, the greater the likelihood that she will fall when she does get up.

Bed Rails and Restraints

Historically, hospitals have considered bed rails a safety device to prevent patients from falling out of bed and sustaining injury. As recently as the 1970s, bed rails were required to be up for all patients 65 or older in many hospitals in the U.S. New reports in the literature and the tighter restrictions on the use of bed rails by JCAHO have caused hospitals to readdress the whole issue of bed rails related to patient safety and patient autonomy.

Recent literature reports on the use of bed rails as restraints reveal that prevention of falls is the most common reason for using bed rails and there is no evidence that bed rails do prevent falls. One study reported in the *Journal of American Geriatrics Society* (JAGS) (1996) stated that 14 of 16 consecutive falls while getting out of bed resulted from climbing over bed rails, often in an attempt to reach the toilet.

It has been suggested that bed rails are most often used with confused, agitated patients and are particularly unsuitable for these patients because they are likely to increase agitation and distress. In addition, confused patients do not interpret rails to define boundaries but rather as barriers to climb over. The resulting fall from the top of a bed rail is much more likely than a simple roll from bed to cause serious damage to a frail patient. Several studies have found that bed rails are up in most falls from bed. Most injuries occur when older persons fall to the floor while climbing over rails. Most patients fell on the evening and night shifts and 50 percent had abnormal cognitive functioning.

In another study reported in *JAGS* (1997), 72 deaths were reportedly caused by bed rails, dispelling the myth that bed rails are a benign safety device. The deaths resulted from entrapments between the mattress and bed rail, entrapment and compression of the neck within rails, and being trapped by rails after sliding partially off the bed and having the neck flexed or the chest compressed.

KEY IDEA

Any protective device that, when asked, the patient/resident cannot release on his own is considered a restraint.

Protective Devices

Physical **restraints** are used as **protective devices** to prevent a patient from harming himself or someone else or to protect him during a medical procedure. Restraints are applied only with the recommendation of a nurse or therapist and *only* with a physician's order (Figure 6–18♦). The nurse or therapist will decide what type of restraint is to be used and the length of time it is to be left in place. Hospitals follow the Joint Commission on Accreditation of Healthcare Organizations (JCAHO) regulations regarding the use of restraints. Never tie or secure a restraint to any movable part of a bed or chair.

restraints Protective measures ordered by a physician to prevent patients from harming themselves or others

protective devices Measures taken to keep a patient safe or to prevent injury

KEY IDEA

Proper documentation is needed to ensure protection of a patient's rights and to record the observation and care of the patient. Care is documented on the restraint flowsheet or unit/division specific documentation form. Depending on the facility, the frequency of checks and documentation standards will vary. Psychiatric patients are checked every 15 minutes while others are checked every 30 or 60 minutes per facility policy.

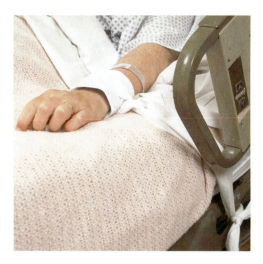

FIGURE 6–18a ◆

Soft protective devices: a soft limb tie

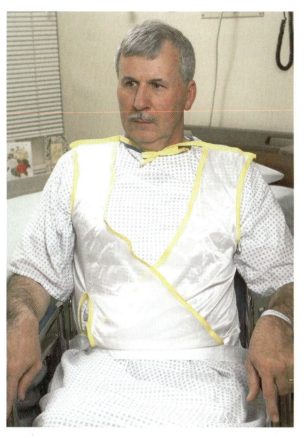

FIGURE 6–18b ◆

Safety vest

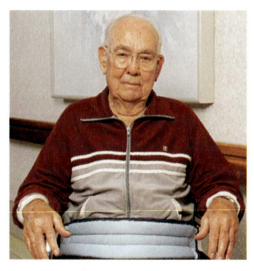

FIGURE 6–18c ◆

Lap or waist restraint

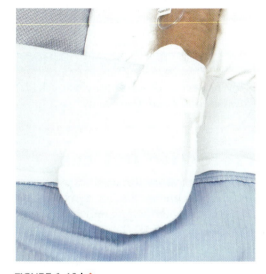

FIGURE 6–18d ◆

Soft cloth mitten

Check the patient per agency policy, usually every 15 minutes for behavior management and every hour for medical surgical patients. Carefully check pressure points on the skin each time. **Release the restraint every 2 hours to offer food and liquids, toilet, exercise, and to reposition the patient.**

APPLYING A WAIST RESTRAINT

RATIONALE: A waist restraint helps a patient sit in a chair safely and comfortably.

PREPARATION

1. Select the appropriate restraint as ordered.
2. Wash your hands.
3. Introduce yourself, identify the patient, and explain what you will do.
4. Provide privacy for the patient.

STEPS

5. Lock the wheels on the chair, commode, or toilet.
6. Wrap the waist restraint or belt around the patient's abdomen and cross the straps behind her back. Follow your institution's guidelines for wrist and ankle restraints.
7. Bring the crossed straps out to the sides and pull through the loops at the sides of the restraints.
8. Secure the restraint and make sure it is not too tight by inserting two fingers between the restraint and the patient's abdomen.
9. Wrap the straps of the restraint once around the metal part of the chair arm near the chair back before securing the straps, out of the resident's reach, at the back of the chair.
10. Your instructor will demonstrate a **clove hitch** tie, which maintains the restraint securely while making sure it can be readily untied in case of emergency.

FOLLOW-UP

11. Make the patient comfortable. Place the call light and personal items within easy reach of the patient before you leave the room, assuring her that you will be available if she needs assistance.
12. Document repeated checks per policy.

CHARTING EXAMPLE: 3/2/04 4pm Waist belt applied to Mr. Star to keep him in his wheelchair. M. White, CNA

Check the patient per agency policy, usually every 15 minutes for behavior management and every hour for medical surgical patients. Carefully check pressure points on the skin each time. **Release the restraint every 2 hours to offer food and liquids, toilet, exercise, and to reposition the patient.**

clove hitch A type of knot that can be easily released in case of emergency

APPLYING A VEST RESTRAINT

RATIONALE: Vest restraints allow confused or demented patients to move around or sit up in bed, but do not allow patients to get up out of their chair or bed.

PREPARATION

1. Select the appropriate restraint.
2. Wash your hands.
3. Introduce yourself, identify the patient, and explain what you will do.
4. Provide privacy for the patient.

STEPS

5. Lock the wheels on the bed or chair.
6. APPLY THE VEST RESTRAINT AS YOU WOULD ANY VEST. THAT OPENS DOWN THE FRONT. MAKE SURE ANY SEAMS OR ROUGH EDGES ARE NOT IN CONTACT WITH THE PATIENT'S SKIN.
7. Wrap the ties around the patient's waist crossing them behind his back pulling them through the loops at the sides.
8. Secure the restraint with a clove hitch or single loop knot out of the patient's reach.
9. Make the patient comfortable. Place the call light and personal items within easy reach of the patient.
10. Check to make sure the restraint is not too tight before you leave the room, assuring the patient that you will be available if he needs assistance.

FOLLOW-UP

11. Document repeated checks per policy.

CHARTING: 3/2/04 9pm Vest restraint applied to Mr. Star as ordered to keep him in his bed. M. White, CNA

Applying Mitts to a Patient

Mitts are thickly padded so that patients cannot close their hands around an object. They often separate the fingers to further reduce the ability to grab and pull. Mitts are used on a short-term basis until the tube, line, or drain is no longer needed or the patient is cognitively aware enough to remember not to pull on the equipment. This device is not used with patients who are of sound mind, because these patients have the right to refuse any type of medical care or treatment that they do not want. Follow your institution's policy on restraints.

APPLYING MITTS

PROCEDURE   OBRA

RATIONALE: Mitts are a medical device that is most often used to prevent a confused patient from pulling on some piece of vital medical equipment, usually a tube, line, or drain.

PREPARATION

1. Assemble the equipment.
2. Identify the correct patient.
3. Explain the procedure to the patient and family. Explain why the mitts are necessary. Tell the patient that the mitts will come off as soon as possible.
4. Wash hands.

STEPS

5. Insert the patient's fingers into one mitt. Separate each finger so that it goes into its own compartment in the mitt. Insert the hand palm side down into the mitt. This is done so that the patient will be unable to grasp the thick padded mitt.
6. Smooth the cloth around the wrist. This avoids wrinkle marks on the skin.
7. Secure the mitt by fastening the fabric fastener at the wrist (Figure 6-19◆). Make it tight enough to prevent the mitt from slipping

over the hand, but not tight enough to harm the skin. You should be able to slip two fingers beneath the fastener.
8. Apply the second mitt to the other hand if medically necessary.

FOLLOW-UP

9. Wash hands and document and report the results of the procedure to the RN or preceptor.

10. Provide care, and continue to monitor the patient every 15 minutes to one hour, according to the institution's policy.

CHARTING EXAMPLE: 1/24/04 10am Mitts applied to Mrs. Smith's hands to prevent her from pulling on her IV line. She will be checked per policy. M. Morize, CNA

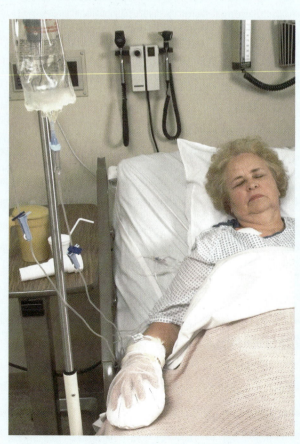

FIGURE 6-19 ◆
Mitts

Always remember:

- Mitts are a restraint device, but they do not guarantee the safety of either the patient or the tube, line, or drain that is to be protected.

- Patients in mitts require frequent visual checks (from every 15 minutes up to every hour, depending on the type of institution).

- Mitts must be removed every 1 to 2 hours to check the skin on the wrist, hands, and fingers for breakdown. Range-of-motion exercises must be performed on the wrists to prevent the joints from becoming immobile. As patients wiggle in the restraints, they might apply additional pressure or tear the skin.

- Patients in mitts must be fed, cleaned, and made comfortable, because they have lost the ability to perform these functions on their own as a result of the restraints. It is very important to maintain the dignity and comfort of patients in restraints. Their lives are in the caregiver's hands.

- Patients and their families must have the rationale for the restraint explained to them.

Patients of all ages must be treated with respect. Children and the elderly might feel as though they are being punished for doing something wrong. If the patient is confused, being restrained often increases anxiety and attempts to "escape." Talk frequently and reassuringly to all patients in restraints. Explain that the mitts are being used to prevent them from accidentally pulling on the line, tube, or drain. Assess the patient frequently: Remove the restraints as soon as the patient's mental capacity has improved or when the medical device is no longer needed.

KEY IDEA

Make sure that patients cannot harm themselves in the mitts by either looping a tube with their hand or removing the restraint too easily. Take the restraints off as soon as possible.

Applying Soft Restraints to a Patient

Soft restraints are medical devices, usually made from cloth, that are used to restrict the movement of the patient's hands (Figure 6–20◆). They are used to prevent patients from injuring themselves or others. Soft restraints are often used in critical care units to prevent patients from pulling out lines, tubes, or drains while they are waking up from anesthetics. They are also used with confused or demented patients when a line, tube, or drain is in place.

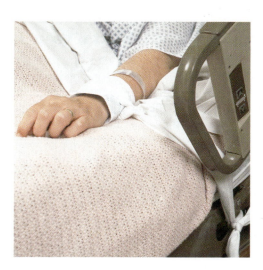

FIGURE 6–20 ◆

Soft restraints

Soft restraints are most commonly applied to the wrists but can be used to restrain a patient who is kicking; in this case, the device is applied bilaterally to the ankles. The device is called a two-point restraint when the wrists are restrained and a four-point restraint when both the wrists and the ankles are restrained.

Effective alternatives that should be attempted before applying restraints include moving the IV pump or pole out of the patient's line of sight (usually closer to the head of the bed) and covering the IV site or tube site with gauze so that it is not as easy to see.

Always remember:

- Always attempt to use alternatives to restraint. Applying a restraint device does not guarantee patient safety or the safety of lines, tubes, or drains.
- Patients in soft restraints require frequent visual checks (from every 15 minutes up to every hour, depending on the type of institution).
- Soft restraints must be removed every 1 to 2 hours to check the skin on the wrist, hands, and fingers for breakdown. Range-of-motion exercises must be performed on the joint to decrease the risks of immobility. As patients wiggle in the restraints, they might apply additional pressure or tear the skin.
- Patients in soft restraints must be fed, cleaned, and made comfortable, because they have lost the ability to perform these functions on their own as a result of the restraints. It is very important to maintain the dignity and comfort of patients in restraints. Their lives are in the caregiver's hands.
- Patients and their families must have the rationale for the restraint explained to them.

Patients of all ages must be treated with respect. Children and the elderly might feel as though they are being punished for doing something wrong. If the patient is confused, being restrained often increases anxiety and attempts to "escape." Talk frequently and reassuringly to all patients in restraints. Explain that the soft restraints are being used to prevent them from accidentally pulling on the line, tube, or drain. Assess the patient: Remove the restraints as soon as the patient's mental capacity has improved or when the medical device is no longer needed.

KEY IDEA

Patients who are in restraints are often more anxious and sensitive to noises than are other patients. Loud noises can be very threatening to them because they often feel "trapped." Reassure patients that they are in a safe place and that you are watching out for them.

Secure soft restraints with a square knot so that they can be released quickly in case of an emergency.

Applying Leather Restraints to a Patient

Leather restraints are used only in emergencies when the patient is a great danger to him- or herself or to others (Figure 6–21♦). Patients requiring leather restraints are usually violently confused or demented due to any number of medical conditions (dementias, head injuries, drug overdose, etc.) and are striking out, hitting, and kicking those around them. Refer to your institution's policy for the application and use of leather restraints.

When the leather restraints are applied to the wrists, it is called two-point restraint. When the restraints are applied to both wrists and both ankles, it is called four-point restraint.

The application of leather restraints usually requires the cooperation of several caregivers to protect the patient from harm. Often, a team approach is used to restrain the patient's limbs and body safely while the leather devices are applied. Even the smallest patient has great strength when agitated to the point of requiring leather restraints. The patient will be frightened and might continue to fight once the restraints are applied. Touching patients in restraints might calm them or make them twice as agitated. Enlist the patient's family to assist in determining strategies to support and calm the patient.

APPLYING SOFT RESTRAINTS

PROCEDURE

OBRA

RATIONALE: Soft restraints are applied to keep a patient from injuring self or others.

PREPARATION

1. Assemble the equipment.
2. Identify the correct patient.
3. Explain the procedure to the patient and family. Explain also why the soft restraints are necessary.
4. Wash hands.

STEPS

5. Place the soft restraint under the patient's wrist.

6. Insert one end of the restraint tie through the slot. Wrap the material around the wrist until the ties meet.

7. Make sure that the material lies smoothly to avoid wrinkles that could damage the patient's skin.

8. Fasten the restraint securely, but not tight enough to impair the skin (see Figure 6–19). You should be able to slip two fingers beneath the soft restraint.

9. Fasten the restraint by making a square knot (left tie over right, and then right tie over left).

10. Loop one of the ties through the bed frame (not the side rail). Fasten both ties together using a square knot.

11. Recheck the circulation and the condition of the patient's skin.

12. Repeat steps 5 to 11 for the other wrist if medically necessary.

13. Check the comfort of the patient, and ensure that the patient's dignity has been maintained.

FOLLOW-UP

14. Wash hands and document and report the results of the procedure to the RN or preceptor.

15. Provide care, and continue to monitor the patient every 15 minutes to 1 hour, according to the institution's policy.

16. Reassess the need for the restraint every 2 hours.

CHARTING EXAMPLE: 11/25/03 11am Soft restraints applied as ordered by Dr. Spinkey. Mrs. Allen told we will be checking her frequently J. Alvarez, CNA

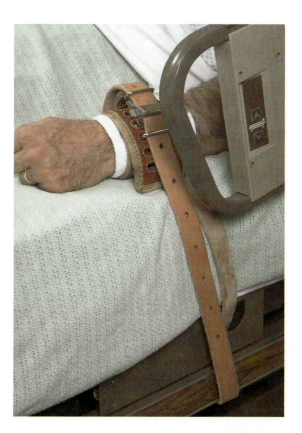

FIGURE 6–21 ◆
Leather wrist restraints (used only in an emergency)

Always remember:

- The need for leather restraints is often emergent. It might not be feasible to try alternatives before applying the leather restraints. However, once the emergency is over and the patient's condition has been assessed, it might be possible to substitute a restraint device that is less restrictive.
- Patients in any type of leather restraint require frequent visual checks (every 15 minutes or continuous observation).

PROCEDURE

APPLICATION AND CARE OF THE PATIENT IN LEATHER RESTRAINTS

OBRA

RATIONALE: Leather restraints are used only in emergencies when a patient is a great danger to himself or others.

PREPARATION

1. Select the appropriate restraint.
2. Wash your hands.
3. Introduce yourself, identify the patient, and explain what you will do.
4. Provide privacy for the patient.

STEPS

5. Lock the wheels on the bed or stretcher.
6. Leather restraints are applied in the following manner:
   a. Apply cuffs with smooth edge toward the patient. Fit snugly to the wrists and ankles.
   b. Draw straps through the slots of the cuff.
   c. Secure straps to the metal portion of bed frame (do not secure straps to side rails) and lock.

Allow 2–3 inches slack to allow for movement.
   d. The key will be placed near the patient and within easy reach of the staff (tape to outside of the foot of the bed).

CARE OF THE PATIENT

- The circulatory status of the restrained limb(s) will be evaluated at least every 15 minutes.
- In the event there is a change in the circulatory condition, the limb will be released immediately and measures taken to improve circulation.
- Wrist and ankle leather restraints are padded, whenever possible, using unsterile ABD pads and tape to prevent abrasions and tensions from occurring.
- Restraints are applied allowing for some patient movement when opposite or all extremities are restrained.
- Restraints are released individually to provide skin care and active or passive range-of-motion exercises at least every 2 hours and prn while the patient is awake.

- When locked restraints are used, the key must be accessible to remove restraints in an emergency situation (keep taped to the outside of the foot of the bed).
- Make sure the patient is as comfortable as possible.
- Assure patient that you or someone else will check on him every 15 minutes and will be available should he need assistance (fluids, blanket, urinal, etc.).

FOLLOW-UP

7. Document repeated checks per policy. Proper documentation is needed to ensure protection of patient's rights and to record the observation and care of the patient. Care is documented on the restraint flowsheet or unit/division specific documentation form.
8. Wash hands.

CHARTING EXAMPLE: 12/12/03 4pm Mr. Blake extremely agitated and combative. Two-point leather restraints applied to Mr. Blake's wrists per order of Dr. Harris. A. Taylor, CNA

Patient Restraint Policy Example

Compliance with individual state patient bills of rights, the public health codes, and the standards of the JCAHO and/or OBRA regulations influence and when revised, require changes in current practice. Patient's rights, dignity, and well-being are supported and maintained. The least restrictive method of restraint and/or seclusion that meets the patient's assessed need is applied. Restraints may be appropriate if the patient shows signs of **dementia**, **delirium**, **confusion**, or impairment of **cognition**. Restraints are the *last resort* of physical management after a thorough assessment of the patient. Note that restraints can have strong, negative psychological and physical effects such as:

- Increased disorganized behavior
- Confused behavior
- Social isolation
- Discomfort
- Demoralization
- Humiliation
- Sense of being punished
- Increased risk of injury or death
- Increased risk of pressure ulcers
- Increased risk of pneumonia
- Increased cardiac load
- Increased risk of disconditioning

Restraint or seclusion may be initiated by a nurse in an emergency situation in response to dangerous patient behavior. Use of restraint as a part of a facility, department, or unit specific approved protocol does not require a doctor's written order. A physician's order is required for use of restraint or seclusion in behavior health areas when a patient's assessed need requires the use of restraint outside a defined, approved protocol.

Alternatives to Restraints

During the past decade, government regulatory agencies and consumer advocacy groups have advocated restraint-free care, through the use of alternative interventions. To protect patient's rights, procedures regarding restraint use have been mandated by the Health Care Financing Administration (HCFA), OBRA of 1990, JCAHO, and the Commission on Accreditation of Rehabilitation Facilities (CARF).

The least restrictive, safe, effective alternative intervention should be considered, before resorting to restraints. The following ideas are one example of a policy. Your supervisor can direct you to your employer's current policy. Additionally, a patient who is in restraints should be monitored and assessed, at least *every 2 hours* to determine if a less restrictive option, or no method of restraints, could occur. Restraints should only be applied if the patient cannot protect himself or others from injury.

Alternative measures include:

- Identifying an underlying clinical problem that can be corrected. This would include medication reactions, hypoxia, pain, infection, or electrolyte imbalance, all of which may cause confusion or depression.
- Frequently reorienting the patient, explaining things to him, conversing with him, even if confused.
- Individualizing your approach by:
  - Offering frequent toileting if the patient is often climbing out of bed—he may be attempting to go to the bathroom
  - Letting the patient stay up later, if his history is that of a late night person
  - Ambulating the patient so that he gets more exercise.

dementia A progressive medical condition characterized by personality change; decline in intellectual capacity, judgment, and memory; and impairment of impulse control

delirium A disordered mental state that develops over a short period of time

confusion Bewilderment; the state of being disoriented to person, place, or time

cognition Awareness; the mental processes by which knowledge is acquired

- Eliminating tubes and drains or making them less apparent to the patient who is pulling at them. This includes:
  - Getting a pulse oximeter on the room air, to determine if oxygen is needed, if the patient pulling at a cannula
  - Capping the IV line, instead of leaving it attached to IV tubing, or placing a sleeve over the site. Place tubing behind the patient, out of sight
  - Discontinuing a Foley catheter or putting underwear on the patient to cover the catheter
  - Placing a loose binder over abdominal tubes and drains.
- Having the patient sit in the hallway for distraction as well as to have more contact with others.
- Giving the patient an activity to do with his hands, such as folding washcloths or giving him something to hold onto such as a stuffed animal, blanket, small ball, etc.
- Using alternative restraint devices where available; these devices are discussed later in Chapter 6
- Family supervision
- Familiar items from home
- Snacks
- Providing reality links: TV, radio, newspaper, open window curtains
- Cushions/pads
- Verbal reminders

When Restraints Are Clearly Indicated

The application of restraints should be initiated only if other measures fail to protect the patient, or others, from possible injury. The least restrictive device should always be utilized. Patient and family education regarding restraints is to be done at the earliest possible time and preferably before restraints are initiated. A RN, LPN, Patient Care Tech or Patient Care Assistant may apply restraints.

Alternatives should be considered prior to the use of restraints unless the patient cannot otherwise be protected from injury to self or others. If a restraint is clinically justified, the least restrictive device should be used.

Available restraint methods include:

- Mitts
- Net bed
- Soft/lap belt
- Soft wrist/ankle restraint
- Leather wrist/ankle restraint

Always assess and consider the type of restraint used for vulnerable patient populations, emergency, pediatric, and cognitively or physically limited patients. A vulnerable patient is one with:

- History of abuse (concentration camp survivor, domestic abuse, political prisoner from a foreign country, etc.) as this creates greater psychological risk
- Underlying physical condition, such as arthritis, where restraints can worsen the symptomology
- Age or cognitive limits

Restraints should be discontinued, or changed to a less restrictive alternative, at the earliest possible time. The patient's change in behavior is to be documented. Additionally, the discontinuation of the restraint order is to be entered into the patient record. A written physician or nursing order is not required.

Key Points for Restraint Orders

Except in an emergency, the verbal or written physician order for restraints is to be obtained before applying restraints and must include:

- Type of restraint and clinical justification. PRN orders are not acceptable.

- If the restraint order was given verbally, *the attending physician must examine the patient and write an order for restraints, within 24 hours* of the initiation of the restraint. *(With Behavior Management standards, the exam and written order are to occur within 1 hour).*

- Subsequently, the physician is to conduct a face-to-face examination of the patient, *every calendar day (every 8 hours for Behavioral Management standards),* and then enter a *written* order if the restraint use is to continue.

- A restraint should be discontinued at the earliest possible time.

- Patient monitoring is essential to ensure the patient's safety, dignity, and well-being.

- Documentation occurs on a new restraint flowsheet, for every calendar day *(every 8 hours for behavioral health),* and is to include:
  - Clinical justification for use of restraint
  - Attempted alternatives
  - Results of patient monitoring, assessment, and reassessment
  - Significant changes in patient condition
  - Patient and family education

Key Points for Behavior Management Patients

- A verbal or written order is to be obtained prior to initiation of a restraint or seclusion.

- A face-to-face physician assessment of the patient is to be completed within 1 hour of seclusion and/or restraint application.

- The physician is to write an order if it is determined that the restraint and/or seclusion is to be continued.

- The patient is to be observed continuously.

- Circulation and skins checks are to occur every 15 minutes.

- The patient is to be *monitored by an RN at least every hour.*

- Restraint and/or seclusion is to be utilized as ordered and *not to exceed:*
  - Adults—4 hours
  - Ages 9–17—2 hours
  - Under age 9—1 hour

- Upon the expiration of the order, a face-to-face assessment is to be completed by the RN (if stated in the order) or a physician is to determine if there is a need for further use of restraints and/or seclusion. If continued use is justified, the order may be written for another time period increment, not to exceed 8 hours total, from the original physician exam:

- Adults—up to 4 hours, not to exceed 8 hours, from the time of the original physician exam

- Ages 9–17—Up to 2 hours, not to exceed 8 hours, from the time of the original physician exam

- Under age 9—Up to 1 hour, not to exceed 8 hours from the time of the original physician exam.

- The physician is to examine the patient, at least every 8 hours and write an order for continuation of the restraint and/or seclusion, if still required by patient.

- Exam results are to be promptly entered into the medical record

Types of Restraints Used

Leather (hard) limb, cloth limb, vest, waist, pelvic, mitts, and net bed.

Restraint and Seclusion Standards Do Not Apply in the Following Situations

Restraint devices may be used for a patient *without a doctor's order* under the following conditions. Individual needs are assessed by appropriate professional staff (where indicated). The assessment is documented and use of the device is added to the patient plan of care.

- A restraint device used during transportation via wheelchair or cart.

- Children (6 months to 4 years) wear vests while in high chairs, wheelchairs, or any transportation vehicle.

- Medical immobilization is customarily employed during medical, diagnostic, or surgical procedures or tests, and is considered a regular part of such procedures or tests, including body restraint during surgery.

- Individual patient needs are assessed for adaptive assistive support mechanisms intended to permit a patient to achieve maximum normative bodily functioning, such as orthopedic appliances, braces, wheelchairs, geri chairs, other appliances, or devices used to posturally support the patient.

- Individual patient needs are assessed for protective devices intended to compensate for a specific physical deficit or to prevent safety incidents not related to cognitive dysfunction, such as bed rails, tabletop chairs, protective helmets, or at times, halter-type devices (i.e., to prevent a cognitively intact patient from falling out of a chair due to a physical inability to support his or her own body).

- A time-out of 15 minutes or less is used with children.

- Forensic and correction officer restriction used for security purposes.

- In home care, if applied by a family member.

- Patient seizure precautions will have four side rails up, with protective seizure pads in place.

- The institution's standard of care for patients who are sedated, recovering from anesthesia, or postoperative/post-procedure may have soft restraints applied to maintain safety for the patient tubes, wounds, and dressings using the following criteria for application and removal of restraints. A nursing assessment determines the individual patient's needs. See table on page "139" regarding criteria for exemption.

Customary patient care and regular hourly observation is performed and documented on the Restraint Flowsheet to ensure safe use (Figure 6–22◆).

RESTRAINT FLOWSHEET
FOR MEDICAL/SURGERY

❏ St. Joseph Mercy Hospital Ann Arbor
❏ Saline Community Hospital
❏ McPherson Hospital
Date: _____   Time: _____

ASSESS OF NEED FOR RESTRAINTS	BEHAVIORS THAT JUSTIFY USE	MD ORDERS
❏ Disoriented and confused ❏ Inability to remember/follow direction ❏ Sedated/unconscious ❏ Attempting to get out of bed or chair ❏ Agitation ❏ Other:	❏ Pulling at tubes/lines ❏ Attempting to D/C equipment ❏ Risk for removal of life sustaining tubes/tx ❏ Attempting to get out of bed when medically not indicated	❏ Order obtained within 1st 12 hours ❏ Order renewed daily

Alternatives Used Before Restraints		**Restraint Devices**
❏ Companion/family at bedside ❏ Increase/decrease stimulation as approp. ❏ Monitor need for tubes/lines and d/c ❏ ASAP as feasible ❏ Tilt recliner chair; move chair into hall if approp. ❏ Camouflage IV sites, dressings, etc. ❏ Diversion activities; folding towels, stacking objects, etc.	❏ Calming, soothing music ❏ Bed/chair alarm ❏ Meds reviewed ❏ Pain management ❏ Wander guard ❏ Physical relocation ❏ Other	**RT** = Right **LT** = Left **B** = Bilateral **L** = Leg **W** = Wrist **G** = Geri Chair **LB** - Lap Belt **M** = Mitt **N** = Net Bed **NN** = No No (pediatric) **V** = Vest (Zipper) **WB** = Waist Belt **SR** = All Side Rails Up **S** = Soft restraint

CARE NEEDS: Document Care Needs Every 2 Hours

Hour	Restraint Type/site	Food/ Fluids	Skin/Circ.	Toilet Q 2 Hrs.	Turn/ ROM	Eval. Q 2 Hrs.	Initials
00							
00							
00							
00							
00							
00							
00							
00							
00							
00							
00							
00							

EVALUATION EVERY 2 HOURS

SB = Same behaviors, continue to restrain
R = Restraints released:
1. Behaviors resolved
2. Family present
3. Trial release
4. Other _____

Care Needs

✔ Observation every hour
✔ Circulation check every 2 hours, warm, dry, cap. refill <3 sec.
✔ Skin check every 2 hrs., dry and intact
✔ ROM and reposition every 2 hrs.
✔ Toilet every 2 hrs.
✔ Offer food/fluids every 2 hrs.
✔ vital signs at least every 4 hours

❏ Info Sheet Given
❏ Explanation Given to Patient or Significant Other

Signature	Initials	Signature	Initials	Signature	Initials

FIGURE 6–22 ◆

Restraint flowsheet for medical/surgery and for behavior management. (Adapted from Patient Restraint Policy, St. Joseph Mercy Hospital, Ann Arbor, MI. Reprinted with permission.)

RESTRAINT FLOWSHEET
FOR BEHAVIOR MANAGEMENT

☐ St. Joseph Mercy Hospital Ann Arbor
☐ Saline Community Hospital
☐ McPherson Hospital
Date:_____   Time: _____

ASSESS OF NEED FOR RESTRAINTS	BEHAVIORS THAT JUSTIFY USE	MD ORDERS
☐ Abusive/threatening behavior presenting imminent risk to self/others/equipment	☐ Emergent application (dander to self or others) ☐ Attempts to strike out at others ☐ Attempts to hurt self ☐ Attempts to destroy property	**18 years and older:** ☐ Physician sees patient within 1 hr face to face Order renewed every 4 hrs. ☐ ⎯⎯ ☐ ⎯⎯ ☐ ⎯⎯ ☐ ⎯⎯ ☐ ⎯⎯ ☐ ⎯⎯ ☐ Physician sees patient face to face every 8 hrs, reassesses and reorders ☐ ⎯⎯ ☐ ⎯⎯ ☐ ⎯⎯

Alternatives Used Before Restraints

☐ Pain management ☐ Other

~~Restraint Devices~~

☐ Companion/family at bedside ☐ Increase/decrease stimulation as approp. ☐ Monitor need for tubes/lines and d/c ASAP as feasible ☐ Use of calm, soothing voice. ☐ Camouflage IV sites, dressings, etc. ☐ Calming, soothing music ☐ use of short Q & A ☐ Wander guard ☐ Meds reviewed ☐ Physical relocation	RT = Right LT = Left B = Bilateral S = soft restraint SR = All Side Rails Up H = Hard (leather)

9 years to 17 years old:
☐ Physician sees patient within 1 hr face to face, reassesses and writes the 1st order.
☐ Order every 2 hrs
☐ ⎯⎯ ☐ ⎯⎯ ☐ ⎯⎯
☐ ⎯⎯ ☐ ⎯⎯ ☐ ⎯⎯
☐ ⎯⎯ ☐ ⎯⎯ ☐ ⎯⎯
☐ ⎯⎯ ☐ ⎯⎯ ☐ ⎯⎯
☐ Physician sees patient face to face every 4 hrs, reassesses and reorders
☐ ⎯⎯ ☐ ⎯⎯ ☐ ⎯⎯
☐ ⎯⎯ ☐ ⎯⎯ ☐ ⎯⎯

Evaluation Every 2 Hours

SB = Same behaviors, continue to restrain
R = Restraints released:
1. Behaviors resolved
2. Family present
3. Trial release
4. Other ⎯⎯⎯

Care Needs - Continual Observation

✔ Circulation check every 15 minutes, warm, dry, cap. refill <3 sec.
✔ Skin check every 15 minutes, dry and intact
✔ ROM and reposition every 2 hrs.
✔ Toilet every 2 hrs.
✔ Offer food/fluids every 2 hrs.
✔ vital signs at least q 2 hrs.

Less than 9 years old:
☐ Physician sees patient within 1 hr face to face, reassesses writes 1st order
☐ Order renewed every hour:
☐ ⎯ ☐ ⎯ ☐ ⎯ ☐ ⎯ ☐ ⎯ ☐ ⎯
☐ ⎯ ☐ ⎯ ☐ ⎯ ☐ ⎯ ☐ ⎯ ☐ ⎯
☐ ⎯ ☐ ⎯ ☐ ⎯ ☐ ⎯ ☐ ⎯ ☐ ⎯
☐ ⎯ ☐ ⎯ ☐ ⎯ ☐ ⎯ ☐ ⎯ ☐ ⎯
☐ Physician sees patient face to face every 4 hrs, reassesses and reorders
☐ ⎯⎯⎯ ☐ ⎯⎯⎯
☐ ⎯⎯⎯ ☐ ⎯⎯⎯
☐ ⎯⎯⎯ ☐ ⎯⎯⎯
☐ Info Sheet Given
☐ Explanation Given To Patient Or Significant Other

CARE NEEDS: Document Care Needs Every 2 Hours

Hour	Restraint Type/site	Food/ Fluids Q 2 Hrs.	Skin/Circ. Observe Q 15 min.	Toilet Q 2 Hrs.	Turn/ ROM Q 2 Hrs.	Eval. Q 2 Hrs.	Initials
24:00							
01:00							
02:00							
03:00							
04:00							
05:00							
06:00							
0:700							
0:800							
0:900							
10:00							
11:00							
12:00							
13:00							
14:00							
15:00							
16:00							
17:00							
18:00							
19:00							
20:00							
21:00							
22:00							

Signature	Initials

FIGURE 6–22 ◆ (*Continued*)

(Adapted from Patient Restraint Policy, St. Joseph Mercy Hospital, Ann Arbor, MI. Reprinted with permission.)

Criteria for Exemption from Policy with Sedated/Anesthetized Patients

APPLICATION CRITERIA	RELEASE CRITERIA
Low level of consciousness. Can be aroused but unable to maintain wakefulness.	Maintains wakefulness.
Exhibits confusion and/or disorientation.	No confusion and/or disorientation.
Unable to remember instructions.	Remembers and repeats instructions.
Grabs at tubes, dressing, etc.	Doesn't grab at tubes, dressing, etc.
Likelihood of falling out of bed or rolling onto an operative site.	Little likelihood of falling out of bed or onto operative site.

Emergency Application for Restraint and/or Seclusion

When the previous situations do not apply, emergency use of restraint and/or seclusion may be initiated before obtaining a physician's order when the assessment of an RN determines the need for immediate intervention to prevent the patient from harming self, others, property, or the treatment environments. The following must be documented by the individuals initiating the emergency application:

- Events leading up to the intervention
- The prior use of alternative measures
- The patient's response to those measures
- The time restraint/seclusion was initiated
- The time restraint/seclusion was terminated
- The physician order for restraint within 2 hours of application or the patient must be released from restraint

Events Preceding and Leading up to Restraint and/or Seclusion

The events leading up to restraint and/or seclusion are documented, along with interventions attempted to prevent the action, and the patient's response to those interventions including (as appropriate):

- Use of positive reinforcement for desired behavior
- Deceleration interventions
- Attempts to obtain the patient's voluntary submission to restraint and/or seclusion/time-out
- Appropriate alternatives

Psychiatry Departments/Behavioral Health

Patients on behavioral care units are observed continuously, or no less than every 15 minutes, while restrained. See restraint policy information in Figure 6–21.

Application of Restraints

The individual caring for the patient is responsible for the correct, safe application of restraints and safety devices, no matter who applies them. Leather restraints are secured with a lock and key. They are secured to the movable frame when an adjustable bed is used.

Patient Care

- Includes correct and safe application of restraints, observation (every 1 hour), offering use of the bathroom, bedpan, or urinal (every 2 hours and as appropriate for the patient's condition), and provision for meals and fluids at least every 2 hours. Care also includes regular hygiene, skin care, color, motion and sensation checks to the restrained extremities, and range of motion (every 2 hours and as needed). Nurses evaluate care every 2 hours.

- When leather restraints are used, the circulatory status of the restrained limb(s) will be evaluated at least every 15 minutes. In the event there is a change in circulatory condition the limb will be released immediately and measures taken to improve circulation.

- Wrist and ankle leather restraints are padded, whenever possible, using unsterile ABD and tape to prevent abrasions and tension from occurring. (See procedure for proper application and care of patients in leather restraints).

Physical Management

1. **Cues of Escalating Behavior**

   a. Difficulty understanding or following directions

   b. Glaring or threatening expression

   c. Rapid breathing, stiff posture

   d. Focusing on leaving, packing bags, can't be redirected

   e. Restlessness, pacing, constantly moving back and forth in bed, or moving extremities if bedridden, w/c bound

   f. Unable to attend to tasks, gets distracted, frustrated

2. **Possible Causes of Agitated Behavior**

   a. Altered thought processes: paranoid, total brain injury (TBI), psychotic

   b. Response to constant internal stimuli

   c. No understanding of the stimuli they are experiencing: unfamiliar faces, sounds (call buttons, phones, TV, beepers, overhead pages, alarms, etc.)

   d. Overstimulated by outside stimuli (call lights, TV, beepers, phones, alarms, voices, etc.)

   e. Physical discomfort: constipated, pain, full bladder, muscle spasms, etc.

   f. Staff may unknowingly contribute to the patient's agitation by ignoring cues, focusing on task, not warning patient when approaching, etc.

3. **Therapeutic Communication**

   a. Only one person talks at a time, decrease as much of background noise as possible (turn off TV, radios, close door to remove outside noise, etc.).

   b. Short concise directions, given one at a time

   c. Be aware of tone of voice, calm and pleasant

   d. Reassure patient, remember: the patient may have memory problems and needs to be reassured that she is safe, her family knows where she is, and that she is getting better.

4. **Helpful Interventions**

   a. For your own safety and to prevent further escalation: Soothing touch to try and calm an agitated patient will not work.

b. Constant and direct eye contact may be interpreted as challenging and confrontive.

c. Remember that agitated patients may not have self-control mechanisms in place and may not be very flexible or open to change. They may demonstrate behaviors that are not appropriate.

d. At times, staff may need to set limits and tell patients directly that their behavior or statements are inappropriate. This must be said in a nondefensive and matter of fact manner.

e. Remember: *verbal* acting out requires *verbal* interventions; *physical* acting out requires *physical* interventions.

f. The goal of prn medications is to help the patient to remain in control of his behavior and also be able to actively participate in therapies.

g. Patients may act out verbally and say things to a caregiver that are offensive. Please do not take this personally and react automatically.

5. **Personal Space**

a. Each individual has his/her own personal space. Personal space consists of an area surrounding our body, about 18 to 36 inches, and we consider this area an extension of our bodies.

b. If a patient starts to be come agitated, back away from her, and out of her personal space. This will put you out of range if she should try to strike or kick you, and will often help to calm her down. Keep yourself between the patient and the door, in case you need an escape route.

c. Be aware that when you are in a patient's intimate space performing care, there is potential for them to feel invaded. To accomplish the tasks needed and keep everyone safe, sometimes two or more staff are needed.

Coping with fear:

a. Fear prevents you from taking charge.

b. Be aware you are afraid. This is a normal response.

c. Don't be afraid to tell a coworker "This patient scares me."

d. Understand rationale for this patient's behavior.

e. The patient is most likely afraid of you.

f. Look beyond outer display: brain injured/psychotic/very afraid.

g. Patients cannot always articulate their fears. We need to anticipate the fear.

h. Patients may be afraid of water, remember this when assisting with personal care. Showers may also overstimulate a patient.

i. Remember that you are not alone. Work as a team. Communicate to others your concerns when a patient's behavior is escalating.

Physical Crisis Management: Team Roles and Responsibilities

KEY IDEA

An organized team approach can minimize or prevent patient assault and injury.

1. **Team Leader**

   a. Person who is the most knowledgeable about the patient or the situation.

   b. Assumes accountability for the outcome of the incident.

2. **Responsibilities**

   a. Communicate to the others that you are assuming the responsibility.

   b. Determine if enough help is available, the group's capabilities and limitations, and the status of the other patients. May delegate someone to call security.

   c. Monitor the emotional status of self, the patient, and the staff throughout the incident. Use verbal/nonverbal techniques to decrease emotion and de-escalate behaviors.

   d. Communicate with the patient: state your role, your intent to help the patient regain control, and acknowledge the patient's distress.

   e. Try to "talk the patient down."

   f. Provide opportunity for patient to ventilate, if he is not posing a physical threat.

   g. Determine when talking has failed and physical intervention is necessary.

   h. If enough staff are present, do not become directly involved. If fewer than four staff are present, control one arm.

   i. Continue explaining to the patient what is happening in a calm, clear voice.

   j. When all limbs are secured, tell staff to release their holds.

   k. Direct a brief debriefing session.

3. **Team Members**

   a. Remove potentially dangerous articles from your clothing and pockets.

   b. Determine who will control each limb, and what each member will do.

   c. Only one person speaks to the patient, it may be the team leader, or someone designated.

   d. Get into position to prepare for physical intervention, blocking escape routes.

   e. Listen to the leader's directions.

   f. Respond stat when the leader signals.

   g. Act in unison with other team members and continue until the limbs are secured. **Never** release a limb until directed by the leader.

   h. Search the patient's pockets and remove belt and glasses.

   i. Participate in the debriefing.

4. **Support Staff**

   a. Be available if team leader needs more staff.

   b. Anticipate the needs of the team, opening or closing doors.

   c. Reassure other patients and visitors.

   d. Cover the unit during the debriefing.

   e. Promote dignity by closing doors. Redirect visitors and, if necessary, other patients.

5. **Threatening Situation: About to Be or Already Been Hit**

   a. Get help (staff, security).

   b. Get medications. Call MD (if no PRNs ordered).

c. Call security. Be specific about what you want them to do.

d. Make sure staff are aware that a patient is threatening or assaultive.

e. If you are going to restrain the patient, make sure one person is in charge.

f. Debrief with all staff involved with physical management of patient after the patient is secured, even if only for 5 minutes. Don't blame self, but try to see what could have been done differently.

g. Remember that sometimes patients strike without warning.

h. Criteria for removing restraints: Know your patient!

Physician Responsibilities: Patient Assessment and Orders

Patient Assessment

The physician (or designee) assesses the individual patient's need for restraint and/or seclusion. Reassessment associated with time-limited orders is used primarily to determine the continuing need for the restraint and/or seclusion. The physician provides clinical oversight or qualified, trained staff to apply or remove restraint and/or seclusion in emergent situations or under written protocols (Table 6–2◆).

TABLE 6–2◆

Restraints: Patient and Family Information Sheet

I.   **What is a restraint?**
     A restraint is any object or device that is used to limit movement or decreases the patient's ability to reach a part of his body. Restraints are used to protect the patient from injuring himself or others.

II. **Why are restraints used?**
     Restraints are applied only when needed to protect a patient or others from injury.

III. **When are restraints used?**
     Restraints are used to protect a patient only after many other methods have been tried. These may include:

     - Taking the patient to the bathroom
     - Changing the patient's position
     - Having someone spend time with the patient (perhaps family)
     - Moving the patient closer to the nurses' station
     - Addressing the patient's pain level

IV. **What to expect while a patient is restrained:**

     - Restraints will be removed as soon as possible.
     - Restraints can sometimes be removed while family is present. It is very important to discuss this with the nurse before the restraint can be removed.
     - A caregiver will check the patient every hour. Every 2 hours, the patient in restraints will be offered something to drink, and asked if he needs to use the restroom.

V.   **How family can help?**

     - Send time with your family member.
     - Talk calmly and provide reassurance.
     - Help caregivers understand the patient's needs and gestures.
     - Help communicate information to the patient.
     - Bring personal reminders/items from home.

SOURCE: Courtesy St. Joseph Mercy Hospital, Ann Arbor, Michigan. Used with permission.

Orders

- Orders are to be obtained from the patient's physician within 2 hours of the application of restraint. If an order is not received in the 2-hour time frame, the restraints must be discontinued.
- **No PRN orders.**
- Order must include type of restraint, reason for restraint, and maximum duration of use not to exceed 24 hours.

OBRA Regulations Federal rules and requirements established by the Omnibus Budget Reconciliation Act of 1987

OBRA Regulations

OBRA, the Omnibus Budget Reconciliation Act of 1987, includes a regulation regarding physical restraints which states, in part, that "any device that limits movement or restricts normal access to one's body" may be used only in circumstances in which a patient may harm himself or someone else or to protect a patient during a medical procedure and only with a physician's order. This regulation applies to nursing facilities that provide long-term care to elderly patients and patients with disabilities. Even when a physician writes an order for a physical restraint, the care team is obligated by law to seek the least restrictive method of maintaining the resident's safety, carefully documenting each step of the process.

The nursing assistant is the care team member who has the greatest amount of contact with the resident and will be more aware of the resident's needs and preferences. A resident who is confused and unable to understand or express his own needs may become restless, agitated, or even aggressive when he is hungry, frightened, or simply needs to go to the bathroom. Long-term care residents cannot be restrained for the staff's convenience— to prevent wandering or getting out of the bed or chair—and all possible causes for unusual or agitated behavior must be investigated prior to considering a restraint for that person. It is very frustrating to be unable to move as you wish; consequently, there is great danger that a restrained person may become injured attempting to do nothing more than gain someone's attention.

KEY IDEA

Any protective device that the patient/resident cannot release on his own is considered a restraint. Lap pillows and trays that a patient cannot remove are restraints.

restraint alternative
Protective measures such as a saddle or wedge cushion, self-releasing belt or lap tray that are used to help prevent falls but do not physically restrain an individual. A lap tray is an alternative only if a patient can remove it.

Restraint Alternatives

A **restraint alternative** is a protective device or technique that prevents the patient or resident from harming himself or others but does not physically restrain the individual. A thorough assessment of each patient by the members of the care team will determine which restraint alternative is appropriate. Documentation of the type of restraint used, why it was used, when it was applied, and when it was removed is important.

Some of the choices are:

- A wedge or saddle cushion, which helps to prevent sliding forward and possibly falling while seated in chair (Figure 6–23◆).
- A self-releasing belt, sometimes preferred by patients who are aware and able to make appropriate choices for themselves (Figure 6–24◆).
- A lap tray, which can help prevent falling out of a chair.

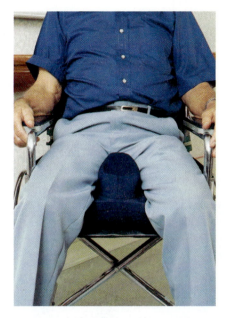

FIGURE 6–23 ◆
Restraint alternatives: a saddle cushion, which prevents sliding forward

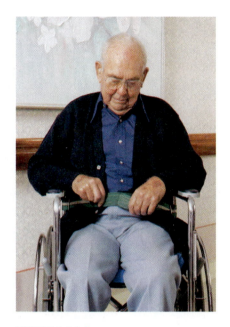

FIGURE 6–24 ◆
Self-releasing safety belt

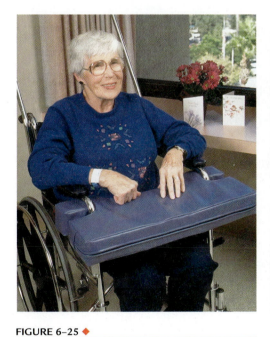

FIGURE 6–25 ◆
Lap pillow

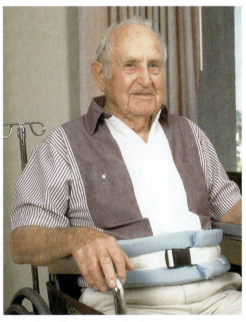

FIGURE 6–26 ◆
Seat-belt–style lap belt with latch

- A lap pillow, which helps to prevent the patient from falling forward and eases the pressure the patient might otherwise experience (Figure 6–25◆).
- Seat-belt–style lap belt with latch (Figure 6–26◆).

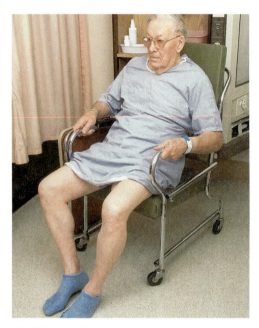

FIGURE 6–27a ◆

Patient slipping in chair

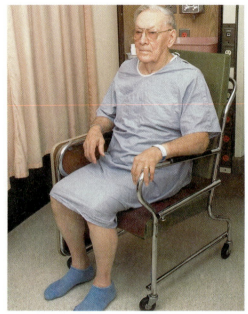

FIGURE 6–27b ◆

Using Posey grip to keep patient from slipping in chair

FIGURE 6–28 ◆

Chair alarm safety device

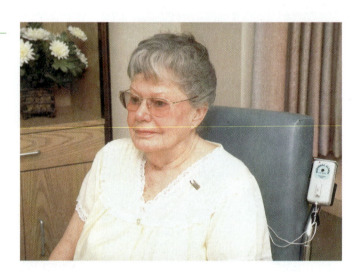

- Using Posey grip or a similar product to keep patient from slipping in chair (Figures 6–27a◆ and Figure 6–27b◆).
- A chair alarm safety device alerts staff to a problem (Figure 6–28◆).
- Patient positioning devices for wheelchair provides support (Figure 6–29a◆ and Figure 6–29b◆).
- A diversion, something of interest to the patient, which can help to take his mind off wandering behavior.
- Any device used as a restraint (including side rails) is to be used only with the order of a physician and only to ensure the physical safety of the patient (Figure 6–30a◆ and Figure 6–30b◆).

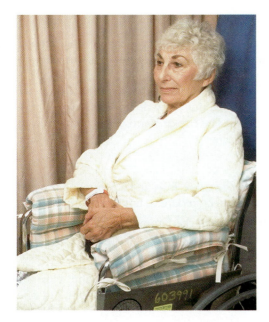

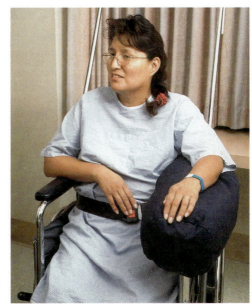

FIGURE 6–29◆

Patient positioning devices for wheelchair

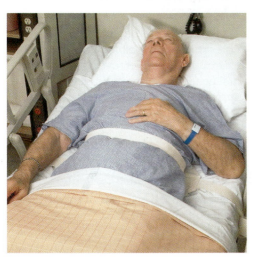

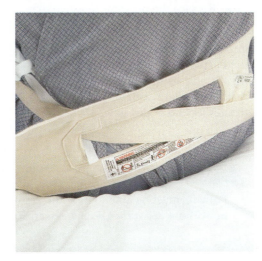

FIGURE 6–30a ◆

Roll belt in bed restraint, front

FIGURE 6–30b ◆

Roll belt in bed restraint, back

- Restraining devices are to be applied correctly and used only according to the policy of the institution.
- Explain the purpose of the restraining device to the patient and family members prior to its use even if the patient is not fully able to understand.
- Check the restrained patient *every 30 to 60 minutes* to be certain the restraint is not too tight and that the resident's needs are being met.
- Release the restraint every two hours, reposition or exercise the patient, offer food and fluids, toilet the patient, and check the patient's skin for redness or irritation. Document all findings including the responses of the patient to the use of the restraint.
- Know the federal (OBRA) guidelines for the use of restraints.
- Use a clove hitch so that the restraint can be easily released in an emergency.

Applying Bed and Chair Alarms

bed alarm A control unit that activates an audible alarm and the nurse call system when the patient's weight leaves a pressure-sensitive mat for a preselected amount of time

chair alarm A battery-operated control unit that activates an audible alarm immediately if the patient tries to get up out of the chair

pressure-sensitive mat A disposable mat that is connected to a bed or chair alarm

Most **bed alarms** and **chair alarms** are used as part of a fall-prevention program and are usually used in conjunction with a patient risk assessment. Both types of alarm work on the principle that the alarm will distract patients, causing them to stop their activity because of the noise. This gives the staff enough time to respond. Bed and chair alarms work well with patients who are impulsive, confused, or forgetful. They do not work well for patients who are paranoid or have psychotic episodes. The use of alarms frees patients from restraints while alerting the nursing staff to patient activity.

Always remember:

- The system consists of a disposable **pressure-sensitive mat** and a control unit. When the patient's weight leaves the mat for a preselected amount of time, the alarm sounds.
- When an alarm is activated, the patient must be checked immediately.
- Alarms should not be used on patients who are hard-of-hearing or who weigh less than 100 pounds.
- Never immerse the mat in water. Instead, wipe it clean with the same cleaning solution used to clean the patient's mattress. Each mat should be used with just one patient.
- Replace the pressure-sensitive mat after 30 days.

Patients of all ages should have the device explained and demonstrated thoroughly. It is important to stress to the patient that the system is a reminder to wait for assistance. When the cognitive status of the patient improves, the alarm should be removed so that the patient is able to function at the highest level of independence. Use of the device requires that the patient weigh at least 100 pounds. Patients with hearing deficits are not good candidates for use of this device.

KEY IDEA

Patients must be able to hear the alarm so they will stop the behavior of trying to get up without assistance. Pressure-sensitive mats should be tested daily.

Restraining the Pediatric Patient

To restrain means to keep someone from doing something or to prevent an action from happening. As with adults, all restraints used for pediatric patients are applied only on the instruction of the nurse or physician. The kind of restraint used for a child depends on why she is being restrained, age, and level of understanding.

- Elbow restraints (Figure 6–31◆) may be applied to a child who has eczema to keep him from scratching himself or to a child who has had surgery on his mouth or eyes, or has an IV, to keep his hands away from those areas. Elbow restraints prevent a child from bending his elbows and, therefore, from reaching or scratching his face.
- Mitten restraints are also used to prevent scratching.

Remember, restraints can cause injury and must be used with extreme care.

Applying Elbow Restraints

- Elbow restraints are made of canvas and tongue depressors or a padded arm-board. They are tied firmly around the child's arm so that they will not slide below the elbow. The child can move the arm but cannot bend the elbow to reach his or her face.

FIGURE 6–31 ◆
Elbow restraint

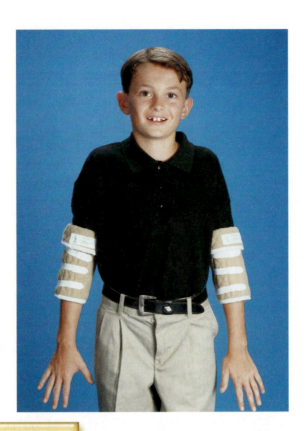

| APPLYING BED AND CHAIR ALARMS | **PROCEDURE** | **OBRA** |

RATIONALE: Alarms are used to distract patients and cause them to stop their activity and alert staff to immediately check on the patient.

PREPARATION

1. Assemble the equipment.
2. Identify the correct patient.
3. Explain the procedure to the patient. Explain also why the alarm is necessary.
4. Wash hands.

STEPS

5. Set up the chair alarm:
   a. Position the pressure-sensitive mat across the back of the chair.
   b. Plug the wire connection from the mat into the control unit.
   c. Attach the control unit to the back of the chair, out of the patient's sight and reach.
   d. Seat the patient in the chair.
   e. Test the alarm system daily.
6. Set up the bed alarm (Figure 6–32◆):
   a. Position the pressure-sensitive mat across the width of the bed, directly on top of the mattress, and under the patient's buttocks.
   b. Plug the wire connection from the mat into the control unit.
   c. Attach the control unit to the bed frame.
   d. Plug the control unit into a wall outlet.
   e. Plug the nurse call light cord into the adapter for the wall call system.
   f. Set the alarm for a 3-second delay.
   g. Place the patient in bed.
   h. Test the alarm system daily.

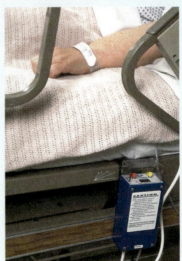

FIGURE 6–32 ◆
Bed alarm attached to the side rails of a patient's bed.

7. Follow the manufacturer's product information guidelines for the on/off and reset mechanisms.

APPLYING BED AND CHAIR ALARMS

PROCEDURE *(continued)*   **OBRA**

9. Provide care, and continue to monitor the patient every 15 minutes to 1 hour, according to the institution's policy. Check the patient immediately if the alarm is activated.

10. When necessary, clean the mat with a damp cloth and sanitizing solution and water. Never use alcohol.

CHARTING EXAMPLE: 11/09/04
3pm Chair alarm set up and tested. Mrs. Jones is aware that the alarm will alert staff if she gets up from the chair. J. Ralston, CNA
11/10/03 9am Bed alarm positioned on Mrs. Jones's bed with alarm set for a 3-second delay. Mrs. Jones reassured it will not go off if she turns to her side. P. Boggs, CNA

FOLLOW-UP

8. Wash hands and document and report the results of the procedure to the RN or preceptor. Include the patient's response to the alarm.

- Such restraints should be removed frequently to prevent muscle cramp and to access the skin. One restraint should be removed at a time, and someone should be present to control the child's arm movements for the time it is off.

- A child may often be frustrated emotionally because of the restraints. His satisfaction must be provided in new ways. Ask your immediate supervisor for guidance in caring for a restrained child.

Ambulation Safety with a Cane, Walker, or Crutches

Various pieces of equipment may be ordered by the physician to assist the patient to ambulate safely. These pieces of equipment include *canes, crutches,* and *walkers.* They support the patient while walking. Each of these pieces of equipment must be adjusted for each individual patient. The hand piece must be level with the patient's hip to accommodate a slight bend of the elbow while the patient is standing and holding the cane, crutches, or walker. The patient must never use these pieces of equipment to help get to a standing position. They are only something to assist the patient to walk.

- **Cane:** Usually used on the patient's stronger side to balance her weight between the cane and the weaker side (Figure 6–33◆).

- **Walker:** Ordered when the patient requires some support when walking due to imbalance or weakness. The walker is safe to push down upon only when all four legs of the walker are on the ground in a level position. When the walker is being moved the patient's feet should be stationary. When the walker is stationary, the patient can move his feet. The walker must be picked up and moved and never slid along the ground unless the walker has wheels. Make sure the walker is the correct size for the patient (Figure 6–34◆).

- **Crutches:** Ordered to decrease weight borne by one or both feet and legs or to provide stability (Figure 6–35◆). Instructions will permit full weight bearing, partial weight bearing, weight bearing to tolerance, or nonweight bearing. Make sure that all pads and grips are securely in place. Check the screws to make sure all hardware is tight. Inspect the rubber tips for wear and make sure they are dry, and free of dirt and/or stones. If the patient is weak, unsteady, or unable to maintain balance, help him to a position of safety and report this to your immediate supervisor.

Ambulation is the action of walking. Gait is the rhythm and movement of the feet and the speed of walking. **Gait training** is done by the physical therapist as the first step toward helping the patient to **ambulate** independently. A gait belt is a device used to hold the patient securely while ambulating him.

ambulation To walk or move about in an upright position

gait training Rehabilitative exercise to help the patient improve his walking ability

ambulate To walk or move about

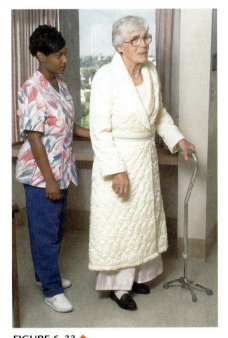

FIGURE 6–33 ◆

CNA assists patient using a cane

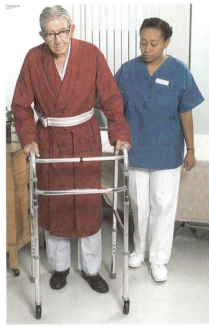

FIGURE 6–34 ◆

Walker

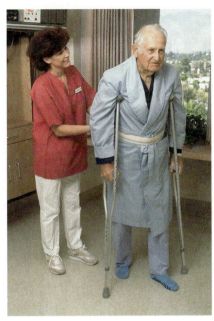

FIGURE 6–35 ◆

Crutches

PATIENT AMBULATION SAFETY	GUIDELINES	OBRA
■ Apply good body mechanics at all times (see Chapter 7). ■ Be sure of the patient's ability to ambulate before you attempt to assist him.	■ If you need help or if you are in doubt, ask your immediate supervisor for assistance.	■ Communicate with the patient by explaining the procedure and telling the patient what you expect of him.

SUMMARY

Safety is a most important consideration. This chapter has reviewed safety measurement precautions to take when caring for patients, listed special considerations and guidelines to follow when oxygen is used, and covered electrical and fire safety. The care and safety of patients requiring protective devices or restraints was also outlined. You are the team member who probably interacts most with the patient, or client. Therefore, your observations and actions are essential to the safety of the patient. Restraint policy and procedures are frequently updated. Follow your employer's current policy.

NOTES

CHAPTER REVIEW

FILL IN THE BLANK Read each sentence and fill in the blank line with a word that completes the sentence.

1. Be sure to lock the _____ on wheelchairs, stretchers, and commode chairs.

2. The special device used with oxygen that controls and regulates the amount of oxygen is called the _____.

3. An _____ extinguisher can be used on all types of fires.

4. _____ is the number one cause of fires in health care institutions.

5. Never tie or secure a restraint device to a _____ part of a bed or chair.

MULTIPLE CHOICE Choose the best answer for each question or statement.

1. All of the following is true about oxygen *except*

   a. it is a colorless, odorless, tasteless gas.

   b. the more oxygen a patient has the better.

   c. oxygen is one of the key elements needed for fire.

   d. room air is 21 percent oxygen.

2. The *P* in the acronym **PASS** means

   a. pass me a fire extinguisher.

   b. panic.

   c. push people out of the way.

   d. pull the safety pin or seal at the top of the extinguisher.

3. All of the following are misuses of electricity *except* which one?

   a. Electrical equipment in contact with water

   b. Use of numerous extension cords

   c. Use of frayed cords and plugs

   d. Use of three-pronged plugs

4. Which of the following is not a restraint alternative?

   a. Chair alarm

   b. Positioning device like a cushion or pad

   c. Lap belt

   d. Constant staff or family supervision

5. When ambulating a patient,

   a. apply good body mechanics.

   b. be sure of the patient's ability to ambulate before you attempt to move him.

   c. always communicate to the patient what you expect of him.

   d. All of the above.

TIME-OUT

TIPS FOR TIME MANAGEMENT

Allow extra time for tasks that slow you down. For example, if you like to take your time, organize your day so that you have the time you need to read assignments and write on charts.

THE NURSING ASSISTANT IN ACTION

Mrs. Smith is an elderly woman with Alzheimer's disease living in an assistive care unit. She frequently wanders into other patients' rooms and then uses their bathrooms or looks in their drawers for belongings she has lost. The other residents are becoming impatient and angry with her. One resident asks you to lock Mrs. Smith in her own room because she is tired of finding her belongings and bathroom messed up by Mrs. Smith. Would locking Mrs. Smith in her room be considered a restraint?

What Is Your Response/Action

CRITICAL THINKING

CUSTOMER SERVICE Try not to rush an elderly person. Doing so can cause increased stress and anxiety or trigger angry outbursts. Do not try to motivate patients by comparing them to their roommate. Avoid comments like "Mr. Sites has finished his meal, why haven't you?" Allow patients to safely take their time to walk or finish whatever they are doing.

CULTURAL CARE Body language, touch, and gestures have various meanings across cultures. Become familiar with gestures that can trigger protective or negative reactions in patients. Approach patients who are frightened with your hands open rather than in fists. Offer reassurance and frequently check patients who have any restraint device in place. If you are unable to speak to patients in their language, check if an interpreter has been found to explain what is happening and ask if there are a few words that you could use to communicate with the patient.

COOPERATION WITHIN THE TEAM In disaster situations or emergencies, do whatever you can to help. This is not the time to worry about whose job it is to do whatever is needed. If you are unsure how to help, check with the person who is taking charge of the situation. Moving patients to safe areas and calling for additional help are priorities.

EXPLORE MediaLink

Additional interactive resources for this chapter can be found on the Companion Website at www.prenhall.com/wolgin. Click on Chapter 6 and "Begin" to select activities for this chapter.

For chapter-related NCLEX-style questions and an audio glossary, access the accompanying CD-ROM in this book.

Video:

■ Activity and Exercise; Assisting clients to use Mechanical Aids for Walking

—Walker

—Cone

7 Body Mechanics: Positioning, Moving, and Transporting Patients

OBJECTIVES

When you have completed this chapter, you will be able to:

- Describe techniques for proper/protective body mechanics.
- Lift, hold, or move an object or patient using techniques for proper/protective body mechanics.
- List the different positions for patients, assist patients into those positions, and drape for privacy.
- List the guidelines for moving and lifting patients.
- Move a helpless patient up in bed.
- Move a patient up in bed with the patient's help.
- Move the mattress to the head of the bed with the patient's help.
- Move a helpless patient to one side of the bed on the patient's back.
- Log roll the patient.
- Turn a patient on either side.
- Transport and reposition a patient in a wheelchair, move the patient from the bed to a wheelchair and back into bed.
- Move the helpless patient using a portable mechanical patient lift.
- Transport a patient by stretcher, and move the patient from the bed to a stretcher and back into bed.
- Assist a patient to ambulate.
- Assist a falling patient.

MediaLink

www.prenhall.com/wolgin

Use the address above to access the free, interactive Companion Website created for this textbook. Get hints, instant feedback, and textbook references to chapter-related NCLEX-style questions. Link to other interesting sites.

AUDIO GLOSSARY:
Use the Companion Website, or the CD-ROM disk enclosed with your textbook, to hear the pronunciation of key terms in the chapter.

The use of proper/protective body mechanics during the positioning, moving, and transporting of patients will help you avoid fatigue and injury as a health care worker. Learning how to apply the techniques correctly will improve safety for you and for the patient.

Proper/Protective Body Mechanics

The term **proper** or **protective body mechanics** refers to the techniques of standing and moving one's body, using the strongest muscles to avoid fatigue or injury. You should understand the techniques of proper/protective body mechanics and learn to apply them to work tasks. As a result, you will feel less tired at the end of the day.

ALERT

For all patient contact, adhere to Standard Precautions (⚭ Chapter 5, pages 83–85). Wear protective equipment as indicated.

proper/protective body mechanics Special ways of standing and moving one's body to make the best use of strength and to avoid fatigue

---

PROPER/ PROTECTIVE BODY MECHANICS	GUIDELINES	OBRA

- When an action requires physical effort, try to use the largest muscles or groups of muscles possible. For example, use both hands rather than one hand to pick up an object.

- Use good posture. Keep your body aligned in front of your work. Maintain the natural curves in your back, keeping ears, shoulders, and hips in vertical alignment. Bend your knees. Keep your weight balanced evenly on both feet.

- Keep your feet slightly more than hip width apart to give you a broad base of support and good balance.

- Position your body close to the load being lifted.

- When you have to move a heavy object, push it or roll it rather than lift and carry.

- Use your arms to support the object. Keep your arms in a fixed position with elbows close to your sides. The muscles of your legs, not the muscles of your back and arms, should do the job of lifting.

- When you are doing work such as giving a back rub, making a corner on a bed, or moving the patient,

align your body in the direction of your work. Avoid twisting at the waist. Always turn or pivot with your feet, or shift your weight from one foot to the other.

- When you lift an object (Figure 7–1a◆):
  - Squat close to the load.
  - Maintain the natural curves in your back.

- Grip the object firmly.
- Hold the load close to your body.
- Keep your arms fixed and close to your sides.
- Lift by pushing up with your strong leg muscles (avoid lifting load with arms to chest and then standing) (Figure 7–1b◆).

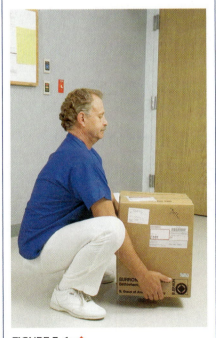

FIGURE 7–1a ◆

Squat close to the load

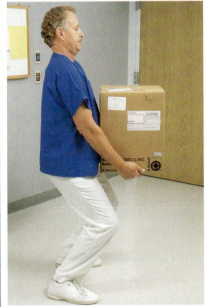

FIGURE 7–1b ◆

With arms fixed close to your sides, lift by pushing up with your strong leg muscles

GUIDELINES *(Continued)*

- Ask for assistance if you think you may not be able to lift the load yourself.
- Lift smoothly; don't jerk. Always count "one, two, three" when working with another person, or say "ready" and "go" so that you work in unison. Do this with both the patient and with other health care workers.

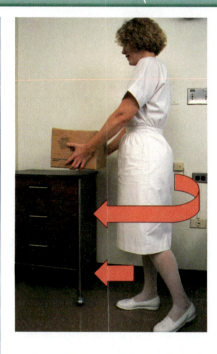

FIGURE 7–2 ◆
Pivot feet

- When you want to change the direction of movement:
  - Pivot (turn) feet (Figure 7–2◆).
  - Use short steps.
  - Turn your whole body using your feet to avoid twisting your back and neck.

Positioning and Draping the Patient

draping Covering a patient or parts of a patient's body with a sheet, blanket, bath blanket, or other material during a physical examination or prior to surgery

drape A covering used to provide privacy during an examination or operation

knee-chest position A bent posture with the knees and chest touching the examining table, sometimes used for examining the rectum or for women who have recently given birth, to allow the uterus to fall forward into its natural position

dorsal lithotomy position The position in which a patient lies on the back, with legs spread apart and knees bent

Fowler's position The position in which the head of the patient's bed is at a 45–90 angle

Draping is the process of covering a patient's entire body or parts of the body with a sheet, blanket, bath blanket, or other material. Draping is usually done during the physical examination of the patient and during surgery. A **drape** is the actual cover used to provide privacy during an examination or an operation.

Many different positions are used for patient comfort or positioning. Certain positions are required for treatment administration, rectal or vaginal examinations, procedures or surgical operations. Patient draping varies for each. Figures 7–3◆ through 7–5◆ show some of the more common positions.

Knee-Chest Position

In the **knee-chest position**, the patient rests on the knees and chest. The head is turned to one side with the cheek on a pillow. The patient's arms are extended slightly, bent at the elbows. Although the arms help support the patient, the main body weight is supported by the knees and chest. The knees are bent so that they are at right angles to the thighs. Draping is done with two sheets, one for the upper part of the body and one for the lower part (Figure 7–4). This position is used in rectal and vaginal examinations.

Dorsal Lithotomy Position

The **dorsal lithotomy position** is the same as the dorsal recumbent position, except that the patient's legs are well separated and the knees are bent more (Figure 7–5). This

BODY POSITIONS

Position

Fowler's
A position for sitting up in bed (while eating, reading, and so on). Also used to allow patients with breathing or heart problems to breathe more easily.

Semi-Fowler's
A gentler angle helps prevent the patient from sliding down in the bed.

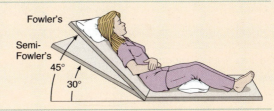

Supine
A position lying flat on the back. (Also called the **dorsal recumbent** or horizontal recumbent position.)

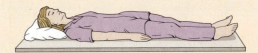

Prone
A position lying flat on the abdomen.

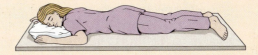

Side-Lying (Lateral)
A side-lying position.

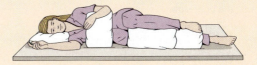

Sims's
A partly side-lying and partly prone position. Often used for rectal exams and enemas.

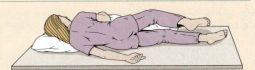

Trendelenburg
The mattress is tilted so that the patient's head is below the level of the feet. May be ordered to promote postural drainage or prevent shock.

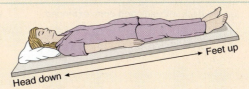

Reverse Trendelenburg
The mattress is tilted so the patient's feet are below the level of the head.

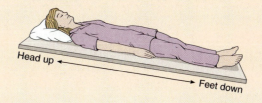

FIGURE 7-3 ◆

semi-Fowler's position The position in which the head of patient's bed is at a 30–45° angle

supine position Lying on one's back

BODY POSITIONS *(Continued)*

Characteristics	Steps to Maintain Good Alignment
Fowler's The head of the bed is raised to a 45° to 60° angle. The patient rests on the back with the knees bent slightly and the arms extended down and flexed. **Semi-Fowler's** The head of the bed is raised to only a 30° to 45° angle.	■ Support the head with a pillow. ■ Place a pillow under the knees. Placing a pillow under each lower arm may also increase comfort. ■ Use a footboard to prevent footdrop if necessary.
The bed is flat. Both arms and legs are extended.	■ Support the patient's head with a pillow. ■ Support arms and hands with pillows if necessary. A small rolled towel or blanket at the small of the back may also give support. Placing a small folded towel under the knees relieves strain on the back. ■ Use a footboard to prevent footdrop, if necessary. ■ To prevent hip rotation outward, make a trochanter roll. ■ Watch pressure points on the elbows, heels, and the tailbone. Lambswool protectors are available that fit heels and elbows.
The legs are extended, the face is turned to one side, and the arms are bent upward at the elbows.	■ Support the patient's head with a pillow. Place another pillow under the abdomen (optional). ■ Reduce pressure on the toes by placing a pillow under the lower legs. You may also move the patient down to allow the legs to hang over the edge of the mattress. No pillow is then needed.
The left-lateral position is when the patient is on the left side, and the right-lateral position is when the patient is on the right side.	■ Place a pillow under the head for support. ■ Place a pillow against the back to maintain the position. ■ Bend the upper leg forward at the knee and hip to help relieve pressure on the back. Placing a pillow between the legs keeps the hip in proper alignment and protects the skin where the legs touch. ■ The lower arm should be flexed. A small pillow or rolled blanket placed under this arm may make the patient more comfortable.
The patient lies on the left side with the left leg and arm extended and the right leg and arm flexed. The left arm rests behind the patient.	■ Support the head and shoulder with a pillow. ■ Support the flexed leg with a pillow. Support the flexed arm and hand with another pillow.
The patient lies on the back with legs and arms extended.	See Supine. Support the patient's body so he or she does not slip out of bed. Place a pillow against the headboard.
See Trendelenburg.	See Trendelenburg.

FIGURE 7–3 *(continued)*

dorsal recumbent position
Lying down or reclining; refers to the back or the back part of an organ

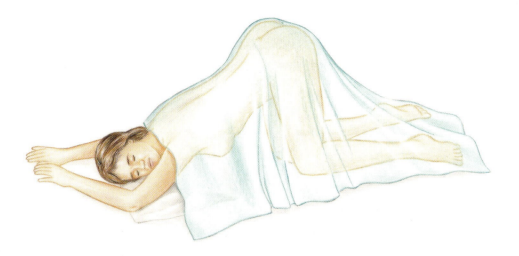

FIGURE 7–4 ◆
Knee-chest position

prone position Lying on one's stomach

side-lying (lateral) positions Lying on one's left or right side

Sims's position Position in which the patient lies on the left side with the right knee and thigh drawn up, often used for a rectal examination

position is used often for examination of the bladder, vagina, rectum, and perineum. If an examination table is being used, the patient's feet are sometimes placed in stirrups.

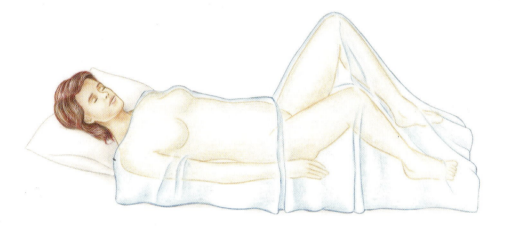

FIGURE 7–5 ◆
Dorsal lithotomy position

Trendelenburg position Position in which the bed or operating table on which a patient is lying is tilted so that the patient's head is about one foot below the level of his or her knees to allow more blood flow to the head and prevent shock; also called *shock position*

Moving and Lifting Patients

KEY IDEA

Moving and lifting patients who cannot assist you can be difficult. For this reason, you must take special care to support and align the patient's body properly.

Many of your tasks require lifting and moving a helpless or **nonambulatory** patient who cannot walk or move himself. A **bedridden** patient must have his position changed often. Proper support and alignment of the patient's body are important.

When moving or lifting a patient, the patient's body should be straight and properly supported; otherwise, the patient's safety and comfort might be affected. The correct positioning of the patient's body is referred to as **body alignment**. Body alignment means the arrangement or adjustment of the patient's body so that all parts of the body are in their proper positions in relation to each other.

Many conditions and injuries, as well as special patient care treatments, make it difficult or even dangerous for a patient to be in a certain position. As a member of the nursing team, you will be responsible for making sure that the patient you are caring for is in the position ordered by the doctor.

nonambulatory Unable to walk

bedridden Unable to get out of bed

body alignment The correct, or anatomical, positioning of a patient's body; also the arrangement of the body in a straight line

MOVING AND LIFTING PATIENTS	GUIDELINES	OBRA

- Before you begin each procedure, identify yourself and explain what you are going to do and encourage the patient to participate and help as much as possible.

- Before moving the patient, place tubing from catheters and IVs where they won't be pulled.
- Give the most support to the heaviest parts of the patient's body.

- Hold the patient close to your body for the most support.
- Move the patient with smooth and steady motions. Avoid sudden jerking movements.

A pull or lift sheet can help you move the patient in bed more easily. A regular extra sheet folded over many times and placed under the patient can be used as a pull sheet. The cotton draw sheet can also be used as a pull sheet. When moving the patient, roll and pull the sheet up tightly on each side next to the patient's body. Grip the rolled portion to slide the patient into the desired position. By using the pull sheet, friction and irritation to the patient's skin are avoided.

AGE-SPECIFIC CONSIDERATIONS

Moving and Lifting Patients

For all lifting and moving procedures: Patients of all ages must be treated with respect. In adolescence, patients are experiencing rapid change in their bodies and in their emotions. Avoid the use of medical jargon to gain their trust and respect. Guard their privacy as you move and transfer these patients. Adults often fear losing control when ill and are prone to feelings of helplessness. Explain clearly what you are doing and encourage them in areas where they may have some control. The older adult experiences numerous physiological changes as the aging process progresses. However, getting older is not a disease process. Allow for a longer response time when giving directions, speak clearly and in lower tones, and make sure the patient is wearing glasses/hearing aides (if applicable) to aid in communication.

KEY IDEA

To avoid trauma to the patient's skin, lift rather than slide the patient when moving her up in bed.

MOVING THE HELPLESS PATIENT UP IN BED	PROCEDURE	OBRA

RATIONALE: Safely lifting and moving a patient avoids injury to caregivers and the patient.

PREPARATION

1. Ask another nursing assistant to work with you.

2. Wash your hands.

3. Identify the patient by checking the identification bracelet.

4. Ask visitors to step out of the room, if this is your hospital's policy.

5. Tell the patient that you and your partner are going to move her up in the bed, even if she appears to be unconscious.

6. Provide privacy for the patient.

STEPS

7. Place the pillow from under the patient's head up against the headboard. This will protect the patient's head.

8. Lock the wheels on the bed.

9. Raise the height of the bed to a comfortable working position.

10. Lower the backrest and footrest, if this is allowed.

PROCEDURE *(continued)*

11. Stand on one side of the bed. The other nursing assistant will stand on the opposite side.

12. Both nursing assistants should stand straight, pivoting with feet slightly toward the head of the bed and hip width apart. The foot closest to the head of the bed should be pointed in that direction. Both should bend their knees and maintain the natural curves in the back.

13. The use of a draw, pull, or turning sheet is always preferred for moving a helpless patient up in bed. This is to avoid friction between the patient's skin and bedding. Roll the sides of the sheet to be used as a pull sheet close to the patient. Each nursing assistant then grasps one side of the rolled portion of the sheet firmly so that, when the patient is moved up, the sheet will stay in place under the patient (Figure 7–6◆).

14. You will be sliding the patient's body when you move her up in bed. Slightly bend your knees as you start to slide the patient shifting your weight from one foot to the other.

15. When you say "one, two, three" in unison, you and your partner will move together to slide the patient gently toward the head of the bed or to the desired position.

16. Make the patient comfortable.

17. Replace the pillow, as per the patient's request.

FOLLOW-UP

18. Lower the bed to a position of safety for the patient.

19. Raise the side rails where ordered, indicated, and appropriate for patient safety.

20. Place the call light within easy reach of the patient.

21. Wash your hands.

22. Report to your immediate supervisor:

- That the patient's position has been changed.
- The time the patient's position was changed.
- How the patient tolerated the procedure.
- Your observations of anything unusual.

CHARTING EXAMPLE: 12/30/04 1 pm Moved Mrs. Jaffe up in bed. She reported that her pain medication is relieving her left leg pain L. Goode, CNA

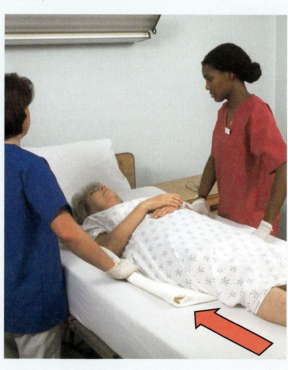

FIGURE 7–6 ◆
Use draw sheet to move helpless patient up in bed

| MOVING A PATIENT UP IN BED WITH THE PATIENT'S HELP | PROCEDURE | OBRA |

RATIONALE: Having the patient assist while being moved provides some muscle exercise for the patient and reduces the weight lifted by the caregiver.

PREPARATION

1. Wash your hands.

2. Identify the patient by checking the identification bracelet.

3. Ask visitors to step out of the room, if this is your hospital's policy.

4. Tell the patient that you are going to move him up in bed. Before you begin, ask your head nurse or team leader if the patient is a cardiac patient and is allowed the necessary exertion for this move.

5. Provide privacy for the patient.

6. Lock the wheels on the bed.

7. Raise the height of the bed to a comfortable working position.

PROCEDURE *(continued)*

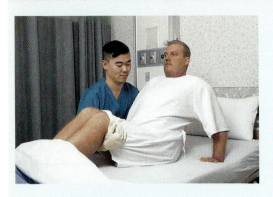

FIGURE 7–7◆
Helping slide the patient toward the head of the bed

8. Lower the backrest and footrest if this is allowed.

STEPS

9. Remove the pillow from under the patient's head. Put the pillow at the top of the bed against the headboard. This will protect the patient's head from hitting the headboard.

10. Put the side rails in the up position on the far side of the bed.

11. Put one hand under the patient's shoulder. Put your other hand under the patient's hip. Provide assistance to the weaker side of the patient.

12. Ask the patient to bend his knees and brace his feet firmly on the mattress.

13. Have your feet hip width apart. The foot closest to the head of the bed should be pointed in that direction.

14. Bend your knees. Maintain the natural curves in your back.

15. Bend your body from your hips and pivot slightly toward the head of the bed.

16. At the signal, "one, two, three," have the patient push toward head of bed with his hands and feet.

17. At the same time, help the patient to move toward the head of the bed by sliding the patient with your hands and arms, as you shift weight from back foot to foot closest to head of bed (Figure 7–7◆).

18. Replace the pillow under the patient's head and shoulders.

FOLLOW-UP

19. Make the patient comfortable.

20. Lower the bed to a position of safety for the patient.

21. Raise the side rails where ordered, indicated, and appropriate for patient safety.

22. Place the call light within easy reach of the patient.

23. Wash your hands.

24. Report to your immediate supervisor:

   - That the patient's position has been changed.

   - The time the patient's position was changed.

   - How the patient tolerated the procedure.

   - Your observations of anything unusual.

CHARTING EXAMPLE: 12/30/04
4pm Moved Mr. Jackson up in bed with her help. M. Jang, CNA

MOVING THE MATTRESS TO THE HEAD OF THE BED WITH THE PATIENT'S HELP

PROCEDURE   OBRA

3. Identify the patient by checking the identification bracelet.

4. Ask visitors to step out of the room, if this is your hospital's policy.

RATIONALE: Having the patient assist while being moved provides some muscle exercise for the patient and reduces the weight lifted by the caregiver.

PREPARATION

1. Wash your hands.

2. Ask another nursing assistant to work with you.

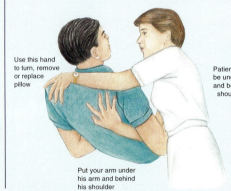

Use this hand to turn, remove or replace pillow

Patient's hand should be under your armpit and behind your shoulder

Put your arm under his arm and behind his shoulder

FIGURE 7–8 ◆
Lock arms with patient

PROCEDURE *(continued)*

5. Tell the patient that you are going to move her mattress to the head of the bed.

6. Provide privacy for the patient.

7. Lock the wheels on the bed.

8. Raise the bed to a comfortable working position.

9. Lower the backrest, if allowed.

STEPS

10. If you are working alone, put the side rail in the up position on the far side of the bed.

11. If you are working with a partner, each of you should stand at opposite sides of the bed and loosen the sheets.

12. Lock arms with the patient and remove the pillow (Figure 7–8◆). Put the pillow on the chair.

13. Ask the patient to grasp the headboard with both hands.

14. Ask the patient to bend her knees and brace her feet firmly on the mattress.

15. Grasp the mattress loops, or grasp the sides of the mattress if there are no loops.

16. At the signal, "one, two, three," have the patient pull with her hands toward the head of the bed and push with her feet against the mattress (Figure 7–9◆).

17. At the same time, both nursing assistants slide the mattress toward the head of the bed, keeping the knees bent and the backs straight.

18. Lock arms with the patient and put the pillow back in place.

FOLLOW-UP

19. Make the patient comfortable.

20. Lower the bed to a position of safety for the patient.

21. Raise the side rails where ordered, indicated, and appropriate for patient safety.

22. Place the call light within easy reach of the patient.

23. Wash your hands.

24. Report to your immediate supervisor:

- That the mattress was moved to the head of the bed with the patient's help.

- The time the mattress was moved to the head of the bed.

- How the patient tolerated the procedure.

- Your observations of anything unusual.

CHARTING EXAMPLE: Moved Mrs. Jackson up in bed with her assistance. L. Goode, CNA

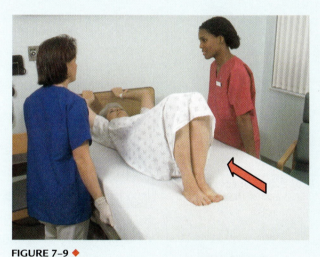

FIGURE 7–9 ◆
On your signal, have patient push with her feet

MOVING A HELPLESS PATIENT TO ONE SIDE OF THE BED ON THE PATIENT'S BACK

PROCEDURE

OBRA

RATIONALE: Safely lifting and turning patients avoids injury to caregivers and the patient.

PREPARATION

1. Wash your hands.

2. Identify the patient by checking the identification bracelet.

3. Ask visitors to step out of the room, if this is your hospital's policy.

4. Tell the patient that you are going to move him to one side of the bed on his back without turning the patient.

5. Provide privacy for the patient.

6. Lock the wheels on the bed.

7. Raise the bed to a comfortable working position.

8. Lower the backrest and footrest, if this is allowed.

PROCEDURE *(continued)*

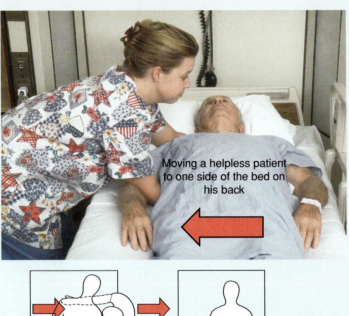

Moving a helpless patient to one side of the bed on his back

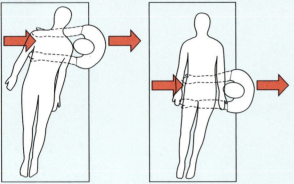

FIGURE 7–10 ◆

Moving a helpless patient to one side of the bed on his back. As a safety measure, this procedure must be done before turning a patient onto his side to ensure that the patient, when turned, is located in the center of the mattress.

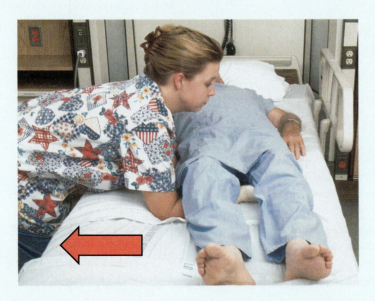

9. Put the side rail in the up position on the far side of the bed.

STEPS

10. Loosen the top sheets, but don't expose the patient.

11. With one leg slightly in front of the other and the front knee slightly bent, slide both your arms under the patient's back to his far shoulder. Slide the patient's shoulders toward you on your arms as you shift weight from the front leg to the back leg while straightening the front leg (Figure 7–10◆).

12. Slide both your arms as far as you can under the patient's hips and slide his hips toward you, again shifting weight from front leg to back leg. Use a pull (turning) sheet whenever possible.

13. Place both your arms under the patient's lower legs and slide them toward you on your arms, again shifting your weight from one leg to the other (Figure 7–11◆).

14. Adjust the pillow, if necessary.

15. Remake the top of the bed.

FOLLOW-UP

16. Make the patient comfortable.

17. Lower the bed to a position of safety for the patient.

18. Raise the side rails where ordered, indicated, and appropriate for patient safety.

19. Place the call light within easy reach of the patient.

FIGURE 7–11 ◆

Using both your arms, slide patient's lower legs toward you

PROCEDURE *(continued)*

20. Wash your hands.

21. Report to your immediate supervisor:
    - That the patient has been moved to one side of the bed on his back.

- The time the patient's position was changed.
- How the patient tolerated the procedure.
- Your observations of anything unusual.

CHARTING EXAMPLE: Documentation usually unnecessary. 12/30/04 4pm Moved Mr. Harp to the left side of his bed. N. Frame, CNA

> **ROLLING THE PATIENT LIKE A LOG (LOG ROLLING)**

PROCEDURE

OBRA

RATIONALE: Safely turning and moving patients avoids injury to caregivers and the patient.

PREPARATION

1. Wash your hands.

2. Identify the patient by checking the identification bracelet.

3. Ask visitors to step out of the room, if this is your hospital's policy.

4. Tell the patient that you are going to roll her to her side like a log.

5. Provide privacy for the patient.

6. Get help, if necessary.

7. Lock the wheels on the bed.

8. Raise the height of the bed to a comfortable working position.

9. Raise the side rail on the far side of the bed.

STEPS

10. Remove the pillow from under the patient's head, if allowed. Put the pillow at the foot of the bed or on a chair. Position the patient's arm across the chest.

11. Position your legs so that one is in front of the other, with the front knee slightly bent.

12. Slide both your arms under the patient's back to her far shoulder; then slide the patient's shoulders toward you on your arms, as you shift your weight from the front leg to the back leg, while straightening your front knee.

13. Grasp the patient under the knees and ankles. Shift your weight from your back foot to the foot closest to the bed as you bend the patient's hips and knees. Place the patient's feet flat on the bed. A pillow may be placed between the patient's legs.

14. Roll the patient onto her side like a log, grasping the patient at her far shoulder and hip/thigh, turning her body as a whole unit. Pull the patient gently toward you (Figure 7–12◆).

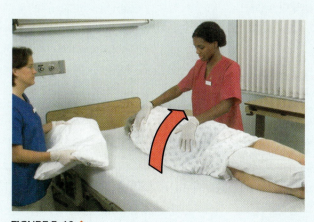

FIGURE 7–12 ◆
Turn patient's body as a whole unit

PROCEDURE *(continued)*

15. Replace the pillow under the patient's head, if allowed.
16. Use pillows against the patient's back to keep her body in proper alignment (Figure 7–13◆).
17. Remake the top of the bed.
18. Reverse the procedure to turn the patient on the opposite side.

FOLLOW-UP

19. Make the patient comfortable.
20. Lower the bed to a position of safety for the patient.
21. Raise the side rails where ordered, indicated, and appropriate for patient safety.
22. Place the call light within easy reach of the patient.
23. Wash your hands.
24. Report to your immediate supervisor:
    - That the patient's position has been changed by log rolling.

- The time the patient's position was changed.
- How the patient tolerated the procedure.
- Your observations of anything unusual.

CHARTING EXAMPLE: 12/30/04 4pm Turned Mrs. Jackson to her right side with assistance. L. Goode, CNA

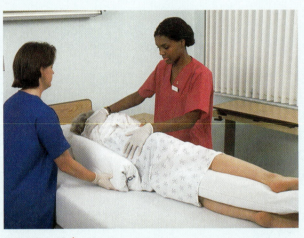

FIGURE 7–13 ◆
Use pillows to maintain proper body alignment

> ### TURNING A PATIENT ONTO THE PATIENT'S SIDE TOWARD YOU

PROCEDURE   OBRA

RATIONALE: Safely turning and moving a patient avoids injury to caregivers and the patient.

PREPARATION

1. Wash your hands.
2. Identify the patient by checking the identification bracelet.
3. Ask visitors to step out of the room, if this is your hospital's policy.

4. Tell the patient you are going to turn her on his side.
5. Provide privacy for the patient.
6. Lock the wheels on the bed.
7. Raise the height of the bed to a comfortable working position.
8. Lower the backrest and footrest, if this is allowed.
9. Put the side rail in the up position on the far side of the bed.

STEPS

10. Loosen the top sheets, but don't expose the patient.

11. When you are turning the patient toward you, cross the patient's arms over the chest, and bend the knees, placing the feet on the bed.
12. With one leg slightly in front of the other and front knee slightly bent, reach across the patient and put one hand behind the far shoulder shifting your weight to the front leg as you do so.
13. Place your other hand behind the far hip; gently roll the patient toward you again as you shift your weight from the front leg to the back leg (Figure 7–14◆).

PROCEDURE *(continued)*

14. Fold a pillow lengthwise and place it against the patient's back for support.
15. Place a pillow under the patient's head.
16. Place the patient's arms and legs in a comfortable position. Be sure the arm nearest the mattress is free from pressure.
17. Remake the top of the bed.

FOLLOW-UP

18. Make the patient comfortable.
19. Lower the bed to a position of safety for the patient.
20. Raise the side rails where ordered, indicated, and appropriate for patient safety.
21. Place the call light within easy reach of the patient.
22. Wash your hands.
23. Report to your immediate supervisor:
    - That the patient's position has been changed.

- The time the patient's position was changed.
- How the patient tolerated the procedure.
- Your observations of anything unusual.

CHARTING EXAMPLE: 12/30/04 4pm Turned and repositioned Mrs. Jackson to her left side. L. Goodman, CNA

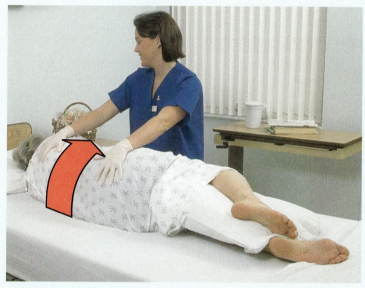

FIGURE 7–14 ◆
Gently roll the patient toward you

TURNING A PATIENT ONTO THE PATIENT'S SIDE AWAY FROM YOU

PROCEDURE

OBRA

RATIONALE: Safely turning and moving a patient avoids injury to caregivers and the patient.

PREPARATION

1. Wash your hands.
2. Identify the patient by checking the identification bracelet.

3. Ask visitors to step out of the room, if this is your hospital's policy.
4. Tell the patient you are going to turn him on the other side.
5. Provide privacy for the patient.
6. Lock the wheels on the bed.
7. Raise the height of the bed to a comfortable working position.
8. Lower the backrest and footrest.
9. Put the side rail in the up position on the far side of the bed.

STEPS

10. Loosen the top sheets, but don't expose the patient.
11. With one leg positioned in front of the other, slide both your arms under the patient's back to the far shoulder as you shift your weight from the back leg to the front leg. Slide the patient's shoulders toward you on your arms as you shift your weight from the front leg to the back leg.

PROCEDURE *(continued)*

12. Slide both your arms as far as you can under the patient's hips and slide the hips toward you again as you shift your weight from the back leg to the front leg. Use a pull (turning) sheet whenever possible.

13. Place both your arms under the patient's lower legs and slide them toward you on your arms as you shift your weight from the front leg to the back leg.

14. Cross the patient's arms over the chest, and bend the patient's knees, placing the feet on the bed.

15. Place one hand on the patient's shoulder near you.

16. Put your other hand along the hip/thigh nearest you.

17. Turn the patient gently on his side, facing away from you (Figure 7–15◆).

18. Fold a pillow lengthwise. Place it against the patient's back for support.

19. Place a pillow under the patient's head.

20. Make sure the patient's arms and legs are in a comfortable position. Put a pillow between the knees if this helps to make the patient comfortable. Be sure the arm nearest the mattress is free from pressure.

21. Remake the top of the bed.

22. Lower the bed to its lowest horizontal position.

FOLLOW-UP

23. Make the patient comfortable.

24. Raise the side rails where ordered, indicated, and appropriate for patient safety.

25. Place the call light within easy reach of the patient.

26. Wash your hands.

27. Report to your immediate supervisor:
    - That the patient's position has been changed.
    - The time the patient's position was changed.

- How the patient tolerated the procedure.
- Your observations of anything unusual.

CHARTING EXAMPLE: 12/30/04 4pm Turned and repositioned Mr. Sausen on his right side. L. Goode, CNA

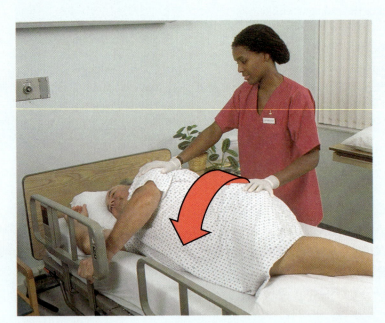

FIGURE 7–15 ◆
Gently turn the patient on his side, facing away from you

REPOSITIONING A PATIENT IN A CHAIR OR WHEELCHAIR

PROCEDURE

OBRA

RATIONALE: Safely repositioning a patient improves body alignment and helps avoids injury to the patient.

PREPARATION

1. Place the patient's feet flat on the floor.

STEPS

2. Bend your knees and place one foot in front of the other.

3. Bend the patient at the waist and gently rock the patient onto the left or right hip, while sliding the other side of the patient's body back into the chair. Repeat for the other side.

4. An alternate technique to adjust the patient's position would be to stand behind the patient in the wheelchair and lift the patient up.

FOLLOW-UP

5. Replace footrests.

CHARTING EXAMPLE: Documentation usually unnecessary. 12/30/04 4pm Repositioned Ms. Jones in her wheelchair. N. Frame, CNA

KEY IDEA

When repositioning a patient in a wheelchair, it is important to remember always to apply techniques for protective body mechanics.

Transporting a Patient by Wheelchair

KEY IDEA

The patient in a wheelchair should be well covered if not dressed in a robe and slippers.

When **transporting** a patient by wheelchair, you may cover the feet as well as the shoulders with a sheet or a blanket, making sure it does not get caught in the wheels. In some institutions the seat of the wheelchair is covered with a piece of linen or with a disposable bed protector if the patient is **incontinent** (unable to control the bowels or bladder). The wheelchair must be wiped off with a disinfectant solution after it has been used by each patient.

When you are transporting a patient in a wheelchair, you should push the wheelchair from behind keeping your body close to the chair, except when entering or leaving elevators. When you are entering an elevator, pull the wheelchair into the elevator backward (Figure 7–16♦). When you are leaving an elevator, ask everyone else to step out first. Push the button marked "open." Turn the chair around, and pull it out of the elevator backward. This may not be necessary with very wide elevators. Take caution not to make contact with other individuals as you push the wheelchair out. Don't move the wheelchair while the elevator is in motion.

When you are moving a patient down a steep incline or ramp, you should take the chair down backward (Figure 7–17♦). To do this, stand behind the chair with your back facing the direction you want to go. Walk backward, holding the chair and moving it carefully down the ramp. Glance back now and then to make sure of your direction and to avoid collisions, as if you were driving a car in reverse.

transporting Moving something or someone from one place to another

incontinent Unable to control the bowels or bladder

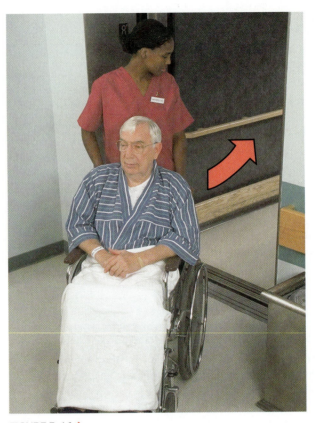

FIGURE 7–16 ◆

Entering an elevator with a patient in a wheelchair

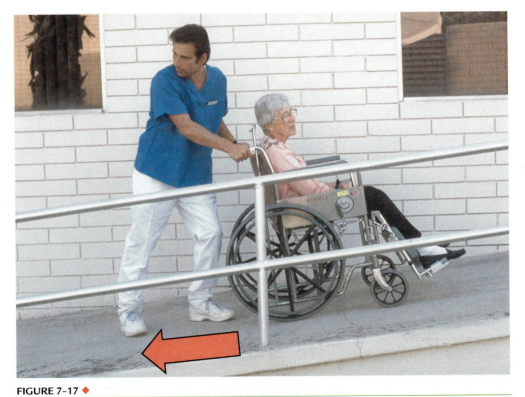

FIGURE 7–17 ◆

Moving down a ramp with a patient in a wheelchair

<table>
<tr><td>

MOVING THE NONAMBULATORY PATIENT INTO A WHEELCHAIR OR ARM CHAIR FROM THE BED

</td><td>

PROCEDURE

</td><td>

OBRA

</td></tr>
</table>

RATIONALE: Safely lifting and moving a patient avoids injury to caregivers and the patient.

PREPARATION

1. Assemble your equipment:

   a. Wheelchair or arm chair

   b. Blanket or sheet

   c. Gait belt, if needed or required

   d. Robe, if desired or needed

2. Wash your hands.

3. Identify the patient by checking the identification bracelet.

4. Ask visitors to step out of the room, if this is your hospital's policy.

5. Tell the patient you are going to help her into a wheelchair.

6. Provide privacy for the patient.

7. Lock the wheels on the bed.

8. Spread a blanket or sheet on the chair. Have the corner of the blanket between the handles over the back so the opposite corner will be at the patient's feet.

9. Ask another nursing assistant to help you (Figure 7–18a-b◆).

STEPS

10. Put the patient's robe and nonskid rubber sole shoes or slippers on while she is in bed.

11. Move the patient to the edge of the bed.

    a. Slide both your arms under the patient's back to the shoulder; then slide the patient's shoulders toward you on your arms.

    b. Slide both your arms as far as you can under the patient's hips and slide the hips toward you.

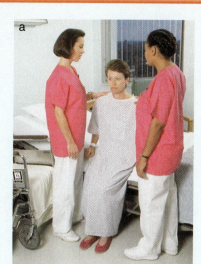

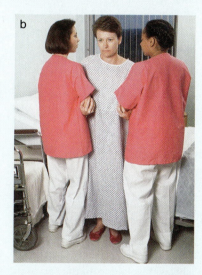

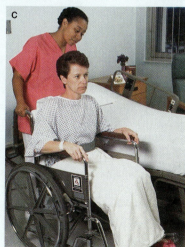

FIGURE 7–18 ◆

Assisting patient to a wheelchair

Use a pull (turning) sheet whenever possible.

   c. Place both your arms under the patient's lower legs and slide them toward you on your arms.

12. Raise the side rail.

13. Lower the bed to its lowest horizontal position so that when you dangle the patient, the feet will touch the floor when she sits up.

14. Raise the back rest so the patient is in a sitting position in bed.

15. Lower the side rail on the side where you and the other nursing assistant will be working.

16. Place both hands under the patient's legs and turn them to the dangling position. The patient's feet should be firmly on the floor. One nursing assistant supports the patient's back and head and raises them at the same time. The other nursing assistant places her arm around the patient's shoulders to support the patient's back while the patient is in the dangling position. Give the patient a minute to adjust. Observe the patient's color.

17. Place a gait belt around the patient's waist her facility policy.

18. Scoot the patient forward to the side of the bed. Place the patient's feet flat on the floor. Support the patient behind the shoulder so that the patient is sitting upright.

19. Place the wheelchair at the bedside with the back of the chair in line with the middle of the bed. Lock the wheels on the chair.

20. Fold up the footrests of the wheelchair so they are out of the way. If the wheelchair has leg rests, adjust them to hang straight down, or remove the footrests/leg rests.

21. Lock the brakes on the wheelchair.

22. Ask patient to hug you in front, around your waist. Then block the

PROCEDURE (continued)

patient's knees between your knees and grasp the gait belt at the patient's sides.

23. The second nursing assistant should be positioned with one knee on the bed.

24. The first assistant, in front, should gently pull the patient forward into the wheelchair while the second assistant guides the patient's hips onto the chair.

25. Fasten the safety straps around the patient to keep her from falling out of the chair (7–18c◆).

26. Arrange the blanket snugly but firmly around the patient. Make sure that no part of the blanket can possibly get caught in the wheels.

27. Adjust the footrests so that the patient's feet are resting comfortably on them.

28. Use the signal cord to call your immediate supervisor and take the patient's pulse and blood pressure if you observe any of the following:

    a. The patient becomes very pale.

    b. The patient seems to be perspiring a lot.

    c. The patient says something like, "I feel weak," "I feel dizzy," or "I feel faint."

29. Adjust the chair to a comfortable angle.

30. Put a pillow behind the patient's back or shoulders, if needed.

FOLLOW-UP

31. Wash your hands.

32. Report to your immediate supervisor:

    ■ That the patient has been moved out of bed into a chair or wheelchair.

    ■ The time the patient's position was changed.

    ■ How the patient tolerated the procedure.

    ■ Your observations of anything unusual.

CHARTING EXAMPLE: 12/30/04 4 pm Moved Mrs. Jackson from her bed to the wheelchair with assistance. B. Gooden, CNA

HELPING A NONAMBULATORY PATIENT BACK INTO BED FROM A WHEEL CHAIR OR ARM CHAIR

PROCEDURE   OBRA

RATIONALE: Safely lifting and moving a patient avoids injury to caregivers and the patient.

PREPARATION

1. Wash your hands.

2. Identify the patient by checking the identification bracelet.

3. Ask visitors to step out of the room, if this is your hospital's policy.

4. Tell the patient you are getting her back into bed.

5. Ask another nursing assistant to help you.

6. Place a pull sheet on the bottom sheets; fan-fold from the top of the bed to the foot.

7. Lock the wheels on the bed.

8. Raise the head of the bed as high as it will go to a sitting position.

9. Lower the bed to its lowest horizontal position.

10. Raise the side rail on the far side of the bed.

STEPS

11. Bring the wheelchair with the patient to the bedside.

12. Position the wheelchair so that the seat of the chair is in line with the middle of the bed. The chair should be positioned so the

patient is transferred from the patient's strongest side.

13. Lock the brakes on the wheelchair.

14. Raise the footrests of the wheelchair, lifting the patient's feet off them and onto the floor at the same time. Remove the footrests if possible.

15. Open up the blanket and safety straps that are on the patient in the wheelchair.

16. Scoot the patient forward in the seat. Place the patient's feet flat on the floor. Support the patient behind the shoulder so that the patient is sitting upright.

17. Place a gait belt around the patient's waist.

PROCEDURE *(continued)*

18. Ask the patient to hug you in front, around your waist. Then block the patient's knees between your knees and grasp the gait belt at the patient's sides.

19. The second nursing assistant should be positioned with one knee on the bed behind the wheelchair.

20. The first assistant, in front, should gently pull the patient forward and up while the second assistant guides the patient's hips onto the bed.

21. Raise that side rail.

22. Raise the bed to waist height.

23. One nursing assistant goes to the far side of the bed.

24. Lower that side rail.

25. Slide both your arms under the patient's back to the shoulder; then slide the patient's shoulders toward you on your arms.

26. Slide both your arms as far as you can under the patient's hips and slide the hips toward you. Use a pull (turning) sheet whenever possible.

27. Keep your knees bent and your back straight as you slide the patient.

28. Place both your arms under the patient's lower legs and slide them toward you on your arms.

29. Both nursing assistants then roll the pull sheet toward the patient and slide the patient up in bed using the pull sheet, using side to side weight shift.

30. Put a pillow under the patient's head.

31. Remake the top of the bed.

FOLLOW-UP

32. Make the patient comfortable.

33. Lower the bed to a position of safety for the patient.

34. Raise the side rails where ordered, indicated, and appropriate for patient safety.

35. Place the call light within easy reach of the patient.

36. Wipe the wheelchair with disinfectant solution and return the chair to its proper place.

37. Wash your hands.

38. Report to your immediate supervisor:
    - That the patient has been put back into bed.
    - The time the patient was put back into bed.
    - How the patient tolerated the procedure.
    - Your observations of anything unusual.

CHARTING EXAMPLE: 12/30/04 4:55pm Moved Mrs. Jackson from the wheelchair back to her bed with assistance. She is resting comfortably. B. Gooden, CNA

HELPING AN AMBULATORY PATIENT WHO CAN STAND, BACK INTO BED FROM A CHAIR OR A WHEELCHAIR

PROCEDURE   OBRA

RATIONALE: Safely lifting and moving a patient avoids injury to caregivers and the patient.

PREPARATION

1. Wash your hands.

2. Identify the patient by checking the identification bracelet.

3. Ask visitors to step out of the room, if this is your hospital's policy.

4. Tell the patient you are getting her back into bed.

5. Provide privacy for the patient.

6. Lock the wheels on the bed.

7. Bring the wheelchair very close to the bed so that the patient's strongest side is closest to bed.

8. Lock the brakes on the wheelchair.

9. Raise the head of the bed to a sitting position.

10. Lower the bed to its lowest horizontal position.

STEPS

11. Raise the footrests of the wheelchair, or remove them. Place the patient's feet on the floor.

12. Open up the safety straps on the wheelchair.

13. Help the patient out of the wheelchair to stand, pivot (turn), and sit on the side of the bed. The patient's feet should be resting firmly on the floor.

PROCEDURE *(continued)*

14. Lean the patient against the backrest.

15. Put one arm around the patient's shoulders for support. Put your other arm under the patient's knees.

16. Swing the patient's body slowly around, helping the patient lift the legs onto the bed.

17. Raise the side rail.

18. Lower the head of the bed.

19. Help the patient move to the center of the bed.

20. Place a pillow under the patient's head.

21. Remove the patient's robe and nonskid shoes or slippers.

22. Remake the top of the bed.

FOLLOW-UP

23. Make the patient comfortable.

24. Lower the bed to a position of safety for the patient.

25. Raise the side rails where ordered, indicated, and appropriate for patient safety.

26. Place the call light within easy reach of the patient.

27. Fold the blanket from the wheelchair and put it in its proper place.

28. Wash the wheelchair with an antiseptic or disinfectant solution and return it to its proper place.

29. Wash your hands.

30. Report to your immediate supervisor:

    - That you have helped the patient back into bed.
    - The time you helped the patient back into bed.
    - How the patient tolerated the procedure.
    - Your observations of anything unusual.

CHARTING EXAMPLE: 12/30/04 8:55pm Moved Mrs. Jackson from the bedside chair back into her bed. She was able to stand and bear her weight with minimal assistance. She is resting comfortably. B. Gooden, CNA

USING A PORTABLE MECHANICAL PATIENT LIFT TO MOVE THE HELPLESS PATIENT

PROCEDURE   OBRA

RATIONALE: Correct use of mechanical lifts to move helpless patients reduces the weight lifted by the caregiver and eliminates back injuries.

PREPARATION

1. Assemble your equipment: mechanical patient lift and sling. (Figure 7–19a-b◆).

2. Wash your hands.

3. Identify the patient by checking the identification bracelet.

4. Ask visitors to step out of the room, if this is your hospital's policy.

5. Tell the patient you are going to get him out of bed by using the portable mechanical patient lift. This kind of lift is sometimes referred to as a Hoyer lift (Figure 7–20◆). (You may need the help of a second nursing assistant as a partner.)

6. Provide privacy for the patient.

7. Position the chair next to the bed with the back of the chair in line with the headboard of the bed.

Lock the wheels of the bed and the mechanical lift.

8. Cover the chair with a blanket or sheet.

STEPS

9. By turning the patient from side to side on the bed, slide the sling under the patient.

10. Attach the sling to the mechanical lift with the hooks in place through the metal frame. Be sure to apply hooks with open, sharp ends away from the patient.

11. Have the patient fold both arms across his chest, if possible.

PROCEDURE (continued)

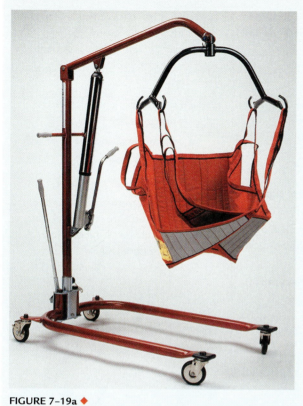

FIGURE 7–19a ◆
(Photo courtesy of Guardian Products, a division of Sunrise Medical)

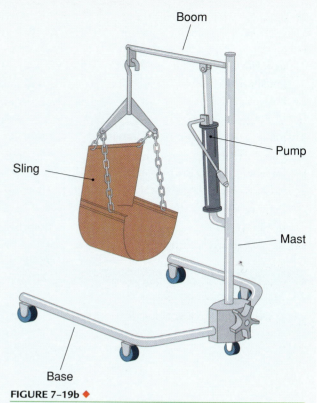

FIGURE 7–19b ◆
Components of a mechanical lift

12. Using the crank, lift the patient from the bed.

13. Have your partner, a second nursing assistant, guide the patient's legs.

14. Lower the patient into the chair.

15. Remove the hooks from the frame of the portable mechanical patient lift.

16. Wrap the patient with the blanket.

17. Secure the patient to the chair with safety straps, if necessary.

18. Leave the patient safe and comfortable in the chair for the proper amount of time, according to your instructions.

19. To get the patient back to bed, put the hooks through the metal frame of the sling, which is still under the patient.

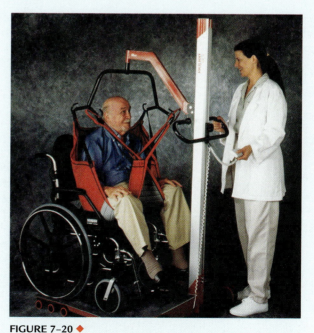

FIGURE 7–20 ◆
Hoyer lift (Photo courtesy of Guardian Products, a division of Sunrise Medical)

PROCEDURE *(continued)*

20. Raise the patient by using the crank on the mechanical patient lift. Lift him from the chair into the bed. Have your partner guide the patient's legs.

21. Lower the patient into the center of the bed.

22. Remove the hooks from the frame.

23. Remove the sling from under the patient by having the patient turn from side to side on the bed.

24. Put a pillow under the patient's head.

25. Remake the top of the bed.

FOLLOW-UP

26. Make the patient comfortable.

27. Lower the bed to a position of safety for the patient.

28. Raise the side rails where ordered, indicated, and appropriate for patient safety.

29. Place the call light within easy reach of the patient.

30. Wash the mechanical patient lift with an antiseptic or disinfectant solution and return it to its proper place.

31. Wash your hands.

32. Report to your immediate supervisor:

    ■ That the patient was taken out of bed by means of the portable mechanical patient lift.

    ■ The time the patient was taken out of bed.

    ■ The prescribed length of time that the patient sat in a chair.

■ That the patient was put back into bed by means of the portable mechanical patient lift.

■ The time the patient was put back into bed.

■ How the patient tolerated the procedure.

■ Your observations of anything unusual.

CHARTING EXAMPLE: 12/30/04 8:55pm Used mechanical lift to move Mr. Trotta from a wheelchair to his bed. He is resting comfortably. L. Slaughter, CNA

Using a Stretcher

stretcher A wheeled cart on which patients are moved from one place to another

A hospital **stretcher** is a wheeled cart on which patients are moved from one place to another. When moving a helpless patient from the patient's bed to a stretcher, you will need a second nursing assistant working as your partner.

KEY IDEA

Whenever you are moving a stretcher, you should stand at the end where the patient's head is and push the stretcher so the patient's feet are moving first. Keep your body close to the stretcher. Be careful to protect the patient's head at all times.

When entering an elevator, push the stop button so the doors of the elevator will not close until you are ready. Pull the stretcher into the elevator with the head-end first (Figure 7–21◆). Stand at the patient's head while the elevator is in motion. When you leave the elevator, press the stop button and push the stretcher out foot-end first.

Use side rails or restraining straps whenever you move a patient on a stretcher. Check the straps before you move the stretcher. Guide the stretcher from the foot-end when going down a ramp.

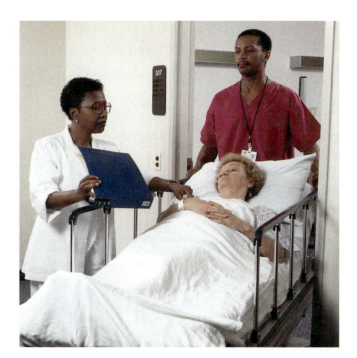

FIGURE 7–21 ◆

Entering an elevator with a stretcher

<table>
<tr><td>

MOVING A PATIENT FROM THE BED TO A STRETCHER

</td><td>

PROCEDURE

</td><td>

OBRA

</td></tr>
</table>

RATIONALE: Safely lifting and moving a patient avoids injury to caregivers and the patient.

PREPARATION

1. Assemble your equipment:
   a. Stretcher
   b. Sheet or blanket
2. Ask another nursing assistant to help you. The two of you should work in unison to move the patient from the bed to a stretcher.
3. Wash your hands.
4. Identify the patient by checking the identification bracelet.
5. Tell the patient you are going to move him from the bed to a stretcher.
6. Ask visitors to step out of the room, if this is your hospital's policy.
7. Provide privacy for the patient.

STEPS

8. Loosen the top sheets.
9. Cover the patient with a blanket or sheet. Remove the top sheets without exposing the patient.
10. Move the stretcher next to the bed.
11. Raise the bed so that it is the same height as the stretcher. Lock the wheels on the bed.
12. Lock the wheels on the stretcher.
13. You will stand on the far side of the bed, using your body to hold the bed in place.
14. Your partner will stand on the far side of the stretcher, using her body to hold the stretcher in place.
15. Position your legs so that one is in front of the other, bend your knees, and maintain the natural curves in your back.
16. At the signal, "one, two, three," push, pull, and slide the patient from the bed to the stretcher, while shifting your weight from the front leg to the back leg (if you are the assistant positioned on stretcher side) or from the back leg to the front leg (if you are the assistant positioned on bed side). Use a pull (turning) sheet whenever possible (Figure 7–22◆).
17. Support the patient's head and feet, keeping the body covered with a loose blanket or sheet.
18. Fasten the stretcher straps around the patient at the hips and shoulders.
19. Put the side rails of the stretcher in the up position for the patient's safety.

FOLLOW-UP

20. Wash your hands.
21. Report to your immediate supervisor:
    - That you have moved the patient from the bed to a stretcher.
    - The time you moved the patient to the stretcher.
    - How the patient tolerated the procedure.
    - Your observations of anything unusual.

PROCEDURE (continued)

CHARTING EXAMPLE: 12/30/04
2pm Moved Mr. Ricard from his bed
to a stretcher with assistance.
P. Allende, CNA

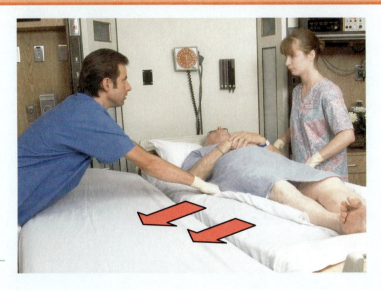

FIGURE 7–22 ◆

Moving the patient from the bed to the stretcher

MOVING A PATIENT FROM A STRETCHER TO THE BED

PROCEDURE   OBRA

RATIONALE: Safely lifting and moving a patient avoids injury to caregivers and the patient.

PREPARATION

1. Assemble your equipment:
   a. Stretcher
   b. Sheet or blanket
2. Ask three other nursing assistants to help you. You should work in unison to move the patient from the bed to a stretcher.
3. Wash your hands.
4. Identify the patient by checking the identification bracelet.
5. Tell the patient you are going to move him from the stretcher to the bed.
6. Ask visitors to step out of the room, if this is your hospital's policy.
7. Provide privacy for the patient.
8. Lock the wheels on the bed.

9. Fan-fold the top sheet to the bottom of the bed.
10. Bring the stretcher next to the bed.
11. Raise the bed so that it is level with the stretcher.
12. Lock the wheels on the stretcher.

STEPS

13. Two nursing assistants stand by the far side of the bed, using their bodies to hold the bed in place.
14. The other two nursing assistants stand by the far side of the stretcher, using their bodies to hold the stretcher in place.
15. Open the stretcher straps.
16. Bend your knees, maintaining the natural curves in your back, and position your legs so that one is in front of the other.
17. At the signal, "one, two, three," slide the patient from the stretcher to the bed. Use a pull (turning) sheet whenever possible.
18. Keep the patient covered with a loose blanket or sheet and support the head and feet.

FOLLOW-UP

19. Make the patient as comfortable as possible.
20. Replace the top sheets, removing the blanket without exposing the patient.
21. Lower the bed to a position of safety for the patient.
22. Raise the side rails where ordered, indicated, and appropriate for patient safety.
23. Place the call light within easy reach of the patient.
24. Wash your hands.
25. Report to your immediate supervisor:
    - That you have moved the patient from the stretcher to the bed.
    - The time you moved the patient from the stretcher to the bed.
    - How the patient tolerated the procedure.

CHARTING EXAMPLE: 12/30/04
7pm Moved Mrs. Jackson from a stretcher to her bed with assistance
B. Gooden, CNA

Assisting the Patient to Ambulate

Ambulation is the act or process of walking. Patients who have been ill, injured, or received surgery and as a result have been in bed for any period of time become weak. They may experience difficulty walking. If the patient has not been out of bed, proceed in steps. First allow the patient to sit on the side of the bed with his feet dangling. If the patient tolerates this well and is not dizzy and does not experience a drop in blood pressure, assist him to a bedside chair. Allow the patient to bear some weight in the transfer process. Next the patient can try walking in his room with or without assistance. Patients who are unsteady on their feet can benefit from having a gait belt in place. Patients may require walkers, canes, or crutches to safely ambulate.

ambulation The act or process of walking

Using a Gait Belt

Use of a gait belt positioned snugly around the patient's waist will help to control the patient while walking. Position yourself slightly behind the weaker side of the patient. Have the patient's stronger side close to a wall if available. Keep one hand on the gait belt at all times (see Chapters 6 and 32).

HELPING A PATIENT TO WALK

PROCEDURE

OBRA

RATIONALE: Patients require assistance to ambulate if they have become weak due to illness, surgery, or injury.

PREPARATION

1. Assemble equipment
   a. Robe, nonskid slippers
   b. Gait belt
2. Identify the patient by checking the identification bracelet.
3. Tell the patient you will assist him to ambulate.
4. Provide privacy for the patient.
5. Wash your hands.
6. Lower bed to lowest position.

STEPS

7. Assist patient to sitting position with feet dangling over the side of the bed.
8. Help patient put on robe and slippers.
9. Observe for dizziness and check for hypotension (decreased blood pressure) if this is the first time the patient has attempted ambulation since the illness or surgery.
10. Apply the gait belt around the patient's waist.
11. Assist the patient to stand.
    a. Stand facing the patient.
    b. Grasp the gait belt with both your hands.
    c. Place your knee against the patient's knee and place your right foot between the patient's feet.
    d. Pull the patient up to a standing position as you straighten your knees.
    e. Keep your hands on the gait belt as you move behind or beside the patient and wait while he gains his balance.
    f. Ask the patient to stand up straight and hold his head up.
12. Assist the patient to walk. Provide support as you walk slightly behind the patient.
13. Walk the required distance or whatever lesser amount the patient can tolerate. Do not rush or hurry the patient and provide encouragement.
14. Return the patient to his bed and assist him back into it.
15. Remove gait belt, robe, and slippers.

FOLLOW-UP

16. Make the patient comfortable.
17. Lower the bed to a position of safety for the patient.
18. Raise the side rails where ordered, indicated, and appropriate for patient safety.
19. Place the call light within easy reach of the patient.
20. Wash your hands.
21. Report to your immediate supervisor:
    - That you have helped the patient back into bed.
    - The time you helped the patient back into bed.
    - How the patient tolerated the procedure.
    - Your observations of anything unusual.

CHARTING EXAMPLE: 12/29/03
2pm Assisted Mr. Curry to ambulate while being supported with a gait belt. He was able to walk to the door of his room and back. After Mr. Curry returned to his bed he said he felt tired but was glad to finally be up out of bed. H. Knight, CNA

FIGURE 7–23 ◆

A walker may be used when the patient requires some support due to imbalance or weakness

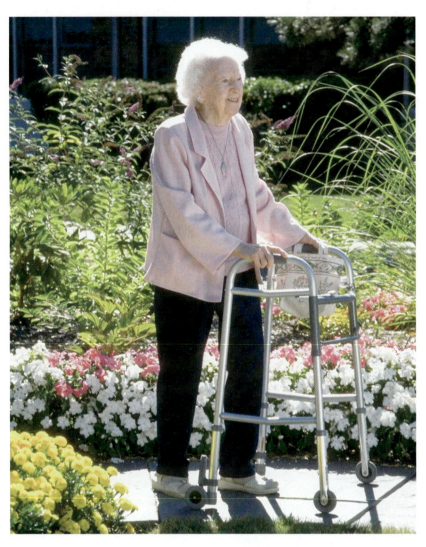

Using a Cane, Walker, or Crutches

Canes, crutches, and walkers (Figure 7–23◆) are pieces of equipment that may be used by the patient to ambulate safely. These pieces of equipment help support the patient while walking and may be ordered by the physician. (See Chapters 6, 16, and 32.)

Assisting a Falling Patient

ASSISTING A FALLING PATIENT	GUIDELINES	OBRA

- If a patient begins to fall, move your feet apart to increase your stability, bend your knees, and lower your body to the floor with the patient. Keep the patient's body close to you.
- Hold onto the patient from behind, placing your arms under the patient's arms and placing your hands on his

transfer or gait belt to help ease him to the floor.
- Maintain the natural curves in your back.
- If the patient is next to a wall when he begins to fall, use the wall to assist in easing the patient to the floor.
- Protect the patient's head from injury.

- Stay with the patient, call for help, and do not move the patient until you are instructed to do so.
- Always ask for assistance to help patient back to a standing position.
- Report the details to your supervisor or charge nurse and complete an incident report.

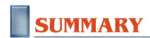

SUMMARY

The use of proper/protective body mechanics during daily work tasks such as positioning, moving, and lifting patients will help you avoid back and shoulder injuries and leave you with more energy at the end of the day. Always ask for assistance when you feel you are unable to perform a task safely on your own.

NOTES

CHAPTER REVIEW

FILL IN THE BLANK Read each sentence and fill in the blank lines with a word that completes the sentence.

1. _____ _____ _____ are special ways of standing and moving to make the best use of strength and to avoid fatigue.

2. A _____ is a covering used to provide privacy during an examination or operation.

3. _____ _____ positions are used to promote comfort and to relieve pressure points.

4. Whenever you are pushing a stretcher, you should be at the end where the patient's _____ is.

5. Use of a _____ _____ positioned snugly around the patient's waist will help you to control the patient while walking.

MULTIPLE CHOICE Choose the best answer for each question or statement.

1. Which one of the following is not a guideline for proper body mechanics?
   a. Position your body close to the load.
   b. Lift and carry rather than push an object.
   c. Use good posture.
   d. Keep your feet slightly apart for better balance.

2. The supine position refers to which patient position?
   a. lying on back
   b. head of the bed up 45–90 degrees
   c. lying down or reclining with the knees bent, soles of the feet flat on the bed
   d. none of the above

3. Trendelenburg's position is used to treat patients who are experiencing
   a. cardiac arrest.
   b. diabetes.
   c. shock.
   d. seizures.

4. The dorsal lithotomy position is used for
   a. shock.
   b. physical exam of the bladder or vagina.
   c. physical exam of the patient's back.
   d. physical exam of the spine.

5. Which of these activities is not a follow-up activity to report to the nurse?
   a. Reporting that the patient's position has been changed.
   b. How many people were required to move the patient.
   c. How the patient tolerated the move.
   d. The time of the position change.

TIME-OUT

TIPS FOR TAKING CARE OF YOURSELF

Ask for help when you need it. It is safer for you and for the patients if you have assistance with procedures that you cannot handle alone. Others with more experience may not require the same amount of help for the same things, but everyone needs help sometimes.

THE NURSING ASSISTANT IN ACTION

You are assigned to assist Mr. Bigg, a helpless 320-pound patient, from a wheelchair to his bed. You bring the mechanical lift to his room and have requested a coworker to help you. When you start explaining what you plan to do, Mr. Bigg resists. He says: "You are not going to use that contraption on me! The last time I was in that thing, the staff person did not know how to work it and frightened me. I am staying right where I am!"

What Is Your Response/Action?

CRITICAL THINKING

CUSTOMER SERVICE When you prepare to assist a helpless patient to the bedside chair, first ask if she needs to use the restroom or if she is in pain. The patient will be more comfortable if her immediate needs are taken care of. Let the patient know you will be checking on her and approximately how long she will be in the chair. Be sure she has a call light within easy reach.

CULTURAL CARE Some patients are very quiet and may not complain of pain. Be sure to check and ask specifically if you think a patient is experiencing pain when you move him or assist him up in bed. Watch for face grimaces, gritting of teeth, increased respirations, or any other sign that indicates the person you are assisting is in pain.

COOPERATION WITHIN THE TEAM Lifting and moving a patient is usually easier with two people. Team up with a coworker and work together to turn, move, or assist patients into chairs for meals. Use the mechanical lifts whenever possible to avoid back injuries.

EXPLORE MediaLink

Additional interactive resources for this chapter can be found on the Companion Website at www.prenhall.com/wolgin. Click on Chapter 7 and "Begin" to seldect activities for this chapter.

For chapter-related NCLEX-style questions and an audio glossary, access the accompanying CD-ROM in this book.

Video:

- Activity and Exercise; Assisting with Ambulation

—One Assistant
—Assisting a Falling Client

8 Admitting, Transferring, and Discharging a Patient

KEY TERMS

admission
assessing
convalescence
discharge
evaluating
holistic
implementing
patient plan of care
physiological
planning
psychological
sociocultural
spiritual
transfer

OBJECTIVES

When you have completed this chapter, you will be able to:

- Explain your role in following the patient plan of care.
- Admit a patient to the nursing unit by following the correct procedure.
- Weigh and measure a patient.
- Follow the correct procedure to transfer a patient to another room or unit within the institution.
- Describe the components of a discharge and patient health education plan and explain the importance of the plan.
- List the discharge planning activities.
- Discharge a patient from the institution following the correct procedure.
- Help make the patient feel comfortable and secure during all activities.

MediaLink

www.prenhall.com/wolgin

Use the address above to access the free, interactive Companion Website created for this textbook. Get hints, instant feedback, and textbook references to chapter-related NCLEX-style questions. Link to other interesting sites.

AUDIO GLOSSARY:

Use the Companion Website, or the CD-ROM disk enclosed with your textbook, to hear the pronunciation of key terms in the chapter.

The admission process is a patient's first glimpse of the individuals who will be providing health care. Nursing assistants can ease the patient's anxiety and help the patient prepare for whatever is ahead. Often, it is necessary for the patient to move from one room in an institution to another. Performing this procedure smoothly will ease anxiety and promote comfort for the patient in the new room. Finally, an expertly performed discharge procedure will increase the patient's confidence at home.

AGE-SPECIFIC CONSIDERATIONS

Admitting, Transferring, and Discharging a Patient

Being admitted to a health care facility or being transferred to a new place in a health care institution is a nervous time for patients of all ages. Children wonder what might happen to them and may be frightened of the equipment and noises of the environment. Allow parents to stay with the child as much as possible. Explain things to the child in simple language. Let the child touch and explore as much equipment as possible. For the adolescent, avoid the use of medical jargon. Maintain privacy, but let them know their parents are available if they want them. For adults and the elderly, allow them to make as many decisions as possible. Explain things in terms that they can understand and allow time for questions and concerns.

At the time of discharge, prepare the patient to go home. For children, this might mean explaining in simple terms the healing process at home and any instructions. Most care needs will be handled by their parents. Adolescents will want to know more about what to do at home and about restrictions. Avoid the use of medical jargon. Answer questions directly with the adolescent and not just with the parents. When discharging the adult and the elderly patient, consider their lifestyles and learning preferences. Emphasize how the information will help them and allow time for questions.

> **ALERT**
>
> For all patient contact, adhere to Standard Precautions (⊙ Chapter 5, pages 83–85). Wear protective equipment as indicated.

Admitting the Patient

A patient coming into a health care institution may be frightened and uncomfortable. The patient may or may not be seriously ill or in pain, but this is a time when you, as a member of the nursing team, are very important to the patient. Being pleasant and courteous from the time the patient enters the institution door until he is settled will make the patient's **admission** process easier.

admission The administrative process that covers the period from the time the patient enters the institution door to the time the patient is settled

KEY IDEA

A nice, relaxed environment and welcome will create a favorable first impression of the health care facility for the patient.

Introduce yourself (Figure 8–1◆). Learn the patient's name and use it often. Do not call an adult patient by the first name unless given permission to do so. Remember that the way you speak and behave will have a lot to do with the patient's impression of the institution. Smile and be friendly. Do not appear to be rushed or busy with other things. Do your work quietly and efficiently.

When admitting a patient to your institution, keep in mind the purpose for the patient's admission. A patient might be having surgery, undergoing a procedure, seeking treatment for an illness, or require long-term assistance with living.

FIGURE 8–1 ◆

Help to make the admission of the patient as pleasant as possible

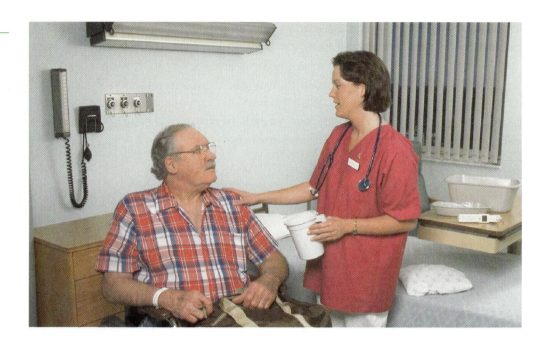

patient plan of care

A written plan stating the nursing diagnosis, the patient goals or expected outcomes, and the nursing orders, interventions, or actions to be taken

assessing Gathering facts to identify needs and problems

planning Deciding what to do and how to do it

implementing Carrying out or accomplishing a given plan

evaluating Determining whether a plan (such as the patient care plan) has been effective

Each institution will have its own policies and procedures for admitting a patient. The nursing team will provide the patient (and the patient's family) with general information to help them to become more familiar with the institution. This information includes a description of the unit's usual activities, usual mealtimes, information about any tests or procedures the patient is to have, and information about the visiting hours of the unit.

Patient Plan of Care

Upon admission or shortly thereafter, an individualized **patient plan of care** is written by the registered nurse. This plan serves as a course of action to assist the patient to achieve optimum wellness (Figure 8–2◆). Patient plans of care are one way for the nursing team to communicate. They provide a structure for **assessing**, **planning**, **implementing**, and **evaluating** individualized care. The assessing and planning stages involve gathering information to identify needs and problems and deciding what to do and how to do it; the implementing and evaluating stages involve carrying out the plan and then determining whether or not the plan worked. Each plan is written to meet the individual needs of the patient. One reason for the written care plan is to ensure that continuous and

FIGURE 8–2 ◆

A sample care plan form

NURSING CARE PLAN				
DATE IDENTIFIED	NURSING DIAGNOSIS	DATE RESOLVED	PATIENT GOAL EXPECTED OUTCOME	NURSING ORDERS INTERVENTIONS/ ACTIONS

consistent care is provided for each patient. The registered nurse will review and discuss the patient's choices and decisions related to the patient's care. These choices and decisions will be reflected in the patient's plan of care.

The admitting registered nurse begins the plan by collecting information for a health history and completing a physical examination. Patient problems and nursing diagnoses are identified, long- and short-term goals are determined, and nursing interventions or actions are planned to help the patient reach these goals. The registered nurse reevaluates the plan of care daily to meet the changing needs of the patient. This reevaluation is continued until discharge and includes patient health education and a discharge plan. All members of the multidisciplinary health care team collaborate on the plan of care and assist the patient to reach the goals by carrying out the interventions written into the plan.

The parts of the plan of care most directly involving the nursing assistant are the activities of daily living, direct bedside care, and making and reporting objective, factual observations. Nursing assistants can observe and report patient progress toward meeting goals. (See Chapter 12 for a checklist of the activities of daily living.) The nursing assistant may read the plan of care for each assigned patient to ensure that the plan is followed. When the plan of care is well developed and used appropriately, it is the single most important tool in providing quality patient care.

ADMITTING THE PATIENT

PROCEDURE

OBRA

RATIONALE: A patient is admitted when he requires care provided in that unit. The process includes collecting, documenting, and sharing information needed to plan the patient's care needs.

PREPARATION

1. Assemble your equipment on the bedside table:

   a. Admission checklist, if used in your institution

   b. Urine specimen container and laboratory requisition slip

   c. Institution gown or pajamas (if part of institutional policy)

   d. Clothing list

   e. Portable scale

   f. Blood pressure cuff and stethoscope

   g. Admission pack (contents vary in each health care institution)

   h. Thermometer

   i. Bedpan and/or urinal, emesis basin, and wash basin (may be in admission pack in some health care institutions)

2. Wash your hands.

3. Fan-fold the bed covers down to the foot of the bed to open the bed.

4. Place the hospital gown or pajamas at the foot of the bed.

5. Put the bedpan, urinal, emesis basin, wash basin, and admission pack in the proper place in the bedside table drawer or stand.

STEPS

6. When the patient arrives on the floor, introduce yourself to the patient and to any visitors. Smile, be friendly. Call the patient by his name. Offer to shake hands and tell the patient your name and job title.

7. Escort the patient to his room. The patient may be escorted to the room by an auxiliary worker. Introduce the patient to any roommates.

8. Ask the visitors to leave the room while you finish admitting the patient, if this is your hospital's policy.

9. Close the door in a private room, or draw the curtain around the bed for privacy.

10. Ask the patient to change into the hospital gown or his own pajamas. If necessary, help the patient get undressed and into the gown. Weigh the patient (see *Procedure: Weighing and Measuring the Height of a Patient Who Is Able to Stand*).

11. Help the patient to get into the bed or allow him to sit in a chair if he is not ordered on bed rest.

12. Raise the side rails on the bed, if necessary.

13. Complete the admission checklist for your institution (Figure 8–3◆).

ADMISSION CHECKLIST
(Fill in every statement and check every appropriate item)

Patient's name _____ Room Number _____

Time of admission _____ a.m./p.m.   Date of admission _____

Admitted by stretcher _____ wheelchair _____ walking _____

Check identification bracelet? Yes ☐ No ☐   Bed tag in place? Yes ☐ No ☐

Side rails up? Yes ☐ No ☐

Bruises, marks, rashes, or broken skin noted? Yes ☐ No ☐

    If yes, describe _____

Weight _____ Height _____   Scale used? Yes ☐ No ☐

Temperature _____ Pulse _____   Respirations _____   Blood Pressure _____

Admission urine specimen collected? Yes _____ ☐ No ☐   Sent to lab? Yes ☐ No ☐

Is the patient allergic to food? Yes ☐ _____ No ☐   Allergic to drugs? Yes ☐ _____ No ☐

Reason for admission _____

Complaints _____

What are your concerns about this hospitalization (Circle all that apply)

    Illness   Test/procedures   Family   Job   Financial

    Surgery   Insurance   Other   None

Have you felt downhearted and blue or see things as hopeless? Yes ☐ No ☐

Do you know why? _____

_____

What is your source of hope and strength? _____

Is there anything else we should know about in order to take care of you? (Dietary, cultural, religious needs or requests?) _____

_____

Highest grade in school completed: _____

How do you learn best? (Check all that apply)

    Reading   Videos

    Verbal instructions   Hands on   With Family Present

                                                           Interpreter needed:

Do you have difficulty with reading? Yes ☐ No ☐

Language spoken if not English: _____

Do you have education needs in any of these areas? (Circle all that apply)   Ability to learn or barriers to learning:

Activity/exercise   Coping/stress   Diet   Disease process

Wound/Incision care   Treatments   Medications   Self Care

Dentures? Yes ☐ No ☐   Partial? Yes ☐ No ☐   Full? Yes ☐ No ☐

    Denture Cup? Yes ☐ No ☐

Vision problems? Yes ☐ No ☐   Does the patient wear glasses? Yes ☐ No ☐   Contacts? Yes ☐ No ☐

Valuables: Money? Yes ☐ No ☐   Describe _____

    Jewelery? Yes ☐ No ☐ Describe _____

Is the patient hard of hearing? Yes ☐ No ☐   Hearing aid? Yes ☐ No ☐

    Artificial limb? Yes ☐ _____ No ☐   Brace? Yes ☐ _____ No ☐

Has the patient been admitted to this hospital before? Yes ☐ No ☐

Is the clothing list complete? Yes ☐ No ☐   Signed by _____

Is the signal cord attached to the bed? Yes ☐ No ☐

Have drugs brought into the hospital by the patient been given to the charge nurse? Yes ☐ No ☐

Name of the nurse drugs were given to _____

Was the patient told not to eat or drink anything until the doctor's visit? Yes ☐ No ☐

Admitted by _____

FIGURE 8–3◆

Admission checklist

PROCEDURE *(continued)*

14. Have the patient place any personal toilet articles and small belongings into or on top of the bedside table. If the patient is unable to do this, you may do it yourself.

15. Ask your immediate supervisor if the patient is NPO or is allowed to have drinking water. If drinking water is allowed, fill the water pitcher.

16. To familiarize the patient with his new surroundings, point out the signal cord or call bell (Figure 8–4◆). Attach the signal cord to the bed where the patient can reach it easily. Test the signal cord, demonstrating and explaining how the intercom system works.

Permit the patient to try the signal cord light.

17. Explain the health care institution's policy on radios, television, newspapers, and mail. Tell the patient at what times his meals will be served. Help the patient to fill out the dietary slip for the next meal, if this is part of your institution's procedure.

18. Make the patient comfortable. Adjust the lights to the patient's preference. Be sure the top sheets and blankets are arranged properly.

19. If the patient is allowed to have the head of the bed elevated and the knee gatch adjusted as high or low

as is comfortable, adjust these to a position of comfort. (Check before gatching the bed as a specific order may be required.) If the bed is self-adjustable, explain how the bed works and show the patient how to adjust it. Lower the bed to a position of safety for the patient.

20. Pull the curtains back to the open position.

21. Raise the side rails where ordered, indicated, and appropriate for patient safety.

FOLLOW-UP

22. Wash your hands.

23. Report to your immediate supervisor:

- That you have completed the admission.
- That the patient is in bed or sitting in a chair.
- That you have completed the admission checklist.
- That the side rails are in the up or down position.
- How the patient tolerated the procedure.
- Your observations of anything unusual.

CHARTING EXAMPLE: 12/12/05 8pm Admitted Mr. Chang to his room, #313. Completed admission checklist and provided information about the room and facility to Mr. Chang. He is resting comfortably in bed. S. Fowler, CNA

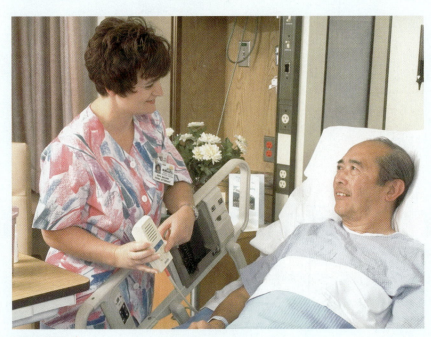

FIGURE 8–4 ◆
Point out the call button to the patient

There are several ways that the patient plan of care can help the nursing assistant provide quality care on a daily basis. The plan of care provides:

- Specific instructions regarding care to be given
- Information needed prior to giving care
- Guidelines for continuity of care
- Information essential for organizing and planning work or special duties

Each health care institution has its own policies and procedures related to the patient's plan of care. Be sure you understand and follow your employer's policies.

Weighing and Measuring

Weights and heights are recorded to provide an important database. Accuracy is important because some medications are ordered based on weight. Nutrition problems are another area where weights are very important and used for comparison and progress evaluation.

FIGURE 8–5 ◆

Types of Scales: (a) standing scale, (b) scale with a mechanical lift, (c) wheelchair scale, (d) bed scale

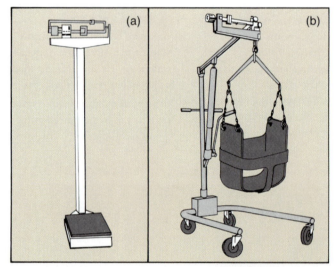

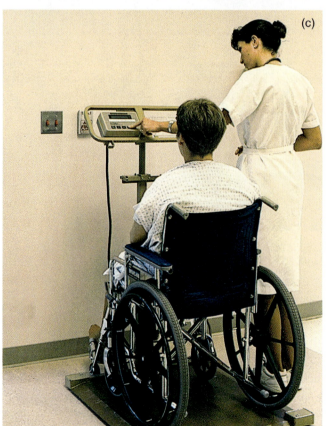

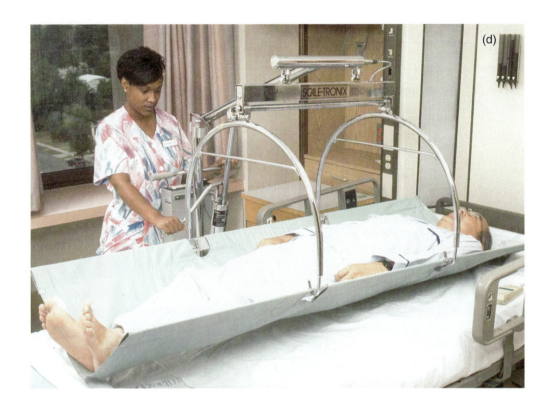

(d)

Many health care institutions have special equipment such as the scale with a mechanical lift for weighing the patient who is unable to stand. Some institutions have special scales with bars on them to assist the patient in standing straight and to keep the patient from falling. For example, a bed scale is used for the patient on complete bed rest. Follow your institution's procedures for these different types of scales (Figure 8–5a-d◆).

WEIGHING AND MEASURING THE HEIGHT OF A PATIENT WHO IS ABLE TO STAND

PROCEDURE

OBRA

RATIONALE: Weight and height are measured to provide accurate data needed to determine medication dosages or treatment needs.

PREPARATION

1. Assemble your equipment:
   a. Portable balance scale
   b. Paper towel
   c. Notepaper
   d. Pen or pencil
2. Wash your hands.

3. Identify the patient by checking the identification bracelet.
4. Ask visitors to step out of the room, if this is your hospital's policy.
5. Tell the patient that you are going to weigh her.
6. Pull the curtain around the bed for privacy.

PROCEDURE *(continued)*

7. Balance the scale. To do this, make sure the scale is standing level. Both weights (poises) must point to zero (0). If they do not, turn the balance screw until the pointer of the balance beam stays steadily in the middle of the balance area. The scale is now balanced.

STEPS

8. Help the patient to stand with both feet firmly on the scale.

9. Ask the patient to place both hands at her side.

10. Adjust the weights (poises) until the balance pointer is again in the middle of the balance area.

11. Note the patient's weight by adding together the numbers on both the large balance and the small balance. Write it down on the notepaper.

12. Raise the measuring rod above the patient's head.

13. Have the patient turn so that her back is against the measuring rod. Be sure that the patient is standing as straight as possible, with her heels touching the measuring bar.

14. Bring the measuring rod down so that it rests horizontally on the patient's head.

15. Note the patient's height. Write it down on the notepaper.

16. Raise the measuring rod. Help the patient to step off the scale.

17. Assist the patient back into bed or help the patient to put on her robe and slippers.

FOLLOW-UP

18. Make the patient as comfortable as possible.

19. Lower the bed to a position of safety for the patient.

20. Pull the curtains back to the open position.

21. Raise the side rails where ordered, indicated, and appropriate for patient safety.

22. Place the call light within easy reach of the patient.

23. Put the scale back where it belongs. Clean if soiled.

24. Wash your hands.

25. Report to your immediate supervisor:

   - That you have weighed and measured the height of the patient.

   - Note if the patient has dressings or braces, as this must be considered for the correct weight.

   - The patients's weight and height.

   - How the patient tolerated the procedure.

   - Your observations of anything unusual.

CHARTING EXAMPLE: 12/12/04
8am Measured Mrs. Briggs'
ht. 5´10´´ and weight 230 lbs.
Assisted back to bed. H. High, CNA

Transferring the Patient

During the patient's stay, a patient may be transferred from one unit or facility to another (Figure 8–6a◆). This may be done for several reasons:

- The patient may have requested a private room, but none was available at the time of admission

- The patient may ask to be transferred from a private room to a semiprivate room

- The patient may be moved to another unit because of a change in the patient's medical condition

transfer Moving a hospital patient from one room, unit, or facility to another

The patient may become alarmed if a doctor orders a **transfer**. In this case, try to calm the patient. Explain that the change is being made for the patient's benefit. Before you help in transferring the patient, be sure his new unit is ready.

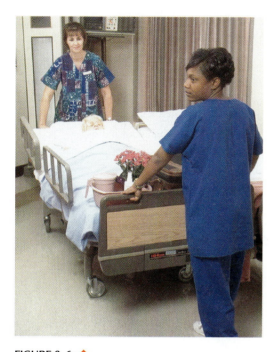

FIGURE 8–6a ◆

Transferring a patient

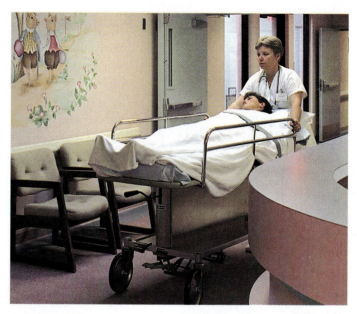

FIGURE 8–6b ◆

Patients are often transferred or admitted by gurney or stretcher

TRANSFERRING THE PATIENT	PROCEDURE	OBRA

RATIONALE: A patient is transferred when there is a change in her condition or when she requires services better provided in a separate facility or unit.

PREPARATION

1. Assemble your equipment, according to the needs of the patient:

   a. Wheelchair

   b. Stretcher or the patient's bed

   c. Cart

2. Check to be sure the new unit is ready to receive the patient.

3. Wash your hands.

4. Identify the patient by checking the identification bracelet.

5. Ask visitors to step out of the room, if this is your hospital's policy.

6. Tell the patient you are going to transfer her to her new room.

7. Collect the patient's personal belongings, patient's record, and equipment that are to be moved with her.

STEPS

8. Transport the patient to the new unit:

   a. The patient can be moved in her own bed from one room to another. Personal belongings can be placed on the bed and moved with the patient. Or, if she has many personal articles, you may use a cart to move them.

   b. You may have to transport the patient by stretcher or wheelchair to her new room (Figure 8–6b◆). Here you will help the patient from the stretcher or wheelchair into her new bed. In these cases, put the patient's belongings and equipment on a cart. Move them

after the patient is settled and safe in the new unit.

9. Follow all safety precautions when wheeling the patient to her new unit. (Some institutions have a transportation service that does this for you.)

10. Give the patient both physical and emotional support (Figure 8–7◆). For example, she may need to be reassured that her family and visitors will be given her new room number.

11. Introduce the patient to her new roommate.

12. Make the patient comfortable in her new room.

13. Introduce her to the nursing staff who will be caring for her. Hand the patient's record to the clerk or nursing caregiver accepting the patient.

14. Arrange the room. Help the patient to put away her personal items or possessions.

PROCEDURE *(continued)*

15. Lower the bed to a position of safety for the patient.

16. Pull the curtains back to the open position.

17. Raise the side rails where ordered, indicated, and appropriate for patient safety.

18. Place the call light within easy reach of the patient.

FOLLOW-UP

19. Wash your hands.

20. Report to the nurse manager or team leader in the new nursing unit that the patient is now in the new unit. Describe how the patient reacted to the transfer.

21. Return to your own floor.

22. Transport the patient's belongings on the cart to the new room if a cart is being used.

23. Strip the bed in the original room on your own floor and take the equipment that was not transferred to the dirty utility room, or follow the procedure used in your institution.

24. Wash your hands.

25. Report to your immediate supervisor:

   ■ That the patient has been transferred to the new unit.

   ■ The time of the transfer.

   ■ The patient's reaction to the transfer.

   ■ Your observations of anything unusual.

CHARTING EXAMPLE: 12/12/05
4pm Transferred Ms. Keller along with her belongings from her assisted living room to the full care unit, Rm 345 on 3 East. M. Mover, CNA

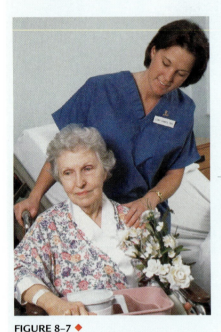

FIGURE 8–7 ◆
Give both physical and emotional support

discharge The official procedure for helping patients to leave the health care institution, including teaching them how to care for themselves at home

Discharging the Patient

Written permission from a doctor is required for the patient to be **discharged**, or officially processed out of the health care institution. Your supervisor will tell you when the doctor has ordered that the patient is to be discharged.

KEY IDEA

If the patient wants to leave and you have not been told that the discharge order has been written by the physician, report this to your immediate supervisor immediately.

In many institutions, the patient must be taken to the business office, cashier, or discharge desk before the patient leaves the facility. (In certain instances a member of the patient's family may do this.)

A patient is sometimes discharged from one health care institution to another, for example, from a hospital to a nursing home. This patient may leave the facility in an ambulance. Your immediate supervisor will give you special instructions for the care of this patient. Some patients may require a caregiver or nurse to accompany them in transfer.

Normally, there is a certain hour by which most patients are discharged. This is so that the room can be cleaned and made ready for new patients, who are often admitted early in the afternoon.

Discharge and Health Teaching

As a result of the DRGs (diagnosis-related groups) system of Medicare payment to health care institutions, patients are staying in health care institutions for shorter periods of time. This means the patients may have a longer **convalescence**, or recovery period, at home.

convalescence The period of recovery after illness or surgery

KEY IDEA

Teaching patients how to care for themselves at home is the responsibility of the entire nursing team.

The nurse will instruct you as to your part in the patient's health teaching as written in the policies of your health care institution. The patient's family should be included in the education process whenever possible. The plan for discharge and health education is of vital importance to the well-being of the patient following discharge from the health care institution.

Four important factors must be included in the discharge and health teaching plan to meet the needs of the whole patient. This is often referred to as the **holistic** approach. It must reflect the four dimensions of the whole person who is the patient. They are:

- **Physiological:** as seen in a person's biological response (physical changes) to alterations in the body's structures and functions
- **Psychological:** as seen in a person's cognitive (level of knowledge) and emotional responses to himself and the surrounding environment
- **Sociocultural:** as seen in a person's noninherited intra-and interpersonal responses to socialization practices learned and transmitted from families and communities
- **Spiritual:** as seen in a person's personal response to inspirational forces

Your immediate supervisor will include the following topics in the discharge instructions and patient health education plan.

Explanation of the patient's disease/disorder:

- History and/or explanation of disease or disorder
- Signs and symptoms expected and those not expected
- What to report to the physician

Explanation of medications as ordered by the physician:

- Name of medication
- Dose: how much the patient is to take
- The correct times to take the medication
- The purpose and expected effects of the medication
- Signs and symptoms of side effects of the medication
- What to report to the physician

Explanation of treatments ordered by the physician:

- Purpose of treatments
- Time of treatments
- How to perform treatments
- Return demonstrations of treatments
- What to report to the physician

Explanation of nutrition and diet:

- Type of diet ordered by physician
- Foods allowed and disallowed on this diet

holistic An approach that reflects the four dimensions of a whole person: physiological, psychological, sociocultural, and spiritual

physiological Referring to a person's biological response to alterations in the body's structures and functions

psychological Referring to a person's cognitive and emotional responses to the self and the surrounding environment

sociocultural Referring to a person's interpersonal responses to socialization practices in the family and community

spiritual Referring to an individual's personal response to inspirational forces

- Amounts of food to be consumed
- Available home health agencies for help; name, phone number, and address

Explanation of care in the home environment:

- Elimination of hazards in the home environment
- Available transportation to the physician's office or clinic
- Available housekeeping services
- Available economic support agencies; name, phone number, and address

Explanation of progression of activities of daily living:

- Outline activities of daily living for the first 2 weeks following hospitalization, with progressive activities
- Signs and symptoms of inability to perform activities
- What to report to the physician

Explanation of future appointments that have been made with the physician or clinic:

- Time and date of appointment
- Name of physician and/or clinic
- Phone number and address of physician or clinic
- The reason why these future appointments are necessary for follow-up care

Explanation of referral agencies:

- Names of agencies
- Address of agencies
- Phone number of agencies
- Name of contact person at the agency

Discharge Planning

Your immediate supervisor is responsible for the following discharge planning activities. You will be instructed on what you should do as your part of this discharge plan. Be sure to follow your immediate supervisor's instructions. Your immediate supervisor will:

- Start discharge planning at the time of admission.
- Work with the physician, health care team members, case manager, social worker, dietitian, family, and significant others.
- Contact the necessary community agencies for referral, if necessary. Include the discharge plan in patient education with family members and/or significant others present when possible.
- Assess the patient's ability for self-care in the home setting.
- Give the patient and/or family members a written plan for all medications (stating time and amount), exercises, and any other pertinent data.
- Make future appointments in the physician's office, clinic, health agency, outpatient department, physical therapy, and social services, as indicated.
- Give the patient and/or family members a written schedule of appointments (date and time). Discuss activities of daily living with the patient and interested family members.
- Give the patient and family members a written outline for any exercises or special activities.
- Advise proper time for continuance of normal activities and lifestyle. Advise patient and/or family members to call, giving the phone number and extension, if they have any questions after they get home.

- Document the entire discharge plan and the patient's reaction to the plan on the permanent record.

- If permitted by your institution's policies, give the patient a copy of the discharge checklist.

PROCEDURE   OBRA

DISCHARGING THE PATIENT

RATIONALE: A patient is discharged when he no longer requires or benefits from the facility or unit's health care services.

PREPARATION

1. Assemble your equipment, according to the needs of the patient:
   a. Wheelchair
   b. Stretcher
   c. Discharge slip, if used in your institution
   d. Cart
2. Wash your hands.
3. Identify the patient by checking the identification bracelet.

STEPS

4. Help the patient collect and pack personal possessions (Figure 8–8◆).
5. Be sure all valuables and medications are returned to the patient.
6. Help the patient get dressed, if necessary.
7. Check that the written instructions are given to the patient by your immediate supervisor, such as:
   a. Doctor's orders to follow at home
   b. Prescriptions

   c. Follow-up schedule of appointments with the doctor or clinic
8. Bring the wheelchair to the patient's bedside and help the patient into it.
9. Before wheeling the patient off the floor, get the discharge slip from your immediate supervisor.
10. Take the patient in the wheelchair to the discharge desk, cashier, or business office, if the patient's family has not already done so. Give the clerk the discharge slip. Get a release form in return.
11. Wheel the patient to the front door. Help the patient out of the wheelchair and into his car (Figure 8–9◆).

12. Say goodbye to the patient.
13. Take the wheelchair and release form back to the floor.

FOLLOW-UP

14. Strip the linen from the bed unless this is done by the environmental services department in your institution. Place it in the dirty linen hamper.
15. Notify the environmental service or housekeeping department that the discharge has taken place and the unit is ready to be cleaned.
16. Wash your hands.
17. Give your supervisor the release form from the business office,

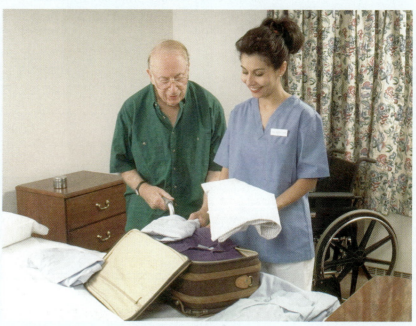

FIGURE 8–8 ◆

Help the patient collect and pack personal possessions

PROCEDURE *(continued)*

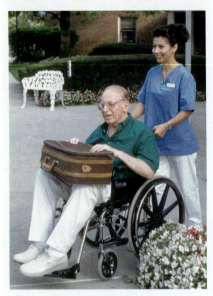

FIGURE 8–9 ◆

Wheel the patient to the door

cashier, or discharge desk. Then report to your immediate supervisor:

- That the patient has been discharged.
- The time of the discharge.
- The type of transportation used for the discharge.
- Who accompanied the patient: husband, wife, daughter, friend.
- That patient was given a copy of the discharge.
- Patient's reaction to the discharge.
- That environmental service has been notified that the unit is ready to be cleaned.

- Your observations of anything unusual.

CHARTING EXAMPLE: 12/14/04 4pm Assisted Mr. Hines to pack his things. Discharged via wheelchair to Ms. Hines, his daughter, who plans to drive him home in her car. Mr. Hines says he is looking forward to feeling less pain in a couple days as he continues to recover from his surgery. M. Rosa, CNA

SUMMARY

Nursing assistants can significantly affect the way the patient experiences the admission, transfer, and discharge processes. By following the patient plan of care as well as proper admitting, transfer, and discharge procedures, the nursing assistant can help the patient to feel comfortable, cared for, and secure in the health care environment.

NOTES

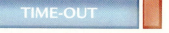

CHAPTER REVIEW

FILL IN THE BLANK Read each sentence and fill in the blank line with a word that completes the sentence.

1. The process that covers the time when the patient enters the institution until she is settled in is called _____.

2. Do not use an adult's first name without first being given _____.

3. Using a _____ lift is often a good idea for patients who cannot stand by themselves.

4. _____ permission is needed from a physician prior to a patient being discharged.

5. The _____ approach to care includes the physiological, psychological, sociocultural, and spiritual aspects of the patient.

MULTIPLE CHOICE Choose the best answer for each question or statement.

1. Which of the following does not create a favorable first impression for a patient being admitted to a facility?
   a. Being greeted warmly
   b. A clean environment
   c. Staff wearing dirty shoes
   d. A quiet relaxed environment

2. The patient plan of care serves as a guide for the care a patient will receive and is written by the:
   a. RN
   b. MD
   c. CNA
   d. RD

3. The weight of the patient is very important because
   a. it will determine the final cost of care.
   b. it will determine who is treated first.

   c. it will be used to determine the dose of some medications.
   d. All of the above.

4. When discharging a patient, do all of the following *except*
   a. wash your hands.
   b. help the patient collect and pack her belongings.
   c. have the patient take his dirty linen home.
   d. make sure the patient takes home all his written instructions.

5. Which of the following is not part of the discharge instructions?
   a. Explanation of medications the patient will take at home
   b. Follow-up appointments
   c. Activity or diet restrictions
   d. How to ignore signs and symptoms of pain

TIME-OUT

TIPS FOR TIME MANAGEMENT

When you help with the discharge or transfer of a patient, use a system, such as beginning at the top drawer of the night stand and emptying all belongings into a bag or suitcase. Progress down the night stand, then empty the closet. Remove the patient's belongings from the trays in the overbed table. Then check the bathroom and under the bed. This will prevent spending time later looking for a belonging that was left behind.

THE NURSING ASSISTANT IN ACTION

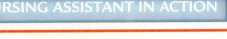

Mr. Jolly has been your patient during the past 4 days. He is now being transferred to a nursing home. He is not looking forward to the move as he feels comfortable with the staff on your unit and is concerned that staff at the new facility will ignore him or be unable to take care of him. He says, "You know I am right!"

What Is Your Response/Action?

CRITICAL THINKING

CUSTOMER SERVICE There are many things patients need to know when they are admitted to a new unit. Some units have printed handouts with details concerning visiting times, usual mealtimes, information about services a patient may require or desire, etc. If the unit where you work has not developed this information, start your own list. You can refer to the list and be sure you have covered the important items for your patients or their families. Add new items as patients ask questions about things you have not mentioned.

CULTURAL CARE Most facilities are treating patients from a variety of cultures. If the information about your unit is not available in a written form, or if the patient cannot read it, ask who can help serve as an interpreter. It can be frightening to be transferred to another unit if you do not have someone who can explain what is happening to you.

COOPERATION WITHIN THE TEAM Some days assignments can become very uneven as patients are admitted and discharged from a given unit. If you help a coworker with an admission or answer her patients' call lights, you will be helping out your coworker as well as the patients.

EXPLORE MediaLink

Additional interactive resources for this chapter can be found on the Companion Website at www.prenhall.com/wolgin. Click on Chapter 8 and "Begin" to select activities for this chapter.

For chapter-related NCLEX-style questions and an audio glossary, access the accompanying CD-ROM in this book.

9 The Patient's Room

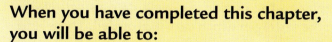

OBJECTIVES

When you have completed this chapter, you will be able to:

- Describe the typical patient's unit and list the equipment it contains.
- Check the unit for convenience to the patient, organization, and safety.
- Describe the purpose of each piece of equipment.
- Create an appropriate environment in the home in which to provide care for the patient.
- Provide a safe environment for the patient by eliminating safety hazards and anticipating safety needs.
- Describe how to contact emergency assistance.

KEY TERMS

alternating-pressure mattress
bed cradle
bedpan
disposable equipment
emesis basin
equipment
flammable
intravenous pole
lamb's wool
patient lift
patient unit
specialty bed
stretcher
urinal
walker
wheelchair

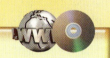

MediaLink

www.prenhall.com/wolgin

Use the address above to access the free, interactive Companion Website created for this textbook. Get hints, instant feedback, and textbook references to chapter-related NCLEX-style questions. Link to other interesting sites.

AUDIO GLOSSARY:

Use the Companion Website, or the CD-ROM disk enclosed with your textbook, to hear the pronunciation of key terms in the chapter.

One of the responsibilities of a nursing assistant is to maintain the patient's room and general environment in a tidy and organized manner. The room arrangement must be convenient for the patient, while affording the space needed for the nursing assistant and others to perform their work. This chapter introduces supplies and equipment commonly used when providing patient care, along with ideas for maintaining the space. You will review the typical room arrangement as well as safety tips to assist you in avoiding accidents while providing a safer environment for the patient. Some health care facilities or agencies refer to the person receiving care as *patient, resident,* or *client* depending on the setting in which care is provided. These references are made from time to time within this chapter when referring to a patient in a hospital, long-term care facility, or home setting.

The Patient's Unit

ALERT

For all patient contact, adhere to Standard Precautions (🔗 Chapter 5, pages 83–85). Wear protective equipment as indicated.

---

patient unit The space for one patient, including the hospital bed, bedside table, chair, and other equipment

equipment Materials, tools, devices, supplies, furnishings, necessary things used to perform a task

The **patient unit** consists of all the room space, furniture, and **equipment** provided by the hospital for one patient. Each unit can be screened off for privacy by draw curtains (Figure 9–1◆).

After a patient has been admitted to the unit for which you are responsible, make sure everything that belongs in the unit is there and in its proper place. If the patient is left handed, put the bedside stand and call light near the left hand; if the patient is right handed, place them near the right hand.

A hospital unit designed for children may be different from an adult unit (Figure 9–2◆). A child's age and the reason for the hospitalization will determine how the unit is arranged and the equipment that will be needed.

The unit should be arranged for the convenience of the patient. The call light system must be easily accessible for the patient, along with items of importance such as eyeglasses and the telephone (Figure 9–3◆). Depending on the patient's needs, other items may need to be close also (such as a urinal or emesis basin). When you straighten the room, consider how it should be arranged in anticipation of what will be happening. For example, the over-bed table should be cleared prior to a meal tray being delivered. Keeping the room tidy and organized is a priority so that the patient and family are comfortable and care can be provided in a safe manner.

Equipment

The modern health care facility has many pieces of equipment needed for patient care and treatment. This equipment might include:

alternating-pressure mattress A pad similar to an air mattress that can be placed beneath the patient to reduce pressure on the head, shoulders, back, heels, elbows, and bony prominences

bed cradle A frame shaped like a barrel cut in half lengthwise used to keep bed linens off a part of the patient's body

- **Alternating-pressure (A-P) mattress:** A device like an air mattress placed beneath a bedridden or elderly patient or a patient at risk for pressure ulcers. It reduces pressure on the head, shoulders, back, heels, elbows, and bony or prominent surfaces.

- **Bed board:** A large board placed beneath the mattress to provide additional support for patients with back, muscle, or bone problems.

- **Bed cradle:** This cradle looks like a half-barrel cut the long way (Figure 9–4◆). It is used to cover a part of the patient's body where she is having great pain, to eliminate pressure and to support the weight of the top linen, to eliminate additional pain in the area, or when you do not want anything to touch that area.

- **Binders:** Strips of heavy cotton cloth with Velcro fasteners. Binders are wrapped securely around the patient's body over the abdomen to give support and comfort following abdominal surgery.

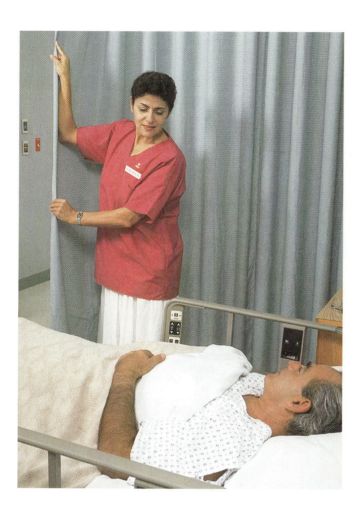

FIGURE 9–1◆
Adjust curtain for the patient's privacy

■ **Foot board:** A small board placed upright at the foot of the bed and used to keep the patient's feet aligned properly to prevent foot drop.

■ **Intravenous poles:** These are called IV poles. They support the bags and tubes used in various treatments. Some IV poles are on casters or rollers for easy movement and may be attached to portable IV pumps. Other IV poles fit into the bed frame.

intravenous pole A tall pole, also called IV pole, which attaches to a bed or is on rollers or casters; this pole is used to hold the containers or tubes needed, for example, during a blood transfusion

FIGURE 9–2 ◆
The pediatric unit

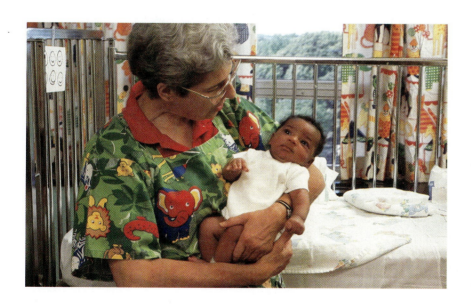

FIGURE 9–3 ◆
Check the patient's unit; place the call light and the patient's personal items within easy reach

lamb's wool A wide strip of lamb's hide with the fleece attached or an imitation material used to increase patient comfort

patient lift A mechanical device with a sling seat used for lifting a patient into and out of such equipment as the hospital bed, bathtub, or wheelchair

specialty bed A bed that constantly changes pressure under the patient. Used to minimize pressure points in the treatment or prevention of pressure ulcers

stretcher A narrow rolling table with or without a mattress or simply a canvas stretched over a frame used to transport patients; the latter may also be called a *litter, gurney,* or *cart*

walker A stable frame made of metal tubing used to support the unsteady patient while walking; the patient holds the walker while taking a step, moves it forward, and takes another step

wheelchair A chair on wheels used to transport patients

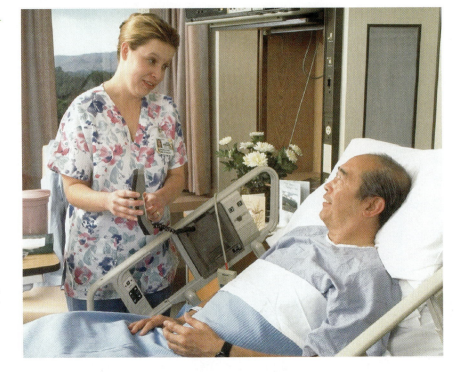

- ■ **Lamb's wool:** Wide strips of lamb's wool cloth (or soft synthetic materials) used to increase patient comfort.
- ■ **Portable patient lift:** A mechanical device used to move the patient from bed to chair and back again when the patient needs full assistance.
- ■ **Specialty bed:** Used to eliminate pressure points and prevent pressure ulcers.
- ■ **Stretcher:** A narrow table with a mattress on wheels used to transport patients. Also called a *litter, gurney,* or *cart.*
- ■ **Walker:** A supportive device used by the patient for help in walking.
- ■ **Wheelchair:** A chair with wheels used to transport patients.

A number of the preceding items are shown in Figure 9–5◆. Other equipment may be used at a particular hospital or health care facility. The nursing assistant will be expected to be familiar with many pieces of equipment and know how to operate, maintain, and clean it. When unfamiliar with the equipment, the nursing assistant must ask for an in-service or review instructions prior to working with the item.

FIGURE 9–4 ◆
The bed cradle is used to keep bed linens off a part of the patient's body

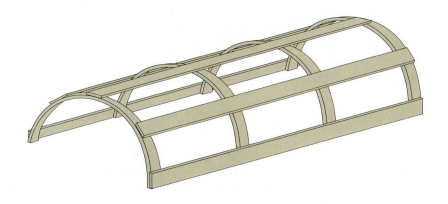

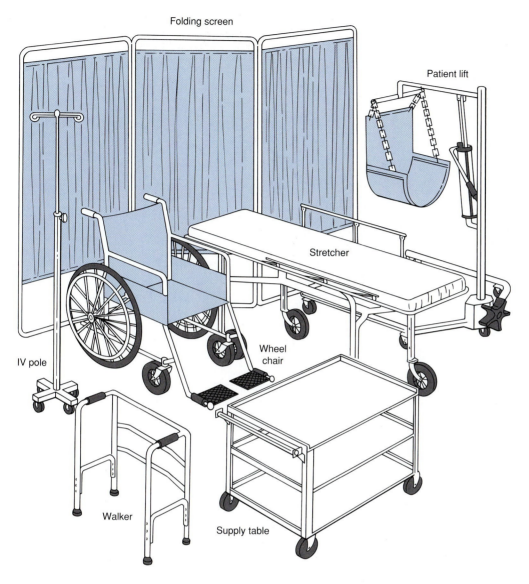

Folding screen

Patient lift

Stretcher

IV pole

Wheel chair

Walker

Supply table

FIGURE 9–5 ◆
Health care equipment

Disposable Equipment

Today, in many health care facilities, reusable equipment has been replaced by **disposable equipment** (Figure 9–6◆). Reusable equipment requires washing and disinfecting. Disposable equipment needs almost no care and is usually prepackaged. It may be made of plastic or paper. Some of this equipment is used only one time and then thrown away. Other disposable equipment may be used several times for one patient only, being cleaned between uses and thrown away when the patient is discharged, or sent home with the patient.

disposable equipment
Equipment that is used one time only or for one patient only and then thrown away

Creating a Safe and Comfortable Patient Room

Patients must be made to feel safe and comfortable. The room temperature, lighting, position of the bed, and the volume of the TV and telephone should be adjusted to suit the patient, unless conditions do not allow it or it interferes with another patient. Always

bedpan A pan used by patients who must defecate or urinate while in bed

emesis basin A pan used for catching material that a patient spits out, vomits, or expectorates

urinal A portable container given to male patients in bed so they can urinate without getting out of bed

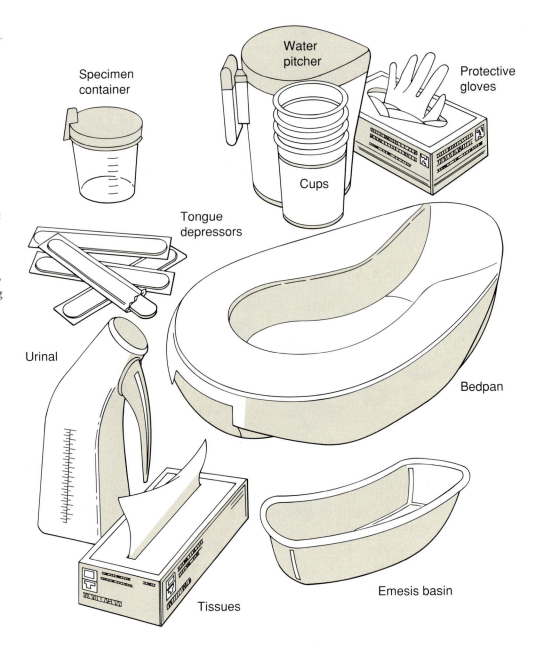

respect the privacy of the patient, realizing that the room is the *patient's* while he is hospitalized. Knock on the patient's door before entering and wait for acknowledgment from the patient (if the patient is able to respond). Provide privacy for the patient by drawing the curtain or closing the door when activity or procedures might expose the patient. Provide comfort for the patient in any way possible such as repositioning, providing extra blankets, refilling the water pitcher, or meeting other needs.

In addition to these considerations, when caring for a patient in a long-term care setting, the nursing assistant will find other ways in which a patient may be made more comfortable. Long-term care patients, referred to as *residents,* bring furniture and personal belongings to the facility to decorate their rooms and make them more like home. As a nursing assistant, you will be responsible for protecting these items on behalf of the resident. To make a resident more comfortable, you may seat him in a favorite chair, play the resident's favorite music on the stereo, or utilize other personal items to aid the resident. In each situation, you will demonstrate respect for the resident's belongings. As in the hospital setting, knock before entering a resident's room. Keep the room uncluttered to prevent trips and falls. Keep only equipment that is needed or in use in the patient's room.

 # Caring for a Patient in a Home Setting

Working in the home environment presents slightly different challenges. The atmosphere and lifestyle will be different in every home in which you work. You must respect the rights of your patient (client) and his family who may have beliefs and opinions, culture, and customs that are different from your own. People of different backgrounds may eat foods you have never seen or tasted; they may behave differently toward their family members than you would; their religious beliefs may seem unusual to you; and their standards of cleanliness or general lifestyle may be different from yours. Accept these differences with respect and understanding, without judging or criticizing. Let your patient, the client, know it is your pleasure, not just your job, to assist him. Recognize you are a guest in your patient's home.

Be careful in the home not to disturb the patient's personal belongings, letters, pictures, and the like. You may suggest they be moved, however, to another place so that you can give better care. It is also important that you not perform heavy cleaning chores, such as moving heavy furniture, waxing floors, shampooing carpets, washing windows, and carrying firewood. You are there to provide care and comfort measures, as you would if the patient were in the hospital. The patient may need equipment or supplies similar to those used in the hospital. If you determine a need for these items, they can be provided in the home to facilitate the patient's care.

Safety

You can create a safe environment for your patient and yourself by eliminating, preventing, or correcting conditions that could cause accidents. Safety includes proper infection control, electrical and fire safety, and accident prevention.

As you go about your work, be alert and look for the hazards listed below. Make a note of these things and bring them to the attention of the patient, family member, or your supervisor, whichever is appropriate. Some of the most common safety hazards in the home are:

- Damaged electrical wiring on large and small appliances or equipment
- Faulty or uneven stairs or loose debris on stairs
- Loose rugs that slip, or those without a nonskid backing
- Poisons (such as cleaning solutions)
- **Flammable** cleaning rags, mops, and brooms (these should be cleaned after each use and stored in a well-ventilated place)
- Sharp objects such as knives, razors, and hypodermic needles
- Wet floor (spills should be wiped up immediately)
- Cluttered hallways or walkways
- Unstable furniture
- Electrical cords that cross a walkway
- Liquids spilled onto equipment
- Wheels on equipment that roll unevenly
- Dimly lit hallways and walkways

flammable Capable of burning quickly and easily

Refer to Chapter 6 for more information on fire safety measures and Chapter 11 for overall safety awareness and accident prevention guidelines to follow while caring for a patient in the home.

Fire Safety and Burn Prevention

- Avoid using flammable liquids.

- Use flame-resistant clothing for the patient and follow the washing instructions on the label inside the clothing to keep them flame resistant.

- Caution the patient against smoking while seated on upholstered furniture or the bed, especially when sleepy.

- If the patient is a smoker, use a deep, wide-rimmed ashtray and set it on a table. Extinguish smoldering butts when the patient is finished smoking.

- Do not use an extension cord or electric cord and plug unless it is in excellent condition. Many facilities require each new piece of equipment to be numbered, checked, and approved by maintenance before it can be used. Equipment that requires electricity is dated and tagged to show when it was last serviced or inspected.

- Arrange furniture with fire safety in mind. Place furniture well away from stoves, space heaters, fireplaces, doorways, and stairs.

- If a fire occurs, get the patient out of the area. Know the exit route.

- Have a fire extinguisher available and a smoke alarm in the home.

- Follow the safety rules of your local fire department; they can train you as to how to use an extinguisher.

- Keep matches away from children and confused adults.

- Check the temperature of water before using it on a patient.

Reporting an Accident or Emergency by Telephone

If an accident or emergency does occur, you must be ready to handle the situation calmly and wisely. Report every accident to your supervisor immediately. It is important to know emergency phone numbers. In the home, keep emergency numbers next to the phone. The list should include:

- Emergency Medical Service (often *911*)

- Police department

- Fire department

- Responsible family member at work

- Your home care supervisor or agency

- Patient's physician

- Nearest hospital

- Ambulance service

- Poison control center

If there is no phone in the home, arrange in advance to use a neighbor's phone in case of an emergency. Some home care agencies provide cellular phones for employees to use in these situations. Remember that a cell phone cannot be traced to an address. When calling for help, it will be important to have the address ready or be able to accurately provide your location. **(Refer to Chapter 13, Emergency Care.)**

In the hospital or long-term care facility, you should know the emergency numbers for fire and medical emergencies. Refer to Chapters 6 and 13 for more information on fire safety and medical emergencies.

By being prepared, you will be better able to handle emergency situations when they arise. Even more important, by observing safety hazards and taking preventive steps you

PROCEDURE

CALLING FOR HELP

OBRA

RATIONALE: It is important to know what information will assist the EMS dispatchers to respond quickly.

PREPARATION

1. Determine what help you require.
2. Have the address or be able to accurately provide your location, room, or apartment number.

STEPS

3. Give your name.
4. Give the name of the patient and identify your location, room number, or address.
5. Clearly state the problem; objectively state exactly what has happened or what help you need. If calling a city emergency number, give the above information, as well as the phone number of the patient's physician to the person who answers the phone call.
6. If you have a phone number for a member of the family, give that number, also.

7. Stay with the individual until help arrives. Follow advice or direction offered by the EMS operator.

FOLLOW-UP

8. Document the time of the emergency and anything unusual that you observed.
9. Discuss the situation with the emergency responders and your immediate supervisor to determine appropriate follow-up.

CHARTING EXAMPLE: 5/3/04 2pm 911 called. EMS responded at 2:20pm. Mrs. Sanchez's daughter and Dr. Morris notified. M. Morrales, CNA

may be able to avert an emergency totally. You should always strive to create and maintain a safe, accident-free environment for every patient.

SUMMARY

The patient's room is important to the recovery or care of the patient in numerous ways. It must provide comfort in order for the patient to rest. It must be perceived as safe for the patient to have peace of mind. For the family, the setting should be presentable and inviting; however, it must also afford staff a clean, safe, adequate space in which to work. It is easy to understand how vital the nursing assistant is in maintaining a safe, comfortable setting. In reviewing the equipment and supplies necessary for patient care, the arrangement of the furniture and equipment, and safety concerns listed, the nursing assistant is able to prepare an efficient, organized, and safe patient setting. Regardless of which setting the patient is in, the nursing assistant, by maintaining the environment as such, enhances the quality of care for each patient.

NOTES

CHAPTER REVIEW

FILL IN THE BLANK Read each sentence and fill in the blank line with a word that completes the sentence.

1. An _____ _____ mattress is a device placed beneath a bedridden patient to decrease the risk for pressure ulcers.

2. Equipment that is used for one patient only is called _____ equipment.

3. A _____ _____ is a frame-shaped device used to keep linens off the bed.

4. Lamb's wool is a piece of material used to increase the patient's _____ .

5. When working in the home, you must respect the patient's beliefs and attitudes even if they are _____ from yours.

MULTIPLE CHOICE Choose the best answer for each question or statement.

1. The unit should be arranged for the convenience of the
   a. patient.
   b. staff.
   c. family.
   d. physician.

2. All of the following are pieces of patient equipment *except*
   a. binders.
   b. foot board.
   c. walkers.
   d. covers.

3. The following are all pieces of disposable equipment *except*
   a. cups.
   b. foot board.

   c. bed pan.
   d. tissues.

4. To create a comfortable room setting for the patient, do all of the following *except*
   a. put the TV on a channel the patient likes.
   b. keep the lights and heat at a level comfortable for the patient.
   c. keep the side rails up at all times.
   d. provide privacy for the patient.

5. Provide a safe environment for your patient by
   a. removing loose rugs that slip.
   b. keeping hallways uncluttered.
   c. cleaning up spills.
   d. All of the above.

TIME-OUT

TIPS FOR TIME MANAGEMENT

Be sure to have emergency contact numbers by the phone and have the address available or be able to accurately provide your location. If you do not know or have trouble remembering the room number, address, or patient's name, write this information on your pad. If you need to report an emergency, you will save time because you will have the information on hand.

THE NURSING ASSISTANT IN ACTION

Mrs. Estes has been admitted for asthma and she has many allergies. She tells you the pillow on her bed neeeds to go because it is bothering her. You are not sure if there is any other type of pillow available for her to use. She tells you to take the pillow out of her room, but you are ordered to have her head elevated.

What Is Your Response/Action?

CRITICAL THINKING

CUSTOMER SERVICE You are assigned to care for an elderly person who has a history of falling. Look carefully at her room to locate any potential safety hazards or items like throw rugs. What actions can you take to reduce hazards or make the room safe? Do not make changes in the patient's room without talking with the patient and letting her know the reason you are moving or removing items.

CULTURAL CARE Many cultures and religions have objects that provide significant comfort or reassurance. Do not touch or remove any photographs, statues, or other objects from a patient's room without his permission. There may be certain items that a family member can bring to a hospital that can be a source of personal or spiritual comfort to the patient or resident. Only by discussing or asking if there are ways to make the patient's room more comfortable will you learn what each individual patient or resident desires.

COOPERATION WITHIN THE TEAM Occasionally you will find patient care items, packaging materials or used supplies that should have been thrown away or properly stored in a patient's room. Clean up the area or throw away the trash even though these items were left by another coworker. Do not complain to the patient about the mess your coworker left for you. If you notice a coworker who frequently leaves things untidy, speak with the person directly or ask your supervisor how to address your concern with the coworker.

EXPLORE MediaLink

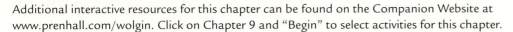

Additional interactive resources for this chapter can be found on the Companion Website at www.prenhall.com/wolgin. Click on Chapter 9 and "Begin" to select activities for this chapter.

For chapter-related NCLEX-style questions and an audio glossary, access the accompanying CD-ROM in this book.

10 Bedmaking

KEY TERMS

closed bed
decubitus ulcers
draw sheet
fan-fold
occupied bed
open bed
postoperative bed

OBJECTIVES

When you have completed this chapter, you will be able to:

- Explain the reason for making the patient's bed with great care.
- Identify and describe the four basic methods of making a bed.
- List the guidelines to follow for bedmaking.
- Make the closed bed.
- Make the open, fanfolded bed.
- Make the postoperative bed (surgical, OR [operating room], stretcher, recovery room bed).
- Make the occupied bed.

MediaLink
www.prenhall.com/wolgin

Use the address above to access the free, interactive Companion Website created for this textbook. Get hints, instant feedback, and textbook references to chapter-related NCLEX-style questions. Link to other interesting sites.

AUDIO GLOSSARY:

Use the Companion Website, or the CD-ROM disk enclosed with your textbook, to hear the pronunciation of key terms in the chapter.

There are four different ways to make a bed. The way it is made depends on the needs of the patient. You will learn how to make a closed bed, open bed, occupied bed, and postoperative bed. Making the bed carefully is very important to the patient's comfort, well-being, and appearance of the environment.

 ## Bedmaking

Some patients are unable or are not permitted to get out of bed. As a result of this, many patients eat, bathe, and use a bedpan in bed. Therefore, it is important to make the patient's bed with great care and to straighten sheets from time to time and adjust the pillow for the patient's comfort.

Whether the patient is in a health care facility or at home, the bed needs to be made without any wrinkles in the sheets. Wrinkles are not only uncomfortable but restrict the patient's circulation and can cause skin breakdown (**decubitus ulcers**).

 ## Four Basic Beds

The **closed bed** is made after environmental service personnel have cleaned the unit following a patient's discharge. The bed is made up closed. The top covers are pulled up to the head of the bed so it will stay clean until a new patient is assigned to it. When a patient is assigned to a unit, the closed bed is made into an **open bed** by fan-folding the top sheets down to the foot of the bed. The **occupied bed** is made with the patient in the bed. The **postoperative bed** may also be called the surgical, OR (operating room), recovery, or stretcher bed. The top sheets are folded lengthwise and positioned on one side of the bed. The postoperative bed allows transfer of the patient from the surgical stretcher to the bed without unnecessary movement.

INTRODUCTION

ALERT

For all patient contact, adhere to Standard Precautions (∞ Chapter 5, pages 83–85). Wear protective equipment as indicated.

decubitus ulcers Tissue breakdown resulting from pressure or reduced blood flow (often called *pressure sores* or *bed sores*)

closed bed Bed made with bedspread in place

open bed Bed made with top sheet folded so as to give patient easy entrance

occupied bed One with a patient in it

postoperative bed Bed made with top sheet folded lengthwise and positioned to one side, allowing transfer of the patient from the surgical stretcher to the bed without unnecessary movement

KEY IDEA

A guideline that protects the patient and the patient's visitors as well as the nursing assistant from germs is to never shake linen and to always hold it away from the uniform.

BEDMAKING | GUIDELINES | OBRA

- Do not shake the bed linen. Shaking spreads germs to everything and everyone in the room, including you.
- Do not allow any linen to touch your uniform.

- Dirty, used linen should never be put on the floor. Place in a laundry bag.
- Fold linen in on itself as you remove it from the bed.
- Do not take extra linen into a patient unit. It is considered contaminated (or dirty) and cannot be used elsewhere.

- Set aside torn linen to send for repair.
- Never use a pin on any item of linen as it may come unfastened and injure the patient.
- Report to your immediate supervisor if you see patients or visitors trying to remove articles of linen from the unit for any reason.

GUIDELINES *(Continued)*

Some health care institutions use melt-away plastic bags for laundry bags. These bags dissolve during the washing process.

- The bottom sheet must be firm, tight, and smooth under the patient. This is very important for the patient's comfort.

- Plastic should never touch a patient's skin. If using a plastic draw sheet, be sure to cover it

entirely with a cotton draw sheet. Small disposable bed protectors may be used with the draw sheet or in place of it.

- By fan-folding the top of the bed, you make it easy for the patient to get back into the bed.

- The cotton **draw sheet** is about half the size of a regular sheet. When cotton draw sheets are not available, a large sheet can be

folded in half widthwise (with small and large hems together). The fold must always be placed toward the head of the bed and the hems toward the foot of the bed.

Remember that you save time and energy by first making as much of the bed as possible on one side before going to the other side. Practice good body mechanics and follow standard precautions when making any bed.

---

draw sheet Small sheet made of plastic, rubber, or cotton placed across the middle of the bed to cover and protect the bottom sheet and assist in moving the patient

Closed Bed

As a nursing assistant, you will have occasion to make many beds. It is important to remember that a clean, comfortable bed has a positive effect on the patient's physical and mental well-being.

| MAKING THE CLOSED, EMPTY BED | **PROCEDURE** | **OBRA** |

RATIONALE: The closed bed is made after discharge cleaning and is ready for a new admission.

PREPARATION

1. Assemble your equipment on a chair near the bed (Figure 10–1◆):

   a. Mattress cover, if used

   b. Bottom sheet

   c. Cotton and plastic draw sheets (or disposable bed protector)

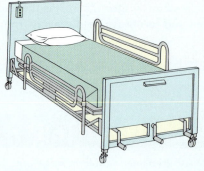

FIGURE 10–1 ◆
The closed, empty bed

   d. Top sheet

   e. Blanket

   f. Bedspread

   g. Pillowcase

   h. Pillow

   i. Pillow protector, if used

2. Place a chair near the bed.

STEPS

3. Wash your hands.

4. Put the pillow on the chair.

5. Stack the bed linen on the chair in the order in which you will use them: first things to be used on top, last things to be used on the bottom.

6. Adjust the bed to the highest horizontal position for comfort while you work (Figure 10–2◆).

PROCEDURE (continued)

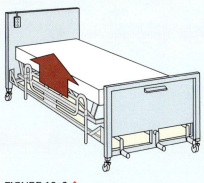

FIGURE 10–2 ◆

Adjust bed to highest horizontal position for comfort

7. Push the mattress to the head of the bed until it touches the headboard.

8. If mattress pads are used in your facility, place the pad on the mattress even with the head edge of the mattress.

9. Fold the bottom sheet lengthwise and place it on the bed:

   a. Place the center fold of the sheet in the center of the mattress from head to foot (Figure 10–3◆).

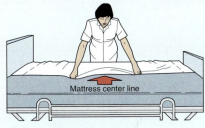

Mattress center line

FIGURE 10–3 ◆

Place the center fold of the sheet in the center of the mattress

   b. Place the large hem to the head of the bed (Figure 10–4◆).

   c. Put the small hem at the foot of the bed, even with the edge of the mattress (Figure 10–5◆).

10. Open the sheet. It should now hang evenly the same distance over each side of the bed. The

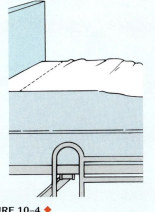

FIGURE 10–4 ◆

Place large hem at the head of the bed

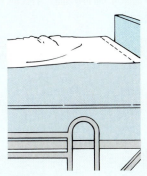

FIGURE 10–5 ◆

Place small hem at the foot of the bed

rough edges of the hem should now face down toward the mattress and away from the patient.

11. There should be 18 inches of the sheet to tuck smoothly and tightly under the head of the mattress.

12. To make a mitered corner:

   a. Pick up the edge of the sheet at the side of the bed 12 inches from the head of the mattress (Figure 10–6◆).

   b. Place the triangle (the folded corner) on top of the mattress (Figure 10–7◆).

   c. Tuck the hanging portion of the sheet under the mattress (Figure 10–8◆).

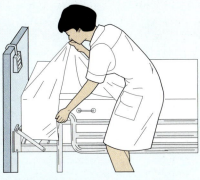

FIGURE 10–6 ◆

Pick up the edge of the sheet 12 inches from the head of the mattress

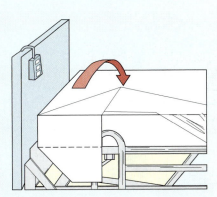

FIGURE 10–7 ◆

Place the triangle on the top of the mattress

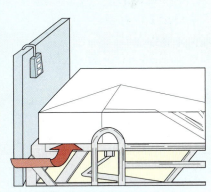

FIGURE 10–8 ◆

Tuck hanging portion of the sheet under the mattress

   d. While you hold the fold at the edge of the mattress, bring the triangle down over the side of the mattress (Figure 10–9◆).

PROCEDURE *(continued)*

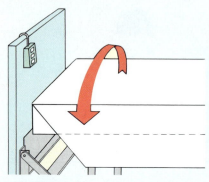

FIGURE 10–9 ◆
Hold fold at the edge as you bring the triangle down over the side of the mattress

e. Tuck the sheet under the mattress from head to foot. Start at the head and pull toward the foot of the bed as you tuck (Figure 10–10◆).

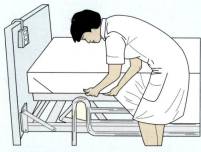

FIGURE 10–10 ◆
Tuck the entire side of the sheet under the mattress

13. Stand and work entirely on one side of the bed until that side is finished.

14. Fold in half and place the plastic draw sheet 14 inches (the length of your forearm) down from the head of the bed. Tuck it in. Be sure each piece of linen is straight and even as you tuck it in (Figure 10–11◆).

15. Cover the plastic draw sheet with the cotton draw sheet and tuck it in.

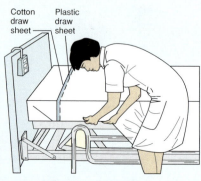

FIGURE 10–11 ◆
Be sure each piece of linen is straight and even as you tuck it in

16. Fold the top sheet lengthwise and place it on the bed:

a. Place the center fold on the center of the bed from the head to foot (Figure 10–12◆).

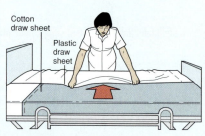

FIGURE 10–12 ◆
Place the center fold of the top sheet in the center of the mattress

b. Put the large hem at the head of the bed, even with the top edge of the mattress.

c. Open the sheet, with the rough edge of the hem up, fan-folding half to the center of the bed.

d. Tightly tuck the sheet under at the foot of the bed (Figure 10–13◆).

e. Make a mitered corner at the foot of the bed (Figure 10–14◆).

f. Do not tuck in at the side of the bed.

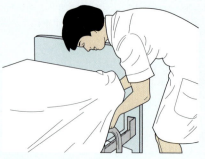

FIGURE 10–13 ◆
Tightly tuck the sheet under the foot of the bed

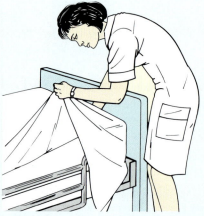

FIGURE 10–14 ◆
Make a mitered corner at the foot of the bed

17. Fold the blanket lengthwise and place on the bed.

a. Place the center fold of the blanket in the center of the bed from head to foot.

b. Place the upper hem 6 inches from the top edge of the mattress.

c. Open the blanket.

d. Tuck it under the foot tightly.

e. Make a mitered corner at the foot of the bed.

f. Do not tuck in at the sides of the bed.

18. Fold the bedspread lengthwise and place it on the bed.

a. Place the center fold in the center of the bed from head to foot.

PROCEDURE *(continued)*

b. Place the upper hem even with the head edge of the mattress.

c. Have the rough edge down.

d. Open the spread.

e. Tuck it under at the foot of the bed tightly.

f. Make a mitered corner at the foot of the bed.

g. Do not tuck in at the sides of the bed.

19. Now go to the other side of the bed. Start with the bottom sheet:

   a. Pull the sheet tight to get rid of all wrinkles.

   b. Miter the top corner (Figure 10–15◆).

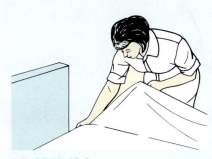

FIGURE 10–15 ◆
Miter the top corner

   c. Pull the plastic draw sheet tight and tuck it in.

   d. Pull the cotton draw sheet tight and tuck it in.

   e. Straighten out the top sheet, making a mitered corner at the foot of the bed.

   f. Miter the corner of the blanket.

   g. Miter the corner of the bedspread.

20. To make the cuff:

   a. Fold the top hem of the spread under the top hem of the blanket.

   b. Fold the top hem of the sheet back over the edge of the spread and the blanket to form a cuff (Figure 10–16◆). The hemmed

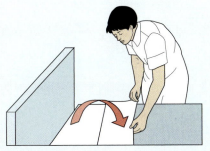

FIGURE 10–16 ◆
Fold the top hem of the sheet over the edge of spread and blanket to form a cuff

side of the sheet must be on the underside so that it does not come in contact with the patient.

21. To put the pillowcase on a pillow:

   a. Hold the pillowcase at the center of the end seam.

   b. With your hand outside the case, turn the case back over your hand (Figure 10–17◆).

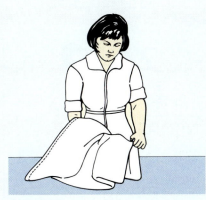

FIGURE 10–17 ◆
With your hand outside the case, turn the case back over your hand

   c. Grasp the pillow through the case at the center of one end of the pillow (Figure 10–18◆).

   d. Fit the corner of the pillow into the seamless corner of the case (Figure 10–19◆).

   e. Bring the case down over the pillow (Figure 10–20◆).

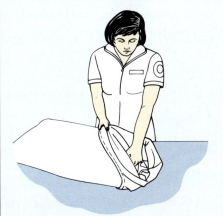

FIGURE 10–18 ◆
Grasp the pillow through the case at the center of one pillow end

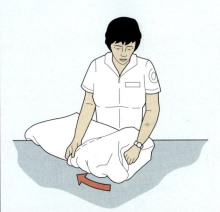

FIGURE 10–19 ◆
Fit the corner of the pillow into the seamless corner of the case

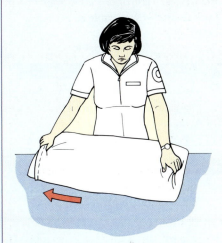

FIGURE 10–20 ◆
Bring the case down over the pillow

PROCEDURE *(continued)*

f. Fold the extra material from the side seam under the pillow.

g. Place the pillow on the bed with the open end away from the door.

22. Adjust bed to its lowest horizontal position (Figure 10–21◆).

FOLLOW-UP

23. Bag and dispose of soiled linen in the laundry hamper.

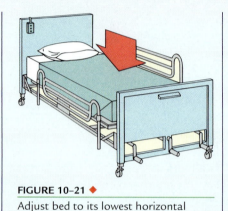

FIGURE 10–21 ◆
Adjust bed to its lowest horizontal position

24. Wash your hands.

25. Report to your immediate supervisor that you have made the closed, empty bed.

Open, Fan-Folded, or Empty Bed

fan-fold Method of arranging bed linens so that the covers and bedspread are folded at the foot of the bed out of the way

You will open the bed when a new patient has been assigned to the unit. You will be making an open bed when a unit is already occupied, but the patient is able to get out of bed and move around while you arrange the unit. The open bed is made exactly like the closed bed except the top sheets are **fan-folded** to the foot of the bed.

MAKING THE OPEN, FAN-FOLDED, OR EMPTY BED

PROCEDURE

OBRA

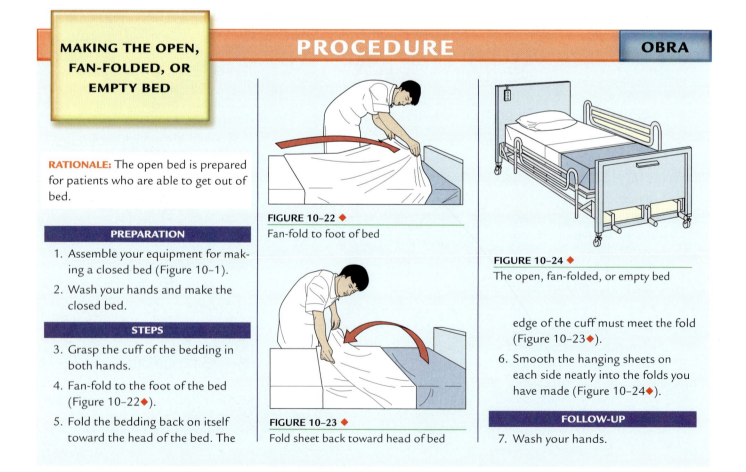

RATIONALE: The open bed is prepared for patients who are able to get out of bed.

PREPARATION

1. Assemble your equipment for making a closed bed (Figure 10–1).

2. Wash your hands and make the closed bed.

STEPS

3. Grasp the cuff of the bedding in both hands.

4. Fan-fold to the foot of the bed (Figure 10–22◆).

5. Fold the bedding back on itself toward the head of the bed. The

FIGURE 10–22 ◆
Fan-fold to foot of bed

FIGURE 10–23 ◆
Fold sheet back toward head of bed

FIGURE 10–24 ◆
The open, fan-folded, or empty bed

edge of the cuff must meet the fold (Figure 10–23◆).

6. Smooth the hanging sheets on each side neatly into the folds you have made (Figure 10–24◆).

FOLLOW-UP

7. Wash your hands.

Postoperative or Surgical Bed

The postoperative bed is also called the surgical, OR (operating room), stretcher, or recovery bed (Figure 10–25◆). The surgical bed is used for patients returning from the postoperative recovery room. The patient is brought in on a stretcher. The surgical bed is positioned to match the stretcher height. The stretcher will be lined up alongside the bed to allow the transfer of the patient from the stretcher to the bed. Some institutions make this bed with bath blankets; others do not. Be sure you follow the policy of the institution that employs you. Bath blankets may be necessary due to the cold surgical environment. In surgery the patient's pulse and blood pressure are lowered. This combined with the patient's lack of movement reduces circulation and reduces the patient's ability to produce body heat.

| MAKING THE POSTOPERATIVE OR SURGICAL BED | **PROCEDURE** | OBRA  |

RATIONALE: The postoperative or surgical bed is prepared for a patient returning from the OR or a procedure.

PREPARATION

1. Assemble your equipment for making a closed bed with the addition of a blanket and two cotton bath blankets.

2. Wash your hands.

STEPS

3. Adjust the bed to the highest horizontal, comfortable working position. Lock the bed in place. Strip

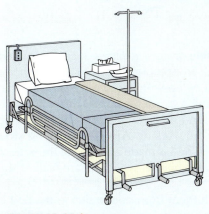

FIGURE 10–25 ◆
The postoperative or surgical bed

all used linen from the bed and place in the laundry bag.

4. Make the bottom part of the bed. Follow the instructions for making a closed bed.

5. Spread one bath blanket across the bed, on top of the draw sheet and bottom sheet. The bottom end of the bath blanket should be even with the foot of the mattress. Tuck the edge under the mattress on your side of the bed (Figure 10–26◆).

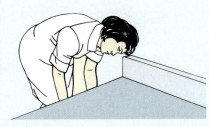

FIGURE 10–26 ◆
Tuck the bath blanket edge under the mattress

6. Go to the other side of the bed. Tuck the bath blanket under the mattress.

7. Spread the second bath blanket across the bed. The upper edge should be about 6 inches from the head of the bed. This blanket gives the patient extra warmth (Figure 10–27◆).

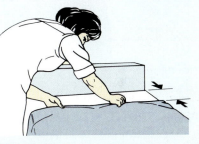

FIGURE 10–27 ◆
The upper edge of second bath blanket should be 6 inches from head of bed

8. Put the top sheet, the regular blanket, and the spread on the bed. Do this the same way as when making the closed bed, but do not tuck them in at the foot of the bed. Instead, all the bedding at the foot end should be folded back on the bed so the folded edge is even with the foot of the mattress (Figure 10–28◆).

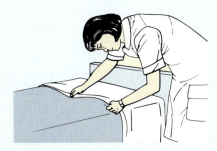

FIGURE 10–28 ◆
Fold bedding even with the foot of the mattress

PROCEDURE *(continued)*

9. Make the cuff the same as for the open bed, except you fold the blanket over the cuff (Figure 10–29◆).

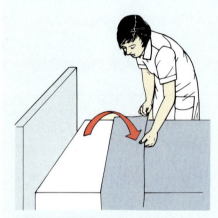

FIGURE 10–29 ◆
Fold blanket over the cuff

10. Go to the side of the bed where the stretcher will be in place.

11. Grasp the top bedding at the side with both hands. Fold the bedding across the bed so the folded edge is even with the far side of the mattress. Again, fold the bedding to the edge so it is twice folded onto itself (Figure 10–30◆).

12. Put the pillow into the pillowcase. Put the pillow upright against the headboard. Place it so as to protect the patient from hitting his or her

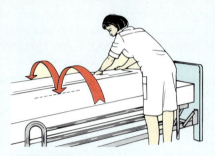

FIGURE 10–30 ◆
Fan-fold bedding to the edge

head on the headboard during the transfer procedure (Figure 10–31◆).

13. Move the bedside table, chair, and any other furniture out of the way to make room for the stretcher.

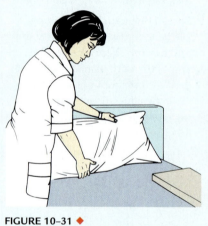

FIGURE 10–31 ◆
Place pillow at headboard

14. Remove everything from the bedside table except a box of tissues and an emesis basin.

15. Bring an IV pole into the room and place near the head of the bed, out of the way (Figure 10–32◆). (This is unnecessary if the facility uses portable IV pumps.)

16. Position the surgical bed to match stretcher height.

FOLLOW-UP

17. Wash your hands.

18. Report to your immediate supervisor that the postoperative, or surgical, bed has been made.

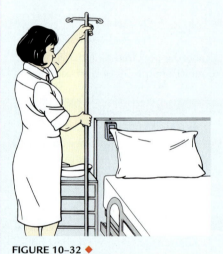

FIGURE 10–32 ◆
Place IV pole near head of bed

Occupied Bed

The occupied bed is made when the patient is not able or not permitted to get out of bed (Figure 10–33◆). The most important part of making an occupied bed is to get the sheets smooth and tight under the patient so that there will be no wrinkles to rub against the patient's skin. When making the bottom of this bed, your job will be easier if you divide the bed into two parts—the side the patient is lying on and the side you are making, so the weight of the patient is never on the side where you are working. **Always keep the side rail up on the patient's side.** Usually, the occupied bed is made after giving the patient a bed bath. The patient should be covered with the bath blanket while you are making the bed. Review the guidelines for bedmaking.

Some patients prefer the pillow to be moved with them from side to side as the bed is being made, and some patients ask you to remove the pillow while making the bed. Either way may be acceptable. However, there may be instances when your immediate supervisor instructs you to keep the patient's head flat, or elevated with a pillow, or in Fowler's position at all times.

MAKING THE OCCUPIED BED

PROCEDURE   **OBRA**

RATIONALE: The occupied bed is made when a patient is unable or not permitted to get out of bed.

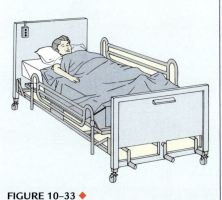

FIGURE 10–33 ◆
The occupied bed

PREPARATION

1. Assemble your equipment in the order in which it will be used, and place on a chair near the bed:

   a. Two large sheets

   b. One plastic draw sheet, if used

   c. One cotton draw sheet, if used

   d. Disposable or reusable bed protectors

   e. One bath blanket

   f. Pillowcase

   g. One blanket (optional per patient preference and room temperature)

   h. One bedspread

   i. One plastic laundry bag

2. Identify the patient by checking the identification bracelet.

3. Tell the patient you are going to make the bed.

4. Provide privacy for the patient.

STEPS

5. Wash your hands and put on gloves. (if linens are soiled).

6. Lower the backrest and knee rest until the bed is flat, if that is allowed. Raise the bed to a comfortable working height and lock in place. Keep side rails up to provide safety for the patient.

7. Loosen all the sheets around the entire bed.

8. Take the bedspread and blanket off the bed and fold them over the back of the chair, leaving the patient covered only with the top sheet.

9. Cover the patient with the bath blanket by placing it over the top sheet. Ask the patient to hold the bath blanket. If the patient is unable to do this, tuck the top edges of the bath blanket under the patient's shoulders. Without exposing the patient, remove the top sheet from under the bath blanket (Figure 10–34◆).

10. If the mattress has slipped out of place, move it to its proper position touching the headboard. Ask another nursing assistant to help.

11. Raise the bedside rail on the opposite side from where you will be working and lock in place (Figure 10–35◆).

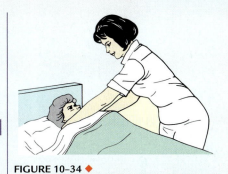

FIGURE 10–34 ◆
Tuck top of bath blanket under patient's shoulders

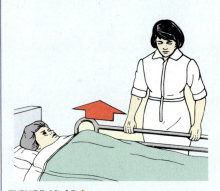

FIGURE 10–35 ◆
Raise and lock the side rail opposite the side on which you will be working

12. Ask the patient to turn onto her side toward the side rail. Help the patient to turn, if necessary. The patient is now on the far side of the bed (Figure 10–36◆).

13. Adjust the pillow for the patient according to instructions. If the patient cannot sit up, lock arms with her and raise her to remove the pillow. If you are leaving the pillow under the patient's head,

PROCEDURE *(continued)*

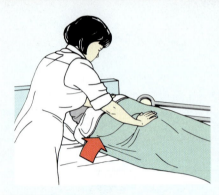

FIGURE 10–36 ◆

Help patient turn toward side rail

then move it over to the side of the bed, adjusting it so that it is comfortable.

14. Fold the cotton draw sheet toward the patient and tuck it against her back.

15. Raise the plastic draw sheet (if it is clean) over the bath blanket and the patient. If the plastic draw sheet is dirty, also fold it toward the patient.

16. Fold the bottom sheet toward the patient and tuck it against her back. This strips your side of the bed down to the mattress (Figure 10–37◆).

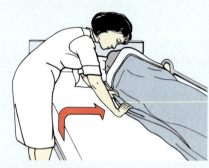

FIGURE 10–37 ◆

Fold and tuck bottom sheet against the patient's back

17. Take the large clean sheet and fold it in half lengthwise. Do not permit the sheet to touch the floor or your uniform.

18. Place the sheet on the bed, still folded, with the fold running along the middle of the mattress. The small hem end of the sheet should be even with the foot edge of the mattress. Fold the top half of the sheet toward the patient. Tuck the folds against her back, below the plastic draw sheet (Figure 10–38◆).

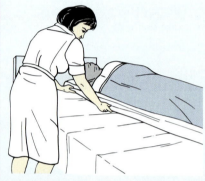

FIGURE 10–38 ◆

Tuck folds of clean sheet against the patient's back below the plastic draw sheet

19. Miter the corner at the head of the mattress. Tuck in the clean bottom sheet on your side from head to foot of the mattress.

20. Pull the plastic draw sheet toward you, over the clean bottom sheet, and tuck in.

21. Place the clean cotton draw sheet over the plastic sheet, folded in half. Fold the top half toward the patient, tucking the folds under her back, as you did with the bottom sheet. Tuck the draw sheet under the mattress.

22. Raise the bedside rail on your side of the bed and lock in place (Figure 10–39◆).

23. Go to the opposite side of the bed.

24. Lower the bedside rail. Ask the patient, or help her, to roll over the "hump" onto the clean sheets away from you. Be careful not to

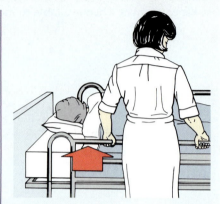

FIGURE 10–39 ◆

Raise and lock side rail on your side of bed

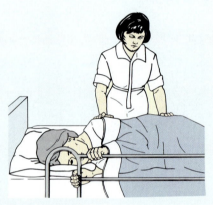

FIGURE 10–40 ◆

Roll or assist patient over hump onto clean sheets

let the patient become wrapped up in the bath blanket while turning (Figure 10–40◆).

25. Remove the old bottom sheet and cotton draw sheet from the bed. Pull the fresh bottom sheet toward the edge of the bed. Tuck it under the mattress at the head of the bed and make a mitered corner (Figure 10–41◆). Then tuck the bottom sheet under the mattress from the head to the foot, pulling firmly to remove any wrinkles (Figure 10–42◆).

26. Pull the plastic draw sheet and clean cotton draw sheet toward you.

PROCEDURE (continued)

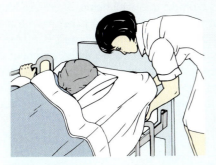

FIGURE 10–41 ◆

Miter the corner

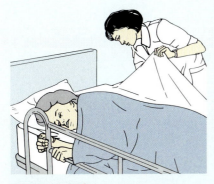

FIGURE 10–42 ◆

Pull bottom sheet tight and miter the corner

27. Then, one at a time, tuck the draw sheets under the mattress along the side.

28. Be sure to pull all the sheets tight as you tuck them in for a tight foundation.

29. Have the patient turn on her back, or turn her yourself, loosening the bath blanket as she turns.

30. Change the pillowcase and place the pillow under the patient's head (Figure 10–43 ◆).

31. Spread the clean top sheet over the bath blanket with the wide hem to the top. The middle of the sheet should run along the middle of the bed. The wide hem should be even with the head edge of the mattress. Remove the bath

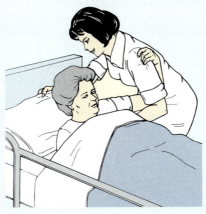

FIGURE 10–43 ◆

Place pillow under patient's head

blanket, moving toward the foot of the bed, without exposing the patient (Figure 10–44 ◆).

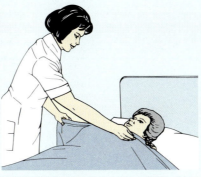

FIGURE 10–44 ◆

Remove bath blanket without exposing patient

32. Tuck the clean top sheet under the mattress at the foot of the bed. Make sure you leave enough room for the patient to move her feet freely. Miter the corners of the sheet.

33. Spread the blanket over the top sheet. Be sure the middle of the blanket runs along the middle of the bed. The blanket should be high enough to cover the patient's shoulders.

34. Tuck the blanket in at the foot of the bed. Make a mitered corner with the blanket.

35. Place the spread on the bed in the same way. Make a mitered corner with the spread.

36. Go to the other side of the bed and pull the top sheet, blanket, and spread over and straighten. Remove bath blanket. Turn the top covers back and miter the top sheet; then miter the blanket, and then miter the spread. Be sure the top covers are loose enough for the patient to move her feet.

37. To make the cuff:

   a. Fold the top hem edge of the spread over and under the top hem of the blanket.

   b. Fold the top hem of the top sheet back over the edge of the spread and blanket to form a cuff. The rough edge of the hem of the sheet must be turned down so the patient does not come in contact with it.

38. Raise the backrest and knee rest to suit the patient, if this is allowed.

39. Make the patient comfortable and replace the call light.

40. Lower the bed to a position of safety for the patient.

41. Raise the side rails when ordered or appropriate for patient safety.

42. Bag and dispose of used linen in the laundry hamper.

FOLLOW-UP

43. Dispose of gloves and wash your hands.

44. Report to your immediate supervisor:

   ■ That you have made the occupied bed.

   ■ How the patient tolerated the procedure.

   ■ Your observations of anything unusual.

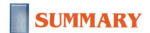 **SUMMARY**

A wrinkle-free bed is very important to the patient's comfort and well-being. There are four basic ways to make a bed. Each serves a special purpose. The closed bed is made with the top covers pulled to the head of the bed. An open bed, which has the top covers fan-folded to the foot of the bed, is made when a patient can be out of the bed. When a patient is bedridden, the occupied bed is made. A postoperative bed is made so the sheets are folded to one side for ease in moving a patient from the recovery stretcher to the bed. One of the guidelines in bedmaking is to never use a safety pin on the linen as it could open and injure the patient.

NOTES

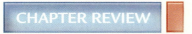

CHAPTER REVIEW

FILL IN THE BLANK Read each sentence and fill in the blank line with a word that completes the sentence.

1. Tissue breakdown resulting from pressure or reduced blood flow is called a _____ _____.

2. A _____ bed is one that is made with the bedspread in place.

3. An _____ bed is one made with the patient in it.

4. _____ should never touch a patient's skin.

5. By _____ a bed, you make it easy for the patient to get in and out.

MULTIPLE CHOICE Choose the best answer for each question or statement.

1. Bedmaking is important because
   a. it increases the patient's comfort.
   b. getting the wrinkles out is good for the skin.
   c. many patients spend a great deal of time in their beds.
   d. All of the above.

2. Never shake the linen when changing the bed in order to
   a. prevent the spread of germs.
   b. avoid knocking things over.
   c. save time.
   d. prevent distracting the patient.

3. When making a patient's bed, you should do all of the following *except*
   a. do not let dirty linen touch your uniform.
   b. avoid taking extra linen in the room.

   c. use pins to fix ripped linen.
   d. fold linen in on itself when removing it.

4. The use of a draw sheet is helpful
   a. to cover and protect the patient's bed.
   b. to move patients in bed.
   c. to increase patient's comfort during moves.
   d. All of the above.

5. Use the open, empty, or fan-folded type of bed when
   a. the patient can get out of bed.
   b. the patient is confined to bed.
   c. the patient is going to surgery.
   d. None of the above.

TIME-OUT

TIPS FOR TIME MANAGEMENT

When discharge cleaning or making up beds is part of your assignment, be sure to start as soon as you can rather than wait until other beds need to be cleaned or made up. Other patients or residents may be waiting to be admitted. You will be less hurried if you space your work rather than trying to get several time-consuming tasks done at the same time.

THE NURSING ASSISTANT IN ACTION

Mr. Jacobs is an elderly man whose bed sheets require frequent changes. You have already changed his bed once on your shift when you notice he has soiled his sheets again. You are already late to leave for your scheduled lunch break. It crosses your mind that you could pretend you did not notice and leave his room.

What Is Your Response/Action?

CRITICAL THINKING

CUSTOMER SERVICE You may encounter patients who have preferences for a particular type of pillow or who may require a hypoallergenic pillow because they are allergic to pillows containing feathers. If there are no other pillows available, suggest that a family member or friend may be able to bring in a pillow to be used by the patient or resident. Be sure to put patients' names on any personal items brought into the facility to reduce the chances they will be lost.

CULTURAL CARE Be aware that time is viewed differently among various cultures. Present-oriented persons may focus on the current moment and be less concerned about things that are scheduled in the future. Your supervisor and your patients may have very different expectations as to when or how soon bed linen should be changed or how quickly you respond to other patients care requests or needs.

COOPERATION WITHIN THE TEAM Check with team members to determine if your assigned patient will be leaving the unit for tests, physical therapy, or procedures. Changing the bed while the patient is away or is required to be up out of the bed is less disruptive for the patient. It is helpful to inform both your team members and the patient that you will be making the bed during that time.

EXPLORE MediaLink

Additional interactive resources for this chapter can be found on the Companion Website at www.prenhall.com/wolgin. Click on Chapter 10 and "Begin" to select activities for this chapter.

For chapter-related NCLEX-style questions and an audio glossary, access the accompanying CD-ROM in this book.

11 *Home Health Care*

OBJECTIVES

When you have completed this chapter, you will be able to:

- Differentiate between working in the home and in the health care institution.
- Describe the four categories of home health care providers.
- Define the role of the home health aide.
- Show respect for the beliefs, opinions, culture, and customs of patients and their families.
- List 26 basic tasks and procedures you may be assigned to perform in the home.
- Assist in the implementation of the discharge plan by communicating with the home care team.
- List nine procedures the home health aide may *not* do in the home.
- Describe 11 potential safety hazards in the home.
- Write a list of the phone numbers that should always be kept next to the phone for use in reporting an accident or emergency.
- List rules to follow for storing infant formula.
- List three types of infant formula.
- Sterilize water, bottles, nipples, and caps.
- Identify eight housekeeping responsibilities the home health aide may be assigned to perform in the home.
- Discuss how to apply at least five principles of infection control to the home setting.
- Discuss nutrition and food service as it applies to the home setting.
- Record your activities and those of the patient during your scheduled home visit.
- Describe the types of patient information that should be reported to the supervisor immediately.

KEY TERMS

bed-bound
caregiver
efficiency
family unit
flammable
formula
hospice care
infection control
long-term supportive care
microorganism
punctuality
responsibility
short-term intermittent skilled
   nursing care
sterilize
time/travel record

MediaLink
www.prenhall.com/wolgin

Use the address above to access the free, interactive Companion Website created for this textbook. Get hints, instant feedback, and textbook references to chapter-related NCLEX-style questions. Link to other interesting sites.

AUDIO GLOSSARY:

Use the Companion Website, or the CD-ROM disk enclosed with your textbook, to hear the pronunciation of key terms in the chapter.

Home health care is a rapidly expanding industry. As health care providers strive to reduce health care costs by decreasing the length of stay, patients are being discharged sooner or receiving services and surgery as outpatients. This chapter will help you discover the uniqueness of home health care and the special role that the nursing assistant or home health aide plays as part of the home care team. Working with patients and their families in their natural home environment presents a different set of challenges and opportunities than may be present in an institutional setting. One noticeable difference is that many agencies refer to individuals receiving care as clients rather than patients. Also, nursing assistants who are trained to work in the home are referred to as home health aides.

The area of home health offers many different types of situations in which you may choose to work. The types and ages of clients served, the hours worked, and the role responsibilities of the home health aide vary from agency to agency across the country. However, all home health aides, through the type of personal care they render, have an opportunity to significantly influence the quality of life of their clients. In this chapter, the qualities and attributes required of someone working in the home care field are discussed. Although the home health aide may be assigned many responsibilities and procedures that are the same as those performed in other settings, such as hospitals, some are unique to the home health care setting and are covered in detail in this chapter.

Working in the Home Health Care Field

ALERT

For all patient contact, adhere to Standard Precautions (⚭ Chapter 5, pages 84–86). Wear protective equipment as indicated.

long-term supportive care
The care of chronically ill patients who are unable to care for themselves and live alone or have limited family support

Home health care allows the patient to remain in her home while receiving an array of services that can encompass short-term intermittent skilled nursing, rehabilitative care, **long-term supportive care**, or hospice care depending on her needs (Figure 11–1◆). Services can be provided on an intermittent basis, such as once a month, or up to 24 hours a day, 7 days a week. The primary purpose of intermittent skilled care is to educate acutely ill patients and their families on how to best meet the patients' specific needs. The goal is to promote maximum independence in self-care and functional ability, encouraging patients' active participation in their own health care. Throughout this chapter the words *client* and *patient* are used interchangeably.

Long-term supportive care is available for chronically ill patients who are unable to care for themselves and live alone or have limited family support. Hospice care is available for patients with terminal conditions who choose to remain at home until their death.

Federal government regulations require home health aides to complete a training program and competency evaluation check to verify skills prior to the time of hire. Additional hours of continuing education are also required yearly. See Chapter 35 for more information about skills competency and continuing education.

For Medicare- and Medicaid-reimbursed agencies, an assessment tool called OASIS is now being utilized at the start of care for each client. OASIS stands for *Outcome and Assessment Information Set* and is used to clearly describe clients' needs, provide data for assessment and care planning, and facilitate information sharing with all caregivers. The OASIS and any other assessment information will be used to determine the home health aide care plan and frequency of visits.

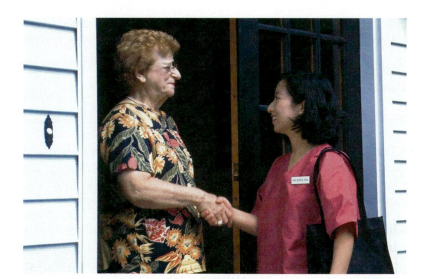

FIGURE 11–1 ◆
The nursing assistant cares for patients in the home

Home Health Care Agencies and Other Employees

Substantial differences can exist among the variety of agencies providing home health care. The four main categories of home health care providers include privately owned, for-profit or not-for-profit agencies; publicly operated health departments; hospital-based home health services; and national networks of investor-owned or not-for-profit agencies. There are state-by-state differences concerning license requirements for home health care agencies. Some agencies may be certified to provide Medicare- and Medicaid-reimbursed services and others may only provide services for patients on a private fee-for-service or insurance-reimbursed basis. The type of services that may be provided are often dependent on the client's health insurance coverage. Medicare and Medicaid typically will pay for home health aides only if the client has a need for a skilled nurse. While the types of home care services provided by agencies vary, all offer basic nursing services. Staffing patterns are determined by the types of services provided. Some agencies offer various levels of home services, including those that do not provide hands-on care. These assistants may be called homemakers or companions, and their duties do not include the personal care that home health aides give. Homemaker and companion's tasks are focused on housekeeping, meal preparing, running of errands, and providing company for the client or someone to assist in obtaining further assistance when needed. In most cases, however, the home care nursing staff will consist of registered nurses, licensed practical/vocational nurses, and home health aides.

The Home Health Aide

With *professional supervision*, the home health aide is able to assist the patient with the activities of daily living and maintain a safe, clean, and comfortable environment. The patient in the home should receive high-quality nursing care. All the nursing skills and principles explained in this textbook must be applied by the home health aide. Adhere to the same high standards of ethical professional behavior outlined in Chapter 2.

Just as the nursing assistant in the health care institution works under the direct supervision of a registered nurse or physician, so does the home health aide in the home. The main difference between working in the home and in the health care institution is that in the home the home health aide may be alone while working. It is essential that the home care aide keep the supervisor and home care nurse informed about any changes observed in the patient's condition.

Helpful Personal Qualities of the Home Health Aide

As a member of the health care team, you are expected to maintain a professional attitude in the home. The same qualities that will make you a successful nursing assistant in a health care institution will be necessary if you are to be successful as a home health aide. The best home health aides are those who are dependable, trustworthy, considerate, tactful, ethical, courteous, self-starters, sympathetic, energetic, polite, careful, observant, sensitive, and good listeners. Communication skills are an essential part of your job. You will be in close contact with the patient, family members, and visitors. Since you will be spending more time in the home than any other team member, patients and families may share important information with you that they may not tell the nurse or therapist.

It is important to respect the privacy and confidentiality of your patient. Do not discuss the patient's condition with visitors in the home. All observations and information obtained from the patient should be shared only with the members of the home care team. You should never discuss your personal problems with the patient.

Demonstrate honesty and accuracy when handling the patient's money and valuables. Show respect by treating the patient's possessions carefully. Display dependability by never leaving before an assignment is completed. Self-discipline, time management, and the motivation to do a good job are especially important qualities, since you are working alone in the home.

The Importance of Efficiency and Punctuality

efficiency Getting all of one's duties completed in an organized fashion within a designated work period

punctuality Arriving at one's planned destination on time

hospice care The care of patients with terminal conditions who choose to remain at home until their death

short-term intermittent skilled nursing care The care provided to acutely ill patients or those with an exacerbated illness with the purpose of educating the patients to become independent in self-care and functional ability

time/travel record Record or log describing how time is spent in a patient's home and/or account of travel time to and from the patient's home or running errands

Efficiency is getting all of your assigned duties completed in an organized and accurate fashion within your designated hours of work. **Punctuality** is arriving at your planned destination on time. The frequency of visits to any one patient may vary from once a week to daily. The length of time spent in the home of a patient can range from 1 to 8 hours on a single visit, depending on whether the home health aide services are part of a short-term, intermittent skilled service or are being provided as part of private duty or **hospice** respite services. If the home health aide is assigned to **short-term intermittent services**, she will be expected to make three to five visits to different patients per day. Usually, the home health aide carries the same patients on her caseload from the time of assignment until the home health aide services are discontinued. Once the home health aide is assigned a caseload of patients, she may be responsible for managing her own visit schedule.

When scheduling the visits for each day, the home health aide must balance individual patient needs and preferences with travel distances to maximize efficient use of her time. The home health aide should always leave a schedule in the home of planned visit dates and times on a weekly basis. Prior to each day's visits, the home health aide should call each patient to confirm the time of the visit. By doing so, the home health aide will ensure that the patient will be at home when she arrives. Once a visit arrival time is agreed on with the patient and/or family, it is important that the home health aide arrive on time. If an unplanned delay occurs, a courtesy call to the patient's home is essential to report the delay and agree on a new arrival time. The number one complaint of home care patients is *the failure of home care staff to adhere to agreed-on arrival times and the lack of communication regarding the change in arrival time.*

You will be shown how to complete a time and/or travel record when one is used by your agency. **Time/travel records** describe the tasks performed in the patient's home and indicate the time required to travel to and from the patient's home or to run errands, for example, to go food shopping.

Transcultural Nursing in the Home

Unlike assignments in a hospital where a unit will have patients with similar conditions or ages such as surgical, orthopedic, or pediatric patients, the home health aide will work in many different types of communities with people of all ages, ethnicities, religious beliefs, economic and educational levels, and medical problems. The home health aide must be able to provide the same unconditional acceptance and compassionate care to all of her patients regardless of these differences. As a member of the home care team, the home health aide is a guest in the patient's home and must behave in a respectful manner.

The atmosphere and lifestyle will be different in every home in which you work. You must respect the rights of the patient and his family to have beliefs and opinions, culture, and customs that might be different from your own. People of different backgrounds may eat foods you have never seen or tasted; they may behave differently toward their family members than you would; their religious beliefs may seem unusual to you; and their standards of cleanliness or general lifestyle may be from yours. Accept these differences with respect and understanding, without judging or criticizing. Let the patient know it is your pleasure, not just your job, to assist him.

 # The Family Unit

A **family unit** is a group brought together by shared needs, interests, and mutual concern for the well-being of all its members. The family may consist of parents, children, and even friends living together with mutual needs (Figure 11–2◆). Every family, regardless of its structure, has unique needs, rules, and customs. When you are working in the home setting, you must be aware and sensitive to the way each particular family functions. Family members can tell you the patient's likes, dislikes, or expectations if the patient is unable to do so.

The family may have values and behaviors that you are not familiar with, or of which you personally disapprove. You may be sent to work in a home where you may feel uncomfortable or unsure of your actions. You should discuss these feelings with your supervisor who can help you understand how to work effectively with the family. Being honest with yourself and recognizing your feelings and reactions can help you provide the best care possible in a given situation. Don't let your feelings keep you from doing the best job you can.

family unit A group brought together by shared needs, interests, and mutual concern for the well-being of all its members

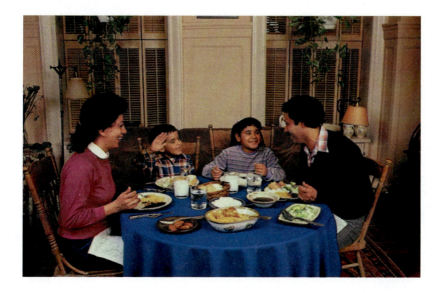

FIGURE 11–2 ◆

A family shares mutual concern for the well-being of its members

Reactions of families to illness, disability, and crisis vary. The loved one's illness or disability may be overwhelming to some family members. A sensitive home health aide can observe some of the problems within the family unit and discuss them with the home care supervisor. Often, when help is offered, a family in crisis can make the necessary changes to cope with illness. Remember, this is a family unit that has set up patterns of coping over a long period of time. You must learn to work with these patterns. Crisis is not a good time to change coping mechanisms. The term **caregiver** refers to the family member who is taking the primary responsibility for the patient. Do not give advice, take sides, make judgments about family members, or get involved in family conflicts and problems.

It is important for you to have a good working relationship with the patient and the family. The patient's family may be unable or unwilling to provide daily health care because they:

- Work outside the home
- Care for small children or older parents or relatives
- Have physical limitations themselves
- Live far away from the patient and as a result they:
    - Cannot help with physical and personal care
    - Cannot provide a safe, clean environment
    - Cannot provide transportation
    - Cannot shop and prepare meals

caregiver The family member or significant other who is taking the major responsibility for the care of the patient

Duties of the Home Health Aide

The basic nursing assistant tasks and procedures you will be accountable for in your work will be found on the job description given to you by your employing agency. Listed here are basic tasks and procedures that you may be asked to perform. While many of the duties are the same as those you would do in any health care institution, there are some differences when working in the home. Seek your supervisor's guidance if you are in a questionable situation. Where the duties are the same, refer to the procedures given throughout this book and follow them carefully when performing them in the home. Do not perform any skill you have not been taught to do, only those tasks you were assigned to do. A home health aide care plan provides direction and a reminder of which tasks need to be done.

While working in the home, be careful not to disturb the patient's or family's belongings. Replace any items you may have moved while providing care for the patient or performing some other required task.

Basic Nursing Assistant Tasks and Procedures

- Keep the patient informed of procedures you perform.
- Observe, record, and report any changes in the patient's condition, and keep records of patient care activities.
- Control the spread of microorganisms in the home by using proper handcleansing techniques; maintain a clean environment for the patient.
- Assist the patient during the use of special equipment such as a wheelchair, walker, commode, or mechanical lift.
- Make the patient's bed and change the linens as often as necessary to maintain a clean, dry, and comfortable bed for the patient.
- Clean any equipment used in the care of the patient.

- Wash the patient's clothing, bed linens, and towels as appropriate.
- Lift, move, and transport the patient and assist with ambulation.
- Assist with passive range-of-motion exercises as ordered.
- Position the patient.
- Assist with personal care, including oral hygiene, bathing, perineal care of females, dressing, shampooing, combing the hair, shaving the beard, nail and foot care, and using the bedpan, urinal, bedside commode, or bathroom facilities.
- Record intake and output as ordered.
- Change simple, nonsterile dressings and apply nonmedicated topical ointments.
- Prepare and serve the patient's food, which might include grocery shopping and cooking; follow prescribed therapeutic diets and feed patients as necessary; offer between-meal nourishment if that is part of the patient's care plan.
- Collect urine specimens, if included in your agency's job description.
- Observe, measure, and record vital signs and weight.
- Apply elastic bandages or antiembolism stockings, external prostheses, and eye prostheses according to agency policy and procedure.
- Assist with ostomy care.
- Provide cast care.
- Prevent pressure ulcers through proper skin care, back rubs, and observation and report of changes.
- Perform basic urine tests for sugar and/or acetone.
- Do light housekeeping tasks related to the direct needs and in the immediate environment of the patient.
- Transport the patient to the physician's office and other appointments after getting permission from the home care supervisor if that is part of your agency's service.
- Report to the home care supervisor or nurse your observations of anything unusual.
- Record all observations about the patient and completed activities of daily living assignments.
- Remind the patient to take any medications that were prescribed by the physician.

Using the Discharge Plan

The home care patient is first evaluated by the home care nurse who develops a care plan based on the patient's needs. If the plan includes assistance with daily living activities such as bathing, dressing, and toileting, the services of a home health aide will be ordered (Figure 11–3◆). Since the primary purpose of home care is to assist the patient and family to become independent in the care of the patient, the types and amounts of services are usually more intense in the beginning and gradually reduced in frequency over the duration of the service period.

The home health aide must understand the outcome goals planned for the patient and the plan of care to support achievement of those goals. The home health aide will generally start out doing more for the patient and gradually encourage the patient to assume more responsibility for his self-care as his condition allows, until he has reached his expected level of independence. When all the goals have been met, the patient will be discharged from home care. The home health aide's communication with the rest of the home care team about the patient's progress and functional ability will assist in the discharge planning process. Home health care provides opportunities to see patients progress and to form supportive relationships.

FIGURE 11–3 ◆

A discharge plan may include assisting a patient with daily living activities

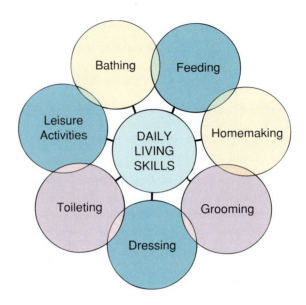

FIGURE 11–3 ◆

A discharge plan may include assisting a patient with daily living activities

Procedures the Home Health Aide May Not Do in the Home

The nursing tasks home health aides are not permitted to do in the home vary from state to state and from agency to agency. In most areas of this country, home health aides may *not* do the following tasks:

- Change sterile dressings.
- Irrigate body cavities (this includes administering enemas and irrigation of ostomies or wounds).
- Perform gastric lavage or gavage.
- Perform catheterization.
- Administer oral medications or apply topical medications.
- Apply heat by any method.
- Care for a tracheotomy tube.
- Perform wound packings.
- Perform heavy cleaning chores such as moving heavy furniture, waxing floors, shampooing carpets, washing windows, and carrying firewood.

Safety in the Home

Patients are prone to having accidents in the home and may be unable to take care of themselves in case of an emergency. As the home health aide, you will be responsible for the patient's safety while you are present in the home. You can ensure a safe environment for your patient and yourself by eliminating, preventing, or correcting conditions that could cause accidents. Safety in the home includes proper infection control, electrical and fire safety, and accident prevention. Refer to Chapter 31 for special precautions regarding infant safety.

Safety Hazards

As you go about your work, be alert and look for the following hazards. Make a note of these hazards and bring them to the attention of the patient, responsible family member, your supervisor, and the home care nurse. Some of the most common safety hazards in the home are:

- Damaged electrical wiring on large and small appliances
- Overloaded electrical outlets
- Faulty or uneven stairs
- Loose rugs that slip
- Poisons (highest incidence in children due to medication and cleaning solutions)
- Flammable cleaning rags, mops, and brooms (these should be cleaned after each use and stored in a well-ventilated place)
- Sharp objects such as knives, razors, and lawn tools
- Wet floors (spills should be wiped up immediately)
- Cluttered walkways
- Unstable furniture
- Ambulatory devices that need repair; for example, replacement of rubber tips on walkers, canes, or crutches

Fire Safety and Burn Prevention

- Avoid using **flammable** liquids. Use flame-resistant clothing for the patient and follow the washing instructions on the label inside the clothing to keep them flame resistant (Figure 11–4◆).

flammable Capable of burning quickly and easily

- Caution the patient against smoking while seated on upholstered furniture or the bed, especially when sleepy.
- Caution the patient and/or family to refrain from smoking when oxygen is being used in the home.
- If the patient is a smoker, use a deep, wide-rimmed ashtray and set it on a table. Extinguish smoldering butts when the patient is finished smoking.

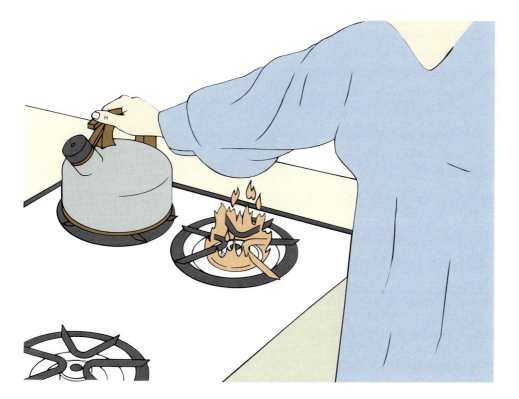

FIGURE 11–4 ◆

Many garment-related fires cause injuries when a loose-fitting portion of a garment, such as a sleeve or skirt hem, comes in contact with a stove burner, lighted candle, space heater, or fireplace fire; flaming liquids also cause serious injuries when they splash onto a garment and ignite its fabric or when the textile is wet with a flammable liquid (such as lighter fluid), which is then ignited by a nearby spark or flame

- Do not use an extension cord or electric cord and plug unless it is in excellent condition.
- Arrange furniture with fire safety in mind. Place furniture well away from stoves, space heaters, and fireplaces, and out of walkways.
- If a fire occurs, get the patient out of the house. If the patient is bedridden, follow your agency's policy regarding fire emergencies. Know the exit route. If the apartment is above the first floor, know where the stairs are.
- To provide a safe, quick exit, make sure the key remains in the lock of any door(s) that lock on the inside with a key.
- Encourage the family to have a fire extinguisher and smoke detector in the home. Make sure smoke detectors are working and batteries are tested monthly.
- Follow the safety rules of your local fire department.
- Keep matches away from children and confused adults.
- Check the temperature of water before using it on a patient.

Reporting an Accident or Emergency by Telephone

If an accident or emergency does occur, you must be ready to handle the situation calmly and wisely. Report every accident to your supervisor immediately.

Phone Numbers to Keep Handy

It is important to have emergency phone numbers written next to the phone. The list should include:

- Emergency Medical Service (often *911*) if available
- Police department
- Fire department
- Responsible family member at work
- Your home care supervisor or agency
- Patient's physician
- Nearest hospital
- Ambulance service
- Poison control center
- Pharmacy

If there is no phone in the home, arrange in advance to use a neighbor's phone in case of an emergency.

Calling for Help

Most states have laws regarding a patient's right to execute an Advance Directive. Make sure you are aware of your agency's policy regarding the types of medical emergencies that are affected by an Advance Directive and how you are to handle them. Many areas have a special phone number to call when an accident or emergency occurs in the home. You may call that number or the physician phone number that you have been given by the family or agency. (See also the procedure on Calling for Help in Chapter 9, pages 210–211.) No matter whom you call, you must be clear in reporting the accident or emergency. Be sure to:

- Give your name and title
- Give the name of the patient
- Clearly state the problem; objectively state exactly what has happened
- Give the address and phone number of where you are
- Clearly state the condition of the patient or person who has had the accident or is in a crisis
- If calling a city emergency number, give the phone number of the patient's physician to the person who answers the phone call
- If you have a phone number for a member of the family, give that number to the emergency answering service
- Remain with the patient until help arrives

Refer to Chapter 6 for additional patient safety information.

 # Care of the Infant in the Home

Home care services to infants may include normal newborn follow-up as well as care of the sick infant. Agencies throughout the country will vary in their policies regarding the types of staff who are assigned to do infant care in the home. If you are employed by an agency that includes infant care in the home health aide job description, refer to Chapter 31 of this textbook regarding the care of infants and pediatric patients. Infant care procedures you may be asked to perform *in the home* are given here in Chapter 11.

If for any reason the mother is unable to feed or care for the baby, you may be asked to do it. Refer to Chapter 31 regarding breastfeeding, burping, bathing, care of the circumcision, and diapering. This is an opportunity to demonstrate to a new mother the newborn's need for handling, affection, and security.

Preparing Formula

If the mother is breastfeeding her baby, you may bring the baby to her when it is time for a feeding. If the baby is being bottle-fed, you may need to prepare the **formula**. The home care nurse will obtain orders from the infant's physician as to the type of formula needed to meet the infant's special needs. Several types of milk-based and milk-free formulas are available. The nurse will provide instructions on the dilution of the formula, number of ounces per feeding, and the number of feedings per day. Be sure to read and follow the directions on the label.

formula A liquid food prescribed for an infant containing most required nutrients

---

STORING FORMULA	GUIDELINES	
■ Formula can be kept refrigerated for 2 days without spoiling. ■ After 2 days, formula must be thrown away. ■ If you are not sure how long formula has been in the refrigerator, discard it.	■ Do not risk the baby's health by feeding her formula that might be spoiled. ■ Formula will begin to spoil within 2 hours when it is left at room temperature.	■ Keep the bottle refrigerated until 10 minutes before the feeding. ■ Do not freeze formula. ■ After feeding, throw away any formula left in baby's bottle.

Different Types of Formula

- Ready-to-feed
- Powdered
- Concentrated liquid

Unopened cans and bottles do not have to be refrigerated. Wash all cans and bottles before opening. Remember to shake all cans of liquid and concentrated formulas before opening them. Use a *clean, sterile can opener* to open all cans. After assembling all needed equipment, wash hands before and after preparation of the formula or sterilization of bottles. Dishwashers provide an easy way to clean baby bottles and nipples. Check with the nurse or the parents to see if special precautions or sterilization is necessary.

Ready-to-feed (Prepared) Formula

While expensive to buy, this type of formula needs no preparation. Shake and open the can and pour the contents into sterile (clean) bottles. Some ready-to-feed formulas come in disposable bottles, to which you attach a sterile nipple and ring, and it is ready to feed the baby. DO NOT ADD WATER.

Powdered Formula

Follow the instructions provided by the nurse regarding the amounts of powder and sterile water to mix together. Be sure to mix the powder with water that you have boiled and allowed to cool. Mix the powder and sterile water in sterile bottles. Once mixed, this formula must be kept refrigerated.

Note: Powder mixes best when you use boiled water that has cooled to a warm temperature. Shake for 5 seconds.

Concentrated Liquid Formula

Follow the instructions provided by the nurse regarding the dilution of the concentrate. You must boil the water before you mix the formula. As with the powdered formula, this must be mixed in sterile bottles or a sterile pitcher. Once mixed, this formula must also be kept refrigerated.

In certain areas, you will not be instructed to boil water to **sterilize** bottles and nipples. Ask your supervisor or the home care nurse for instructions for your area.

sterilize Destroying all microorganisms

PROCEDURE   OBRA

STERILIZING TAP WATER

RATIONALE: Water in some homes may contain harmful microorganisms best destroyed by boiling the water.

PREPARATION

1. Wash your hands.
2. Assemble your equipment:

   a. Saucepan
   b. Water
   c. Timer, watch, or clock

STEPS

3. Fill the saucepan two-thirds full with water and place on burner.
4. When the water comes to a full boil, begin timing. Allow the water to remain at a full boil for 20 minutes in covered pan.
5. Allow the water to cool before using it to mix the formula.

CHARTING EXAMPLE: 11/30/04
8 am Sterilized water. M. Clean, CNA

| STERILIZING BOTTLES | PROCEDURE | OBRA |

RATIONALE: Some water supplies contain harmful microorganisms. Bottles and water require sterilization to kill these microorganisms.

PREPARATION

1. Wash your hands.
2. Assemble your equipment:
   a. Bottles
   b. Nipples, caps, and jar
   c. Bottle brush
   d. Dishwashing detergent
   e. Hot water from the tap
   f. Large pot with cover or a special sterilizing pot for baby bottles
   g. Small towel
   h. Tap water
   i. Timer, watch, or clock
   j. Tongs

STEPS

3. Scrub bottles, nipples, and caps with hot soapy water. Use the bottle brush to clean inside the bottles. Always squirt hot, soapy water through the holes in the nipples to clean out any dried-on formula.
4. Rinse thoroughly with hot water.
5. Fold the small towel to fit the bottom of the pot and lay it in the pot to prevent the bottles from breaking (this is not necessary when using a bottle rack).
6. Stand the washed bottles on the towel in a circle around the inside of the pot (Figure 11–5◆).

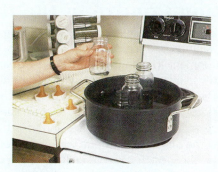

FIGURE 11–5 ◆
Sterilizing bottles

7. Place the caps and nipples into the clean, empty jar and place it into the pot at the center of the bottles.
8. Pour water into and around the bottles and into the jar with the nipples until two-thirds of each bottle is under water. Place the tongs upright in the pot to sterilize them.
9. Cover the pot and place on the stove.
10. When the water comes to a full boil, begin timing. Allow the water to remain at a full boil for 20 minutes.
11. Using the sterile tongs, remove the nipples and caps in the jar 10 to 15 minutes after the full boil began. With the nipples still inside the jar, stand the jar on the table to cool.
12. Take the cover off the pot and allow it to cool.
13. Remove the sterile bottles from the pot with sterile tongs.

FOLLOW-UP

14. Empty the water out of the pot. The pot is now sterilized and can be used for mixing the formula, if needed.

CHARTING EXAMPLE: 11/30/04 4pm Bottles and water sterilized M. Clean, CNA

Housekeeping Responsibilities in the Home

The tasks expected of you will vary from home to home depending on the availability and ability of family members. If the home care nurse asks you to do the shopping for the patient, keep an accurate written account of the amount of money given to you by the patient. Be sure to save the register receipts for the total amount spent. Return the correct amount of change. Include this information, along with the date and time, in your written report.

It is best to clarify any questions with your supervisor as to what will be expected of you before you make your first visit to the home. This will avoid future misunderstandings. Patients and their family members will sometimes request you to do tasks that are not appropriate or allowed by your agency. It is helpful to be open and honest when communicating with the patient and family members. Refusal of these tasks should be done in a firm but tactful manner. If problems arise, notify your supervisor and request that she or the nurse explain your role to the family.

Cleaning Responsibilities May Include:

- Washing linens and clothing used by the patient only
- Sweeping the floor or vacuuming the carpet in the patient's immediate area of use
- Straightening up and dusting the patient's immediate area
- Cleaning the bathroom, including tub, toilet, sink, floor, and mirror after assisting the patient with his bath
- Returning used items to their proper places
- Disposing of soiled, disposable items, following your agency's policy on the handling and disposal of waste materials; refer to Chapter 5 for information on waste management
- Cleaning spills and crumbs from the stove, counters, sink, and floor following preparation of meals for the patient
- Washing dishes used by the patient only

infection control Restraining or curbing the spread of microorganisms

responsibility A duty or obligation; that for which one is accountable

microorganism A living thing so small it cannot be seen with the naked eye but only through a microscope

Infection Control in the Home

It is your **responsibility** to assist in preventing the spread of **microorganisms** in the home by using proper handwashing techniques, standard precautions, and maintaining a clean environment for the patient. Refer to Chapter 5 for detailed instructions on handwashing and standard precautions. Wash fruits and vegetables before cooking or serving. Refrigerate or freeze all perishable foods as appropriate. You should use hot water and detergent when washing dishes. Wash dishes and cooking vessels immediately after using. Be sure to rinse well. Dispose of garbage and soiled supplies promptly.

Cleaning the tub and commode with a disinfectant will help to eliminate odors and will cut down on the growth of bacteria. If there is more than one person using the bathroom, encourage them to use their own towels. Never place soiled linen or clothing on furniture or carpets. Place them in a plastic bag until the family can wash them, unless the nurse has asked you to do the laundry. Laundry bleach is an inexpensive and effective disinfectant that can be found in most homes. Be careful not to allow bleach to come in contact with carpets and materials that could become damaged by the bleaching action.

If there are no cleaning supplies available, discuss this with your supervisor or the home care nurse. In some homes, cleaning supplies and even patient care supplies may be limited. You will have to be flexible and improvise with what is available. For example, you may substitute baking soda on a wet toothbrush or a solution of mouthwash and water if there is no toothpaste.

Nutrition and Food Service

Prior to mealtime, assist the patient to wash his face and hands. Some patients, especially those with dentures, will find the meal more appetizing if they rinse their mouths out with mouthwash and water. Assist with oral hygiene as desired by the patient. Position the patient for maximum comfort and to reduce risk of choking or aspiration.

Some patients may have prepared meals delivered to their homes if they live alone and are unable to prepare their own meals. The delivered meals usually consist of one warm meal and one cold meal. The nurse may ask you to set up the meal and assist the patient as needed. In some cases, you may have to prepare a light meal or snack for the patient (Figure 11–6a◆). The kind of written instructions left in the home by the nurse will vary from agency to agency; however, most will leave basic instructions or a home health aide assignment sheet in the home.

If the patient's special diet needs are not included on the instruction sheet, check with your supervisor or the nurse before preparing the meals. When preparing foods, consider

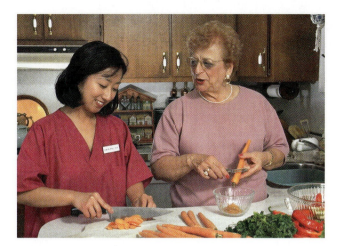

FIGURE 11–6a ◆

The home health aide can assist the client with snack or meal preparation.

the patient's likes and dislikes, including cultural preferences and religious practices, allergies to foods, and ability to chew and swallow. Some patients have difficulty in chewing because dentures do not fit well, their own teeth are in poor condition, or because they have mouth sores. If you notice this, report it to your supervisor or the nurse and try to provide softer, more easily chewed foods. The food should always be prepared and arranged in an attractive manner and served on a clean surface. Check all foods for spoilage before serving.

If you are assigned to stay with the patient for a full 8-hour shift, inquire as to when the patient prefers to have her meals. If you will be in the home for a shorter period of time to render care and are to prepare a meal for the patient, schedule your visit so you will be in the home during mealtime. If you have to leave the home before the meal is to be served, a cold meal may be prepared and left in the refrigerator or within reach of the patient.

The **bed-bound** patient's appetite may be small. Even if the meals are small, they must be well balanced and contain enough fluids.

bed-bound Unable to get out of bed

Refer to Chapter 21 for nutritional information. When purchasing and preparing food, it is important to read the food product labels to be certain that the food is allowed on the patient's prescribed diet (Figure 11–6b◆).

Reporting And Recording

A carefully written record of your activities and those of the patient must be kept. These notes help you and other team members monitor any changes in the client's status. The format of written home health aide assignments will vary from agency to agency. Some agencies combine the assignment sheet and the patient's daily record on the same form. You will receive charting expectations and information from your agency.

Regardless of the type of record form, it is very important that you document everything you do while in the home, including how the patient tolerated activities and procedures. It is important to record the patient's orientation to time, place, and person. Record the patient's food intake, activity level, vital signs, and urine sugar and acetone results.

Be sure your handwriting is neat and legible. It is best to write each activity down as soon as it is completed, while you are still in the home. Do not rely on your memory. If you are to report to your supervisor before you leave the home or after you have completed all of your patient home visits for the day, be sure this is done. However, observations of any problems or changes in the patient's condition should be reported to the supervisor or home care nurse immediately.

Figure 11–7◆ shows a sample of a home health aide daily progress record. To document the activities of daily living on a flow sheet see Chapter 12.

Not a Low Calorie Food		
Nutrition Facts		
Serving Size 1 cup (49g)		
Servings Per Container about 10		
Amount Per Serving	Cereal	Cereal with 1/2 cup Skim Milk
Calories	170	210
Calories from Fat	5	5
		% Daily Value**
Total Fat 0.5g*	1%	1%
Saturated Fat 0g	0%	0%
Polyunsaturated Fat 0g		
Monounsaturated Fat 0g		
Cholesterol 0mg	0%	0%
Sodium 0mg	0%	3%
Potassium 200mg	6%	11%
Total Carbohydrate 41g	14%	16%
Dietary Fiber 5g	21%	21%
Insoluble Fiber 5g		
Sugars 0g		
Other Carbohydrate 36g		
Protein 5g		
Vitamin A	0%	4%
Vitamin C	0%	2%
Calcium	2%	15%
Iron	8%	8%
Thiamin	8%	10%
Riboflavin	2%	10%

FIGURE 11–6b ◆

Reading labels will help you select foods suited to the patient's diet

Tasks to be performed. (Each visit or as specified) ✓

*Do per Patient request

Frequency of visits: _____

Estimated length of visits: _____

PERSONAL CARE	NUTRITION / MEAL PREPARATION	TREATMENTS
Bed Bath	Fluid Restriction	❏ Change Ostomy Appliance (specify): _____
Sponge Bath	Nothing by Mouth	_____
Shower	Diet (specify)	_____
Tub Bath	Assist with Meal Prep. / Snack	_____
Backrub	Encourage Fluid	_____
Shampoo	Assist / Feed Pt.	_____
Shave	**HOME SUPPORT ACTIVITIES**	_____
Comb / Brush Hair	Assist with Meds / Supp.	❏ Decubitus Care (specify): _____
Oral Hygiene	Maintain Clean, Sale Environment	_____
Nail Care (clean & file only)	Linen Change	_____
Pori Care	Essential Laundry	_____
Skin Care powder / lotion	Wash Dishes	_____
Apply Ted Hose	Encourage Pt. Independence	_____
ACTIVITIES	Relieve Family Member	Wound Care (specify): _____
Bedrest with Position Changes	Role Model	_____
Bedrails Up	**PRECAUTIONS**	_____
Use of Transfer / Gait Belt	Diabetic	_____
Use of Hoyer Lift	Oxygen O2 @ _____ / _____	_____
Ambulation Assisted Unassisted	Fall	_____
Cane	Seizure	_____
Walker	Bleeding	_____
Wheelchair	Sale Transfer	Foot Soak (specify): _____
No weight bearing Rt. Lt.	Other	_____
ELIMINATION	**SPECIAL CONDITIONS**	_____

ELIMINATION	SPECIAL CONDITIONS		TREATMENTS
Incontinent Care	Alert	Smoking	_____
Foley/SP Catheter Care	Oriented	Cats / Dogs	_____
Date Last BM	Confused	Vision	_____
Assist with Toileting	Lives Alone	HOH	_____
BRP / BSC / Bedpan / Urinal	DNR	Deal	Home Exercise Program (specify): _____
Empty Drainage / Ostomy Pouch	**Dx:**		_____
Change / Date Foley Bag			_____
Administer Enema (specify)	_____		_____
Check / Remove Fecal Impaction	_____		_____

VITALS

	ABOVE	BELOW
Pain		N/A
BP		
Temp.		
Pulse		
Resp.		
Wt.		

Dx: _____

Allergies: _____

Home Exercise Program (specify): _____
_____

Orthopedic / Support Device (specify): _____
_____

Nurse's Signature: _____   Date: _____

SAINT JOSEPH MERCY
HEALTH SYSTEM
A MEMBER OF TRINITY HEALTH

**SAINT JOSEPH MERCY LIVINGSTON
HOME CARE AND HOSPICE**
907 Fowler Street
Howell, Michigan 48843-2320
517-540-9000

Patient Name: _____

Patient Number: _____

Cert: Period: _____

HOME HEALTH AIDE ASSIGNMENT SHEET

6789-05 R 5/02 (M) D   WHITE–Chart • CANARY–Home • PINK–HHA Coordinator

FIGURE 11–7 ◆

The home health aide daily progress note. (Courtesy St. Joseph Mercy Hospital, Ann Arbor, MI. Reprinted with permission.)

❏ DIABETIC PRECAUTIONS

- DO NOT trim nails or allow patient to ambulate without footwear.
- During cleansing of feet. inspect for blisters. sores or open areas and report to SN/Therapist if they develop.
- Observe for signs and symptoms of hypoglycemia (low blood sugar) or hyperglycemia (high blood sugar).

HYPOGLYCEMIA – Rapid Onset:
Cold, clammy skin, shaking, nervousness, woakness, confusion, rapid heartbeat, sweating, dizziness, hunger, blurred vision, fatigue headache, irritability, pallor, sleepiness, numbing of fingers, toes, or mouth, slurred speech.

Treatment:
1. Give patient simple carbohydrates immediately (i.e., cranberry juice, apple juice, fruit punch, regular soft drink, etc.).
2. Call office to report patient's condition and receive further instructions.

If patient is unconscious, CALL 911. Initiate CPR, if appropriate.

HYPERGLYCEMIA – Slow Onset:
Extreme thirst, frequent urination, flushed, dry skin, nausea, increased appetite, blurred vision, numbness, fatigue, difficulty breathing, "fruity" smelling breath, abdominal pain, vomiting, headache, drowsiness leading to possible loss of consciousness.

Treatment:
1. Call office and report patient's condition and receive further instructions.
2. If loss of consciousness occurs CALL 911 and initiate CPR, if appropriate.

❏ OXYGEN PRECAUTIONS

When Oxygen is in use:
DO NOT:
- Allow smoking or the use of any open flame (gas stove, fireplace, candles) near where oxygen is being used or stored.
- Store oxygen near radiators, space heaters, heat ducts, steam pipes or other sources of heat.
- Use electric equipment (electric razors, radios, vaporizers, electric blankets, heating pads) within five feet of oxygen source.
- Leave cylinders in a closed car during warm weather.
- Place oxygen cylinders in closets with clothes and no ventilation.
- Use heavy coatings of oily lotions, lace creams or hair dressings while receiving oxygen (use only water soluble products such as K-Y Jelly).
- Use aerosol sprays in the vicinity of oxygen equipment.
- Put oil or grease on or near the oxygen equipment.
- Set liquids on top of the concentrator.
- Block the inlet or outlet filters.

DO:
- Post the warning sign stating that oxygen is in use.
- Have an all-purpose fire extinguisher readily available and visible.
- Store cylinders securely so they can't topple over or lay them flat.

❏ FALL PRECAUTIONS

- Keep floors dry
- USE assistive devices
- Use Bed rail
- Keep passage ways clear of clutter
- Allow appropriate rest periods
- Change positions slowly

❏ SEIZURE PRECAUTIONS

Report promptly to SN/Therapist anytime a patient has a seizure.

DO:
- Pad side rails if the patient has them
- Protect patient from injury by moving furniture or objects but DO NOT restrain patient (let him move freely)
- Loosen any tight clothing
- Stay with patient

Symptoms patient may have:
- May know when he is about to have a seizure (says he sees lights or "feels different")
- Muscles become stiff and begin to twitch or jerk
- Becomes incontinent of bowels or bladder
- Tired or confused after a seizure

After a seizure occurs:
1. Check level of consciousness.
2. CALL 911 and initiate CPR, if appropriate.
3. Patient may be confused. Tell him where he is and who you are.
4. Place patient on his side to prevent choking.
5. Report to SN/Therapist the time of the seizure, how long it lasted, and the patient's status.

❏ BLEEDING PRECAUTIONS

Causes:
- Patient is on Coumadin, Heparin, or another medication, which may cause bleeding.
- Trauma (i.e., cuts, falls, wound or disease complications, etc.)

DO NOT:
- use straight edge razors, trim nails, or use sharp tools or utonsils on patient unless authorized by SN/Therapist.

DO:
- use electric razors, use soft toothbrushes.
- Report to office all signs and symptoms of bleeding.

Report to RN:
- Nosebleeds
- Abnormal brulsing
- Blood in urine
- Blood in stool / tarry stools
- Coughing or spitting up blood
- Vomiting blood / coffee ground vomit
- Joint or abdominal pain
- Bleeding into the whites of the eyes
- Trauma induced bleeding

Immediate Treatment for Active Bleeding:
1. Apply direct pressure to site for 5 minutes, if possible.
2. Place patient in a lying down position.
3. Elevate site of bleeding, if possible.
4. If bleeding continues, call the office and receive further instructions.

❏ SAFE TRANSFER

- Speak clearly. Allow time for patient to follow directions
- Assess for dizzy / light headedness / balance with position changes
- Non-skid footwear
- Use good body mechanics
- Use assistive devices

❏ OTHER

SAINT JOSEPH MERCY LIVINGSTON HOME CARE AND HOSPICE
907 Fowler Street
Howell, Michigan 48843-2320
517-540-9000

SAINT JOSEPH MERCY HEALTH SYSTEM
A MEMBER OF TRINITY HEALTH

Patient Name: _____

Patient Number: _____

Cert. Period: _____

Date: _____

RISK FACTOR INSTRUCTION SHEET

FIGURE 11–7 (*Continued*)◆

The home health aide daily progress note.

AGE-SPECIFIC CONSIDERATIONS

Caring for patients in the home requires the same attention to the age-specific care needs of the patient as in a health care institution. The ages of the family members also become important, because they provide physical and emotional care for the patient. Keep in mind safety features for all age groups, such as choking hazards for small children, gun safety for older children, and tripping hazards and oxygen safety for the elderly (Figure 11–8♦). Elderly patients will often require reinforcement of the proper use of new assistive equipment (Figure 11–9♦). Infection control issues include proper mixing of formula for infants and proper food preparation and storage of leftovers.

FIGURE 11–8 ♦

Practice oxygen safety with an elderly patient with COPD

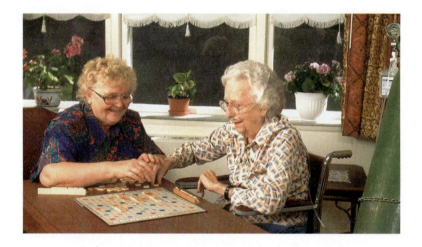

FIGURE 11–9 ♦

CNA reinforcing the proper use of assistive equipment

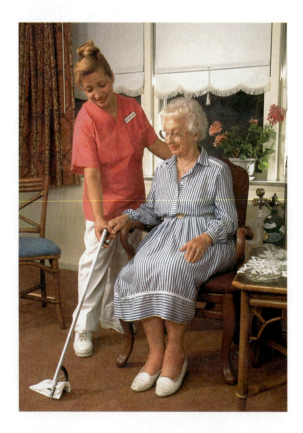

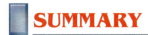 **SUMMARY**

The primary purpose of home health care is to allow the patient to remain in his natural environment while being restored to his maximum level of independence in self-care and functional ability. The frequency and duration of services may vary from once a month to 24-hour care. The role of the home health aide is to assist the patient with activities of daily living and maintenance of a clean, safe, and comfortable environment. The home health aide must be able to work independently and effectively with patients and families regardless of age, ethnicity, cultural or religious beliefs, and medical problems.

NOTES

CHAPTER REVIEW

FILL IN THE BLANK Read each sentence and fill in the blank line with a word that completes the sentence.

1. A group of people brought together by shared needs, interests, and mutual concerns for the well-being of all its

   members is a _____ .

2. _____ _____ involves the restraining or curbing the spread of microorganisms.

3. A patient who is unable to get out of bed is _____ _____ _____ .

4. If an accident or medical emergency occurs in the home, call _____ .

5. One of the principal concerns of the home health aide is patient _____ .

MULTIPLE CHOICE Choose the best answer for each question or statement.

1. When caring for a person in his or her home, home health aides generally refer to that person as

   a. client.

   b. patient.

   c. sir or madam.

   d. diagnosis.

2. Which of the following is not a helpful characteristic of a home health aide?

   a. Polite

   b. Trustworthy

   c. Inconsiderate

   d. Careful

3. Which of the following is not a reason why a person may need home health assistance?

   a. Family works outside the home.

   b. Patient does not want help.

   c. The client cannot shop and prepare meals.

   d. The client cannot provide transportation.

4. Which of the following is not a duty of the home health aide?

   a. Preparing bottles

   b. Shopping for food for the client

   c. Changing sterile dressings

   d. Collecting specimen samples

5. Which of the following phone numbers does not need to be kept handy?

   a. Fire station

   b. Police station

   c. Pizza delivery

   d. Pharmacy delivery

TIME-OUT

TIPS FOR TIME MANAGEMENT

Take time to see, hear, and appropriately touch a patient when you are giving care. You may
observe or detect a problem in the early stages, so it can be prevented from becoming worse.
Prevention or early detection results in better care and usually saves time in the long run.

THE NURSING ASSISTANT IN ACTION

You are assigned to care for Mr. McCollum in his home. He is an elderly man dying from lung cancer. Your supervisor informed you that he is not supposed to smoke because he is receiving oxygen. Mr. McCollum asks you to please bring him cigarettes and let him smoke anyway because he is already dying so why not give him the one thing he really needs to make him feel better?

What Is Your Response/Action?

CRITICAL THINKING

CUSTOMER SERVICE When working in a client's home you may get to know the client well and be asked to address him by his first name. You may do so if this is the client's choice. When discussing the client with you supervisor or other caregivers, refer to the client as Mr. _____ .

CULTURAL CARE You may be assigned to work in the home of a client with strict personal preferences or religious prohibitions regarding food they consume or bring into their homes. If you are aware that the client is Jewish, Muslim, or vegetarian, check first to see if there are foods they prefer you do not bring into or eat while in their home.

COOPERATION WITHIN THE TEAM Working in the home allows you to learn much about the client and her family. The client may be confused about certain care and she may discuss it with you. You can help reinforce why certain treatments are needed, if you know the reason. When unsure, offer to inform other care providers that the client needs additional information or would like some aspect of her care explained again.

EXPLORE MediaLink

Additional interactive resources for this chapter can be found on the Companion Website at www.prenhall.com/wolgin. Click on Chapter 11 and "Begin" to select the activities for this chapter.

For chapter-related NCLEX-style questions and an audio glossary, access the accompanying CD-ROM in this book.

12 Personal Care of the Patient

OBJECTIVES

When you have completed this chapter, you will be able to:

- Establish a schedule of personal care.
- Record what you have done for the patient on the activities of daily living (ADL) flow sheet (or other appropriate form).
- Care for the patient's mouth using good oral hygiene techniques.
- Bathe the patient.
- Give perineal care.
- Care for the patient's nails and feet as instructed.
- Give a back rub.
- Change the patient's gown.
- Care for the patient's hair.
- Shave the patient's beard; remove facial hair.
- Help the patient use a bedpan, a urinal, or a bedside commode.
- Care for the incontinent patient.

MediaLink

www.prenhall.com/wolgin

Use the address above to access the free, interactive Companion Website created for this textbook. Get hints, instant feedback, and textbook references to chapter-related NCLEX-style questions. Link to other interesting sites.

AUDIO GLOSSARY:

Use the Companion Website, or the CD-ROM disk enclosed with your textbook, to hear the pronunciation of key terms in the chapter.

This chapter provides you with the knowledge and skills needed to provide daily care for patients. This includes giving or assisting with oral hygiene, bathing, perineal care, care of nails and feet, back rub, changing the patient's gown, hair care, shaving, and elimination. Special care for patients who are incontinent is also presented.

INTRODUCTION

Daily Care of the Patient

Each patient is an individual with a special set of needs. Care must be unhurried and personalized to meet each patient's special needs. The tasks that are listed here may seem very routine, but the nursing assistant can greatly increase the comfort of patients by performing them.

ALERT

For all patient contact, adhere to Standard Precautions (⚭ Chapter 5, pages 83–85). Wear protective equipment as indicated.

KEY IDEA

One example of a special need would be a patient who is going to surgery. Patients scheduled for surgery are usually NPO (nothing by mouth). You would not give any drinking water but you would provide oral hygiene to increase comfort.

AGE-SPECIFIC CONSIDERATIONS

When performing personal care for small children, keep in mind that they may experience stranger anxiety. Try to have the parent assist or remain close by to comfort the child. Babies lose body heat more quickly than adults, so dry their skin quickly. Adolescents value privacy and are generally very modest. Allow them as many choices as possible when assisting with or providing personal care. Adults and geriatric patients may have concerns over loss of control and feelings of helplessness if they cannot perform their own care. Try to maintain as many personal habits and practices as possible.

Early Morning Care: Before Breakfast (Sometimes called Early A.M. Care)

- Offer the bedpan or urinal or assist ambulatory patient to bathroom or commode.
- Wash the patient's hands and face.
- Help with oral hygiene.
- Pass fresh drinking water, if permitted.
- Clean the overbed table and position it to receive food tray.
- Raise the head of the bed, if permitted.
- Reposition patient as needed, if permitted.

Morning Care: After Breakfast (Sometimes called A.M. Care)

- Before giving personal care, provide privacy for the patient.
- Offer the bedpan or urinal.
- Assist with oral hygiene.

ACTIVITIES OF DAILY LIVING CHECKLIST

SELF —Done by patient
ASSIST —Patient assisted by nursing staff
TOTAL —Done by nursing staff
✔ —Check procedure performed.
Include time if appropriate.

DATE															
DIET	B'fast	Dinner	Supper	B'fast	Dinner	Supper	B'fast	Dinner	Supper	B'fast	Dinner	Supper	B'fast	Dinner	Supper
Ate all food served															
Ate approx. ½ food served															
Refused to eat															
PROCEDURE	11-7	7-3	3-11	11-7	7-3	3-11	11-7	7-3	3-11	11-7	7-3	3-11	11-7	7-3	3-11
A.M. or H.S. Care															
Oral Hygiene															
Bath–Bed bath complete															
Bed bath partial															
Shower															
Tub															
Self Care															
Back Care															
Bed Made															
ELIMINATION															
Bowel movement															
Involuntary B.M.															
Voided															
Incontinent															
Foley cath.															
Sitz Bath @															
ACTIVITY															
Bed rest complete															
Dangle															
Bed rest–B.R.P.															
Up in chair															
Up in room															
Walk in hall															
Ambulatory															
POSITION CHANGED															
Flat in bed															
Semi–Fowler's															
Deep breathe, cough															
Range of motion															
Turn from side to side															
Side Rails–Up															
Down															
Fresh Water @															
SIGNATURE & TITLE															

FIGURE 12–1 ◆

The activities of daily living checklist

- Help the patient to bathe—follow instructions from your immediate supervisor.
- Give the patient a complete bed bath, partial bed bath, shower, or tub bath.
- Change the patient's gown.
- Help the male patient to shave his face, if allowed.
- Make the bed.
- Straighten the unit.
- Reposition patient as needed, if permitted.

Afternoon Care: After Lunch

- Offer the bedpan or urinal.
- Wash the patient's hands and face.
- Assist with oral hygiene.
- Change the patient's gown, if necessary.
- Straighten the unit.
- Pass fresh drinking water.

Evening Care: After Supper, Before Bedtime (Sometimes called P.M. Care)

- Offer the bedpan or urinal.
- Wash the patient's hands and face.
- Assist with oral hygiene.
- Give a back rub, if allowed.
- Change the draw sheet, if necessary or at patient's request.
- Smooth and tighten the sheets.
- Offer the patient an extra blanket.
- Pass fresh drinking water.

Activities of Daily Living: The Flow Sheet

In many health care facilities, the nursing assistant is required to record—check off (✓) or initial—what has been done for the patient on an **activities of daily living (ADL) flow sheet** (Figure 12–1◆) or a *patient care flow sheet* (Figure 12–2◆). Follow the nurse's instructions regarding this documentation.

 Oral Hygiene

Care of a person's mouth and teeth is called **oral hygiene**. A sick person's mouth often has a bad taste because of medications or the illness. The tongue may be covered with a grayish coating that spoils the appetite. With good care, the patient's mouth will feel fresh and clean and may increase the desire to eat. Giving oral hygiene is an essential part of daily patient care (Figure 12–3◆). Teeth should be brushed every morning, every evening, and after eating (Figure 12–4a◆). Flossing teeth once a day is desirable to promote healthy gums (Figure 12–4b◆ and 12–4c◆). In your work, you will be giving oral hygiene to

activities of daily living (ADL) The activities or tasks usually performed every day, such as toileting, washing, eating, or dressing

flow sheet A checklist or chart for recording the activities of daily living

oral hygiene Cleanliness of the mouth

Catherine
McAuley
Health System

St. Joseph Mercy Hospital
5301 East Huron River Drive
P.O. Box 995
Ann Arbor, Michigan 48106

8765-004 N 4/93

Patient Care Flow Sheet

Admission Date	OP Date	POD

Date		MIDNIGHTS								DAYS								AFTERNOONS							
		24	01	02	03	04	05	06	07	08	09	10	11	12	13	14	15	16	17	18	19	20	21	22	23
VITAL SIGNS	Temperature																								
	Pulse																								
	Respiratory Rate																								
	Blood Pressure																								
	CVP																								
FLUID INTAKE	Oral																								
	Feeding/NG					CREDITS					CREDITS								CREDITS						
	IV/IVPB																								
	Hyperal/Lipids																								
	Blood																								
	Total 8°																	24° Total							
FLUID OUTPUT	Urine																								
	Emesis																								
	Nasogastric Tube																								
	Total 8°																	24° Total							
ACTIVITY	Safety Code																	EVENING SHIFT							
	Progression Weight																								
	SCDs / TEDs																								
SAFETY / RESTRAINT	Type of restraint and																	DAY SHIFT							
	Location of restraint																								
	Observation q1°																								
	Turn/ROM q2°																								
	Fluids offered																	MIDNIGHT SHIFT							
	Toilet patient q2°																								
	Skin status under restraint checked																								
	Circulation checked																								

FIGURE 12–2 ◆

The patient care flow sheet (Chart adapted with permission of St. Joseph Mercy Hospital, Ann Arbor, Michigan)

Date		24	01	02	03	04	05	06	07	08	09	10	11	12	13	14	15	16	17	18	19	20	21	22	23
	Diet and Amount	BREAKFAST								LUNCH								SUPPER							
	Weight																								
	Stool character and number																								
GI / GU	Guaiac and date of last stool																								
	Bowel sounds																								
	Bladder																								
RESPIRATORY	Assessment																								
	Cough / Deep Breathe																								
INTEGUMENT	Surgical incision / Dressing																								
	Drains / characteristics																								
	Wound Care																								
TESTS AND SPECIMENS	Test results (mg/dL)																								
	Treatment/Medications																								
BLOOD GLUCOSE	Patient response																								
	ACCU-CHECK Instrument No.																								
	Date of last quality check																								
	CHEMSTRIP Lot No.																								
	Same as Calibration Lot (Yes, No)																								
	Sample type (cap, venous)																								
	Initials																								
NEUROLOGICAL	Assessment																								
	Best Eye Opening																								
	Best Verbal Response																								
	Best Motor Response																								
	Total Score																								
	Grasp																								
	Leg Lift / Foot Presses																								
	Pupils R																								
	L																								
HYGIENE	AM Care / HS Care																								
	Foley Care / Perineal Care																								
	Oral Care																								

KEY

Bowel Sounds:
✓ = Present in all 4 quadrants

Bladder:
✓ = Able to empty bladder Urine clear and yellow
F = Foley to DD
F✓ = Foley to DD, urine clear and yellow

Respiratory Assessment:
✓ = Bilateral breath sounds clear and respirations quiet and regular
☆ = See description

Surgical incision:
I✓ = incision well approximated no drainage
D✓ = dressing dry / intact
★ = See description

Best Motor Response:
6 = Obeys commands
5 = Localizes pain
4 = Flexion withdrawal
3 = Flexion abnormal
2 = Extension abnormal
1 = No response

Grasp and Leg Lift
R = L, R > L, or R < L and
W = Weak
S = Strong

Pupils
Record size in mm and
R = reactive to light
NR = nonreactive to light

Neurological Assessment:
✓ = Alert and oriented X3
☆ = See description

Best Eye Opening:
4 = spontaneous
3 = to speech
2 = to pain
1 = no response

Best Verbal Response:
5 = Oriented to time, person, place
4 = Confused
3 = Inappropriate words
2 = Incomprehensible sounds
1 = no response

FIGURE 12–2 (continued)
The patient care flow sheet

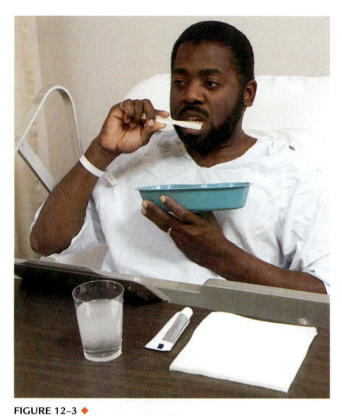

FIGURE 12–3 ◆

Oral hygiene is an essential part of daily patient care

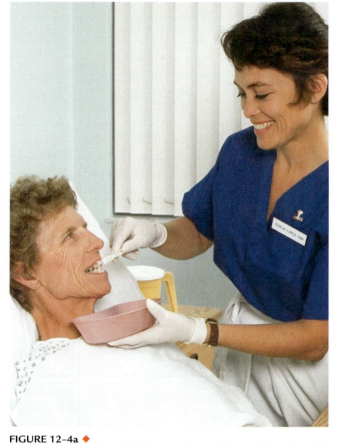

FIGURE 12–4a ◆

In your work as a nursing assistant, you will be giving oral hygiene to patients

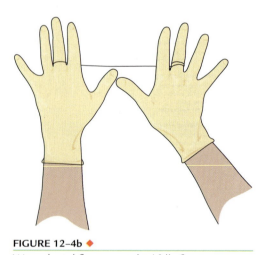

FIGURE 12–4b ◆

Wrap dental floss around middle fingers

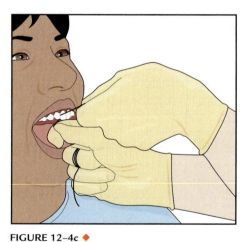

FIGURE 12–4c ◆

Hold dental floss firmly between each thumb and forefinger to properly floss around each tooth

dentures Artificial teeth. Dentures may replace some or all of a person's teeth; they are described as being partial or complete and upper or lower

conscious and unconscious patients. When necessary, you will be cleaning their **dentures** (false teeth).

Oral hygiene is given to unconscious patients and patients who are NPO (nothing by mouth) every 2 hours. The purpose is to keep the lips and oral tissues moist. Unless this is done, the lips and oral tissues tend to dry out, split, and bleed, and may develop a mucous coating much more rapidly.

KEY IDEA

A person's mouth and teeth need more care when a person is ill than when he or she is well. Always wear gloves when performing oral hygiene. Oral hygiene can be performed at the bedside or in the bathroom. Look at the mouth and gums for redness or skin breakdown.

PROCEDURE   **OBRA**

ORAL HYGIENE

RATIONALE: Oral hygiene is performed to freshen the patient's mouth, clean the teeth, provide moisture, and reduce bacteria in the mouth.

PREPARATION

1. Assemble your equipment on the bedside table:
   a. Mouthwash
   b. Fresh water
   c. Disposable cup
   d. Straw (optional)
   e. Toothbrush
   f. Toothpaste
   g. Emesis basin
   h. Face towel
   i. Disposable gloves
   j. Dental floss and disposable face mask
2. Identify the patient by checking the identification bracelet.
3. Tell the patient you will help her clean her teeth and mouth.
4. Provide privacy for the patient.
5. Wash your hands and put on gloves.
6. Raise bed to a comfortable working height.

STEPS

7. Position patient to a sitting position, if possible.
8. Spread the towel across the patient's chest to protect the gown and top sheets.
9. Mix one-half cup of water with one-half cup of mouthwash in the disposable cup.
10. Let the patient take a mouthful of the mixture if allowed and rinse her mouth.
11. Hold the emesis basin under the patient's chin so she can spit out the mouthwash solution.
12. Put toothpaste on the wet toothbrush.
13. If the patient can do it, let her brush her teeth. If she cannot, brush her teeth for her. Brush the tongue to freshen breath and remove bacteria.
14. Help the patient rinse the toothpaste out of her mouth, using the mouthwash solution or fresh water.
15. Floss the patient's teeth using a 12- to 14-inch piece of dental floss. Wear a disposable face mask while flossing a patient's teeth as there is potential for gum bleeding and your face will be in close proximity when flossing teeth.
    Wrap ends of the dental floss around your middle fingers (see Figure 12–4b). Ask the patient to open her mouth. As you hold the dental floss between your thumb and forefingers, gently insert the floss between each tooth, down to but not into the gum (see Figure 12–4c). When finished, offer water or mouthwash so the patient can rinse her mouth.
16. Clean and put your equipment in its proper place. Discard disposable equipment.

FOLLOW-UP

17. Make the patient comfortable and replace call light.
18. Dispose of your gloves and wash your hands.
19. Lower the bed to a position of safety for the patient.
20. Raise the side rails when ordered or appropriate for patient safety.
21. Report to your immediate supervisor:
    ■ That you have assisted the patient with oral hygiene.
    ■ How the patient tolerated the procedure.
    ■ Your observations of anything unusual.

CHARTING EXAMPLE: 12/02/04
7am Brushed and flossed Mrs. Ehnis' teeth. L. Hill, CNA (or check oral hygiene box on flow sheet)

CLEANING DENTURES (FALSE TEETH)	PROCEDURE	OBRA

RATIONALE: Dentures are cleaned to freshen the patient's mouth, clean the teeth, and reduce bacteria in the mouth.

PREPARATION

1. Assemble your equipment on the bedside table (Figure 12–5◆):

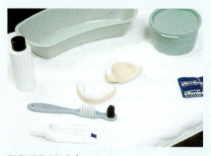

FIGURE 12–5 ◆
Preparation for cleaning dentures

   a. Paper towel

   b. Mouthwash

   c. Disposable denture cup

   d. Emesis basin

   e. Toothbrush or denture brush

   f. Towel

   g. Denture toothpaste

   h. Disposable gloves

2. Identify the patient by checking the identification bracelet.

3. Tell the patient you wish to clean his dentures.

4. Provide privacy for the patient.

5. Wash your hands and put on gloves.

6. Raise bed to a comfortable working height.

STEPS

7. Position patient to a sitting position, if possible.

8. Spread the towel across the patient's chest to protect the gown and top sheets.

9. Ask the patient to remove his dentures. (Have paper towel in the emesis basin ready to receive them.) Assist the patient who is unable to remove his own dentures.

10. Take the dentures to the sink in the lined emesis basin (Figure 12–6◆).

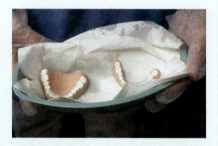

FIGURE 12–6 ◆
Place dentures in a lined emesis basin

11. Place a paper towel or washcloth in the bottom of the sink to guard against breaking dentures if you drop them accidentally. Fill the sink with water.

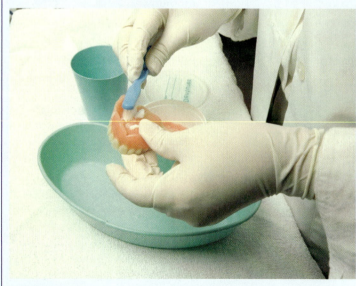

FIGURE 12–7 ◆
Brush all surfaces of the dentures

12. Apply toothpaste or denture cleanser to the dentures. With the dentures in the palm of your hand, brush all surfaces until they are clean (Figure 12–7◆).

13. Rinse dentures thoroughly under cool running water (Figure 12–8◆).

14. Fill the clean denture cup with cool water, some mouthwash and water, or dental solution. Place the dentures in the cup and close the lid.

15. Help the patient rinse his mouth with water and/or mouthwash.

16. Have the patient replace the dentures in his mouth if this is what he wants. Be sure dentures are moist before replacing them.

17. Leave the labeled denture cup with the clean solution on the bedside table where the patient can reach it easily. Some patients remove dentures between cleanings.

18. Clean and replace all your equipment. Discard disposable equipment in the proper container.

PROCEDURE *(continued)*

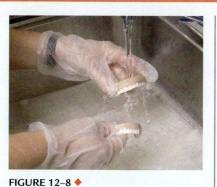

FIGURE 12–8 ◆
Rinse dentures thoroughly

FOLLOW-UP

19. Make the patient comfortable.

20. Dispose of your gloves and wash your hands.

21. Lower the bed to a position of safety.

22. Raise the side rails when ordered or appropriate for patient safety.

23. Place the call light within easy reach of the patient.

24. Report to your immediate supervisor:

   ■ That you have cleaned the patient's dentures.

   ■ Your observations of anything unusual.

CHARTING EXAMPLE: 12/02/04
7:30am Mouth care given; brushed and cleaned Mr. Black's dentures. L. Hill, CNA (or check oral hygiene box on flow sheet)

ORAL HYGIENE FOR THE UNCONSCIOUS PATIENT (SPECIAL MOUTH CARE)

PROCEDURE   OBRA

RATIONALE: Oral hygiene is performed to freshen the patient's mouth, clean the teeth, provide moisture, and reduce bacteria in the mouth.

PREPARATION

1. Assemble your equipment on the bedside table:

   a. Towel

   b. Emesis basin

   c. Special disposable mouth care kit of commercially prepared swabs. Or if such a kit is not available:

      ■ Tongue depressor to hold mouth open or teeth apart, if necessary

      ■ Applicators or gauze sponges

      ■ Lubricant such as glycerin, petroleum jelly, or a solution of lemon juice and glycerin

   d. Disposable gloves

2. Identify the patient by checking the identification bracelet.

3. Tell the patient what you are going to do. Even though a patient seems to be unconscious, he still may be able to hear you.

4. Provide privacy for the patient.

5. Wash your hands and put on gloves.

6. Raise the bed to a comfortable working height.

STEPS

7. Stand at the side of the bed. Turn the patient's head to the side facing you.

8. Put a towel on the pillow under the patient's head and partly under the face.

9. Lower head of bed, if possible. Gravity causes saliva to automatically run out of the mouth and prevents drainage into lungs.

10. Put the emesis basin on the towel under the patient's chin.

11. Tell the unconscious patient you are going to open his mouth. Press on his cheeks or open the mouth using gentle pressure with hand on chin. **Never** put your fingers into the mouth of an unconscious or uncooperative patient.

12. Open the commercial package of swabs, if available. Wipe the patient's entire mouth to remove debris and dried mucus (roof, tongue, and inside the cheeks and lips) with the prepared swab (Figure 12–9◆).

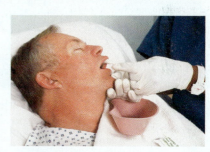

FIGURE 12–9 ◆
Wipe the entire inside of the patient's mouth, including the inside of the cheeks and lips

13. Put used swabs into the emesis basin. Some commercial swabs leave a coating of glycerin solution on the entire inside of the mouth, tongue, and teeth.

14. If a disposable mouth care kit of commercially prepared swabs is not available:

   a. Moisten the applicators with mouthwash solution.

PROCEDURE *(continued)*

b. Use your free hand to insert the applicator in the patient's mouth. **Never** put your fingers in the unconscious patient's mouth.

c. Thoroughly wipe the roof of the mouth, the teeth, and the tongue.

d. Change applicators when soiled.

e. Place the used applicators and other supplies in the emesis basin.

f. Use clear water on more applicators to rinse out the patient's mouth.

15. Dry the patient's face with the towel.

16. Using an applicator, put a small amount of water-soluble lubricant on the patient's lips and tongue.

17. Clean and return your equipment to its proper place. Discard disposable equipment.

FOLLOW-UP

18. Raise head of the bed if it was lowered. Make the patient comfortable.

19. Dispose of your gloves and wash your hands.

20. Lower the bed when ordered or appropriate for patient safety.

21. Raise the side rails when ordered or appropriate for patient safety.

22. Place the call light within easy reach of the patient.

23. Report to your immediate supervisor:

   ■ That you have given the patient oral hygiene.

   ■ How the patient tolerated the procedure.

   ■ Your observations of anything unusual.

CHARTING EXAMPLE: 12/08/04
6am oral care given to Mr. Kelly.
F. Cooper, CNA (or check oral hygiene box on flow sheet)

Helping the Patient to Bathe

Patients who are able to manage their own daily personal care—oral hygiene and bathing—should be encouraged to do so. There are several important reasons for bathing the patient. Bathing gets rid of dirt on the patient's body. It eliminates body odors and cools and refreshes the patient. The bath stimulates circulation, helps to prevent skin breakdown, and can be relaxing.

KEY IDEA

self-care Activities or care tasks performed by the patient

Patients who are ordered to be on **self-care** should be encouraged to do as much as possible for themselves.

The physician may order one of four types of baths, based on the patient's condition. The patient may be given a complete bed bath, a partial bed bath, a tub bath, or a shower.

Bathing requires movements of certain parts of the body; the patient's legs and arms are lifted and the head and torso are turned. This activity exercises muscles that might otherwise remain unused. (Range-of-motion exercises are covered in Chapters 33, *Rehabilitation and Return to Self-Care.*) At this time, the nursing assistant has the opportunity to observe the patient for any unusual body changes such as skin rashes, pressure ulcers, or reddened areas. (Refer to Chapters 17, *The Integumentary System and Related Care,* for a discussion of skin disorders associated with confinement to bed.)

KEY IDEA

Change the bath water from time to time as it appears soapy or gets cool.

Types of Baths

Complete bed bath	The patient who is too weak or ill is given a complete bed bath. When you are giving this bath, you will get little or no help from the patient. Sometimes the doctor will write an order placing the patient on complete bed rest. In this case, the patient is not permitted to do anything.
Partial bed bath	Patients may be able to take care of most of their own bathing needs. In this case you bathe only the areas that are hard for the patient to reach, such as the back or feet.
Tub bath	The tub bath might be ordered by the doctor for therapeutic reasons.
Shower	Showers may be permitted for patients who are recovering from their illness (convalescent patients). These patients have been judged by their doctor to be strong enough to get out of bed and walk around.

BATHING THE PATIENT — GUIDELINES — OBRA

- Usually the complete bed bath is given as part of morning care. After the bath, the hair is combed, the gown changed, and the occupied bed is made.

- Use good body mechanics. Keep your feet separated, stand firmly, bend your knees, and keep your back straight.

- Raise the patient's bed to a comfortable working position with the side rails up on the far side of the bed.

- Change the water during the bed bath as necessary. For example, change the water whenever it becomes soapy, dirty, or cold.

- Only one part of the body is washed at a time. Wash, rinse, and dry each part or area very well. Then cover it right away with the bath blanket.

- Soap has a drying effect on the patient's skin. Be sure to rinse off all the soap.

- When you are not using the soap, keep it in the soap dish instead of the basin. In this way, the water will not dissolve the soap and get too soapy.

- Putting the patient's hands and feet into the water makes the patient feel relaxed.

- Observe the condition of the patient's skin when you are giving the bath. Report any redness, rashes, broken skin, or tender places you see on the patient's body.

- Never trim or cut fingernails or toenails without special instructions from the nurse.

- At the beginning of the bath, put the patient's bottle of lotion for the back rub in the basin of water to keep it warm or put lotion on your hands and rub your hands together to warm it up.

- Deodorant should be used if the patient asks for it. It should be applied after the bath has been completed and before the clean gown is put on.

- Check the patient's gown and bed linens for personal items or valuables and return them to the patient before putting the gown in the laundry hamper.

THE COMPLETE BED BATH — PROCEDURE — OBRA

RATIONALE: Bathing is done to cleanse the patient's skin.

PREPARATION

1. Assemble your equipment on the bedside table (Figure 12–10◆):
   a. Soap and soap dish
   b. Washcloths
   c. Wash basin
   d. Bath thermometer, if available
   e. Face and bath towels
   f. Talcum powder or corn starch (optional)
   g. Clean gown
   h. Bath blanket

PROCEDURE *(continued)*

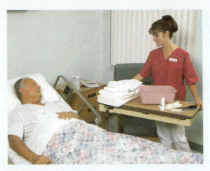

FIGURE 12–10 ◆

Preparation for the complete bed bath

    i. Orange stick for nail care, if used by your institution

    j. Lotion

    k. Comb or hair brush

    l. Disposable plastic or cloth laundry bag for dirty linen (whichever is used by your institution)

    m. Clean bed linen, stacked on the chair in order of use, if the bed is to be made following the bed bath

    n. Disposable gloves

2. Identify the patient by checking the identification bracelet (Figure 12–11◆).

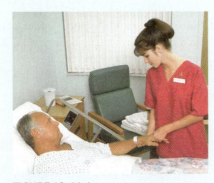

FIGURE 12–11 ◆

Identify the patient

3. Wash your hands (Figure 12–12◆) and put on gloves.

4. Tell the patient you are going to give him a bed bath.

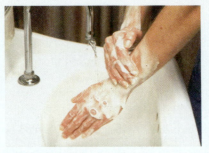

FIGURE 12–12 ◆

Wash hands and forearms

5. Provide privacy for the patient (Figure 12–13◆).

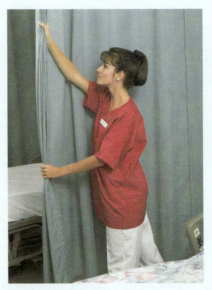

FIGURE 12–13 ◆

Provide privacy for the patient

STEPS

6. Assist the patient with oral hygiene.

7. Offer the bedpan or urinal.

8. Place the laundry bag on a chair near the bed.

9. Raise the bed to a comfortable working position and lock it in place (Figure 12–14◆).

10. Pull out all the bedding from under the mattress. Leave it

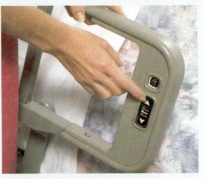

FIGURE 12–14 ◆

Raise bed to a comfortable working position

hanging loosely at all four sides of the bed (Figure 12–15◆).

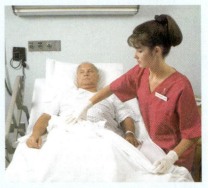

FIGURE 12–15 ◆

Pull out all bedding from under the mattress

11. Take the bedspread and regular blanket off the bed. Fold them loosely over the back of the chair, leaving the patient covered with the top sheet.

12. Place the bath blanket over the top sheet.

13. Remove the top sheet from underneath without uncovering (exposing) the patient. Fold the sheet loosely over the back of the chair if it is to be used again; if not, put it in the laundry bag.

14. Lower the headrest and knee rest of the bed, if permitted. The patient should be in a flat position, as flat as is comfortable and as is permitted.

PROCEDURE *(continued)*

15. Remove the patient's gown and ornamental jewelry. (It is not necessary to remove wedding rings.) Keep the patient covered with the bath blanket. If the gown belongs to the patient, put it away as requested. Place the hospital gown in the laundry bag. Put the jewelry into the drawer of the bedside table.

16. Fill the wash basin two-thirds full of warm water (115°F; 46.1°C).

17. Help the patient to move to the side of the bed closest to you. Use good body mechanics.

18. Put a towel across the patient's chest and make a mitten with the washcloth (Figure 12–16◆). Wash

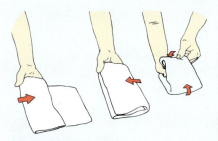

FIGURE 12–16 ◆
Make a mitten with the washcloth

the patient's eyes from the nose to the outside of the face. Ask the patient if he wants soap used on his face. Wash the face, ears, and neck. Be careful not to get soap in his eyes. Rinse and dry by patting gently with the bath towel (Figure 12–17◆).

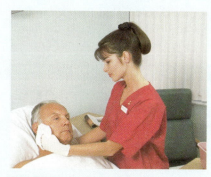

FIGURE 12–17 ◆
Wash face, ears, and neck

19. Put a towel lengthwise under the patient's arm farthest from you. This will keep the bed from getting wet. Support the patient's arm with the palm of your hand under his elbow. Then wash his shoulder, armpit (axilla), and arm. Use long, firm, circular strokes. Rinse and dry the area well (Figure 12–18a-b◆ and 12–19◆).

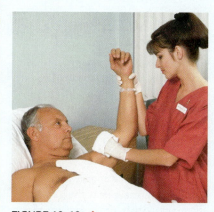

FIGURE 12–18a ◆
Wash his shoulder

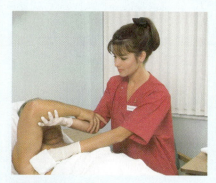

FIGURE 12–18b ◆
Wash his armpit

20. Place the basin of water on the towel. Put the patient's hand into the water. Wash and rinse it well. Clean beneath the patient's fingernails with an orange stick. Dry the hand well and place it under the bath blanket.

21. Repeat Steps 19 and 20 for the shoulder, axilla, arm, and hand closest to you.

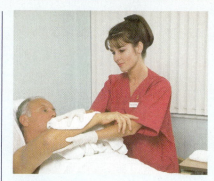

FIGURE 12–19 ◆
Wash his forearm

22. Place a towel across the patient's chest. Fold the bath blanket down to the patient's abdomen. Wash and rinse the patient's chest. Take note of the condition of the skin under the patient's breasts. Dry the area thoroughly.

23. Cover the patient's entire chest with a towel. Fold the bath blanket down to the pubic area. Wash the patient's abdomen (Figure 12–20◆). Be sure to wash the navel (umbilicus) and in any

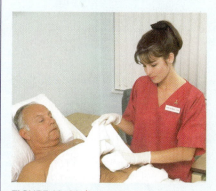

FIGURE 12–20 ◆
Wash patient's abdomen

creases of the skin. Dry the patient's abdomen (Figure 12–21◆). Apply warm lotion and look for any reddened areas. Then pull the bath blanket over the abdomen and chest and remove the towels.

24. Water may need to be changed at this time. Empty basin, rinse, and fill as before.

PROCEDURE *(continued)*

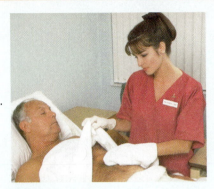

FIGURE 12–21 ◆

Dry patient's abdomen

25. Fold the bath blanket back from the patient's leg farthest from you.

26. Put a towel lengthwise under that leg and foot.

27. Bend the knee and wash, rinse, and dry the leg and foot. Take hold of the heel for more support when flexing the knee or place your hand under the knee (Figure 12–22◆). If

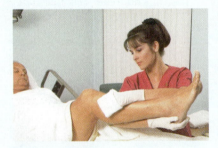

FIGURE 12–22 ◆

Provide support by taking hold of the patient's foot

the patient can easily bend his knee, put the wash basin on the towel. Then put the patient's foot directly into the basin to wash it.

28. Observe the toenails and the skin between the toes for general appearance and condition. Look especially for redness and cracking of the skin. Take away the basin. Dry the patient's leg and foot and between the toes (Figure 12–23◆). Cover the leg and foot with the bath blanket and remove the towel.

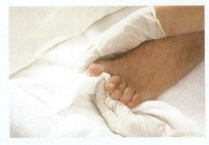

FIGURE 12–23 ◆

Dry between the toes

29. Repeat Steps 25–28 for the leg and foot closest to you.

30. Ask the patient to turn on his side with his back toward you. If he needs help in turning, assist him. Raise the side rail to the up position so the patient is safe. Return to your working side of the bed.

31. Put the towel lengthwise on the bottom sheet near the patient's back. Wash, rinse, and dry the back of the neck, back, and buttocks with long, firm, circular strokes (Figure 12–24◆). Give the

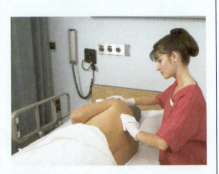

FIGURE 12–24 ◆

Wash the back using long, firm, circular strokes

patient a back rub with warm lotion. The patient's back should be rubbed for at least a minute and a half. Give special attention to bony areas (for example, shoulder blades, hips, and elbows). Look for reddened areas. Remove the towel and turn the patient on his back.

32. Water should be changed before giving perineal care. (See perineal care later in this chapter.)

33. Put a clean gown on the patient (Figure 12–25◆).

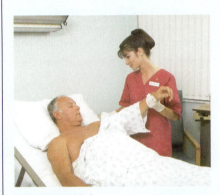

FIGURE 12–25 ◆

Put a clean gown on the patient

34. Comb the patient's hair if he cannot do this for himself (Figure 12–26◆).

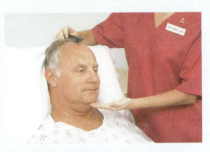

FIGURE 12–26 ◆

Comb the patient's hair

35. Make the patient's bed. Straighten the bedside table. Remove any unneeded articles. Replace the items the patient wants on the table.

FOLLOW-UP

36. Help position the patient in good body alignment.

37. Clean and return your equipment to its proper place. Discard disposable equipment.

38. Wipe off the bedside table. Check linen for any personal items. Bag

PROCEDURE *(continued)*

and discard soiled linen in the hamper (Figure 12–27◆).

39. Raise the backrest and knee rest to suit the patient, if this is allowed

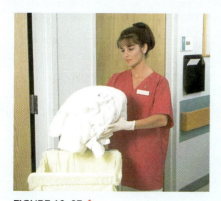

FIGURE 12–27 ◆
Discard soiled linen in the hamper

(Figure 12–28◆). Lower bed to a position of safety for the patient.

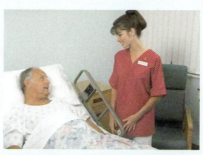

FIGURE 12–28 ◆
Raise back rest to suit the patient when allowed

40. Raise the side rails when ordered or appropriate for patient safety.

41. Dispose of your gloves and wash your hands.

42. Replace jewelry.

43. Place the call light within easy reach of the patient.

44. Report to your immediate supervisor:

   ■ That you have given the patient a bed bath.

   ■ How the patient tolerated the procedure.

   ■ Your observations of anything unusual.

CHARTING EXAMPLE: 12/08/04
7:45am Complete bed bath given to Mr. Kelly. Lotion applied to dry skin on his arms, legs, and back.
F. Cooper, CNA (or check bath or AM care box on flow sheet)

THE PARTIAL BED BATH (PARTIAL SELF-CARE)

PROCEDURE   **OBRA**

RATIONALE: A partial bed bath is done to cleanse areas of the patient's skin and body where the patient is unable to reach.

PREPARATION

1. Assemble your equipment on the bedside table:

   a. Soap and soap dish

   b. Washcloth

   c. Wash basin

   d. Bath thermometer, if available

   e. Face and bath towels

   f. Talcum powder or corn starch (optional)

   g. Clean gown

   h. Bath blanket

   i. Orange stick for nail care, if used by your institution

   j. Lotion for back rub

   k. Comb or hair brush

   l. Disposable plastic or cloth laundry bag for dirty linen (whichever is used by your institution)

   m. Clean bed linen, stacked on the chair in order of use, if the bed is to be made following the bed bath

   n. Disposable gloves

2. Identify the patient by checking the identification bracelet.

3. Wash your hands and put on gloves.

4. Provide privacy for the patient.

5. Tell the patient you are going to help her with a bath.

6. Raise the bed to a comfortable working height.

STEPS

7. Assist the patient with oral hygiene.

8. Offer the bedpan or urinal or assist patient to bathroom.

9. Place the laundry bag on a chair near the bed.

10. Pull out all the bedding from under the mattress. Leave it hanging loosely at all four sides of the bed.

11. Take the bedspread and regular blanket off the bed. Fold them loosely over the back of the chair, leaving the patient covered with the top sheet.

12. Place the bath blanket over the top sheet. Remove the top sheet from underneath without uncovering the patient. Fold the sheet loosely over the back of the chair if it is to be used again. Or put it in the laundry bag.

PROCEDURE *(continued)*

13. Remove the patient's gown and ornamental jewelry. (It is not necessary to remove wedding rings.) Keep her covered with the bath blanket. If the gown belongs to the patient, put it away as requested. Place the jewelry into the drawer of the bedside table. Put the hospital gown into the laundry bag.

14. Fill the wash basin two-thirds full of warm water (115°F; 46.1°C).

15. Ask the patient to wash the areas of her body that she can reach easily.

16. Place the call light where the patient can easily reach it. Instruct her to signal when she has finished washing herself.

17. Dispose of gloves and wash your hands.

18. Leave the room.

19. When the patient signals that she is finished, go back into the room.

20. Wash your hands and put on gloves.

21. Empty the water, rinse the basin, and fill it with clean warm water (115°F; 46.1°C).

22. Wash the areas of the body that the patient was unable to reach. Follow the procedure you learned for a complete bed bath. The body parts washed by the patient plus the body parts washed for the patient by the nursing assistant should equal a complete bed bath.

23. Put a clean gown on the patient without exposing her.

24. Lower the bed to a position of safety for the patient.

25. If allowed out of bed, assist the patient to a chair.

26. Make the empty bed.

27. Raise the side rails when ordered or appropriate for patient safety.

28. Place the call light in its proper place.

29. Clean and return your equipment to its proper place. Discard disposable equipment.

30. Wipe off the bedside table. Bag and discard used linen in the laundry hamper.

FOLLOW-UP

31. Dispose of your gloves and wash your hands.

32. Make the patient comfortable and replace jewelry.

33. Report to your immediate supervisor:

    ■ That you have given the patient a partial bath.

    ■ How the patient tolerated the procedure.

    ■ Your observations of anything unusual.

CHARTING EXAMPLE: 12/09/04 7:45am Assisted Mrs. Allan with her bath. Lotion applied to dry skin on her arms, legs, and back. F. Cooper, CNA (or check bath or AM care box on flow sheet)

PROCEDURE　　OBRA

THE TUB BATH

RATIONALE: The tub bath is done to relax a patient and cleanse the patient's skin.

PREPARATION

1. Assemble your equipment on a chair near the bathtub.

   a. Bath towels

   b. Washcloths

   c. Bath mat, if available

   d. Soap

   e. Bath thermometer, if available

   f. Wash basin

   g. Clean gown

   h. Disinfectant solution

   i. Disposable gloves

   j. Disposable plastic or cloth laundry bag for dirty linen (whichever is used by your institution)

   k. Place a chair near the tub

2. Wash the bathtub with the disinfectant solution (Figure 12–29◆).

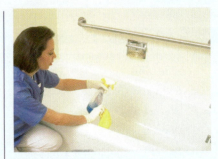

FIGURE 12–29 ◆

Wash the tub with disinfectant solution

You may do this before you get the patient up.

PROCEDURE *(continued)*

3. Identify the patient by checking the identification bracelet.

4. Tell the patient you are going to give him a tub bath.

5. Wash your hands and put on gloves.

6. Provide privacy for the patient.

STEPS

7. Help the patient out of bed. Get him into a bathrobe and slippers and to the room with the bathtub, either by walking or by wheelchair.

8. For safety, remove all electrical appliances from near the bathtub.

9. Place the chair next to the bathtub. Assist the patient into the chair.

10. Fill the bathtub half full of warm water (105°F; 40.5°C).

11. Place one towel in the bathtub for the patient to sit on (Figure 12–30◆).

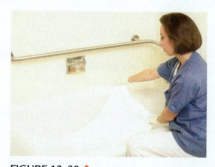

FIGURE 12–30 ◆
Place towel in the bathtub

12. Place one towel or bath mat on the floor where the patient will step out of the tub. This will prevent him from slipping.

13. Assist the patient with getting undressed and into the bathtub. A towel may be used to cover the genitals.

14. Let the patient stay in the bathtub as long as permitted, according to your instructions. Do not leave patient unattended.

15. Help the patient wash himself, if help is needed (Figure 12–31◆).

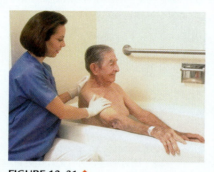

FIGURE 12–31 ◆
Assist patient to wash himself

16. Put one towel across the chair.

17. Drain the water from the tub.

18. Help the patient out of the bathtub. Seat him on the towel-covered chair, if he needs assistance.

19. Dry the patient well by patting gently with a towel (Figure 12–32◆). Assist the patient in putting on pajamas or gown, bathrobe, and slippers.

20. Dispose of gloves.

21. Help the patient return to his room and into bed.

FOLLOW-UP

22. Make the patient comfortable and replace the call light.

23. Lower the bed to a position of safety for the patient.

24. Raise the side rails when ordered or appropriate for patient safety.

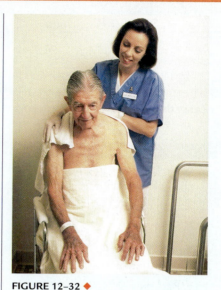

FIGURE 12–32 ◆
Dry the patient well

25. Return to the tub room.

26. Put on clean gloves. Clean the bathtub with disinfectant solution.

27. Bag and discard soiled linen in the laundry hamper.

28. Dispose of your gloves and wash your hands.

29. Report to your immediate supervisor:

   ■ That you have given the patient a tub bath.

   ■ How the patient tolerated the procedure.

   ■ Your observations of anything unusual.

CHARTING EXAMPLE: 12/12/04 8:45am Assisted Mr. Crawford with his tub bath. Lotion applied to dry skin on his arms, legs, and back. F. Copper, CNA (or check bath or AM care box on flow sheet)

| HELPING THE PATIENT TAKE A SHOWER | PROCEDURE | OBRA |

RATIONALE: Showering is done to cleanse the patient's skin.

PREPARATION

1. Assemble your equipment on a chair near the shower:
   a. Bath towels
   b. Soap
   c. Showercap
   d. Washcloth
   e. Bath mat
   f. Clean gown
   g. Disinfectant solution
   h. Disposable plastic or cloth laundry bag for dirty linen (whichever is used in your institution)
   i. Disposable gloves
2. Wash the floor of the shower with disinfectant solution (you may do this before you get the patient up).
3. Identify the patient by checking the identification bracelet.
4. Tell the patient that you will assist her with taking a shower.
5. Wash your hands and put on gloves.
6. Provide privacy for the patient.

STEPS

7. Help the patient out of bed and into a bathrobe and slippers. Help her to the bathroom with shower, as necessary.
8. For safety, remove all electrical appliances from the shower room.
9. Place one towel on the floor outside the shower.
10. Place one towel on a chair close to the shower. Assist the patient into the chair.
11. Turn on the shower and adjust the water temperature.
12. Assist the patient into the shower.
13. Give the patient soap and washcloth so that she can wash herself, but wait beside the shower in case the patient needs assistance.
14. Turn off the water and assist the patient out of the shower when she is finished. Seat her on the towel-covered chair.
15. Dry the patient well by patting gently with the towel.
16. Dispose of gloves and wash your hands.
17. Assist patient with pajamas or nightgown, bathrobe, and slippers.
18. Help the patient return to her room and into bed, or a chair if permitted.

19. Make the patient comfortable and replace the call light.
20. Lower the bed to a position of safety for the patient.
21. Raise the side rails when ordered or appropriate for patient safety.

FOLLOW-UP

22. Return to the shower room.
23. Put on gloves. Bag and discard soiled linen in the laundry hamper.
24. Remove the gloves and wash your hands.
25. Report to your immediate supervisor:
    - That you have helped the patient take a shower.
    - How the patient tolerated the procedure.
    - Your observations of anything unusual.

CHARTING EXAMPLE: 12/12/04 8:45am Assisted Mrs. Crawford with her shower. She enjoyed the shower and did not become weak or dizzy today. Towel dried and lotion applied to dry skin on her arms, legs, and back. F. Copper, CNA (or check bath/shower or AM care box on flow sheet)

Perineal Care

perineum (perineal area)
The body area between the thighs (external genitalia and rectal area)

Perineal care is specific care given to the **perineum** or **perineal area** (the external genitalia and rectal area) during the daily bath and after voiding or defecating. Cleansing is always done anterior to posterior (front to back).

Perineal care provides cleanliness and comfort for both the male and female patient. It helps to prevent irritation and infection. Special perineal care is given following childbirth. In some institutions perineal care may be done in the shower, tub, on the toilet, or in bed. Follow the instructions of your immediate supervisor in your institution. The following is instruction in giving perineal care in the bed.

KEY IDEA

Incontinent pads rather than a bedpan should be used when providing perineal care for an elderly person or individual with existing skin breakdown. It will reduce the possibility of skin tears and be less uncomfortable for the patient.

PROCEDURE

PERINEAL CARE FOR THE MALE PATIENT

OBRA

RATIONALE: Perineal care is done to cleanse the perineal area of the patient's skin and body where they are unable to reach or to prevent skin breakdown on incontinent patients. It provides comfort, promotes healing, and allows for observation of the area.

PREPARATION

1. Assemble your equipment:
   a. Bath blanket
   b. Bedpan and cover or urinal and cover
   c. Soap
   d. Basin with warm water (115°F; 46.1°C)
   e. Bath thermometer
   f. Disposable gloves
   g. Disposable bed protector
   h. Washcloth and towel
   i. Disposable plastic or cloth laundry bag for dirty linen (whichever is used by your institution)
2. Identify the patient by checking the identification bracelet.
3. Tell the patient you are going to provide perineal care.
4. Provide privacy for the patient.
5. Provide safety with the side rail up on the opposite side of the bed.
6. Lower the side rail on the side nearest you.

STEPS

7. Position the patient on his back (a side-laying position is also used with some patients).
8. Remove the bedspread and blankets and place on a nearby chair or table for use after the bath.
9. Cover the patient with the bath blanket.
10. Being careful not to expose the patient, slide the sheet out from under the bath blanket and leave fan-folded at the foot of the bed.
11. Ask the patient to raise his hips, and then slide the bed protector under him.
12. Put on gloves. Offer the patient a bedpan or urinal. If used, raise the side rail, measure output if necessary, and discard the contents in the bathroom. Remove and dispose of gloves and wash your hands.
13. Ask patient to flex his knees and separate his legs. If the patient is on his side, use a pillow or folded bath blanket between the knees to separate the legs comfortably and to allow easier access to the perineal area.
14. Slide down the bath blanket to expose the perineal area only, keeping the legs covered.
15. Put on gloves.
16. Wet the washcloth in the basin, form it into a mitt, and add a small amount of soap. Too much soap will be difficult to rinse off, and may be drying or irritating to the skin.

17. Grasp the penis gently in one hand and apply soap with the washcloth. Start at the meatus and wash in a circular motion down to the base on each side of the penis.
18. Uncircumcised patients require that the foreskin be pulled gently down to expose the end of the penis, which can then be washed. If the foreskin is very tight and cannot be retracted with gentle effort, continue with the bath, but be sure to report this to your immediate supervisor.
19. Wash the scrotum, lifting it to wash the perineum.
20. Rinse the washcloth, using the mitt to rinse the area washed. More than one rinse, or wash, may be necessary to clean the area thoroughly.
21. Dry the area with the towel. Place the foreskin back in position for the uncircumcised patient.
22. Turn the patient on his side away from you, and flex the knee of his upper leg slightly, if this is permitted depending on his restrictions.
23. Wet the washcloth, form into a mitt, and apply soap.
24. Wash the anal area, using gentle front (perineum) to back (coccyx) strokes.
25. Rinse carefully as before. Repeat the wash and rinse if necessary.
26. Dry gently.
27. Reposition patient on his back.
28. Remove the protective pad from the bed and dispose of it.
29. Dispose of gloves and wash your hands. Apply clean disposable gloves.

PROCEDURE (continued)

30. Pull the sheet over the top of the bath blanket. Slide the bath blanket out from under the sheet. Bag and discard in laundry hamper.

31. Place the spread and blanket back on the patient. Tuck in as required.

FOLLOW-UP

32. Empty the basin of water, clean according to policy, place in proper storage, dispose of washcloths and towel. Dispose of gloves and wash your hands.

33. Document the procedure (and output if appropriate). Remember to document any redness, sores, rashes, swelling, bleeding, discharge, or discomfort the patient may have in that area.

CHARTING EXAMPLE: 12/12/04 10:45am Perineal care given to Mr. Crane after he was incontinent of urine and feces. Skin dry, intact, no red areas. F. Cooper, CNA (or check perineal care or partial bath on flow sheet, as well as incontinent, if it applies)

PERINEAL CARE FOR THE FEMALE PATIENT

PROCEDURE

OBRA

RATIONALE: Perineal care is done to cleanse the perineal area of the female patient's skin and body where she is unable to reach, clean the stitches in the perineal area following vaginal delivery of a baby, or to prevent skin breakdown on incontinent patients. It provides comfort, promotes healing, and allows for observation of the area.

PREPARATION

1. Assemble your equipment:
   a. Bath blanket
   b. Bedpan and cover
   c. Soap
   d. Basin with warm water (115°F; 46.1°C)
   e. Bath thermometer
   f. Disposable gloves
   g. Disposable bed protector
   h. Washcloth and towel
   i. Disposable plastic or cloth laundry bag for dirty linen (whichever is used by your institution)

2. Identify the patient by checking the identification bracelet.

3. Tell the patient that you are going to provide perineal care.

4. Provide privacy for the patient.

5. Provide safety with the side rail up on the opposite side of the bed.

6. Lower the side rail on the side nearest you.

STEPS

7. Position the patient on her back (a side-laying position is also used with some patients).

8. Remove the bedspread and blankets and place on a nearby chair or table for use after the bath.

9. Cover the patient with the bath blanket.

10. Being careful not to expose the patient, slide the sheet out from under the bath blanket and leave fan-folded at the foot of the bed.

11. Ask the patient to raise her hips, and then slide the bed protector under her.

12. Put on gloves. Offer the patient a bedpan. If used, raise the side rail, measure output if necessary, discard the contents in the toilet, and clean the bedpan. Remove gloves. Wash your hands.

13. Ask patient to flex her knees and separate her legs. If the patient is on her side, use a pillow or folded bath blanket between the knees to separate the legs comfortably and to allow easier access to the perineal area.

14. Slide down the bath blanket to expose the perineal area only, keeping the legs covered.

15. Put on gloves.

16. Wet the washcloth in the basin, form it into a mitt, add a small amount of soap. Too much soap will be difficult to rinse off, and may be drying or irritating to the skin.

17. Separate the vulva with one hand.

18. To wash gently:

   ■ Using the mitt, stroke the outer labia *once* from top downward to the perineum.

   ■ Rinse the washcloth, and repeat this *one* stroke to rinse the area.

   ■ Using the soaped mitt, stroke the other outer labia *once* from top, downward to the perineum.

   ■ Rinse the washcloth, and repeat this *one* stroke.

   ■ Repeat the above steps for both inner labia.

   ■ Separate the labia with one hand.

   ■ Wash and rinse with the same *one* downward stroke.

PROCEDURE *(continued)*

19. Rinse the washcloth, using the mitt to rinse the area washed.
20. More than one rinse, or wash, may be necessary to clean the area thoroughly.
21. Dry the area with the towel.
22. Turn the patient on her side away from you, and flex the knee of her upper leg slightly, if this is permitted depending on her restrictions.
23. Wet washcloth, form into a mitt, and apply soap.
24. Wash the anal area, using gentle front (perineum) to back (coccyx) strokes.
25. Rinse carefully as before. Repeat the wash and rinse if necessary.
26. Dry gently.

27. Reposition patient on her back or her side.
28. Remove the protective pad from the bed and dispose of it.
29. Dispose of gloves and wash your hands. Apply clean disposable gloves.
30. Pull the sheet over the top of the bath blanket. Slide the bath blanket out from under the sheet. Bag and discard in laundry hamper.
31. Place the spread and blanket back on the patient. Tuck in as required.

FOLLOW-UP

32. Empty the basin of water, clean according to policy, place in proper storage, dispose of

washcloths and towel. Dispose of gloves and wash your hands.
33. Document the procedure (and output if appropriate). Remember to document any redness, sores, rashes, swelling, bleeding, discharge, or discomfort the patient may have in that area.

CHARTING EXAMPLE: 12/17/04 10:45am Perineal care given to Mrs. Byrd after she was incontinent of urine and feces. Skin dry, intact, no red areas. F. Cooper, CNA (or check perineal care or partial bath on flow sheet, as well as incontinent if it applies)

Care of Nails and Feet

Follow your health care facility's policy regarding care of nails and feet, specifically that of cutting nails. Always receive specific instructions from your supervisor before cutting a patient's nails. Routine and proper nail and foot care can help prevent infections and foot odor. For the elderly, those with poor circulation, and patients with diabetes, the lack of nail and foot care could result in an infection and even cause the patient to have a foot amputated.

CARE OF NAILS AND FEET — GUIDELINES — OBRA

- Have ambulatory patients sit in a bedside chair with the over-bed table positioned to more easily soak their fingers in the emesis basin and each foot separately in the bath basin filled with warm water (105°F; 40.5°C).
- For toenails and feet, follow the same procedure as for a partial bath.

- Allow the feet to soak for 10 minutes in the warm (105°F) water.
- Using the washcloth, rub the dry skin from the heels of the feet and wash well between the toes.
- Dry the feet thoroughly, especially between the toes.
- An orange stick can be used to gently remove any dirt from under the nails.
- If you have permission to do so, trim the nails straight across.

(Many institutions will not allow you to use an emery board or file because it may damage the soft tissue around the nails.)
- Fingernails can be soaked in the emesis basin and then trimmed if needed. Be very careful not to trim any nail too short.
- Apply lotion or petroleum jelly after drying the hands and feet.
- Report any redness or problems noted.

The best time to observe the nails and feet is during the bath. If the nails are dirty or need trimming, this is a good time to do it. Nails should be trimmed at least weekly.

The Back Rub

Back rubs are usually given during morning care, right after the patient's bath. They also are given (1) as part of evening care, (2) when changing the position of a bedridden patient, (3) for very restless patients who need relaxing, and (4) on a doctor's orders for "special back care" (Figure 12–33a-c◆).

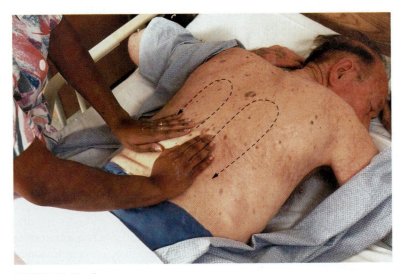

FIGURE 12–33a ◆

Back rubs are usually given during morning care, right after the patient's bath

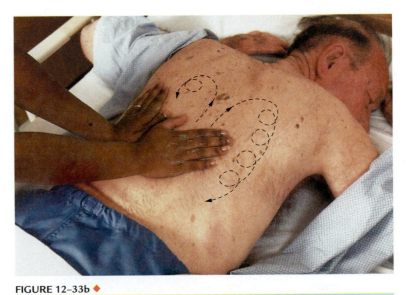

FIGURE 12–33b ◆

Use firm circular motions with hands and fingertips over each bony area

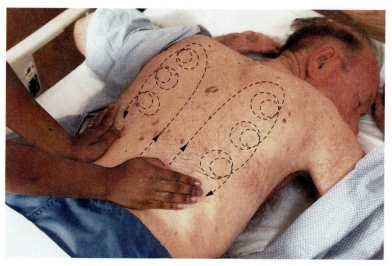

FIGURE 12–33c ◆

Repeat firm circular motions covering the entire back

<table>
<tr><td>

GIVING THE PATIENT A BACK RUB

</td><td>

PROCEDURE

</td><td>

OBRA

</td></tr>
</table>

RATIONALE: The back rub is given to relax the muscles, stimulate circulation, or refresh a patient.

PREPARATION

1. Assemble your equipment on the bedside table:
   a. Towels
   b. Lotion
   c. Basin of warm water (115°F; 46.1°C)
2. Identify the patient by checking the identification bracelet.
3. Tell the patient you are going to give him a back rub.
4. Provide privacy for the patient.
5. Wash your hands. (It is necessary to wear gloves to provide a back rub when you or the patient has any skin rashes, cuts, or open sores.)
6. Raise the bed to a comfortable working position.

STEPS

7. Ask the patient to turn on his side or abdomen so his back is toward you. Use the position that is most comfortable for the patient and for yourself.
8. The side rail should be in the up position on the far side of the bed.
9. Lotion may be warmed by placing the container in a basin of warm water (Figure 12–34◆).

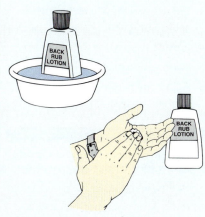

FIGURE 12–34 ◆

Apply warm lotion to your hands

10. Open the ties on the patient's gown or remove pajama top.
11. Pour a small amount of lotion into the palm of your hand.
12. Rub your hands together using friction to warm the lotion.
13. Keep your knees slightly bent and your back straight.
14. Apply lotion to the entire back with the palms of your hands. Use firm, long strokes from the buttocks to the shoulders and back of the neck.
15. Exert firm pressure as you stroke upward from the buttocks toward the shoulders. Use gentle pressure as you stroke downward from shoulders to buttocks (Figure 12–33a).
16. Use a circular motion on each bony area (Figure 12–33b).
17. This rhythmic rubbing motion should be continued from 1.5 to 3 minutes (Figure 12–33c).
18. Dry the patient's back by patting gently with a towel.
19. Close and retie the gown.

PROCEDURE *(continued)*

20. Assist the patient in turning back to a comfortable position and replace the call light.

FOLLOW-UP

21. Arrange the top sheets of the bed neatly.

22. Lower the bed to a position of safety for the patient.

23. Raise the side rails when ordered or appropriate for patient safety.

24. Put your equipment back in its proper place. Discard disposable equipment.

25. Wash your hands.

26. Report to your immediate supervisor:

    ■ That you have given the patient a back rub.

    ■ The time it was given.

    ■ How the patient tolerated the procedure.

■ Your observations of anything unusual.

CHARTING EXAMPLE: 12/12/04 9:45pm Mr. Crawford was given a back rub at 9pm with lotion as he was feeling stiff and uncomfortable. He now is resting comfortably. D. Copperfield, CNA (or check back rub or AM or PM care box on flow sheet)

A back rub relaxes the muscles, stimulates circulation, and refreshes the patient. Because of pressure caused by the bedclothes and the lack of movement to stimulate circulation, the skin of a bedridden patient needs special care to prevent skin breakdown.

Changing the Patient's Gown

When you change a patient's gown be careful not to expose the patient's body unnecessarily. It is important to prevent the patient from feeling any embarrassment or sudden chill from exposure to cool air.

PROCEDURE   OBRA

CHANGING THE PATIENT'S GOWN

RATIONALE: The gown is changed when dirty, wet, or soiled.

PREPARATION

1. Assemble your equipment on the bedside table:

   a. A clean gown

   b. Disposable gloves

   c. Disposable plastic or cloth laundry bag for dirty linen (whichever is used in your institution)

2. Identify the patient by checking the identification bracelet.

3. Tell the patient you are going to change his gown.

4. Provide privacy for the patient.

5. Wash your hands and put on gloves.

6. Adjust the bed to a comfortable working height.

STEPS

7. Ask the patient to turn on his side with his back toward you so you can untie the tapes.

8. If the patient cannot be turned, you will have to reach under his neck to untie the tapes.

9. Loosen the soiled gown around the patient's body.

10. Get the clean gown ready to put on the patient. Unfold it and lay it across the patient's chest on top of the bath blanket or top sheets.

11. Take off one sleeve at a time, leaving the old gown in place on the patient.

12. Slide each arm through one sleeve of the clean gown (Figure 12–35◆).

13. If the patient cannot hold his arm up, put your hand through the sleeve. Take his hand in yours and slip the sleeve up the patient's wrist and arm. Do this for both

PROCEDURE *(continued)*

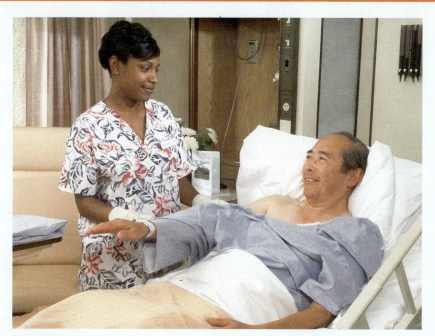

FIGURE 12–35 ◆
Slide each arm through one sleeve of the patient's clean gown

arms. Then pull the gown down over the patient's chest. If the patient has a sore arm, remove the sleeve on the unaffected arm first. Then remove the sleeve on the sore (affected) arm. To put the clean gown on, put the sleeve on the sore (affected) arm first. Then slide the unaffected arm through the second sleeve.

14. Remove the soiled gown from under the bath blanket or top sheets.

15. Tie the tapes on the clean gown. Some patients want only the tapes at the neck tied so they will not be lying on knots.

16. Put the soiled gown in laundry bag and place in hamper.

FOLLOW-UP

17. Make the patient comfortable and replace the call light.

18. Lower the bed to a position of safety for the patient.

19. Raise the side rails when ordered or appropriate for patient safety.

20. Remove the gloves and wash your hands.

21. Report to your immediate supervisor:

  - That you have replaced the patient's soiled gown with a clean one.

  - Your observations of anything unusual.

CHARTING EXAMPLE: 12/12/04 9:45pm Gown changed and PM care was given to Mr. Lee. He now is resting comfortably. V. James, CNA (or check PM care box on flow sheet)

 # Hair Care

Patients who will be in the health care institution for a long time may occasionally need to have their hair shampooed. Often the doctor must write the order for a shampoo. The nurse must give you instructions for giving the shampoo. For patients on bed rest, the patient must be in bed when the shampoo is given. Other patients may be allowed to shampoo in the tub or shower.

| SHAMPOOING THE PATIENT'S HAIR | PROCEDURE | OBRA |

RATIONALE: The hair is washed to clean the hair, stimulate scalp circulation, or refresh a patient.

PREPARATION

1. Assemble your equipment on the bedside table:

    a. Basin of warm water (105°F; 40.5°C)

    b. Pitcher of warm water (115°F; 46.1°C)

    c. Bath thermometer

    d. Large basin

    e. Water trough (shampoo tray) or plastic sheet

    f. Disposable bed protector

    g. Pillow with waterproof case

    h. Face and bath towels

    i. Washcloth, to cover the patient's eyes

    j. Paper cup

    k. Bath blanket

    l. Cotton

    m. Disposable gloves

    n. Disposable plastic or cloth laundry bag for dirty linen (whichever is used in your institution)

2. Identify the patient by checking the identification bracelet.

3. Tell the patient you are going to give her a shampoo.

4. Provide privacy for the patient.

5. Wash your hands and put on gloves.

6. Raise the bed to its highest horizontal position.

STEPS

7. Brush the patient's hair. Have her turn her head from side to side so the hair can be brushed one exposed side at a time.

8. Place a chair at the side of the bed near the patient's head. The chair should be lower than the mattress. The back of the chair should be touching the mattress.

9. Place the small towel on the chair. Put the large basin on the chair.

10. Put small amounts of cotton in the patient's ears for protection.

11. Ask the patient to move across the bed so that her head is close to where you are standing.

12. Remove the pillow from under the patient's head. Cover the pillow with the waterproof case. Place the pillow between the shoulder blades, so that the head tilts back when the patient lies down.

13. Put the bath blanket on the bed. From underneath, fan-fold the top sheets to the foot of the bed without exposing the patient.

14. Place the disposable bed protector on the mattress under the patient's head.

15. Place the shampoo trough under the patient's head. A trough can be made by rolling over the three sides of the plastic sheet three times. This makes a channel for the water to run off. Put the end of the channel under the patient's head. Have the other open end hanging over the side of the bed. This free end of the plastic sheet should be put into the large basin on the chair.

16. Loosen the patient's gown at the neck.

17. Dampen the washcloth and ask the patient to hold the damp washcloth over her eyes (Figure 12–36◆).

18. Fill the basin with warm water. Put the basin on the bedside table with the paper cup.

19. Fill the pitcher with warm water. Have the pitcher on the bedside table, for extra water, if needed.

20. Fill the paper cup with water from the basin. Pour it over the hair; repeat until completely wet.

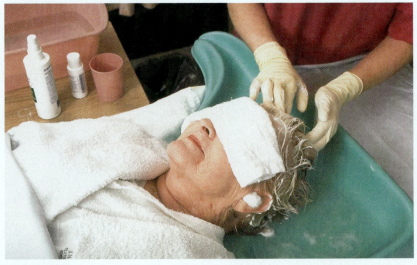

FIGURE 12–36 ◆
Apply a damp washcloth over patient's eyes. Use both hands to carefully shampoo hair

PROCEDURE (continued)

21. Apply a small amount of shampoo and, using both hands, wash the hair and massage the patient's scalp with your fingertips. Avoid using fingernails as they could scratch the scalp.

22. Rinse the soap off the hair by pouring water from the cup over the hair. Have the patient turn her head from side to side. Repeat this until the hair is free of shampoo.

23. Dry the patient's forehead and ears with the face towel.

24. Remove the cotton from the ears.

25. Raise the patient's head and wrap the head with a bath towel.

26. Rub the patient's hair with the towel to dry it as much as possible.

27. Remove your equipment from the bed. Change the patient's gown, if necessary.

28. Comb the patient's hair. Leave a towel wrapped around the head or spread a towel out over the pillow under the head until the hair is completely dry. If a dryer is available, use it to dry the patient's hair. Use low or warm setting and move dryer to avoid burning the scalp.

29. Remove the bath blanket and at the same time bring the top sheets back up to cover the patient.

FOLLOW-UP

30. Make the patient comfortable and replace the call light.

31. Lower the bed to a position of safety for the patient.

32. Raise the side rails when ordered or appropriate for patient safety.

33. Clean and return your equipment. Discard disposable equipment.

34. Remove the gloves and wash your hands.

35. Report to your immediate supervisor:

    ■ That you have given the patient a shampoo.

    ■ How the patient tolerated the procedure.

    ■ Your observations of anything unusual.

CHARTING EXAMPLE: 12/12/04 9:45am Washed Ms. Howell's hair with shampoo and conditioner. Afterward she said she is feeling much better. D. Copperfield, CNA (or check Hair wash or AM care box on flow sheet)

KEY IDEA

As with other types of personal care, a patient may be too weak or ill to take care of her own hair. It may be difficult for her to raise her arms. Combing and brushing a patient's hair almost always leaves the patient looking and feeling better.

COMBING THE PATIENT'S HAIR

PROCEDURE

OBRA

RATIONALE: Hair is combed to remove tangles or assist a helpless patient to look and feel better.

PREPARATION

1. Assemble your equipment on the bedside table:

   a. Towel

   b. Comb or brush

   c. Hand mirror, if available

   d. Disposable gloves

   e. Disposable plastic or cloth laundry bag for dirty linen (whichever is used by your institution)

2. Wash your hands and put on gloves.

3. Identify the patient by checking the identification bracelet.

4. Provide privacy for the patient.

5. Tell the patient you are going to brush or comb her hair.

6. Raise the bed to a comfortable working height.

STEPS

7. If possible, comb the patient's hair after the bath and before you make the bed.

8. Lay a towel across the pillow under the patient's head. If the patient can sit up in bed, drape the towel around her shoulders.

9. If wearing glasses, ask the patient to remove them before you begin.

PROCEDURE *(continued)*

Be sure to put the glasses in a safe place.

10. Part the hair down the middle to make it easier to comb.

11. Brush or comb the patient's hair carefully, gently, and thoroughly, combing small amounts of hair at a time.

12. For the patient who cannot sit up, separate the hair into small sections. Comb each section separately, using a downward motion. Ask the patient to turn her head from side to side or turn it for her so you can reach the entire head (Figure 12–37◆).

13. Comb the patient's hair into the style the patient requests.

14. If the patient has very long hair, suggest braiding it to keep it from getting tangled.

15. Be sure you brush the back of the head. Observe any breaks in skin or abnormal findings.

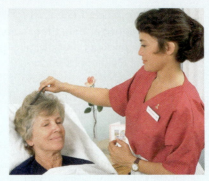

FIGURE 12–37 ◆
Comb each section of hair separately

16. Remove the towel when you are finished.

FOLLOW-UP

17. Let the patient use the mirror.

18. Make the patient comfortable and replace the call light.

19. Lower the bed to a position of safety for the patient.

20. Raise the side rails when ordered or appropriate for patient safety.

21. Clean and return your equipment to its proper place.

22. Remove the gloves and wash your hands.

23. Report to your immediate supervisor:

   ■ That you have combed the patient's hair.

   ■ How the patient tolerated the procedure.

   ■ Your observations of anything unusual.

CHARTING EXAMPLE: 12/12/04 9:45am Combed and styled Ms. Howell's hair. Afterward she said she is feeling much better. D. Copperfield, CNA (or check AM care box on flow sheet)

Shaving the Patient's Beard

A regular morning activity for most men is shaving their beard. A patient is often well enough to shave himself. In this case, you will give him only the help that is necessary, such as being sure he has the equipment he needs. Sometimes patients are too ill or weak to shave themselves. In such cases, you will do it. Before shaving any patient's face, be sure to get permission from your immediate supervisor. Certain patients may not be permitted to shave or be shaved.

Shaving can be done with an electric razor or a safety razor. Often, the patient will have his own electric razor which you will be able to use.

KEY IDEA

Many hospitals have special rules and policies regarding electrical equipment being brought into the hospital. Follow the nurse's instructions regarding electric razors. Due to bleeding precautions certain patients should not be shaved with a safety razor.

| SHAVING THE PATIENT'S BEARD | **PROCEDURE** | **OBRA** |

RATIONALE: Shaving is done to remove unwanted facial hair and to assist a helpless patient to look and feel better.

PREPARATION

1. Assemble your equipment on the bedside table:
   a. Face towel
   b. Basin of warm water (115°F; 46.1°C)
   c. Shaving brush, shaving cream, and safety razor, or
   d. Electric razor
   e. Disposable gloves
   f. Disposable plastic or cloth laundry bag for dirty linen (whichever is used by your institution)
2. Identify the patient by checking the identification bracelet.
3. Tell the patient you are going to shave his beard (Figure 12–38a◆).
4. Provide privacy for the patient.

5. Wash your hands and put on gloves.
6. Raise the bed to a comfortable working height.

STEPS

7. Adjust a light so that it shines on the patient's face.
8. Raise the head of the bed, if allowed.
9. Spread the face towel under the patient's chin. If the patient has dentures, be sure they are in his mouth.
10. Pat some warm water or use a damp, warm washcloth on the patient's face to soften his beard if using a safety razor.
11. Apply shaving soap generously to the face if using a safety razor.
12. With the fingers of one hand, hold the skin taut (tight) as you shave in the direction that the hairs grow. Start under the sideburns and work downward over the cheeks (Figure 12–38b◆). Continue carefully over the chin. Work upward on the neck under the chin. Use short, firm strokes.

13. Rinse the safety razor often.
14. Areas under the nose and around the lips are sensitive. Take special care in these areas.
15. If you nick the patient's skin, report this to your supervisor.
16. Wash off the remaining soap when you have finished.
17. Pat on aftershave lotion or powder, as the patient prefers.

FOLLOW-UP

18. Make the patient comfortable and replace the call light.
19. Lower the bed to a position of safety for the patient.
20. Raise the side rails when ordered or appropriate for patient safety.
21. Clean and return your equipment. Bag soiled towel and place in hamper. Discard disposable equipment. Razor blades or disposable razors should be discarded in sharps containers.
22. Dispose of gloves and wash your hands.
23. Report to your immediate supervisor:
    - That you have shaved the patient's beard.
    - How the patient tolerated the procedure.
    - Your observations of anything unusual.

CHARTING EXAMPLE: 12/12/04 9:45am Shaved Mr. Yacks. Afterward he said he is feeling much better. D. Copperfield, CNA (or check shave or AM care box on flow sheet)

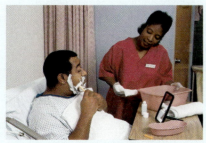

FIGURE 12–38a ◆
Assisting the patient with shaving

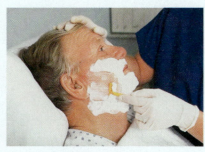

FIGURE 12–38b ◆
Work downward over the cheeks

Elimination Needs

Some patients are unable to get out of bed to use the bathroom. For these patients a **urinal** and a **bedpan** are required. The urinal is a container into which the male patient **urinates**. The bedpan is a pan into which he **defecates** (moves his bowels). The

urinal A portable container given to male patients so they can urinate without getting out of bed

bedpan A pan used by patients who must defecate or urinate while in bed

urinate To discharge urine from the body; other words for this function are *void, micturate,* and *pass water*

eliminate (defecate) To rid the body of waste products; to excrete, expel, remove, put out (to have a bowel movement; to excrete waste matter from the bowels)

fracture pan A bedpan with a flat end that goes under the patient

fracture pan is slightly smaller and shallower than the regular bedpan. It is used by the patient whose illness or injuries don't allow the patient sufficient movement to utilize a bedpan. The female patient uses the bedpan for urination and defecation.

Wear gloves whenever handling a bedpan or urinal after use. You should always cover the bedpan and remove it from the patient's bedside to the bathroom as quickly as possible after use. At this time you would collect a specimen if required. You would also measure the urine if the patient is on intake and output.

PROCEDURE

OFFERING THE BEDPAN

OBRA

RATIONALE: The bedpan provides a means of collecting urine or stool output of bedridden patients.

PREPARATION

1. Assemble your equipment on the bedside table (Figure 12-39◆):

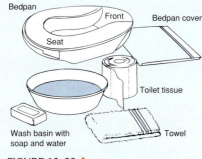

FIGURE 12-39 ◆
Assemble equipment

  a. Bedpan and cover, or fracture pan and cover (may be placed on chair) (Figure 12-40◆)
  b. Toilet tissue
  c. Wash basin with warm water (115°F; 46.1°C)
  d. Soap
  e. Hand towel
  f. Powder

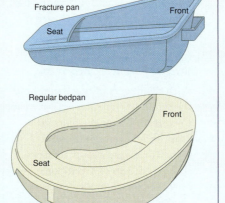

FIGURE 12-40 ◆
Choose appropriate type of bedpan and cover

  g. Disposable bed protector
  h. Disposable gloves

2. Identify the patient by checking the identification bracelet.
3. Ask the patient if she would like to use the bedpan.
4. Provide privacy for the patient.
5. Wash your hands and put on gloves.
6. Raise the bed to a comfortable working position.

STEPS

7. Take the bedpan out of the bedside table. Warm the bedpan if necessary by running warm water inside it and along the rim. Dry the outside of the bedpan with paper towels. Put powder on the bedpan to decrease friction.
8. Fold back the top sheets so that they are out of the way.
9. Raise the patient's gown, but keep the lower part of her body covered.
10. Ask the patient to bend her knees and put her feet flat on the mattress if she is able. Then ask the patient to raise her hips. If necessary, help the patient to raise her buttocks by slipping your hand under the lower part of her back. Place the protective pad and then the bedpan in position with the seat of the bedpan (smooth round rim) under the buttocks (Figure 12-41a◆). (Place the fracture pan

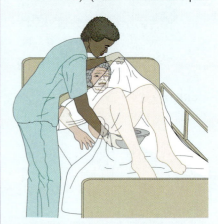

FIGURE 12-41a ◆
Position bedpan under the buttocks

PROCEDURE *(continued)*

with the flat end under the patient's buttocks.)

11. Sometimes the patient is unable to lift her buttocks to get on or off the bedpan. In this case, turn the patient on her side with her back to you. Put the bedpan against the buttocks. Then turn the patient onto the bedpan (Figure 12–41b◆).

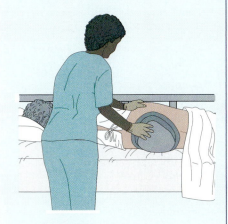

FIGURE 12–41b ◆
Assist the patient to roll over onto the bedpan if necessary

12. Replace the covers over the patient.

13. Raise the backrest and a knee rest, if allowed, so the patient is in a sitting position (Figure 12–41c◆).

14. Put toilet tissue and the call light where the patient can reach them easily.

15. Ask the patient to signal when she is finished.

16. Raise the side rails to the up position.

17. Dispose of gloves and wash your hands. Leave the room to give the patient privacy, if her condition allows.

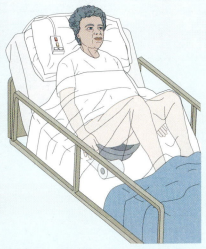

FIGURE 12–41c ◆
Raise patient to a comfortable sitting position

18. When the patient signals, return to the room.

19. Wash your hands and put on gloves.

20. Help the patient to raise her hips so you can remove the bedpan.

21. Cover the bedpan immediately with a disposable pad or a paper towel if no cover is available.

22. Help the patient if she is unable to clean herself. Turn the patient on her side. Clean the anal area with toilet tissue or a warm washcloth, if necessary.

23. Take the bedpan to the patient's bathroom.

24. If a specimen is required, collect it at this time. Measure the urine if the patient is on intake and output.

25. Check the excreta (feces or urine) for abnormal (unusual) appearance.

26. Empty the bedpan into the patient's toilet.

27. Health care institutions have different equipment in the bathroom for cleaning the bedpan. Follow your institution's instructions for cleaning the bedpan.

28. Put the clean bedpan and cover back into the bedside table.

29. Help the patient to wash her hands in the basin of water.

FOLLOW-UP

30. Dispose of your gloves and wash your hands.

31. Make the patient comfortable and replace the call light. Lower the backrest as necessary.

32. Lower the bed to a position of safety for the patient.

33. Raise the side rails when ordered or appropriate for patient safety.

34. Report to your immediate supervisor:

- That the patient has urinated or defecated.

- If a specimen was collected.

- How the patient tolerated the procedure.

- Your observations of anything unusual.

CHARTING EXAMPLE: 12/12/04 9:45am Assisted Mrs. Warren to use the bedpan. She had a bowel movement and voided 450cc of urine. M. Madden, CNA (or check or document output box on flow sheet)

PROCEDURE

OFFERING THE URINAL

OBRA

RATIONALE: The urinal provides a means of collecting urinary output of male bedridden patients.

PREPARATION

1. Assemble your equipment on the bedside table:
   a. Urinal and cover
   b. Basin with warm water (115°F; 46.1°C)
   c. Soap
   d. Towel
   e. Disposable gloves
2. Identify the patient by checking the identification bracelet.
3. Ask the patient if he would like to use the urinal.
4. Provide privacy for the patient.
5. Wash your hands and put on gloves.

STEPS

6. Give the urinal to the patient (Figure 12–42◆).
7. Place the call light within easy reach.

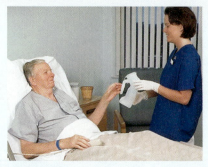

FIGURE 12–42 ◆
Give urinal to the patient

8. Ask the patient to signal when he is finished.
9. Dispose of your gloves and wash your hands. Leave the room to give the patient privacy, if his condition allows.
10. When the patient signals, return to the room, wash your hands, and put on gloves.
11. Cover the urinal and take it to the patient's bathroom.
12. Check the urine for abnormal (unusual) appearance.
13. Measure the urine if the patient is on intake and output. Collect a specimen at this time, if required.
14. Empty the urinal into the toilet. Wash and rinse.

15. Put the clean urinal back in the patient's bedside table.
16. Remove the gloves and wash your hands.
17. Help the patient to wash his hands in the basin of water.

FOLLOW-UP

18. Make the patient comfortable and replace the call light.
19. Lower the bed to a position of safety for the patient.
20. Raise the side rails when ordered or appropriate for patient safety.
21. Report to your immediate supervisor:
    - That the patient has urinated.
    - If a specimen was collected.
    - How the patient tolerated the procedure.
    - Your observations of anything unusual.

CHARTING EXAMPLE: 12/12/04 9:45am Offered Mr. Waxman the urinal. He voided 450cc of urine. M. Madden, CNA (or check or document urine output box on flow sheet)

PROCEDURE

OFFERING THE PORTABLE/BEDSIDE COMMODE

OBRA

RATIONALE: The bedside commode provides a means of collecting urine or stool output of patients.

PREPARATION

1. Assemble your equipment on the bedside table:

   a. Portable bedside **commode** next to the bed (Figure 12–43◆)
   b. Bedpan and cover, or the container used in your institution
   c. Toilet tissue
   d. Basin of warm water (115°F; 46.1°C)
   e. Soap
   f. Towel
   g. Disposable gloves

2. Identify the patient by checking the identification bracelet.
3. Tell the patient you will assist him onto the bedside commode.
4. Provide privacy for the patient.
5. Wash your hands and put on gloves.

STEPS

6. Put the commode next to the patient's bed. Open the cover and

commode A movable chair enclosing a bedpan with an opening that can fit over a toilet

PROCEDURE *(continued)*

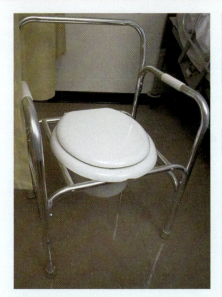

FIGURE 12–43 ◆
Portable bedside commode

insert a bedpan under the toilet seat if a pan is not already in place.

7. Help the patient put on his slippers and then help him out of bed and onto the commode.

8. Put toilet tissue and the call light where the patient can reach them easily.

9. Ask the patient to signal when he is finished.

10. Dispose of your gloves and wash your hands. Leave the room to give the patient privacy, if his condition allows.

11. When the patient signals, return to the room. Wash your hands.

12. Put on gloves and help the patient clean himself.

13. Assist the patient back to bed.

14. Close the cover on the commode.

15. Help the patient to wash his hands in the basin of water.

16. Make the patient comfortable.

17. Remove the bedpan from under the commode. Cover it and carry it to the patient's bathroom.

18. Check the excreta (feces or urine) for abnormal (unusual) appearance.

19. Measure output if patient is on intake and output. If a specimen is required, collect it at this time.

20. Empty the bedpan into the toilet.

21. Health care institutions have different equipment in the bathroom for cleaning the bedpan. Follow your institution's instructions for cleaning the bedpan.

22. Dispose of your gloves and wash your hands.

23. Put the clean bedpan back in the bedside table. Put the commode in its proper place.

FOLLOW-UP

24. Lower the bed to a position of safety for the patient.

25. Raise the side rails when ordered or appropriate for patient safety.

26. Place the call light within easy reach of the patient.

27. Report to your immediate supervisor:

   ■ That the patient has voided or defecated.

   ■ If a specimen was collected.

   ■ How the patient tolerated the procedure.

   ■ Your observations of anything unusual.

CHARTING EXAMPLE: 12/12/04 9:45am Assisted Mr. Warren up out of bed to use the bedside commode. He had a bowel movement and voided 450cc of urine. M. Madden, CNA (or check or document output box on flow sheet)

 # The Incontinent Patient

Some patients are not able to control their bladder or bowels. This condition is called **incontinence**. A draw sheet and a reusable or disposable bed protector are used on the bed. These patients should be checked frequently to make sure they are clean and dry. Follow the procedure for a partial bed bath each time the patient is soiled. (See perineal care earlier in this chapter.) For urinary incontinence in some patients, the physician may order an indwelling catheter. Due to the increased risk of a urinary infection with an indwelling catheter, an external condom catheter may be ordered for males. For some patients, bowel and bladder retraining will be ordered. Your supervisor will instruct you on the procedures for retraining each individual patient.

incontinence The inability to control the bowels or bladder

KEY IDEA

Washing and drying the patient thoroughly will decrease the probability of the patient getting decubitus ulcers and infections.

SUMMARY

Meeting the needs of your patients in regard to their activities of daily living is a major responsibility. Assisting patients with oral hygiene, bathing, perineal care, care of nails, feet, and hair, and elimination in a skillful manner will increase their comfort and well-being. Following each procedure correctly will provide for safety for you and the patient. Each patient is to be treated as an individual. Your observations while helping patients are important to other members of the health care team as they evaluate care needed.

NOTES

CHAPTER REVIEW

FILL IN THE BLANK Read each sentence and fill in the blank line with a word that completes the sentence.

1. Care of a person's mouth and teeth is called _____ _____.

2. Activities that can be performed by the patient are called _____ _____ activities.

3. _____ is the inability to control the bowels or bladder.

4. You would give your patients a _____ or a _____ if they needed to urinate in bed.

5. Providing _____ _____ helps a patient feel better and look better.

MULTIPLE CHOICE Choose the best answer for each question or statement.

1. Helping the patient with oral hygiene, bathing, and making the bed are all part of
   a. early A.M. care.
   b. A.M. care.
   c. afternoon care.
   d. evening care.

2. Helping a patient with oral hygiene, offering a bedpan, and giving a back rub are all part of
   a. early A.M. care.
   b. A.M. care.
   c. afternoon care.
   d. evening care.

3. Which of the following will not allow you to accurately measure urine output?
   a. Urinal
   b. Bedside commode

   c. Toilet
   d. Bedpan

4. When cleaning dentures, do all of the following except
   a. wear gloves.
   b. provide privacy.
   c. take the dentures to the sink in your hands.
   d. moisten the dentures to put them back in place.

5. Which of the following is not a type of bath?
   a. Complete bed bath
   b. Partial bed bath
   c. Shower
   d. All of the above are types of baths.

TIME-OUT

TIPS FOR TIME MANAGEMENT

If you arrive at work and find that your unit is understaffed, the best approach is to carefully plan your work to accomplish the most you can in the least amount of time. Resist the urge to waste precious time complaining, waiting for more help, or acting defeated before you begin.

THE NURSING ASSISTANT IN ACTION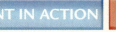

You are assigned to wash and style the hair of Mrs. Williams, an African American woman. You have never seen or used the hair products she has on hand for you to use. You want Mrs. Williams to think you know what you are doing, and are unsure what she will think if you tell her the truth. You attended a class at the beginning of your orientation, but today you do not remember anything now that you need the information! She says, "Well what are you waiting for? I thought you came in here to help me do my hair?"

What Is Your Response/Action?

CRITICAL THINKING

CUSTOMER SERVICE Patients will have different preferences for when they wish to shower or bathe or receive personal care. When possible try to accommodate them. Forcing a patient to comply with your schedule will not leave the patient with a positive view of your consideration or customer service.

CULTURAL CARE You may care for patients who use hair care or skin products different from those you use. Learn to use common products frequently used by patients you encounter in your workplace. Be aware that members of some cultures believe it is inappropriate for a caregiver to provide perineal care to or bathe a patient of the opposite sex. Whenever possible, accommodate the patient's preferences.

COOPERATION WITHIN THE TEAM If there is a caregiver of the same sex as the patient qualified to perform a personal care procedure that person should be assigned to assist with that patient care procedure. A notation should be made on the care plan alerting staff of this preference. Your supervisor can assist you in problem solving when you encounter patient preferences that you are unsure how to handle.

EXPLORE MediaLink

Additional interactive resources for this chapter can be found on the Companion Website at www.prenhal.com/wolgin. Click on Chapter 12 and "Begin" to select activities for this chapter.

For chapter-related NCLEX-style questions and an audio glossary, access the accompanying CD-ROM in this book.

Video:

- Activity and Exercise; Bathing an Adult Client

13 Emergency Care

OBJECTIVES

When you have completed this chapter, you will be able to:

- List the guidelines to follow in an emergency.
- Describe the signs of shock and guidelines for care of a patient in shock.
- Explain the purpose of CPR and list its three basic elements.
- List the signs of heart attack, cardiac arrest, and stroke, and explain what should be done to help the person in crisis.
- Explain the purpose of the Heimlich maneuver.
- Demonstrate how to assist someone who is having a seizure.
- Demonstrate the most effective way to control bleeding.
- Demonstrate first aid for a burn victim.
- Explain what to do for someone who has been poisoned.

KEY TERMS

bioterrorism
cardiac arrest
cardiopulmonary resuscitation (CPR)
cardiovascular system
emergency
first aid
heart attack
hemorrhage
poison
seizure
shock
stroke

MediaLink

www.prenhall.com/wolgin

Use the address above to access the free, interactive Companion Website created for this textbook. Get hints, instant feedback, and textbook references to chapter-related NCLEX-style questions. Link to other interesting sites.

AUDIO GLOSSARY:

Use the Companion Website, or the CD-ROM disk enclosed with your textbook, to hear the pronunciation of key terms in the chapter.

This chapter provides an overview of common emergencies that require immediate action and the guidelines to follow for each emergency situation. These emergencies include shock, chest pain, heart attack or myocardial infarction, cardiopulmonary resuscitation, stroke, seizures, hemorrhage, burns, and poisoning.

The main goals in dealing with emergencies are handling the immediate crisis, preventing further harm or injury, and providing security and comfort until help arrives. Never leave a person who needs immediate help. Have someone else call for additional assistance.

What to Do in an Emergency

emergency Events that call for immediate action

first aid The first action taken to help a person who is in crisis

---

ALERT

For all patient contact, adhere to Standard Precautions (Chapter 5, pages 83–85). Wear protective equipment as indicated.

---

bioterrorism Terrorist attacks using chemical or biological materials

Emergencies are events that call for immediate action! **First aid** is the immediate care or first action taken to help a person in crisis, which may range from a small cut or trauma resulting from an accident to a sudden illness. First aid provides care until additional help arrives. Protect yourself using Standard Precautions and follow the procedures or policies provided by your employing health care institution. As a health care worker you will be expected to provide first aid and respond to emergencies. A course in basic first aid and basic life support serves as a useful foundation because emergencies can occur anywhere at any time. First aid courses are available through the National Safety Council or the Red Cross. Basic life-support courses are offered by the American Red Cross and the American Heart Association.

Emergency responders, police and fire departments, hospitals, and public health agencies work to defend the public against biological and chemical terrorism. They are putting plans in place to integrate their efforts to respond to **bioterrorism**, that is, biological and chemical attacks. The terrorist attacks and anthrax exposures of September 2001 demonstrated the difficult challenges faced by our hospitals and public health systems in responding effectively to such incidents. As a health care worker, it is important for you to be aware of your community's plan for disseminating public health information in the event of a biological or chemical attack. Your employer will include orientation and ongoing training in the use of protective equipment needed to safely respond to emergencies.

Legal Issues

In your place of employment, your responsibility is to stay with the patient, call for help or notify the nurse, and begin first aid. Once the nurse arrives you may be asked to assist. Outside of work you are not legally required to provide first aid. If you decide to render help, you must perform correctly within the limits of your training. Once begun, you must continue your first aid until you are exhausted, other help arrives, or it is no longer needed. Many states have Good Samaritan laws that protect the legal rights of persons offering first aid. As long as you operate within the guidelines of your training, you are usually safe from legal judgments.

KEY IDEA

When responding to an emergency situation, the basic rules of first aid include remaining calm, providing reassurance, and not moving the individual unless absolutely necessary to protect the person from further harm or danger.

Each employing agency should have written procedures for emergency and first aid care that you should follow. When caring for a person in the home, an emergency plan should be available to the caregiver (family member) or the employee of an agency to follow. This plan should include phone numbers (in many areas, 911) of the police, fire rescue squads, emergency medical help, and for physicians, emergency rooms, the nearest hospital, telecommunication services for the deaf, and the regional poison control center.

Before you take any action, you must determine

- What the problem or emergency is (look at the entire situation)
- If anyone is available to help you
- What must be done immediately to maintain life for the person in crisis
- What you, the nursing assistant, are capable of doing
- If the person in crisis can be moved

Once these determinations are made, follow the guidelines in the box.

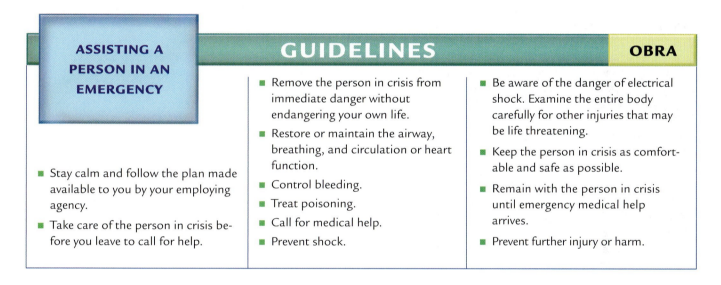

ASSISTING A PERSON IN AN EMERGENCY

GUIDELINES

OBRA

- Stay calm and follow the plan made available to you by your employing agency.
- Take care of the person in crisis before you leave to call for help.

- Remove the person in crisis from immediate danger without endangering your own life.
- Restore or maintain the airway, breathing, and circulation or heart function.
- Control bleeding.
- Treat poisoning.
- Call for medical help.
- Prevent shock.

- Be aware of the danger of electrical shock. Examine the entire body carefully for other injuries that may be life threatening.
- Keep the person in crisis as comfortable and safe as possible.
- Remain with the person in crisis until emergency medical help arrives.
- Prevent further injury or harm.

Emergency Medical Services

Most areas have emergency medical services (EMS) systems, where you dial a given phone number (usually 911) and tell the operator the following information:

- Address of the emergency, including the nearest cross street
- Phone number from which you are calling
- How many people need assistance
- The type of emergency
- What is being done for the victims

The operator will give you instructions as to when you can hang up and what you should do until assistance arrives (Figure 13–1◆). If needed, perform cardiopulmonary resuscitation (CPR) until emergency medical rescue help arrives.

All local emergency phone numbers should be written on or near your telephone. By knowing your local emergency number and calling for help when an emergency arises, you can take responsibility for the rescue of the victims.

Recognition and management of foreign body airway obstruction are covered in basic CPR courses. It is recommended that you enroll in one of these courses or gain CPR instruction through your institution or employer.

FIGURE 13–1 ◆

Most areas have emergency medical service systems

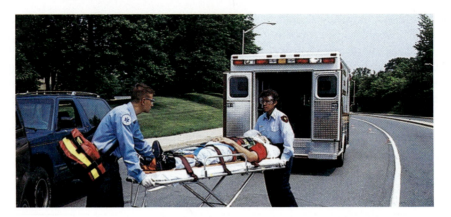

Shock

shock The failure of the cardiovascular system to provide sufficient blood circulation to every part of the body

cardiovascular system Circulatory system which includes heart, arteries, veins, and capillaries

Shock may occur in those individuals who experience a medical or trauma emergency. **Shock** is the failure of the **cardiovascular system** to provide sufficient blood circulation to every part of the body. Diagnostic signs of shock are

- Eyes are dull and lack luster
- Pupils may be dilated
- Face is pale and cyanotic (blue)
- Respirations are shallow, irregular, or labored
- Pulse is rapid and weak
- Skin is cold, clammy (moist), and pale

The shock patient may be:

- Nauseated
- Anxious and restless
- Thirsty

The shock patient may:

- Collapse
- Vomit

Types of Shock

Shock may be caused by many factors, such as

- Excessive blood loss
- Any severe injury
- Insufficient oxygen
- Spinal cord damage
- The reaction of the nervous system to fear, the sight of blood, and so on
- Inadequate heart function
- Infection
- Loss of body fluid or changes in body chemistry
- Extreme allergic reaction

Hemorrhagic shock is caused by blood loss. The reduction of blood volume means that circulation is impaired; this may occur for several reasons:

- External bleeding
- Internal bleeding
- Loss of plasma (the straw-colored liquid component of blood) due to burns or crushed tissues

Respiratory shock is caused by insufficient oxygen in the blood. The inability to fill the lungs completely is the result of impaired breathing. This may happen because of

- A chest wound
- Broken ribs
- A collapsed lung
- Airway obstruction
- Spinal cord damage that has paralyzed the muscles of the chest

Neurogenic shock is caused by loss of control of the nervous system. This may occur because of

- Trauma to the spinal cord
- Infection

Psychogenic shock or fainting is caused by a reaction of the nervous system to fear, bad news, the sight of blood, or a minor injury. Sudden dilation of the blood vessels occurs and the blood flow to the brain is reduced. The person faints, and unless other problems are present, fainting is usually self-correcting. When the head is lowered, blood circulates to the brain and normal function is restored. However, injury due to fainting, such as falling and injuring a body part, can occur.

Cardiogenic shock is caused by inadequate functioning of the heart. When the heart does not continuously operate due to disorders that weaken the heart muscle, the heart may no longer have the strength to pump blood to all parts of the body.

Septic shock is caused by infection. Toxins released into the bloodstream have a harmful effect on the blood vessels, causing them to dilate (get larger), which results in incomplete filling of the circulatory system.

GUIDELINES

ASSISTING THE PATIENT IN SHOCK

- Call for medical help.
- Maintain an open airway to ensure breathing.
- Keep the person quiet and lying down with the feet and legs slightly higher than the body and head unless contraindicated (Figure 13–2◆). Maintain normal body temperature.
- If a broken bone is suspected, keep the person in crisis flat. Do not move the person.

- Control bleeding.
- Do not offer any food or drink.
- Talk to the person in crisis and offer reassurance.
- Stay with the person in crisis until emergency medical rescue help arrives.

FIGURE 13–2 ◆

Keep the person quiet and lying down with the feet and legs slightly higher than the body and head; maintain normal body temperature

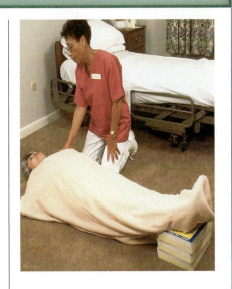

Metabolic shock is caused by loss of body fluids and changes in body chemistry. This happens because of

- Loss of body fluids through diarrhea, vomiting, or urination
- Severe disturbance of body salts or the acid-base balance in diseases

Anaphylactic shock or allergic reaction occurs when a person comes in contact with something to which he or she is extremely sensitive or allergic. This may be caused by

- Insect stings (bees, yellow jackets, wasps, and hornets)
- Inhaled substances (dust, pollen)
- Injected substances (drugs such as penicillin)
- Ingested substances (foods, medications)

Heart Attack, Chest Pain, and Cardiac Arrest

heart attack Interruption or damage to the blood supply to the heart muscle; myocardial infarction

The heart muscle has its own blood supply. Interruption or damage to this blood supply is a **heart attack**, or myocardial infarction, which may cause damage to the heart muscle. Since it is difficult to determine if chest pain is really a heart attack, all chest pain is treated as if it could be a heart attack.

Signs and symptoms of a heart attack include

- Chest pain or discomfort, with lightheadedness
- Shortness of breath
- Lowered blood pressure
- Shallow and difficult respirations
- Profuse perspiration or sweating
- Wet, clammy, cold skin
- Rapid, weak, irregular pulse or lack of a pulse
- Pale color
- Nausea and vomiting
- Loss of consciousness or fainting

If there is chest pain, it is severe and crushing and may radiate to the inner left arm, the jaw, or the neck; the person in crisis may refer to the chest pain as a belt around his chest or heaviness in his chest. Sharp, stabbing, or short twinges of chest pain are usually not signs of a heart attack.

cardiac arrest The unexpected stopping of the heartbeat and circulation

Cardiac arrest is the unexpected stopping of the heartbeat and circulation (loss of heart function). This situation calls for immediate emergency care.

Signs and symptoms of cardiac arrest include

- Loss of consciousness
- Absence of pulse
- Absence of heart sounds
- Absence of breath sounds
- Enlargement of the pupils of the eye
- Ashen gray color of the skin
- Lips and nailbeds may turn blue

ASSISTING THE PERSON HAVING CHEST PAIN, A HEART ATTACK OR MYOCARDIAL INFARCTION	GUIDELINES	OBRA

- Call for medical help or activate the EMS system.
- Help the person in crisis into a comfortable position that allows the easiest breathing.

- Loosen clothing if it is tight.
- Encourage the person in crisis to remain quiet.
- Measure respiration and pulse at frequent intervals.
- Talk to the person in crisis; offer reassurance to him.
- Do not offer any food or drink.

- Stay with the person in crisis until emergency medical rescue help arrives.

Cardiopulmonary Resuscitation (CPR)

Cardiopulmonary resuscitation (CPR) is a basic lifesaving procedure for sudden cardiac or respiratory arrest. The technique of CPR provides basic emergency life support until emergency medical help arrives. CPR keeps oxygenated blood flowing to the brain and other vital body organs until medical treatment can be given to restore normal heart function.

cardiopulmonary resuscitation (CPR) An emergency procedure used to reestablish effective circulation and respiration in order to prevent irreversible brain damage

KEY IDEA

Only a person who has been trained in CPR can safely perform the rescue techniques. The only way of learning CPR is to enroll in an approved, supervised program.

Note: The following material is not intended to be a CPR course. An authorized CPR course includes practice on mannequins supervised by a certified trained instructor to direct you in CPR with written and performance examinations. The American Heart Association and the American Red Cross, as well as other community service organizations, offer classes in CPR. Most health care institutions require all employees to be certified in CPR and to complete periodic recertification. Only a person who has been trained in CPR should perform the rescue techniques. Different techniques are required for adults versus pediatric patients and must be learned.

There are three basic rescue skills to CPR. These are referred to as the ABCs of CPR:

- A, airway
- B, breathing
- C, circulation

Airway

The first action to take is to check the person for unresponsiveness. Tap or gently shake the person and shout "Are you OK?" If there is no response, call for assistance now (call for another individual or 911) so you can proceed to start CPR.

The American Heart Association has identified four situations or exceptions in which you should "phone fast" (perform 1 minute of CPR on adults before calling 911) for help.

These include:

1. Submersion or near drowning
2. Poisoning or drug overdose
3. Trauma
4. Respiratory arrest

The most important factor in successful resuscitation is the immediate opening of the airway. There are many possible causes of an obstructed airway. The most common cause in an unconscious person is the tongue.

The recommended technique for opening the airway must be simple, safe, easily learned, and effective. Since the head-tilt/chin-lift method meets these criteria, it is considered the method of choice. (Appropriate training should be obtained in an approved course before applying in practice. You may also be taught the jaw-thrust technique.)

To accomplish the head-tilt maneuver, one hand is placed on the victim's forehead and firm backward pressure is applied with the palm to tilt the head back. To complete the head-tilt/chin-lift maneuver, the fingers of the other hand are placed under the bony part of the lower jaw near the chin to gently lift the chin up (Figure 13–3◆). This supports the jaw and helps to tilt the head back. Do not use this technique if there is a possibility of injuries to the head, neck, or spine because it is possible to do further injury to the patient.

■ Look to see if there is any chest movement.
■ Listen for any breath sounds.
■ Feel for the victim's breath on your cheek (Figure 13–4◆).
■ If the victim does not spontaneously begin breathing after you have opened the airway, then begin rescue breathing.

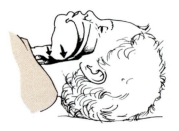

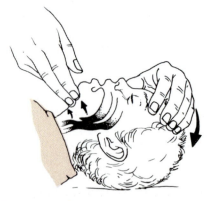

FIGURE 13–3 ◆

The head-tilt/chin-lift maneuver

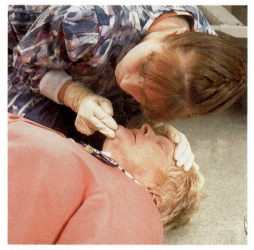

FIGURE 13–4 ◆

Open the airway and look, listen, and feel

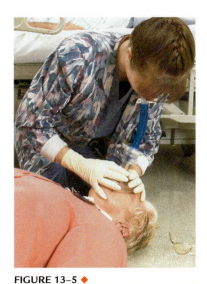

FIGURE 13–5 ◆

One-way valve face mask

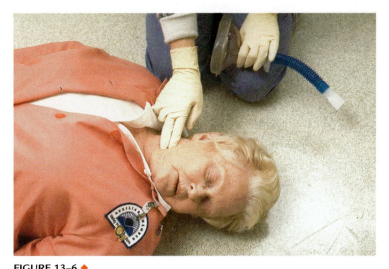

FIGURE 13–6 ◆

With the tips of your fingers find the groove next to the Adam's apple and feel for a carotid pulse

Breathing

Mouth-to-mouth rescue breathing is the most effective way of getting oxygen into the lungs of the victim. The American Heart Association teaches mouth-to-mouth, mouth-to-nose, mouth-to-stoma, Ambu bag-valve mask and mouth-to-barrier device breathing. The Ambu bag-valve mask or mouth-to-barrier methods are preferred to reduce the risk of contact exposure.

The barrier device or mask should have a one-way valve so that exhaled air does not enter the rescuer's mouth (Figure 13–5◆). Barrier devices often have a short tube that is placed between the patient's teeth and allows the rescuer to breathe through it. If rescue breathing is deemed necessary, the barrier device is positioned over the victim's mouth and nose, ensuring an adequate seal. Mouth-to-barrier device breathing is then initiated using slow inspiratory breaths (1 ½ to 2 seconds), as described next.

Keeping the airway open by the head-tilt/chin-lift maneuver, you should gently pinch the nose closed with the thumb and index finger of the hand on the forehead. Open your mouth wide and place it tightly over the victim's mouth, creating a tight seal. Blow two slow breaths lasting 1 ½ to 2 seconds and then remove your mouth. Turn your head to the side with your ear close to the victim's mouth and listen for a return of air. If there is no return of air, or if you met resistance while trying to blow air into the patient, you must recheck the head and neck position. If the airway is obstructed, no air can flow to the lungs. (See the guidelines on performing the Heimlich maneuver under Choking.)

After you have given the victim two breaths, check to see if the heart is beating. To feel the carotid pulse, use your hand that has been lifting the chin. With the tips of your fingers, find the groove next to the Adam's apple and feel for a pulse for 5 to 10 seconds (Figure 13–6◆). Check the pulse after the first minute and then every few minutes thereafter. If the heart is beating, you must breathe for the victim at a rate of 12 breaths per minute (one breath every 5 seconds) for an adult while maintaining the open airway. If the heart is not beating (no pulse), you will then have to artificially pump the heart and circulate the victim's blood using external chest compressions.

For both one-rescuer and two-rescuer CPR, deliver 10 to 12 breaths per minute and pause after every 15th chest compression for two ventilations. When performing two-rescuer CPR, once the patient is intubated and the airway is secured, the rate changes to a 5:1 ratio. Pause after every 5th chest compression for one ventilation.

Note: To protect both the victim and yourself when performing CPR, a pocket face mask or other protective device must be used as a barrier. The barrier will protect the victim and yourself from transferring any communicable diseases either individual may be carrying.

There are many types of protective barrier devices; your instructor and the facility where you are working will determine which device you will use to reduce your risk of exposure to infectious disease. No device, however, can guarantee 100% protection from transmission of germs. Whenever available, use an Ambu bag or similar bag-valve mask to provide the highest level of protection and rescuer safety.

Circulation

External chest compression along with mouth-to-mouth resuscitation will allow oxygenated blood to circulate to the brain and other organs. To perform external chest compression, kneel next to the victim's chest. Place the heel of one hand on the lower one-third of the sternum, place your other hand on top; the fingers may be either interlaced or extended but should be kept off the chest wall (Figure 13–7◆). As you compress downward, your shoulders should be directly over the victim's midline and your arms kept straight (Figure 13–8◆). For an adult victim you will depress 1½ to 2 inches. When you release this pressure, do not remove your hands from the sternum. These compressions should be rhythmic so that compression and release are of equal duration. Deliver 15 compressions for every two breaths when you are providing rescue breathing. Deliver a rate of 100 compressions per minute.

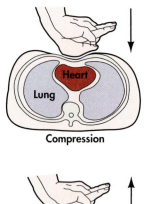

Compression

Release

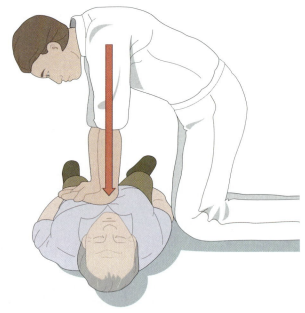

FIGURE 13–7 ◆

Compression and release should be of equal duration

FIGURE 13–8 ◆

Your shoulders should be directly over the victim's midline and your arms kept straight

ADULT CPR WITH ONE RESCUER

RATIONALE: CPR is a lifesaving measure performed only when cardiac arrest has occurred. The person must be unresponsive, not able to breathe, and have no pulse.

PREPARATION

1. First determine unresponsiveness by tapping or gently shaking the person. Shout "Are you OK?" If there is no response, the person is considered unconscious.

2. Have an available bystander activate the EMS system by calling 911. If alone, you do it now or after completing 1 minute of rescue support (see section titled *Airway*).

STEPS

3. Position the person on his back. Logroll the person and avoid twisting the spine. Place the person on a flat hard surface with his arms alongside his body.

4. Open the airway using the head-tilt/chin-lift or jaw-thrust maneuver.

5. Check for breathing. **Look** to see if the person's chest is raising and falling. Lean close to the person's mouth and **listen** for the escape of air during expiration. Position your cheek near the person to **feel** any air coming from the person's nose or mouth.

6. If the person is not breathing, place your bag-valve mask device, pocket face breathing mask, or barrier device on the patient's mouth.

7. Give two effective rescue breaths lasting 1½ to 2 seconds each. Watch for the chest to rise as you ventilate. Allow the chest to deflate between breaths.

8. Check for carotid pulse. Check for the carotid pulse on the side of the patient's neck. Use your other hand to keep the person's airway open using the head-tilt maneuver. Check the brachial pulse and observe for any signs of movement, breathing, or coughing in response to the two breaths. If signs of circulation are present, but breathing is absent or inadequate, provide rescue breathing (one breath every 5 seconds)

9. Begin chest compressions if the person has **no circulation (pulse).** At the rate of 100 compressions per minute, begin cycles of 15 compressions followed by two breaths.

   a. Count out loud—"1 and 2 and 3 and 4,"—continuing up to 15.

   b. Open the airway and give two breaths.

   c. Repeat the cycle of compressions until you have finished a total of four whole cycles of 15 compressions each followed by two breaths.

10. Check 3 to 5 seconds for the carotid pulse. Activate the EMS system if this has not been done.

11. If no pulse, continue CPR using cycles of 15 compressions followed by two breaths. Check for breaths every 2 to 3 minutes.

12. Continue CPR until help arrives to relieve you, the patient resumes breathing and has a heart rate, or you become too exhausted to continue.

FOLLOW-UP

13. Wash hands.

14. Document and report the results to your supervisor or the EMS responder.

CHARTING EXAMPLE: 12/1/04 9am Mr. Jones was walking to the bathroom when he slumped to the floor. He had no signs of responsiveness, pulse, or respirations. I called 911. CPR initiated at 9:03am and continued until EMS arrived at 9:15am. Mr. Jones was placed on oxygen and his heart rate resumed while the EMS team treated him. He was transported to Mercy Hospital Emergency Room at 9:40am. I called his daughter, Ms. Marietta Jones, and she is also on her way to the hospital. J. Flores, CNA

Choking

Choking occurs when the airway is closed or blocked. If the airway is blocked, the person cannot breathe or speak. As discussed, the lack of oxygen can result in cardiac arrest and death. Choking is always a serious situation. The "universal sign for choking" is the clutching of the throat (Figure 13–9◆).

When a person is choking on a foreign object, for example a piece of poorly chewed food, it is important to assess whether the person requires help. Ask "Are you choking?" If

FIGURE 13–9 ◆
The universal sign of choking

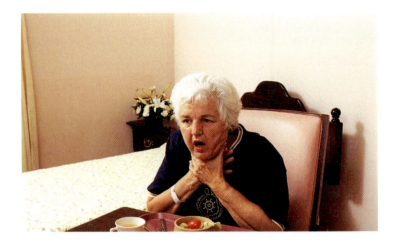

the person is able to breathe, speak, or cough effectively, don't interfere. Otherwise, offer assistance immediately. The Heimlich maneuver is used to dislodge an object and open the airway of a conscious or an unconscious victim. Like so many first aid procedures, the Heimlich maneuver can cause injuries if not performed properly. Use it when you are absolutely certain it is necessary to save life. Use Standard Precautions when performing the Heimlich maneuver.

PERFORMING THE HEIMLICH MANEUVER

GUIDELINES

For a conscious person:

- Determine if there is partial or complete airway obstruction. Ask "Are you choking?" If the person is able to breathe, speak, or cough effectively, don't interfere. Offer assistance if the person cannot speak or make a sound.

- Stand behind the person and put your arms around the waist allowing the person's arms to hang free.

- Make a fist with one hand and place the thumb side of your hand on the abdomen between the umbilicus (belly button) and the sternum (Figure 13–10a◆).

- Grasp this hand with your other hand and press it into the abdomen with a quick upward movement (Figure 13–10b◆).

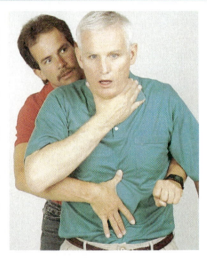

FIGURE 13–10a◆

Place the thumb side of your fist against the victim's abdomen just below the ribs and above the umbilicus or navel.

- Be sure each thrust is a separate movement. Check the patient after five thrusts.

- Repeat and continue these steps until the object is successfully dislodged.

For an unconscious adult:

- Determine unresponsiveness by gently shaking the person and asking "Are you OK?"

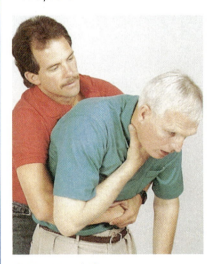

FIGURE 13–10b ◆

Use a quick upward thrust.

GUIDELINES *(continued)*

- If there is no response, call for help or send someone to activate EMS (dial 911).
- Position head and neck to open the airway using the head-tilt/chin-lift method. Tilt the head back with one hand while you lift the chin with the other.
- Place your cheek near the victim's face as you spend a few seconds listening and seeing if you feel any air movement against your cheek.
- Attempt to ventilate the victim with two quick breaths. If unsuccessful, reposition the head and try to give the breaths again.

- Straddle the victim's legs while on your knees.
- Position one hand on top of the other and give three to five firm upward thrusts in the upper abdomen above the umbilicus but below the sternum (Figure 13–11◆).
- Move to the patient's head and sweep the mouth with your finger to try to remove the object.
- Repeat and continue until the object is dislodged.
- Once the object is removed, ventilate or do CPR if necessary.

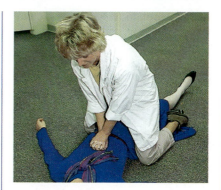

FIGURE 13–11 ◆
Straddle the unconscious victim to administer the Heimlich maneuver.

Stroke or Cerebrovascular Accident

Stroke or cerebrovascular accident occurs when there is damage to a blood vessel in the brain. See Chapter 26 for details. If you suspect that someone is having a stroke, treat him until emergency medical help arrives.

Signs and symptoms of a stroke include

- Seizures
- Difficulty breathing
- Headache
- Change in state of consciousness
- Difficulty with speech or vision
- Paralysis on one side, most evident in an extremity
- Unequal pupils
- Puffing of the cheeks on exhalation
- Drooling (unable to control oral secretions)

stroke Interruption or damage to the blood supply to the brain; a cerebrovascular accident

ASSISTING A PERSON WHO IS SUSPECTED OF HAVING A STROKE

GUIDELINES

- Call for medical help.
- Maintain an open airway to ensure breathing.

- Keep the person in crisis warm.
- Do not offer any food or drink.
- Protect paralyzed extremities.
- Stay with the person in crisis until emergency medical rescue help arrives.

- Provide CPR if needed (to be performed by a qualified individual).

■ Seizures

seizure An episode either partial or generalized, which may include altered consciousness, motor activity, or sensory phenomena and convulsions

A **seizure** is an episode, either partial or generalized, caused by abnormal brain activity, which may include alteration of consciousness, motor activity, or sensory phenomena and convulsions. The length and severity of the seizure vary. In more severe seizures, the patient may have fallen to the floor, will be unconscious and unable to respond. See Chapter 26 for care of the simple partial seizure, complex partial seizure, and generalized tonic-clonic seizure patient.

KEY IDEA

Protecting an individual from injury and maintaining a patient's airway are primary considerations when caring for a patient experiencing a seizure.

AGE-SPECIFIC CONSIDERATIONS

Seizures may occur at any age. All patients will be concerned that a seizure will occur at school, at work, or in public and will cause them embarrassment. They need reassurance and education about compliance to a medication schedule. When a seizure activity is related to trauma or a bad prognosis related to a brain tumor, adults of all ages will need time to adjust to their medical condition. Parents of children will need reassurance of the cause of the seizure and want to know the likelihood of its reoccurrence. They may be very frightened and anxious if an unexpected seizure occurs in the children's presence.

ASSISTING A PERSON WHO IS HAVING A SEIZURE

GUIDELINES

- Call for medical help.
- Turn the head of the person having a seizure to the side to promote the drainage of saliva or vomitus. (May be difficult to maintain if complex partial. DO NOT force the mouth open!)
- Loosen clothing around the neck.
- Do not try to pry (force) the teeth apart or place anything in the mouth.
- Maintain a patent airway (open).
- Protect the person from injury.
- Pad any areas that may be dangerous to the patient (for example, the corners of furniture) and move any object that might cause injury.
- Do not attempt to restrain the patient.
- Report observations to the immediate supervisor.

Hemorrhage

During a **hemorrhage**, an extreme and unexpected loss of blood occurs, which has several effects on the body:

■ The loss of red blood cells, which carry oxygen to the body cells, causes a lack of oxygen.

■ The loss of blood volume results in lower blood pressure.

■ The force of the heartbeat is reduced since there is less blood to pump.

If the bleeding or hemorrhage is not stopped, the body goes into shock. Death may occur in a matter of several minutes if the hemorrhage is due to arterial bleeding. Pressure to the site must be primary and constant to stop arterial bleeding. The control of bleeding is secondary only to the maintenance of an airway and the restoration of breathing in first aid. Arterial blood, which is pumped away from the heart through arteries, can be bright red in color. The bright red color is due to the high oxygen concentration. The blood returning to the heart through the veins is a darker color because the oxygen has been exchanged for carbon dioxide and other waste materials.

Bleeding may be classified according to its source:

■ Arterial bleeding from an artery usually occurs in spurts.

■ Venous bleeding from a vein appears as a steady flow of blood.

■ Bleeding from capillaries is characterized by the slow oozing of blood and is more easily controlled.

The most effective method of controlling external bleeding is direct pressure on the wound and elevation of the area, if possible. Direct pressure should be applied with the palm of the hand (Figure 13–12◆). (*Note:* Follow Standard Precautions—wear gloves and maintain body substance isolation to avoid contact with body fluids.) When the bleeding is in spurts, the application of pressure at a pressure point may control the bleeding and is applied simultaneously with direct pressure and elevation of the bleeding body part.

A pressure point is a site where a main artery lies near the surface of the body, directly over a bone. The use of pressure points requires skill on the part of the rescuer and should be used only after direct pressure and elevation have failed. If pressure on the pressure

hemorrhage The extreme or unexpected loss of blood; heavy bleeding

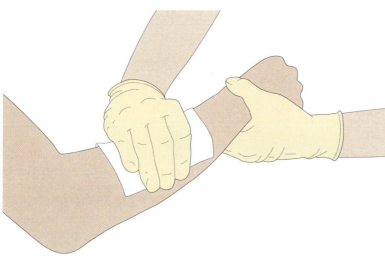

FIGURE 13–12 ◆

Direct pressure should be applied with the palm of the hand

points does not effectively control the bleeding, then a tourniquet must be applied. The application of a tourniquet is very dangerous unless adequate measures are available to control shock. The loosening of the tourniquet may prove fatal. The prolonged use can cause the loss of a limb. A tourniquet should be used only as a last resort to control life-threatening bleeding or hemorrhaging that cannot be controlled by any other means. Follow the instructions of your immediate supervisor.

When the classic signs of shock are present but there is no obvious injury, suspect internal bleeding. Internal bleeding can occur within the body's tissues (swelling or bruising), from an organ (chest, liver), or into a body cavity or organ (abdomen, pelvis). The signs and symptoms of internal bleeding are:

- Rapid and weak pulse
- Shallow and rapid respirations
- Weak and helpless feeling
- Dilated pupils
- Vomiting blood that has the appearance of coffee grounds (stomach)
- Pale, moist, and cold skin
- Thirst
- Shaking and trembling
- Coughing up bright red blood (lungs)
- Blood in the urine (bladder, kidneys) or stool (GI system)

ASSISTING THE PERSON WHO IS HEMORRHAGING	GUIDELINES	
■ Apply direct pressure over the bleeding area. (*Note:* Use Standard Precautions and appropriate dressings.)	■ Elevate the bleeding limb. ■ Call for medical help. ■ Apply a dressing and secure it with a bandage or adhesive tape. Observe for bleeding.	■ Remain with the person in crisis until emergency medical rescue help arrives. ■ Keep the person warm (cover with a blanket).

Burns

Tissue damage caused by excessive heat, regardless of the source, is a burn. Steam, electricity, sun, chemicals, or fire can all cause excessive heat and a burn. Burns are classified as superficial, partial, or full thickness. A superficial burn is a minor or the least severe burn, and full thickness is the worst burn. All first aid and treatment for burns are intended to prevent complications and further injury to the body part(s) and to speed up the healing process. Complications of a burn may include infection, shock, pain, loss of body heat and fluid, swelling of breathing passages, and death.

ASSISTING THE PERSON WHO HAS BEEN BURNED

GUIDELINES

For a minor, superficial burn:

- Flush the area with cold water for 1 minute.
- Cover the area with a clean or sterile moist pad.

For a partial or full thickness burn:

- Call for medical help.
- Stop the burning process—smother or douse the fire. Remove heat source.
- Do not remove clothing stuck to the burned area.
- Keep the airway open to ensure breathing.

- Cover the area with a clean or sterile dressing.
- Stay with the person in crisis until medical help arrives.
- Observe and provide care for signs of shock.

Poisoning

Poison is any substance that is toxic to the body. Immediate action and good observation skills are necessary if poisoning or an overdose of medication is suspected. Poisons can enter the body by several means (Figure 13–13◆). Table 13–1◆ lists common poisons and the reactions they might cause.

poison Any substance ingested, inhaled, injected, or absorbed into the body that will interfere with normal physiological functions

INHALATION

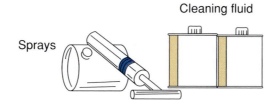

Sprays

Cleaning fluid

INJECTION

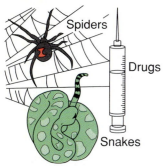

Spiders

Drugs

Snakes

INGESTION

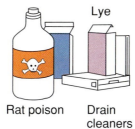

Lye

Rat poison

Drain cleaners

ABSORPTION

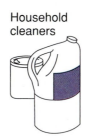

Household cleaners

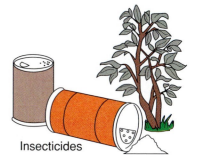

Insecticides

FIGURE 13–13 ◆

Poisons can enter the body by several means

TABLE 13–1

Common Poisons

POISON	SYMPTOMS AND SIGNS
Acetaminophen	Nausea, vomiting, heavy perspiration. The victim is usually a child.
Acids	Burns on or around the lips. Burning in mouth, throat, and stomach, often followed by heavy vomiting.
Alkalis (ammonia, bleaches, detergents, lye, washing soda, certain fertilizers)	Check to see if mouth membranes appear white and swollen. There may be a "soapy" appearance in the mouth. Abdominal pain is usually present. Vomiting may occur, often full of blood and mucus.
Arsenic (rat poisons)	"Garlic breath," with burning in the mouth, throat, and stomach. Abdominal pain can be severe. Vomiting is common.
Aspirin	Delayed reactions, including ringing in the ears, rapid and deep breathing, dry skin, and restlessness.
Corrosive agents (disinfectants, drain cleaners, household acids, iodine, pine oil, turpentine, toilet bowl cleaners, styptic pencil, water softeners, strong acids)	(See Acids)
Food poisoning	Difficult to detect since symptoms and signs vary greatly. Usually you will note abdominal pain, nausea and vomiting, gas, loud, frequent bowel sounds, and diarrhea.
Iodine	Upset stomach and vomiting. If a starchy meal has been eaten, the vomitus may appear blue.
Metals (copper, lead, mercury, zinc)	Metallic taste in mouth, with nausea and abdominal pains. Vomiting may occur. Stools may be bloody or dark.
Petroleum products (some deodorizers, heating fuel, diesel fuels, gasoline, kerosene, lighter fluid, lubricating oil, naphtha, rust remover, transmission fluid)	Note characteristic odors on patient's breath, on clothing, or in vomitus.
Plants—contact (poison ivy, poison oak, poison sumac)	Swollen, itchy areas on the skin, with quickly forming "blister-like" lesions.
Plants—ingested (azalea, castor bean, elderberry, foxglove, holly berries, lily of the valley, mistletoe berries, mountain laurel, mushrooms and toadstools, nightshade, oleander, rhododendron, rhubarb, rubber plant, some wild cherries)	Difficult to detect, ranging from nausea to coma. Always question in cases of apparent child poisoning.
Strychnine (rat poisons)	The face, jaw, and neck will stiffen. Strong convulsions occur quickly after ingesting.

Babies, toddlers, and small children will likely put things in their mouths. Parents need to install childproof locks on cabinets containing medications, toxic cleaning products, or other poisonous substances. Teens may experiment with toxic substances such as sniffing glue, or getting high or binge drinking, which can result in alcohol poisoning or death. Parents need to caution teens and young adults to be alert at parties or on dates to avoid leaving their drinks unattended or consuming punches because there has been an increase in use of "date-rape" drugs, which can be lethal in large doses. Adults may ignore warning labels and use cleaning or toxic chemicals in inadequately ventilated places. Elderly persons with poor eyesight may accidentally injest a toxic substance or, in confusion, overdose on prescribed medications.

ASSISTING THE PERSON WHO HAS BEEN POISONED

GUIDELINES

- Observe the person in crisis.
- Check the mouth for signs of burns.
- Check the breath for a significant odor.
- Ask questions of the person in crisis and other persons present to gather as many facts as possible before you act. Look for a medication container or bottle that may have been holding the poison.
- Call the regional poison control center immediately. The number is always found on the inside cover or on the first page of the telephone book.
- Call for medical help.
- Follow the directions given to you from the poison control center. If you have been instructed to induce vomiting, save any vomitus from the person in crisis.
- If the person in crisis is unconscious:
  - Do not give anything by mouth.
  - Position the person on his or her back with the head facing you.
  - Maintain a clear airway.
- If the person stops breathing, perform artificial respiration, using a pocket face mask or other barrier device to protect yourself. *Note:* This should be done only on the directions from the poison control center. There are times when you should not perform mouth to mouth resuscitation due to the type of poison ingested.
- If it is necessary to move the person in crisis to a safe area, do so, but remember not to injure yourself while you are doing this.
- Keep the person in crisis warm and comfortable.
- Do not leave until emergency medical rescue help arrives.

SUMMARY

This chapter has provided an overview of common emergencies and guidelines to follow for situations requiring immediate action. These situations include shock, heart attack (myocardial infarction), chest pain, cardiopulmonary resuscitation, stroke, seizures, hemorrhage, burns, and poisoning. The Chapter Review will help you evaluate what you have learned from the contents of this chapter.

CHAPTER REVIEW

FILL IN THE BLANK Read each sentence and fill in the blank line with a word that completes the sentence.

1. An _____ is a situation or event that requires immediate action.

2. Failure of the cardiovascular system to provide sufficient blood circulation to every part of the body results in _____.

3. _____ _____ is the unexpected stopping of the heartbeat and circulation.

4. The "A" in ABC stands for _____.

5. Apply _____ pressure with the palm of the hand over an area that is bleeding.

MULTIPLE CHOICE Choose the best answer for each question or statement.

1. All of the following may be signs of shock *except*
   a. eyes appear dull and lackluster.
   b. pupils may be dilated.
   c. the patient is not breathing.
   d. face appears pale and cyanotic.

2. Signs of a cardiac arrest may include all of the following *except*
   a. loss of consciousness.
   b. absence of pulse.
   c. bleeding.
   d. absence of breathing.

3. When initiating CPR, you first determine unresponsiveness and then
   a. call for assistance.
   b. open the airway.
   c. check for breathing.
   d. check for pulse.

4. If a choking person can still speak a little
   a. go ahead and perform the Heimlich maneuver.
   b. wait before performing CPR.
   c. wait before performing the Heimlich maneuver.
   d. leave and come back and check on the person in 10 minutes.

5. If your patient is having a seizure, you should
   a. try to force a tongue blade between his teeth.
   b. ask "Can you speak?"
   c. not attempt to restrain the patient's movements.
   d. leave the patient and go get help.

TIME-OUT

TIPS FOR TIME MANAGEMENT

Do the most important tasks first, not necessarily the tasks you enjoy the most. Leaving a patient who wants to chat may be difficult, but if another patient or staff member is waiting for your help, you must prioritize. End your conversation with a chatty patient with a smiling promise to return when you have some time to talk.

THE NURSING ASSISTANT IN ACTION

You have wheeled Mrs. Raja, a postsurgical patient who has just been discharged, to the lobby exit. As you are helping her into the car, you notice some bright red blood on the front of her dress. You suspect there may be a serious problem as the stain is getting larger. Her husband tells you, "She is fine, she wants to leave. Don't worry, I'll drive her home and we will call her doctor if necessary."

What Is Your Response/Action?

CRITICAL THINKING

CUSTOMER SERVICE In emergency situations patients may have belongings or valuables that are left behind in their room if they are transferred to receive lifesaving care. Make a list of the items and secure them in a safe, preferably locked place. Offer to have someone contact a family member or friend if the patient tells you no one is aware he has come for treatment.

CULTURAL CARE Be aware some patients may have religious prohibitions regarding blood transfusions or prefer not to be subjected to extreme lifesaving measures. It is important to know which patients have Do Not Resuscitate (DNR) orders and to not start CPR on them if they stop breathing or go into cardiac arrest. Respect their documented personal choices and decisions.

COOPERATION WITHIN THE TEAM When a patient experiences an unexpected event or emergency, the caregiver assigned to that patient will need to give the patient his full attention. If your assistance is not directly needed, check other patients assigned to that caregiver. Reassure the patients that you will meet their immediate needs during the time you are relieving your colleague.

EXPLORE MediaLink

Additional interactive resources for this chapter can be found on the Companion Website at www.prenhall.com/wolgin. Click on Chapter 13 and "Begin" to select activities for this chapter.

For chapter-related NCLEX-style questions and an audio glossary, access the accompanying CD-ROM in this book.

14 The Human Body

KEY TERMS

anatomy
anterior
blood and lymph tissue
cardiac muscle tissue
cell
connective tissue
deep
dorsal
epithelial tissue
inferior
muscle tissue
nerve tissue
organ
physiology
posterior
superficial
superior
system
tissue
ventral

OBJECTIVES

When you have completed this chapter, you will be able to:

- List the things all living cells have in common.
- Relate the parts of a cell to their functions.
- Explain the process of cellular division.
- List the basic groupings of cells that build a human body.
- Name the primary kinds of tissues, their functions, and examples of their location in the human body.
- Identify the organs and basic functions of each body system.
- Describe the body in anatomical position.

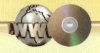

MediaLink
www.prenhall.com/wolgin

Use the address above to access the free, interactive Companion Website created for this textbook. Get hints, instant feedback, and textbook references to chapter-related NCLEX-style questions. Link to other interesting sites.

AUDIO GLOSSARY:
Use the Companion Website, or the CD-ROM disk enclosed with your textbook, to hear the pronunciation of key terms in the chapter.

This chapter presents a basic review of the structures and functions of the human body. An explanation of the reproduction and structure of cells and the grouping and organization of cells, tissues, and organs is given. Understanding of the functions and relationships among the many organs and systems in the human body is essential for the nursing assistant. One such system is the respiratory system—nose, pharynx, larynx, trachea, bronchi, and lungs. The respiratory system gives the body air to supply oxygen to the cells through the blood and eliminates carbon dioxide. A table lists all the body systems, the functions of each system, and the organs that comprise each system. Anatomical position is discussed in relationship to care of the patient.

INTRODUCTION

Anatomy and Physiology

Anatomy is the study of the body structure and the relation of its parts. **Physiology** is the science that deals with the physical and chemical processes of cells, tissues, and organs of living organisms. The study of anatomy and physiology is the basis for understanding the clinical procedures that you will perform as a nursing assistant.

anatomy The study of the structure of an organism

physiology The study of the functions of the body dealing with the physical and chemical processes of cells, tissues, and organs of living organisms

Cells, Tissues, and Organs

This section provides descriptions of the structure and relationship of cells, tissues, and organs in the human body. *Cells* describes the structure of the cell and the process of cell division. *Tissues* identifies the various type and function of tissues found in the body. *Organs* explains the relationship of various tissues to specific organs and organs to specific body systems.

Cells

The **cell** is the fundamental building block of all living matter. Cells are microscopic in size. They are the living parts of organisms. The human body is made up of millions of cells. There are many kinds of cells and each has a special task within the body. Living cells have many things in common:

cell The basic unit of living matter

- They come from preexisting cells.
- They use food for energy.
- They use oxygen to break down food.
- They use water to transport various substasnces.
- They grow and repair themselves.
- Most reproduce themselves. (Only mature neural cells do not reproduce themselves.)

Structure of the Cell

Cells consist of three main parts: the nucleus, the cytoplasm, and the cell membrane (Figure 14–1◆).

The nucleus is important to the process of heredity, growth, and cell reproduction. It contains chromosomes that control cell activity. Chromosomes are threadlike structures that contain deoxyribonucleic acid (DNA) and control heredity factors. They control physical and chemical traits a person inherits, for example eye color, skin color, and height.

FIGURE 14-1 ◆

The cell

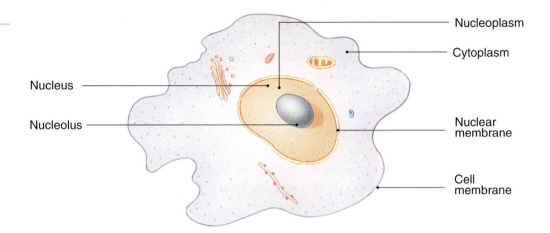

The cytoplasm is the substance surrounding the nucleus and is where the activities of the cell take place. Messenger RNA molecules pass from the nucleus into the cytoplasm and direct the formation of the protein molecules necessary to maintain life. Through messenger RNA, the nucleus controls the kinds of chemical reactions carried out by the cell. The cell membrane keeps the cytoplasm within cell bounds and allows certain substances to pass in and out of the cell.

Cell Division

Cells reproduce by division. In any cell preparing for division, the nucleus initially duplicates its chromosomes exactly. As the cell continues to divide, the duplicate chromosomes, or chromosome pairs, divide and move to opposite sides of the nucleus. Then the rest of the cell contents divide and go with one or the other pair of chromosomes. After a new cell membrane forms between the two sides, division is complete. The new cells are identical.

KEY IDEA

Current research to discover the causes of many diseases involves studying the cell and its immediate environment. With today's explosion of scientific knowledge about the cell, it is hoped that scientists will more readily find ways to cure or prevent many diseases.

tissue A group of cells of the same type

epithelial tissue Tissue that lines, protects, secretes, absorbs, and receives sensations

connective tissue Tissue that connects, supports, covers, lines, pads, or protects other body structures

Tissues

Individual cells usually do not work alone. Groups of cells of the same type that work together to perform a particular function are called **tissues** (Figure 14–2◆). Some of the primary kinds of tissues (Table 14–1◆) in the human body are:

- **Epithelial tissue:** The function of this tissue is to protect, secrete, absorb, and receive sensations. Examples are skin, linings of the intestines, and linings of the glands and organs.

- **Connective tissue:** The function of this tissue is to connect, support, cover or line, and pad or protect. Examples are bone, blood, ligaments, and tendons.

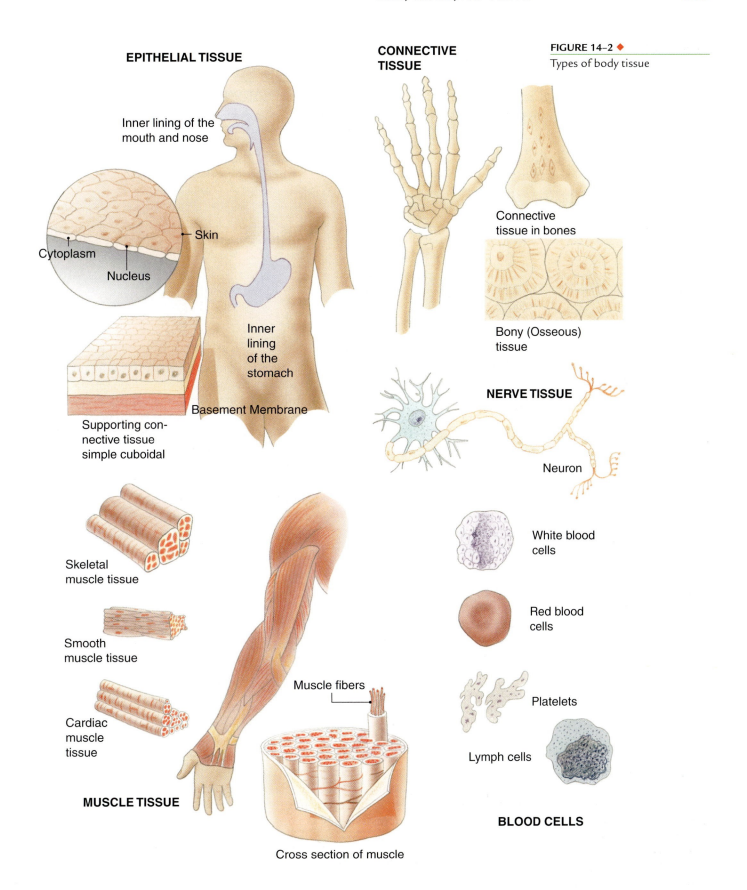

FIGURE 14–2 ◆

Types of body tissue

EPITHELIAL TISSUE

Inner lining of the mouth and nose

Skin

Cytoplasm

Nucleus

Inner lining of the stomach

Basement Membrane

Supporting connective tissue simple cuboidal

CONNECTIVE TISSUE

Connective tissue in bones

Bony (Osseous) tissue

NERVE TISSUE

Neuron

Skeletal muscle tissue

Smooth muscle tissue

Cardiac muscle tissue

Muscle fibers

MUSCLE TISSUE

Cross section of muscle

White blood cells

Red blood cells

Platelets

Lymph cells

BLOOD CELLS

TABLE 14–1

Primary Kinds of Tissue

TYPE OF TISSUE	FUNCTION	LOCATION IN THE BODY
Epithelial tissue	Protect, secrete, absorb, receive sensations	Lining of mouth and nose, skin, lining of stomach
Connective tissue	Connect, support, cover	Tendons, bones, layer of fatty tissue under skin
Muscle tissues (a) striated (b) smooth (c) cardiac	Movement—stretch, contract	Muscle groups in arms, legs, abdomen, back and internal organs
Nerve tissue	Transmit impulses to and from the central nervous system and to and from the body systems	Throughout the body
Blood and lymph tissue	Circulate nutrients, oxygen, and antibodies throughout the body; remove waste products	Circulatory system

muscle tissue Tissue that ensures movement; it is capable of stretching and contracting

cardiac muscle tissue Involuntary muscle tissue found only in the heart

nerve tissue Tissue that carries nervous impulses between the brain, the spinal cord, and all parts of the body

blood and lymph tissue Tissue composed of singular cells that move within a fluid to every part of the body, circulating nutrients, oxygen, and antibodies and removing waste products

organ A part of the body made of several types of tissue grouped together to perform a certain function; examples are the heart, stomach, and lungs

- **Muscle tissue:** The function of this tissue is movement. Striated tissue is found in voluntary muscles, those you can move consciously. Smooth tissue is found in the involuntary muscles, such as those that push food and water through the gastrointestinal tract or those that allow actions such as dilation (making opening larger) or contraction (making opening smaller) of the pupil of your eye and blood vessels. **Cardiac muscle tissue** is specific smooth muscle tissue found only in the involuntary muscles of the heart.

- **Nerve tissue:** The function of this tissue is to carry nervous impulses from a portion of the brain or spinal cord to all parts of the body and vice versa. The body cannot renew nerve tissue.

- **Blood and lymph tissue:** In this type of tissue the cells are singular and move within a fluid to every part of the body (technically these are in the family of connective tissue).

Organs

Tissues are grouped together to form **organs**, such as the heart, lungs, and liver. Each organ has a specific function. Figure 14–3◆ shows the organs of the body and their approximate locations. The prefixes associated with the organs (cardio, pneumo, gastro, and so on) are combined with roots and suffixes to form the medical terminology discussed in the Appendix.

The body has two major cavities, the dorsal cavity and the ventral cavity (Figure 14–4◆). The dorsal cavity is divided into the cranial and the spinal cavities. The ventral cavity is divided into the thoracic and abdominal cavities. Some organs are located in body cavities. For example, the brain is found in the cranial cavity in the head. The heart and lungs are found in the thoracic cavity. The stomach, spleen, liver, pancreas, kidneys, small and large intestines, urinary bladder, and, in the female, the ovaries and uterus are located in the abdominal cavity. The abdominal cavity is lined with a membrane called the peritoneum which protects organs from rubbing together when they move. This membrane also keeps organs in place within the abdominal cavity.

FIGURE 14–3 ◆

Organs of the body

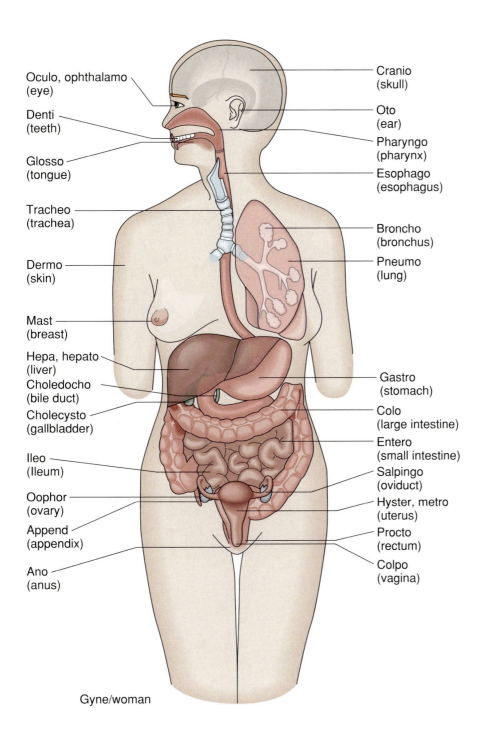

Oculo, ophthalamo (eye)

Denti (teeth)

Glosso (tongue)

Tracheo (trachea)

Dermo (skin)

Mast (breast)

Hepa, hepato (liver)

Choledocho (bile duct)

Cholecysto (gallbladder)

Ileo (Ileum)

Oophor (ovary)

Append (appendix)

Ano (anus)

Cranio (skull)

Oto (ear)

Pharyngo (pharynx)

Esophago (esophagus)

Broncho (bronchus)

Pneumo (lung)

Gastro (stomach)

Colo (large intestine)

Entero (small intestine)

Salpingo (oviduct)

Hyster, metro (uterus)

Procto (rectum)

Colpo (vagina)

Gyne/woman

FIGURE 14-3 *(continued)*
Organs of the body

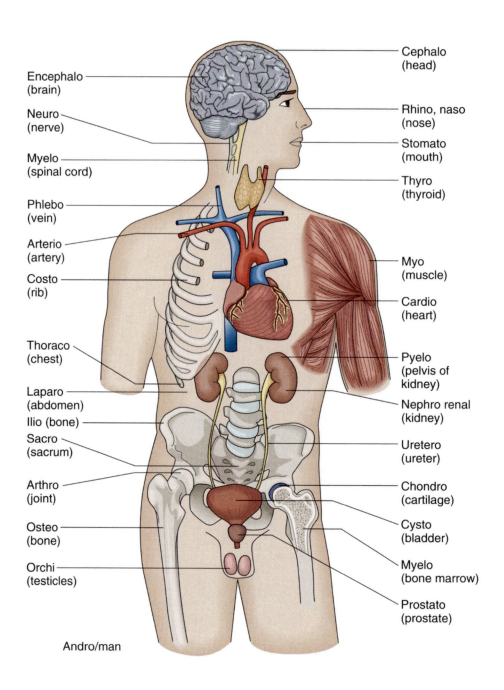

Encephalo
(brain)

Neuro
(nerve)

Myelo
(spinal cord)

Phlebo
(vein)

Arterio
(artery)

Costo
(rib)

Thoraco
(chest)

Laparo
(abdomen)

Ilio (bone)

Sacro
(sacrum)

Arthro
(joint)

Osteo
(bone)

Orchi
(testicles)

Cephalo
(head)

Rhino, naso
(nose)

Stomato
(mouth)

Thyro
(thyroid)

Myo
(muscle)

Cardio
(heart)

Pyelo
(pelvis of
kidney)

Nephro renal
(kidney)

Uretero
(ureter)

Chondro
(cartilage)

Cysto
(bladder)

Myelo
(bone marrow)

Prostato
(prostate)

Andro/man

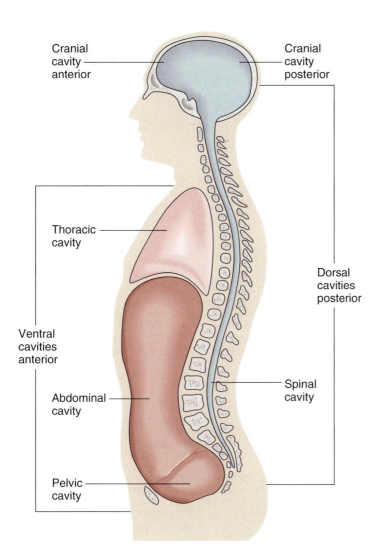

FIGURE 14–4 ◆
Body cavities

Cranial cavity anterior

Cranial cavity posterior

Thoracic cavity

Dorsal cavities posterior

Ventral cavities anterior

Abdominal cavity

Spinal cavity

Pelvic cavity

 # Body Systems

Cells, tissues, and organs make up the body systems that keep the human body healthy and functioning normally. Figure 14–5◆ shows an example of three types of tissue combining to form an artery. Arteries are organs found in the circulatory system. Organs that work together to perform similar tasks make up body **systems**. It is easier to study anatomy and physiology by body systems (Table 14–2◆). Always remember that systems cannot work by themselves but are dependent on each other.

system A group of organs acting together to carry out one or more body functions

Anatomical Position

As part of the study of each system, it is helpful to take an overall look at the body and to become familiar with the names given to body areas. In any demonstration or diagram, the body or body part shown is in the anatomical position (Figure 14–6◆). The person is standing up straight, facing you, palms out and feet together. When you look at a person in the anatomical position, remember that the left side is always on your right side. This is especially important in studying diagrams. The front of a person is referred to as the **anterior**

anterior Located in the front; opposite of posterior

FIGURE 14–5 ◆

Three types of tissue combine to form an artery

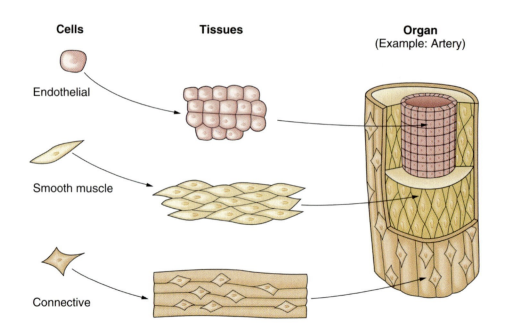

TABLE 14–2

Body Systems

SYSTEM	FUNCTION	ORGANS
Skeletal	Supports and protects the body	Bones; joints
Muscular	Gives movement to the body	Muscles; tendons; ligaments
Digestive (gastrointestinal)	Takes in and absorbs nutrients and eliminates wastes	Mouth; teeth; tongue; esophagus; salivary glands; stomach; duodenum; small and large intestines; liver; gallbladder; ascending, transverse, and descending colon; rectum; anus; appendix
Nervous	Controls activities of the body	Brain; spinal cord; nerves
Urinary (excretory)	Removes wastes from the blood, produces urine, and eliminates urine	Kidneys; ureters; bladder; urethra
Reproductive	To reproduce; allows a new human being to be born; for sexual fulfillment and expression of sexuality	**Male:** testes, scrotum, penis, prostate glands **Female:** ovaries, uterus, fallopian tubes, vagina
Respiratory	Gives the body air to supply oxygen to the cells through the blood and eliminates carbon dioxide	Nose; pharynx; larynx; trachea; bronchi; lungs
Circulatory	Carries food, oxygen, and water to the body cells and removes wastes	Heart; blood; arteries; veins; capillaries; spleen; lymph nodes; lymph vessels
Endocrine	Secretes hormones directly into the blood to regulate body functions	Thyroid and parathyroid glands; pineal gland; adrenal glands; testes; ovaries; breasts; thymus; pancreas; and pituitary gland
Integumentary	Provides first line of defense against infection, maintains body temperature, provides fluids, and eliminates waste	Skin; hair; nails; sweat and oil glands

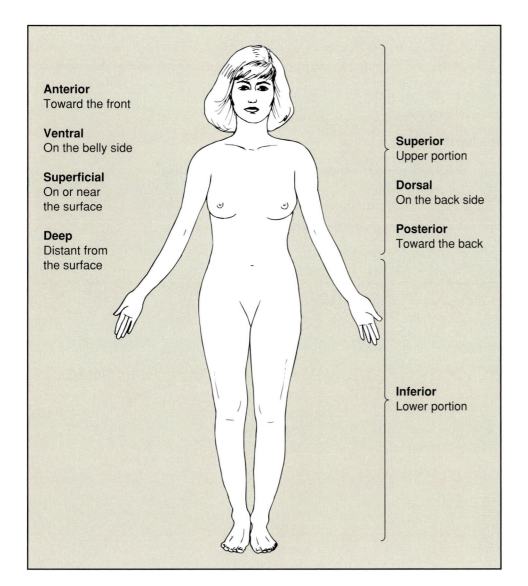

FIGURE 14–6 ◆
The body in anatomical position

superficial On or near the surface of the body

deep Distant from the surface of the body

---

or **ventral** side. The back, containing the spine (backbone), is called the **posterior** or **dorsal** side. The areas of the body closer to the head are called **superior**. Those closer to the feet are called **inferior**. These terms may also be used to describe the position of an organ in the body.

 ## SUMMARY

The study of anatomy and physiology forms the basis for understanding the clinical procedures performed by nursing assistants. The cell is the basic building block of the human body. Cells combine to form tissues, and tissues combine to form organs. Organs that perform similar tasks work together as systems. When a person becomes ill or is involved in an accident, body structures may be damaged and their functions disrupted. Remember when you look at a patient in anatomical position your right is the patient's left. The terms anterior or ventral, posterior or dorsal, superior, and inferior are used to describe areas of the body and the position of organs.

ventral On the abdominal, anterior, or front side of the body

posterior Located in the back or toward the rear

dorsal Refers to the back or to the back part of an organ

superior The upper portion of the body

inferior The lower portion of the body

CHAPTER REVIEW

FILL IN THE BLANK Read each sentence and fill in the blank line with a word that completes the sentence.

1. The study of the structure of an organism is called _____.

2. The basic unit of living matter is called the _____.

3. The function of _____ tissue is to protect, secrete, absorb, and receive sensations.

4. Tissues that are grouped together form _____.

5. A group of organs acting together to carry out one or more body functions is called a _____.

MULTIPLE CHOICE Choose the best answer for each question or statement.

1. Cells do all of the following *except*
   a. use food for energy.
   b. use carbon dioxide to break down food.
   c. grow and repair themselves.
   d. use water to transport various substances.

2. Which of the following carries impulses from a portion of the brain or spinal cord to all parts of the body?
   a. White blood cells
   b. Red blood cells
   c. Platelets
   d. Nerve tissue

3. Which of the following is not an organ?
   a. Stomach
   b. Liver
   c. Hand
   d. Brain

4. All the activities of the body are regulated by the
   a. endocrine system.
   b. digestive system.
   c. urinary system.
   d. circulatory system.

5. The front side of a person is called the
   a. posterior.
   b. anterior.
   c. dorsal.
   d. superior.

TIME-OUT

TIPS FOR TAKING CARE OF YOURSELF

Be aware that your body requires adequate rest to maintain proper functioning. You may be asked to work on your scheduled day off due to understaffing. You also may be called at home and asked to come to work on your day off. Strike a balance between helping out when you are needed and having some time away from the workplace to rest and relax.

THE NURSING ASSISTANT IN ACTION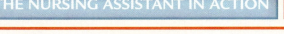

You are assigned to work with patients whose disease conditions are different from those you are most familiar with. How can you prepare to increase your knowledge of the most important body systems' functions and the conditions which are being treated in the unit?

What Is Your Response/Action?

CRITICAL THINKING

CUSTOMER SERVICE There are times when patients will tell you they did not understand what their nurse or doctor was talking about when they were answering questions. If you can provide the information to the patient in a way they can understand, you can do so. Often it is most helpful to tell the nurse or doctor that the patient still has concerns or questions and needs to review the information again with them. Remember that when patients are ill, stressed, and confused they may find it difficult to remember what was told to them. Patients may be uncomfortable saying they have no idea what was said to them, do not remember, or that they need more information.

CULTURAL CARE There are many individual and cultural differences in body size, proportions, and what are considered to be signs of beauty. Tattoos, body art or piercing, hairstyles, or clothing choices will vary and may be unlike those you prefer. Your patients may believe the way you look or dress is not acceptable within their cultures. Try to accept and appreciate the differences in others and do not convey to patients the feeling that you think there is something wrong with their body or culture because it is different.

COOPERATION WITHIN THE TEAM You will recognize times when a new coworker or fellow student has less information than they need to take care of the patients assigned to them. How you offer to help them or provide information makes a big difference. Do not comment to patients that your coworker has no idea what she is doing. Tell your coworker you would like to speak with her privately and use that opportunity to see how you can assist her to find resources she needs to increase her knowledge. Remember to thank people who help you learn new things.

EXPLORE MediaLink

Additional interactive resources for this chapter can be found on the Companion Website at www.prenhall.com/wolgin. Click on Chapter 14 and "Begin" to select activities for this chapter.

For chapter-related NCLEX-style questions and an audio glossary, access the accompanying CD-ROM in this book.

15 Growth and Development

KEY TERMS

chronological age
circumference
cognitive
development
fine motor
gross motor
growth

OBJECTIVES

When you have completed this chapter, you will be able to:

- Describe typical growth patterns in infants, toddlers, preschoolers, school-aged children, and adolescents.

- Identify the developmental skills used to describe the various stages of development of human beings over their life spans.

- Describe the developmental tasks characteristic of each stage of development.

- Describe age-based factors, or situations, you must keep in mind as you care for your patient: infant, toddler, preschooler, school-age child, adolescent, young adult, middle-aged adult, or older adult.

MediaLink

www.prenhall.com/wolgin

Use the address above to access the free, interactive Companion Website created for this textbook. Get hints, instant feedback, and textbook references to chapter-related NCLEX-style questions. Link to other interesting sites.

AUDIO GLOSSARY:

Use the Companion Website, or the CD-ROM disk enclosed with your textbook, to hear the pronunciation of key terms in the chapter.

This chapter reviews normal growth and development from infancy to death. Typical growth patterns and developmental stages based on chronological age are described, including the effects of injury and illness on the ability of individuals to perform at their age-appropriate level of development. Nursing assistant behaviors corresponding to, or based on, the patient's chronological age and typical task masteries or competencies that can be expected at that age are presented.

 INTRODUCTION

Growth and Development

The terms *growth* and *development* are often used together to indicate the sum of the changes—physical, intellectual, emotional, and social—that occur in a person over the course of the life span. Though related, growth and development are not the same. **Growth** refers to the quantitative physical changes human beings experience throughout their lives. These physical changes—growth—can be measured in pounds and inches (kilograms and centimeters). **Development** refers to the acquisition of and the increase in the ability to use motor, language, cognitive, and social skills that people acquire over their life span.

growth The physical changes that take place in a person's body over the life span

development The motor, language, cognitive, and social skills that are acquired over the course of the life span

KEY IDEA

Growth and development usually follow patterns and stages, although both may occur at different rates for different individuals. In each developmental stage, there are tasks that must be mastered before the person matures into the next stage. The boundaries between each stage overlap, but there are general characteristics that describe the typical person within that stage.

Growth

Growth begins at conception and extends through all stages of life. Growth from a single cell to a human being capable of life outside the womb occurs rapidly during the 40 weeks of a woman's pregnancy. Once the infant is delivered, the infant continues to grow rapidly for the first year of life.

Infants: Birth–1 Year

Usually, the infant gains about 1½ pounds (0.689 kg) per month for the first 6 months, thereby doubling the infant's birth weight. See Table 15–1◆ to determine how to convert pounds to kilograms. During the next 6 months, the growth rate begins to slow down so the weight gain is approximately 1 pound per month. By the time the infant is a year old, the infant birth weight will have tripled. Infants grow in length at a rate of about 1 inch per month for the first 6 months, then the growth rate slows to about 1/2 inch per month for the next 6 months. At 1 year, the birth length has usually increased by 50%. See Table 15–1 for converting inches to centimeters.

The measurement of the **circumference** of the head of an infant is very important. This measurement is necessary because the size of the skull reflects the growth and the size of the cranial contents. If the brain is not growing properly, the head circumference is usually small. At birth, the head circumference of normal full-term infants is usually 13½ inches (35 cm). The rate of growth of the head circumference during the first 6

circumference The distance around an object or body part, such as the head

TABLE 15–1

Conversion Equivalents

1 kilogram (kg) = 2.2 pounds (lb)
1 centimeter (cm) = 2/5 inch (0.3937 in.)

FIGURE 15–1 ◆

Measuring an infant's head

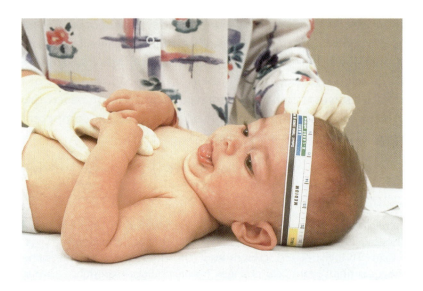

months is 1/2 inch per month, slowing to 1/4 inch per month for the rest of the first year. If the infant's weight, length, and head circumference are all within the same range (percentile), the infant is said to be growing normally (Figure 15–1◆).

Toddlers: 1–2 Years

Toddlers grow at a slower rate than they did as infants. The average weight gain is 4 to 6 pounds (1.8 to 2.7 kg) per year from 1 to 3 years. The rate of increase in height slows to 3 inches (7.5 cm) per year. Increase in height occurs mainly in elongation of the legs, rather than the trunk. Another trend is that the adult height is approximately twice the child's height at age 2. Head circumference is not usually measured after the first year unless a problem had already been identified in the infant's first year of life.

Preschoolers: 2–5 Years

Preschoolers continue to gain 4 to 6 pounds and 3 inches per year just as in the toddler period. However, since growth in the 2- to 5-year-old is focused mainly in the elongation of the trunk, rather than in the legs, the preschooler appears taller and thinner when compared to the toddler.

School-Age Children: 5–12 Years

School-age children gain 4 to 6 pounds and grow 2 inches per year. Girls and boys differ very little in size during this period, but just prior to their teenage years girls begin to surpass boys in height and weight. During late childhood or preadolescence, boys grow about 1 inch per year, while girls grow an average of 2 inches per year. Many girls will experience body changes with the onset of puberty between 10 and 12 years of age.

Adolescence: 12–18 Years

Adolescence is a period of rapid growth almost as dramatic as the growth seen during infancy. Adolescence begins and ends at different ages for each person and is typically assigned a wide range of chronological ages—usually 12 to 18 years of age. This growth period is characterized by physical and sex-specific changes in girls and boys. Rapid increases in height and weight generally occur 2 years earlier in girls than in boys. Boys

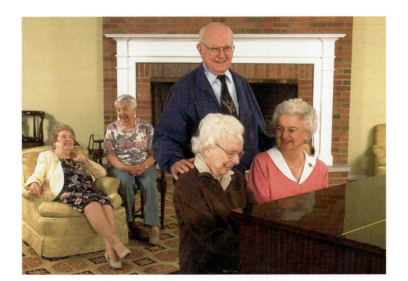

FIGURE 15–2 ◆

Socialization with others is important for older adults

grow an average of 2 to 8 inches per year and gain 15 to 65 pounds during adolescence. Girls grow 4 to 12 inches and gain 15 to 55 pounds during adolescence. The development of other physical changes such as secondary sex characteristics—breasts and pubic hair in girls and genitalia and pubic hair in boys—is significant during this period.

Young, Middle, Older Adult: 18–75+ Years

Changes during this period are significant in that the physical changes that occur are fewer and more subtle. By age 18, most of the biological growth is complete. Following adolescence the body enters a period when the body's growth and restorative powers focus on healing in response to illness and injury. Eventually, the effects of the aging process begin to take a toll on the various bodily systems. Knowledge of the human body and increased benefits and availability of modern science allow for a healthier aging population.

Old Age: 76–100+ Years

Physical changes are more pronounced with failing physical health and growing dependency on others. Most significant others and friends die, and the extent of emotional and physical support available influences this final stage. Individuals who have good coping skills and ability to socialize with others are more likely to have more satisfying lives (Figure 15–2◆).

Development

As noted earlier in this chapter, *development* refers to the accomplishment of and the increase in the ability to use motor, language, cognitive, and social skills that people acquire over their life span. **Cognitive**, language, social, **fine motor**, and **gross motor** skills are necessary for performance of the tasks that all humans must master. Newborns have few of these skills at birth. However, they seem to be born with the uncanny ability to capture the hearts of their parents—the initial caregivers. Parents move instinctively toward their newborn infant at the slightest signal that the infant is in distress. As humans age chronologically from infant to toddler, then from toddler to

cognitive The mental processes by which knowledge is acquired

fine motor Refers to the movement of small muscles, such as those in the hands and fingers

gross motor Refers to the movement of large muscles, such as those used in walking or hitting a ball

TABLE 15–2

Developmental Tasks and Chronological Age

SKILL AREA	INFANT: BIRTH–1 YEAR	TODDLER: 1–2 YEARS	PRESCHOOL: 2–5 YEARS	SCHOOL AGE: 5–12 YEARS
Cognitive	Learns about new things by feeling and working with objects encountered in the immediate environment and by placing or trying to place those objects in the mouth	Expands knowledge of things by learning words associated with objects in the environment	Comprehends tired, hungry, and other bodily experiences Recognizes colors	Learns relationship of objects to other objects and to self Learns relationship between objects and feelings
Social	Attaches to primary caregiver(s) Infant begins by recognizing faces and smiling; at about 6 months the infant begins to recognize primary caregiver(s) and expresses fear of strangers Plays simple interactive games like peek-a-boo and pat-a-cake	Learns self and primary caregiver(s) are different or separate from each other Undresses self Imitates and performs tasks seen in environment Expresses needs or indicates wants without crying	Begins to separate easily from caregiver(s) Dresses with supervision Washes and dries hands Plays interactive games (tag)	Acts independently, but emotionally close to caregiver Performs work and gets rewarded for it Dresses without supervision Forms same-sex play groups and clubs
Language	Vocalizes, squeals, and imitates sounds Says "dada" and "mama"	Says three words other than dada and mama Follows simple instructions	Names one picture Follows directions Combines words to make simple sentences of two or three words; uses plurals Gives first and last names	Defines words Knows and describes what things are made of
Gross Motor	Lifts head first, then chest Rolls over, pulls to sit, crawls, and stands alone	Walks well, kicks, stoops and jumps in place Throws balls	Runs well, hops, pedals tricycle Balances on one foot	Skips, balances on one foot for 10 seconds Overestimates physical abilities
Fine Motor	Reaches for objects and rakes up small items Grasps rattles Feeds self crackers	Unbuttons clothes Builds tower of four cubes Scribbles Uses spoon Picks up very small objects	Buttons clothes Builds tower of eight cubes Copies simple figures or letters, for example "o" Begins to use scissors	Draws man with six parts Copies detailed figures and objects

preschooler, and so on, they learn to think, to "coo" or talk, to socialize, to pick up small objects, and to walk. Human beings develop skills in each of these areas in a particular pattern, or sequence. Most people, as the old saying reminds us, learn to crawl before they learn to walk. Humans build on skills they have developed at a previous stage of development (Table 15–2◆).

Chronological Age

chronological age Actual age in years and months

Chronological age is linked to developmental skill acquisition, but not exactly in a lock-step fashion. For example, most children start walking by their first birthday. However,

ADOLESCENT: 12–18 YEARS	YOUNG ADULT: 18–40 YEARS	MIDDLE ADULT: 40–65 YEARS	OLDER ADULT: 65–75 YEARS	OLD AGE: 75–100+
Understands abstract concepts like illness and death	Fully developed; continues to develop knowledge-base related to school or job	Fully developed	Fully developed	Fully developed May be impaired
Experiences turmoil with rapidly changing moods and behavior Demonstrates interest in peer group almost exclusively Distances from parents emotionally Expresses concern with body image Experiences falling in and out of love	Establishes independence from parents Forms an individual lifestyle Adjusts to companions Selects a career Copes with career, social and economic constraints Chooses a mate Learns to live cooperatively with mate Becomes a parent	Builds socioeconomic status Assists younger and older to cope Fulfilled by work, family, or by giving or caring for others Copes with physical changes of aging Relates to grown children and the empty nest Deals with aging parents Copes with the death of parents	Develops mutually supportive relationships with grown children Adjusts to loss of friends and relatives Copes with loss of spouse Adjusts to retirement Forms new friends Adjusts to new role in the family Copes with dying	Develops mutually supportive relationships with grown children and grandchildren Copes with loss of spouse, friends, and sometimes children Forms new friends/withdraws Adjusts to new role in the family Copes with dying
Vocabulary increases Understands more abstract concepts, for example, grief	Fully developed	Fully developed	Fully developed	Fully developed
Awkwardness may be apparent as individuals learn to deal with rapid increases in size due to growth spurts	Fully developed	Beginning physical changes of aging such as decreased energy and endurance	Physical changes associated with the aging process are more significant	Pronounced physical changes associated with the aging process Stamina, sight, and hearing diminished
Fully developed	Fully developed	Fully developed	Physical changes associated with the aging process begin to appear	Physical changes associated with the aging process present

some start to walk as early as 8 months, and still others wait until they are 16 months old. The normal chronological-age range given (for walking) is from 8 months to 16 months, so the children cited in this example have all developed the ability to walk within the usual chronological-age range. Once development skills are mastered, the person is able to perform them most of the time.

Illness

Illness can have a profound effect on a person's ability to use skills that are already developed. When people are ill, they often behave at a lower developmental stage than their chronological age would suggest. For example, parents of a hospitalized 4-year-old may express concern that their child, who is toilet-trained, is once again wetting the bed. The nursing assistant's role is to reassure the parents that such a behavioral change is not unusual. Sometimes children cope with the anxiety and pain often accompanying hospitalization by reverting to behaviors that kept them anxiety- and pain-free at an earlier age. Support the child, parents, and other family members by addressing their anxieties and fears, and the temporary setback will usually resolve itself.

Injuries

Injuries such as head injuries or a stroke can necessitate the relearning of skills from earlier stages of development. For example, a stroke could mean that a person would have to relearn how to walk or talk. Frustration limits one's ability to cope with such difficult situations and may cause them to revert back to an earlier developmental level as well. Instead of thinking logically and realizing that with rehabilitation their walking may improve, they throw something across the room in exasperation at their inability to walk as they had before.

Chronological-Age Considerations

Knowledge of developmental-task masteries associated with chronological age is key to your ability to relate appropriately with patients and to provide needed nursing care. You must also be aware that illness and injury may sometimes impact negatively on a person's performance. The approach, or technique, you will use in delivering care to patients in the Infant: Birth–1 year range will be different from the approach you will use with patients in the School-Age: 5–12 year range. Your behavior will be based on chronological-age considerations of the patient (Figure 15–3◆). Table 15–3◆ lists typical nursing assistant behaviors that correspond to or are based on the patient's chronological age and typical task masteries or competencies to be considered as you provide care. Chapter 32 addresses many specific age considerations for older adults.

FIGURE 15–3 ◆
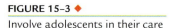

Involve adolescents in their care

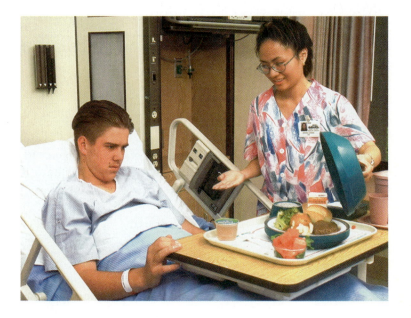

TABLE 15–3

Appropriate Nursing Assistant Behaviors for Various Age Groups

INFANT: BIRTH–1 YEAR	TODDLER: 1–2 YEARS	PRESCHOOL: 2–5 YEARS	SCHOOL-AGE CHILD: 5–12 YEARS
Keep child with parent(s). Use parents to comfort rather than restrain child during hurtful or scary experiences. Explain procedures to parents so they can calm patient. Keep small objects (such as IV tube caps and safety pins) out of child's reach. Ensure that the side of the bed is up. Place visually interesting objects where child can observe them. Provide age- and disease-appropriate toys.	Keep child with parent(s). Use parents to comfort rather than restrain child during hurtful or scary experiences. Explain procedures to parents so they can calm patient. Keep small objects (such as IV tube caps) out of child's reach. Ensure that the side of the bed is up. Toddlers are accustomed to being "on the go." Efforts to interfere with their movements may provoke negative displays, obstinacy, even temper tantrums. Interact with children on their terms, which may mean moving about with them.	Keep child with parent(s). Use parents to comfort rather than restrain child during hurtful or scary experiences. Explain procedures in simple words, describing only what patients will see, what things will look like outside the body. For example, if child will have an IV, demonstrate the tubing and IV needle hub. Don't show or talk about things that will not be visible to the child, such as the needle. Provide activities that engage the child and lessen anxiety when appropriate.	Allow independent movement as appropriate. Explain procedures in greater detail. Offer choices, when possible, to allow children to experience some control over their bodies and environment. For example, ask if patient would like you to make the bed now or after breakfast. Explain how long a painful procedure will take. This will avoid or shorten the child's attempts to stall the experience. When possible, give a tour before hospitalization to acquaint child with the environment.

ADOLESCENT: 12–18 YEARS	YOUNG ADULT: 18–40 YEARS	MIDDLE ADULT: 40–65 YEARS	OLDER ADULT: 65–75 YEARS AND OLD AGE: 75–100+
Show interest in visits by the patient's peers, supporting and complimenting positive behavior. Involve adolescents fully in decisions about their health care. Express interest in and support adolescents who exhibit concern about scars or imperfections, even if they are minor. Body image is very important at this age.	Involve patient in decision making about all aspects of health care. Review with patient what treatments are scheduled, including when they will take place, and so on. Knowing what to expect next helps the patient adapt to unfamiliar surroundings and routines. Listen to patient's concerns about the effect illness will have on progress toward lifelong goals like meaningful relationships, offspring, and employment.	Involve patient in decision making about all aspects of health care. Ask if patient would like a family member or other person present to provide support, help with hearing and clarifying information when needed, or making a health care decision. Provide information when the family member or other person arrives. Review with patient what treatments are scheduled, including when they will take place, and so on. Knowing what to expect next helps the patient adapt to unfamiliar surroundings and routines.	Ask patient about the routine followed at home, and adapt the hospital routine as much as possible to the patient's at-home routine. Review with patient what treatments are scheduled, including when they will take place, and so on. Knowing what to expect next helps the patient adapt to unfamiliar surroundings and routines. Ask if patient would like a family member present to provide support in making a health care decision. Provide information needed when the family member arrives.

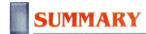

SUMMARY

Growth and development refer to the physical, intellectual, emotional, and social changes that occur over the life span of every human being. Although both may occur at different rates for different individuals, there are general principles and characteristics that describe the typical person within each stage of development. Illness and injury impact individuals' abilities to use their developed skills; however, human beings continue to adapt to triumphs and adversities throughout their entire lives. Consideration of specific developmental capabilities based on chronological age of patients is key to determining your role. Basic knowledge and understanding of the general principles of normal growth and development, including chronological-age differences, provide nursing assistants with a sound basis for delivering informed patient-centered care.

NOTES

CHAPTER REVIEW

FILL IN THE BLANK Read each sentence and fill in the blank line with a word that completes the sentence.

1. In each developmental stage, there are _____ that have to be mastered.

2. A measurement of the _____ of a child's head provides important information about growth.

3. _____ motor control refers to the movement of small muscles, such as those in the feet and hands.

4. _____ age is the person's actual age in years and months.

5. _____ and _____ can have a profound effect on a person's ability to use skills that they have already developed.

MULTIPLE CHOICE Choose the best answer for each question or statement.

1. Growth and development usually follow patterns and stages and
   a. are always the same in all cultures.
   b. are identical in both boys and girls.
   c. may occur at different rates in different people.
   d. are only different in old age.

2. Growth and development of infants
   a. is not predictable.
   b. usually follows predictable patterns.
   c. is about 5 pounds a month.
   d. is slower than other age ranges.

3. Growth and development in adolescence is
   a. more rapid than in infancy.
   b. unpredictable.
   c. faster for boys than for girls.
   d. characterized by development of secondary sex changes.

4. Development in a person includes learning skills such as
   a. cognitive skills.
   b. language skills.
   c. gross motor and fine motor skills.
   d. All of the above.

5. A developmental task of old age is
   a. coping with the death of parents.
   b. selecting a career.
   c. coping with the loss of friends.
   d. building socioeconomic status.

TIME-OUT

TIPS FOR TIME MANAGEMENT

When other staff members interrupt you while you are giving patient care, continue to work as you listen to them. Give an answer or appoint a time and place to meet when you will be able to give assistance to them.

THE NURSING ASSISTANT IN ACTION

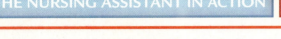

You are working with a colleague who appears disrespectful when she talks to her patients. Her answers are short and curt. Sometimes she speaks to teenagers or older adults like they are small children. So far you have not said anything. Today your patient complains to you about your coworker's attitude.

What Is Your Response/Action?

CRITICAL THINKING

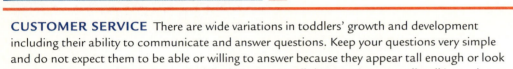

CUSTOMER SERVICE There are wide variations in toddlers' growth and development including their ability to communicate and answer questions. Keep your questions very simple and do not expect them to be able or willing to answer because they appear tall enough or look like they should be able to do so. Avoid asking parents all the questions as well, talking only to them as if the toddler is not in the room. Both parent and child are your customers.

You should understand that when caring for older adults, extra time may be required. Many older adults have difficulty seeing or hearing and will tire easily. Avoid trying to rush them when assisting them to walk or eat. Older adults may feel upset or become agitated when they feel rushed. Go slowly and proceed at a pace comfortable for the individual patient.

CULTURAL CARE As a nursing assistant you will encounter many variations and cultural differences related to the onset of puberty in young girls. African American girls may experience changes in their breasts and begin menstruation 1 to 3 years earlier than Caucasian girls. Teenage girls who have been malnourished, have had little food to eat, or have eating disorders tend to have fewer or no periods and underdeveloped breasts.

COOPERATION WITHIN THE TEAM Most facilities have patients whose ages vary considerably. Some team members will be more skilled communicating with one group of patients than others. If you are young, some patients closer to your age may confide in you because they find it difficult to talk to others old enough to be their parents. More experienced caregivers may be comfortable relating to patients of any age. If you encounter problems relating to older or younger patients, observe who among your coworkers has fewer problems. Talk with them and ask for advice or ideas to improve your approach. It is helpful to add information to the patient's care plan when you identify the patient's preferences or specific things that work well.

EXPLORE MediaLink

Additional interactive resources for this chapter can be found on the Companion Website at www.prenhall.com/wolgin. Click on Chapter 15 and "Begin" to select activities for this chapter.

For chapter-related NCLEX-style questions and an audio glossary, access the accompanying CD-ROM in this book.

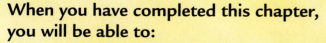

16 The Musculoskeletal System and Related Care

OBJECTIVES

When you have completed this chapter, you will be able to:

- Identify the functions of the muscular system.
- Explain how groups of muscles work together to perform body motion.
- List the functions of the skeletal system.
- List the four general types of bones and give examples of each.
- Name four major types of joints and give examples of each.
- Label a diagram of the skeletal and surface muscles.
- Describe how aging affects the musculoskeletal system.
- List common diseases and disorders of the musculoskeletal systems.
- Describe the scope of orthopedic nursing care and the purposes of orthopedic equipment.
- Describe and explain the reasons for special skin care for the orthopedic patient.
- List important points to observe while performing any nursing task involving patients in traction.
- List important points to observe while performing any nursing task involving patients in plaster casts.
- Identify several types of supportive devices and the nursing assistant's role in caring for patients who use such devices.
- Identify the different patient care and positioning needs of individuals with hip versus knee replacements.

KEY TERMS

abduction
adduction
arthritis
atrophy
contract
contracture
extension
flex
flexion
fracture
joint
ligament
orthopedics
osteoarthritis
relax
rheumatoid arthritis
traction
trapeze
walker

MediaLink

www.prenhall.com/wolgin

Use the address above to access the free, interactive Companion Website created for this textbook. Get hints, instant feedback, and textbook references to chapter-related NCLEX-style questions. Link to other interesting sites.

AUDIO GLOSSARY:
Use the Companion Website, or the CD-ROM disk enclosed with your textbook, to hear the pronunciation of the key terms in the chapter.

The human body works most efficiently when a person is physically active. Thus, proper care of the musculoskeletal system plays an important role in maintaining overall good health. The nursing assistant can have a positive impact by helping patients care for themselves and encouraging them to be as active as possible. This chapter provides the background necessary for carrying out these responsibilities. It describes the musculoskeletal system, common diseases and disorders affecting it, and the nursing assistant's role in orthopedic nursing care.

The Muscular System

ALERT

For all patient contact, adhere to Standard Precautions (⊂⊃ Chapter 5, pages 83–85). Wear protective equipment as indicated.

flex To bend; the act of bending a body part

The muscular system makes possible all the body's motion: that of the whole body and that which occurs inside the body. Besides moving the body, muscles help to keep the body warm, especially during activity. Muscles have an exceptionally rich blood supply, so they are the most infection-free of all the body's basic tissues (see Figure 16–1a◆ and Figure 16–1b◆).

Groups of muscles work together to perform a body motion. Other groups perform the opposite motion. These pairs of muscle groups are called *antagonistic groups*. For example, when you **flex** your arm (bring it toward your shoulder), your biceps muscle contracts and

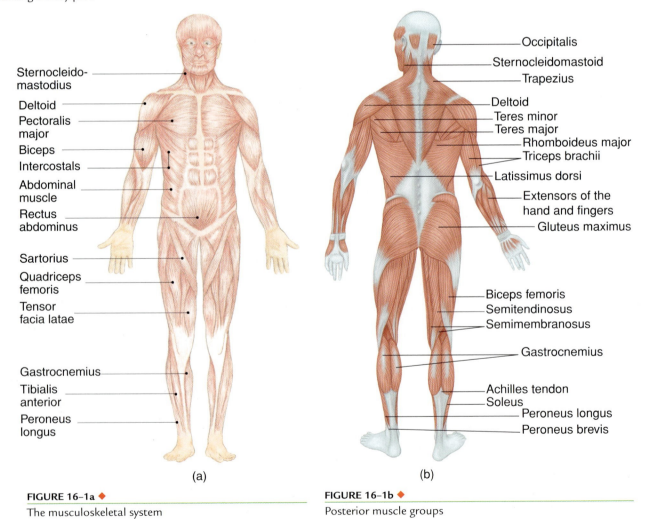

Sternocleido-mastodius
Deltoid
Pectoralis major
Biceps
Intercostals
Abdominal muscle
Rectus abdominus
Sartorius
Quadriceps femoris
Tensor facia latae
Gastrocnemius
Tibialis anterior
Peroneus longus

Occipitalis
Sternocleidomastoid
Trapezius
Deltoid
Teres minor
Teres major
Rhomboideus major
Triceps brachii
Latissimus dorsi
Extensors of the hand and fingers
Gluteus maximus
Biceps femoris
Semitendinosus
Semimembranosus
Gastrocnemius
Achilles tendon
Soleus
Peroneus longus
Peroneus brevis

(a)

(b)

FIGURE 16–1a ◆

The musculoskeletal system

FIGURE 16–1b ◆

Posterior muscle groups

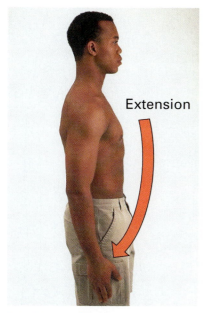

FIGURE 16–2a ◆
Extension

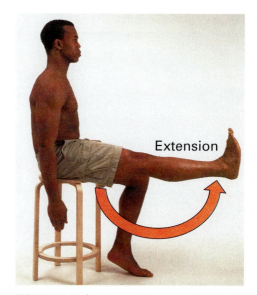

FIGURE 16–2b ◆
Flexion

FIGURE 16–2c ◆
Extension

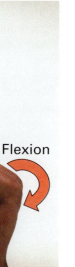

FIGURE 16–2d ◆
Flexion

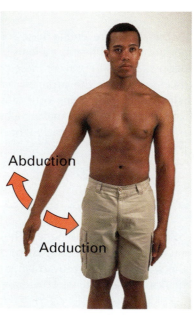

FIGURE 16–2e ◆
Abduction and adduction

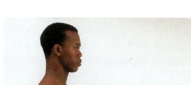

relax To place in a resting position, in which muscle tension decreases and fibers lengthen

flexion Bending of a joint (elbow, wrist, knee)

extension Straightening or lengthening a muscle, thereby making the angle formed by bones and muscles greater

abduction Movement of an arm or leg away from the center of the body

adduction Movement of an arm or leg toward the center of the body

atrophy Wasting away of muscles; decrease in muscle size

contracture An abnormal shortening of a muscle

the triceps muscle **relaxes**. When you extend your arm (straighten it), the biceps relax while the triceps contract.

You should know the terms for the basic ways in which muscles can move parts of the body. **Flexion** is bending at a joint, such as the elbow (Figure 16–2b◆ and 16–2d◆), wrist, or knee. Its opposite is **extension**, or straightening (Figure 16–2a◆ and 16–2c◆). **Abduction** means moving a part away from the body midline. Conversely, **adduction** means moving it toward the body (Figure 16–2e◆ and 16–3◆).

If a muscle is kept inactive for too long, it tends to shrink and waste away. This is called **atrophy**. In addition, immobility (remaining perfectly still) can lead to **contracture**, a

FIGURE 16–3 ◆

(a) Abduction, moving a body part away from the midline (b) adduction, moving a body part toward the midline

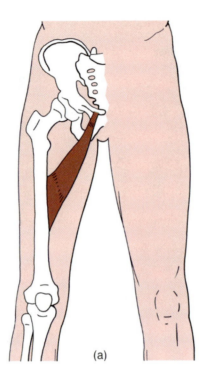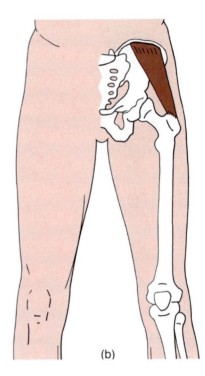

(a)   (b)

permanent muscle shortening. Preventing these conditions is among the reasons why regular exercise is important to good health. Patients who cannot be physically active may be given range-of-motion exercises to prevent these problems.

The largest muscle groups are the strongest ones. Using your large muscle groups for heavy tasks can help you avoid straining your other muscles and hurting yourself. For example, when helping to lift a patient or making a bed, remember to use the strong muscles of your legs rather than those of your back. (For more information on moving and lifting patients, see Chapter 7.)

The Skeletal System

The skeletal system is made up of 206 bones. The bones act as a framework for the body, give it structure and support, and are the passive organs of motion. In other words, bones do not move by themselves but are moved when a nerve impulse stimulates a muscle to **contract** (shorten). Bones also store vital minerals that are necessary for many other body activities.

Another function of the bones is to protect the vital organs. The bones of the head are designed to protect the very delicate tissue of the brain (Figure 16–4◆). They are joined by *sutures,* similar to a zigzag pattern, and totally surround the brain and cranial nerves. Two other kinds of bones that protect vital organs are the vertebrae of the spinal column, which protect the spinal nerve cord, and the ribs, which guard the heart and lungs.

There are four types of bones (Figure 16–5◆):

1. *Long bones,* such as the big bone in your thigh, the femur
2. *Short bones,* like the bones in your fingers, the phalanges
3. *Irregular bones,* such as the vertebrae that make up the spinal column
4. *Flat bones,* like the bones of the rib cage

Bone cells grow and reproduce slowly. Therefore, **fractures** (broken bones) can mend, but the process is slow and gradual. The new bone hardens gradually as calcium is

contract Get smaller; shortening the length of muscle, thereby making the angle formed by bones and muscles smaller

fracture A break in a bone

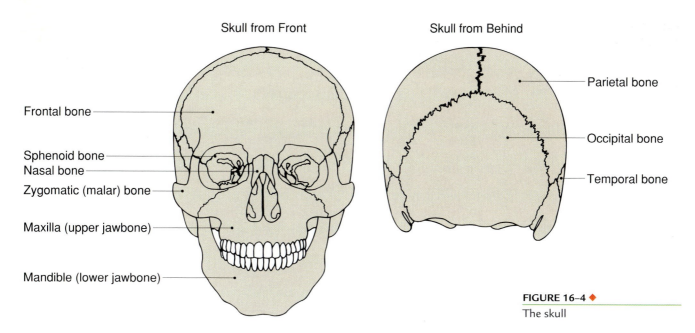

Skull from Front

Skull from Behind

Frontal bone

Sphenoid bone
Nasal bone
Zygomatic (malar) bone

Maxilla (upper jawbone)

Mandible (lower jawbone)

Parietal bone

Occipital bone

Temporal bone

FIGURE 16–4 ◆

The skull

deposited. Blood supply to bone tissue is poor in comparison to other areas of the body. Therefore, bone has relatively low resistance to infection.

Joints (Motion)

In a healthy human body, all the systems of the body work together. No one system can stand alone. During each body movement, the skeletal system, muscular system, nervous

FIGURE 16–5 ◆

Types of bones

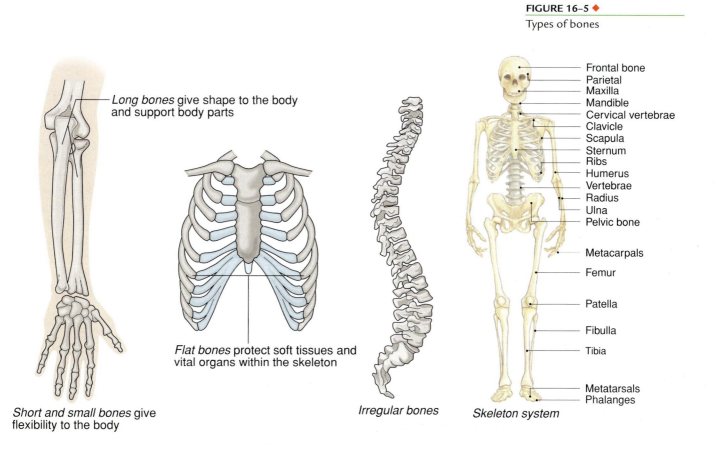

Long bones give shape to the body and support body parts

Flat bones protect soft tissues and vital organs within the skeleton

Short and small bones give flexibility to the body

Irregular bones

Skeleton system

Frontal bone
Parietal
Maxilla
Mandible
Cervical vertebrae
Clavicle
Scapula
Sternum
Ribs
Humerus
Vertebrae
Radius
Ulna
Pelvic bone
Metacarpals
Femur
Patella
Fibulla
Tibia
Metatarsals
Phalanges

FIGURE 16–6 ◆

Types of joints

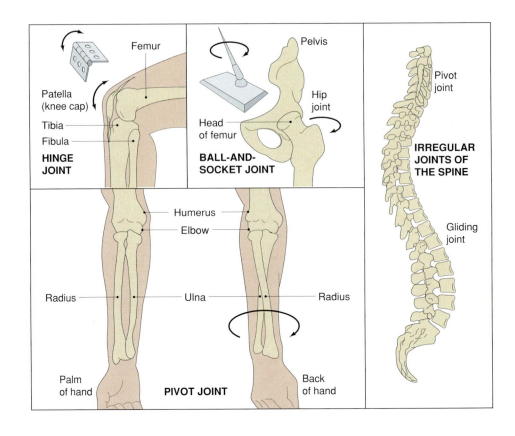

system, and circulatory system are all interacting. This body movement occurs at the joints, a perfect example of how several systems must work together.

joint A part of the body where two bones come together

ligament Tough, white fibrous cord that connects bone to bone

Joints are the meeting place where one bone connects with one or more other bones. They are the necessary levers for all motion. Joints are made up of many structures. The tough, white fibrous cord, the **ligament**, connects bone to bone. The *tendons* connect muscle to bone. Joints—especially those in the shoulder, hip, and knee—are enclosed in a strong capsule lined by a membrane that secretes a fluid called *synovial fluid*. This fluid acts as a buffer, very much like a waterbed, so that the ends of the bones do not get worn out from too much motion. Other structures that protect the bone include the pad of cartilage at the end of the bone, a sac of synovial fluid (which is known as a *bursa*), and a disk of cartilage called the *meniscus*. Many such safeguards are built into the body. The human body has several kinds of joints (Figure 16–6◆). The hinge joint, such as in the knee, is freely movable. There are also less movable joints, such as those between the vertebrae. Some joints do not move at all, such as the joints between the bones of the head, which protect the brain.

The Musculoskeletal System and the Normal Aging Process

The musculoskeletal system undergoes changes as a person gets older. Unless the person remains physically active, muscles become weaker and lose their tone. The body therefore loses strength and endurance. Such changes affect many parts of the body, including the organs. For example, weakening muscles may cause heart function to decrease and breathing to become more difficult.

Cartilage deteriorates with age, and tissue hardens. As a result, joints become stiff, making movement more difficult. A person may react to this difficulty by being less active. If so, the reduced activity can bring about further loss of muscle tone.

Bones become porous and brittle with age; they do not remain as hard as they once were. The body's absorption of calcium decreases. Some older people lose calcium, especially if they do not bear weight (stand). This makes the bones even weaker. Therefore, bones in an older person break more easily.

The spinal column (bones of the spine) may also change, bringing about a stooped posture and loss of height. Some people become as much as 2 inches shorter than they were as a young adult.

Common Diseases and Disorders of the Musculoskeletal System

The changes of aging can make a person more likely to be injured as one gets older, but diseases and disorders of the musculoskeletal system can occur at any age. Following are the most common conditions:

- **Bursitis:** inflammation of the bursa (sac of synovial fluid)
- **Contusion:** injury to soft tissue
- **Sprain:** strain of a ligament or tendon surrounding a joint; ligaments may be partially torn
- **Joint dislocation:** injury in which a bone end that forms part of a joint is displaced (pulled out so that it is no longer in anatomic position)
- **Fracture:** break in a bone (Figure 16–7◆)
  - **Simple fracture:** broken bone with no external wound
  - **Compound fracture:** broken bone with an external wound or fragment of bone protruding through the skin

FIGURE 16–7 ◆

Types of bone fractures

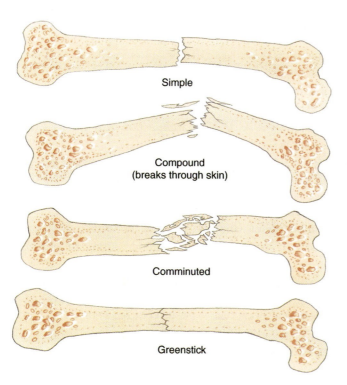

Simple

Compound
(breaks through skin)

Comminuted

Greenstick

arthritis Chronic condition of inflammation of the joints

osteoarthritis A degenerative, painful bone disease affecting the spine, hips, finger joints, or knees

rheumatoid arthritis A chronic disease condition affecting the connective tissue of the body, especially the joints

■ *Surgical amputation:* removal of a portion of a limb

■ *Low back pain:* pain that often is accompanied by muscle spasms

■ **Arthritis:** the inflammation of one or more joints. Arthritis is a common, chronic condition found most often in older and/or very obese individuals.

■ **Osteoarthritis:** a degenerative, painful bone disease affecting the spine, hips, finger joints, or knees. This condition is seen most often in the elderly, especially women or individuals who are obese or who have had joint injuries. Pain can be very severe and, for many sufferers, is felt more often in cold or damp weather. Treatment involves taking aspirin or pain relievers, with local heat or cold treatments if they relieve the patient's pain. Obese persons are encouraged to diet and reduce their weight. Many elderly persons with osteoarthritis require a cane or walker for ambulation. Fall prevention measures are particularly important to prevent further pain and debilitation.

■ **Rheumatoid arthritis:** a chronic disease condition affecting the connective tissue of the body, especially the joints. This condition occurs more often in women than men and can occur at any age. The joints in the hand are affected first. Over time this progressive disease causes painful inflammation and swelling in other body joints: the wrists, shoulders, elbows, ankles, knees, and hips. Changes in organs evidently affect the lungs, heart, eyes, kidneys, and/or skin. The person will often have joint stiffness when she awakens, progressive finger or foot deformities, limited range of motion, feel easily exhausted, have weight loss from decreased appetite, and can have fever. Treatment includes ongoing pain medications, rest, localized hot or cold treatments, and joint replacement in many cases.

■ *Osteogenic sarcoma (cancer):* malignant bone tumor

■ *Osteoporosis:* a bone condition wherein the bone becomes brittle, porous, and easily broken. This disease affects primarily women after menopause and older persons who have lacked calcium in their diets. Persons at risk are those who are inactive, smokers, and heavy alcohol drinkers. Calcium intake requires that bones bear weight. Many women take estrogen replacement to help prevent osteoporosis. Long-term estrogen replacement has become more controversial. Calcium supplements, vitamins, and weight-bearing exercise are ways to improve bone density. Signs of osteoporosis include low back pain, loss of height, stooped posture, and low bone density. Fractures can occur very easily, and protecting the person from falls or injuries is important. Frail individuals can suffer fractures by being roughly pulled up from a chair or turned in bed.

■ *Muscular dystrophy:* a condition characterized by a progressive atrophy of muscular tissue

■ *Osteomyelitis:* inflammation of or an infection in the bone caused by bacteria introduced by trauma or surgery

■ *Tuberculosis:* an infectious disease that usually affects the lungs, but can affect bone tissue. TB can invade the spinal vertebrae, destroying the disks and resulting in the collapse and wedging of the vertebrae and shortening of the spine. If pressure in the spinal cord occurs, paralysis may result. The patient may require some of the same orthopedic care discussed later in this chapter.

■ *Poliomyelitis:* (not seen often) viral infection causing an inflammation of the gray matter of the spinal cord, resulting in partial or complete paralysis

■ *Trauma to spinal cord:* accidental injury damaging the spinal cord and resulting in paralysis of some area of the body. Trauma to the spinal cord may result in paralysis of the arms, legs, and body below the level of the injury. This immobility causes the patient to require a lot of supportive care.

■ *Guillain-Barré syndrome:* a disease of the nervous system resulting in ascending paralysis

Care of the Orthopedic Patient

Orthopedics (also spelled *orthopaedics*) is the science of the prevention and correction of deformities and the treatment of diseases of the bones, muscles, joints, and fasciae (supporting membranes) either by manipulation, special apparatus, or surgery. Orthopedic nursing requires special knowledge and skills in addition to routine patient care. To care for the orthopedic patient, the nursing assistant needs knowledge of body mechanics and specialized procedures related to the treatment of this type of patient. Nursing assistants will need to be familiar with special equipment such as splints, casts, traction devices, and walkers.

Modern science is constantly developing new ways and means to help the orthopedic patient. In the past, traction and bed rest were the method of treatment for most patients with orthopedic problems. Today, improved methods of surgery, lighter casting materials, shortened hospital stays, and the identified physiological benefits of early ambulation (walking or moving about while standing) have led to changes in the care of orthopedic patients. A patient who is put in traction remains there for a shorter period of time than in past years. Early ambulation using assistive devices such as canes and walkers promotes faster healing with fewer circulatory side effects such as blood clots.

The emphasis on early ambulation requires the nursing assistant to provide both ambulatory and nonambulatory orthopedic care. Both types of orthopedic care pose special challenges:

- Routine nursing care is difficult to give when a patient is in a cast or traction. It will often be necessary to carry out some procedures with the least possible disturbance to these orthopedic devices.

- Especially if the patient must endure a long period of restricted mobility, he may become unduly discouraged. Encouraging independence through the use of special devices for walking or retrieving objects out of reach promotes muscle tone and a positive mental outlook for the patient.

Orthopedic Equipment

Orthopedic care may involve the use of special equipment. These orthopedic devices are used for several purposes:

1. To provide support for the injured part until it heals
2. To prevent deformity and weakness in the injured muscles and joints
3. To help the patient to ambulate with safety as early as possible in the healing process

Support for the injured part may be provided by bandages, adhesive strapping, splints, or plaster casts applied externally. Support may also be applied directly to a bone by using pins, metal plates, or prosthetic devices (for example, the replacement of a joint). These specialized *prostheses* (artificial aids) are applied in the operating room, using specialized surgical procedures. To prevent stiffness or deformity, the patient will be asked to use the affected part within limits ordered by the doctor. Frequently, the patient needs the support of a brace, crutches, or a walker.

When a patient must wear a brace, there are often specific restrictions. Some braces must be worn continually, while others must be applied before getting out of bed. It is important to check the patient's plan of care to see if any specific instructions are included.

To promote early ambulation, the physician often prescribes a **walker** for the patient to use. A walker is a metal frame device with handgrips and four legs. It is open on one side. This device provides stability and security for a patient who is weak on one side or restricted in the amount of weight he can put on one foot. The use of the walker will

orthopedics The medical specialty that covers the treatment of broken bones, deformities, or diseases that attack the bones, joints, and muscles

walker A metal frame device with handgrips and four legs that is open on one side; provides stability and security for the patient who is weak on one side or restricted in the amount of weight he can put on one foot

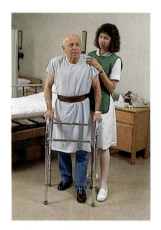

FIGURE 16–8 ◆

Assisting a patient to use a walker

trapeze A triangle-shaped bar attached to the overbed frame of a traction setup which enables the patient to pull himself up in bed

traction Exertion of pull by means of weights or pulleys, often used for realignment of bones or other limb tissues

depend on what kind of surgery or injury the patient had. Always check with your supervisor before assisting a patient to use a walker (Figure 16–8◆).

Special Skin Care for the Orthopedic Patient

Besides routine nursing care, the orthopedic patient may need special skin care. In the early stages of an injury or after surgery, the patient may be confined to bed because of traction. Even a casted patient will have restricted mobility. This type of patient is particularly susceptible to pressure ulcers.

The nursing assistant should change the patient's position every 2 hours following the doctor's instructions, give special back care, and change the area of pressure as often as is possible to prevent pressure ulcers. Providing a smooth, clean, dry bed and keeping the cast clean can promote patient comfort and prevent pressure ulcers. A **trapeze**, suspended from an over-the-bed frame, allows the patient to move or lift himself, to aid in back care, and to use the bedpan.

Care of the Patient in Traction

Traction means the exertion of pull by means of weights and pulleys. Countertraction (exertion of pull in the opposite direction) must be present to maintain body alignment. Traction is used to promote and maintain the alignment of broken (fractured) bones and for other orthopedic conditions and treatment. It may be applied to the skin externally or to the bone internally through surgery. It is maintained by the use of a special frame on the bed (Figure 16–9◆).

The patient will be taught to use a trapeze to raise or pull up his head or upper body (Figure 16–10◆). If the patient is uncomfortable, tell your immediate supervisor. Never change the patient's body position without permission from your immediate supervisor. A nursing assistant will never set or adjust any of the equipment in use on a patient in traction. This is strictly a function of the physician, registered nurse, physical therapist, or orthopedic technician. The nursing assistant, however, is expected to check periodically as instructed on the traction apparatus and to report any observed problem to the immediate

FIGURE 16–9 ◆

A patient in traction

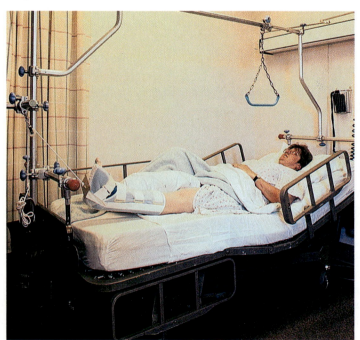

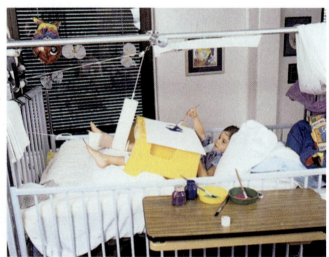

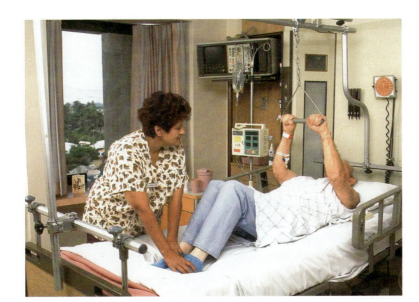

FIGURE 16–10 ◆

Patient learning to use trapeze

supervisor. The following questions concern points that the nursing assistant should observe while performing any nursing task involving a patient in traction.

- Are the weights resting on the floor or against the bed?
- Is a cable off its pulley?
- Has the patient slid down in the bed?
- Is the casted body part painful?
- Is the skin blue in color on the body part where the cast ends?
- Is the part cold to the touch?
- Does the patient complain of pain?

If the answer to any of these questions is yes, report the situation to your immediate supervisor at once: None of these conditions should exist, and all should receive prompt attention.

Care of Patients in Casts

Casts are, in effect, a form of splint. They are used as a support to hold injured bones in alignment while they are healing. Casts are wet when applied and then allowed to dry. Casts are made from Gortex, fiberglass, plastic, or plaster of paris. They harden as they dry, and the whole cast becomes rigid. Plastic or fiberglass casts perform the same task as plaster casts but are lighter, cleaner, and easier to use and remove. These lighter casts are more commonly used because they make it easier for the patient to move about and ambulate. These casts come in a variety of colors. Gortex casts are designed to allow patients to bathe or shower while wearing the cast. Water does not damage this type of cast.

While a cast is drying, the patient's position must be maintained and the cast left uncovered. Pillows are placed to support the cast so it will not bend or move while still soft. Often ice packs are applied to the cast at the area of incision to reduce swelling.

Casts are confining and can be very uncomfortable. The skin area near the edges of the cast can become irritated and develop skin breakdown from chafing.

Casts should not restrict circulation. The nursing assistant should observe patients in casts for signs of pain, pallor, bluish color, loss of sensation, and coldness to the touch. Ask the patient whether he is experiencing any tingling or numbness, which are signs of poor circulation. Compare the extremities for size, color, and warmth. Feel the exposed part of the limb to note whether it is cold. Any symptom of circulatory impairment should be reported immediately to the nursing assistant's supervisor.

The nursing assistant should be sure that the patient's cast does not become soiled while he is using a bedpan or urinal. Keeping the cast clean helps greatly to avoid discomfort and other skin irritations.

Any unusual odors coming from the cast or stains on the cast should be reported to the nurse manager or supervisor at once. An odor or stain could be a sign that a pressure ulcer or infection is forming under the cast. Itching should also be reported, and the patient instructed not to try to scratch the body part with foreign objects.

Supportive Devices

An orthopedic patient may require special supportive devices to help her maintain a position that is comfortable and prevent problems such as contractures. The following are some common supportive devices:

- *Pillows* of appropriate sizes and shapes may be placed where they support joints and provide comfort.

- A *trochanter* roll is a rolled-up towel or small blanket placed next to the tip of the thigh bone (the greater trochanter). This supportive device prevents external rotation of the hip, which could interfere with ambulation and cause permanent disability.

- An *abduction splint* is a device designed to keep the thighs apart. This position maintains proper alignment of the hip joints and prevents skin-to-skin contact.

- An *abductor pillow* or *abductor wedge* is a special pillow or foam wedge that keeps an injured leg abducted (away from the center of the body), preventing strain on a fracture site or hip prosthesis (artificial joint).

- A *Palmer splint* keeps the hand in a functional position. It prevents contractures in patients with paralysis of the hand or wrist.

- A *hand roll* is a round device made up of different materials and placed in the palm of the hand. It prevents or treats contractures of the hand and prevents fingernails from pressing into the palm.

- A *foot board* is a padded board placed at (or affixed to) the foot of the patient's bed. It is designed to exert slight pressure against the bottom of the feet of a patient lying in the supine position (on her back), thereby preventing contracture of the foot.

- A *foot stool* is used when the angle of the hip must be maintained within certain prescribed limits when a patient is sitting; for example, a postoperative total hip replacement patient.

When a patient uses supportive devices such as these, the nursing assistant should observe how the devices are placed. If the device or patient is repositioned, report the change to the immediate supervisor. Also, the nursing assistant may be directed to observe, massage, or clean the skin where it comes into contact with the supportive devices. Report to your immediate supervisor any signs of skin irritation or pressure in the area of the supportive device.

Total Hip Replacement (THR)

Arthroplasty is the term used when a joint is replaced or refashioned. Another term is "total joint replacement." This procedure may be performed on the elbow, hip, knee, or shoulder. Most frequently, these joints are replaced due to osteoarthritis or degenerative joint disease, which occurs with aging. Arthroplasty may also be performed on younger adults whose joints have been damaged by falls, accidents, trauma, or congenital malformations.

In a total hip replacement, the diseased head of the femur is surgically removed. It is replaced with a stainless steel ball on a stem. The stem is cemented into the canal of the femur using a special type of surgical glue. The curved area where the head of the femur fits against the pelvic bone is called the acetabulum. A cup made of specialized plastic is cemented into the surgically smoothed acetabulum. The replaced femur head and acetabulum fit together perfectly, providing a new joint that moves without friction.

Normally, the muscles and ligaments of the hip hold the femur in the acetabulum and prevent hip dislocation. The muscles and ligaments of the hip are not attached to these plastic and stainless steel devices, however. For several months after surgery, a patient with a hip replacement cannot move his or her leg in certain directions because dislocation could occur. The patient might then need another surgery to correct the dislocation.

Patient Care

When you care for a patient who has had a recent total hip replacement, you must keep a wedge-shaped foam piece, called an abduction pillow, between the legs to keep the hip abducted. Adduction of the operative leg, especially past the midline of the body, can cause dislocation.

You will turn the patient with the abduction pillow in place. Turn the patient every 2 hours, but turn only to the back and to the unoperated side. Place pillows at the patient's back to maintain the side position.

When you assist a patient with a total hip replacement out of bed, you will remove the abduction pillow. The patient will either bear no weight or only partial weight on the operative leg, depending on how recently the hip was replaced. You will assist him or her to pivot on the unoperated leg.

A reclining wheelchair with elevating leg rests must be used for a patient with a recent hip replacement. The patient must not bend further than 60 degrees at the hip for the first 10 days after surgery and must not bend more than 90 degrees for several months because further flexion can cause dislocation of the femur. The reclining wheelchair back is placed at the appropriate angle. During transfer in or out of bed, you must take care to prevent adduction of the affected leg.

Once the patient is in the wheelchair, elevate the leg rests and place pillows between the legs to maintain abduction. Place the call signal and other needed items within reach so the patient does not flex at the hip in an attempt to obtain some item out of reach.

When you care for a patient with a total hip replacement who is in bed, be sure to place blankets within reach so the patient does not bend at the hip to pull blankets from the foot of the bed.

CARING FOR PATIENTS WITH THR	GUIDELINES	
■ Turn every 2 hours to back and inoperative side with abduction pillow in place. ■ Use a fracture pan when a bedpan is necessary.	■ Use a raised toilet seat to prevent flexion greater than 90 degrees when sitting. ■ Keep the affected leg abducted at all times. ■ Use a reclining wheelchair with elevated leg rests.	■ Do not allow the patient to bend over to pick up something or to put on shoes and socks. ■ Do not allow the patient to sit or lie with the legs crossed. ■ Assist the patient to stand from a chair without flexing more than 90 degrees at the hip.

Total Knee Replacement

A total knee replacement surgery involves smoothing the lower end of the femur and cementing a smooth stainless steel covering over it. The top end of the tibia is surgically removed, and a notched stainless steel plate is cemented to the top of the tibia. The covering on the lower end of the femur and the plate on the top of the tibia fit perfectly and glide easily against one another, creating a friction-free joint. A plastic piece, called a patellar button, is cemented to the back of the kneecap to prevent friction when the knee bends and straightens.

Patient Care

When you care for a patient with a total knee replacement you will see a continuous passive range-of-motion machine, called CPM, in use. The patient's operative leg is placed in the CPM, which then gently exercises the knee to promote flexibility. The CPM is set for different amounts of flexion and extension, according to the physician's orders. The patient should use the machine as much as can be tolerated, up to 22 hours per day. When the operative leg is not in the CPM, extend the leg on the bed, without pillows beneath it.

Use a wheelchair with elevating leg rests for a patient with a recent total knee replacement. When you assist the patient out of bed, he or she will pivot on the unoperative leg. Elevate the affected leg at all times when the patient is out of bed.

Anti-embolism stockings may be ordered for patients who have had recent total knee replacements. Exercise care when you apply the stockings over the surgical incision to avoid injury to the area. See Chapter 29, section titled *Elastic Stockings and Elastic Bandages*.

When the patient begins to ambulate, a knee immobilizer should be placed on the operative leg. The patient will also use an assistive device such as crutches or a walker until full weight bearing is allowed, approximately 2 months after discharge.

SUMMARY

It is important to understand how the human musculoskeletal system appears and functions. When this body system is injured, the patient will have decreased mobility. This decreased mobility will require special care of the involved body part, the skin, and the equipment. There has been an increased emphasis on getting the patient to resume normal activity as soon as possible. This helps to avoid complications of immobility, such as pressure ulcers, contractures, and blood clots. Infections can cause serious complications for patients who have had surgery. Use Standard Precautions and report any signs of infection.

NOTES

CHAPTER REVIEW

FILL IN THE BLANK Read each sentence and fill in the blank line with a word that completes the sentence.

1. _____ is the exertion of pull by weights or pulleys, often used for realignment of bones or other limb tissues.

2. The wasting away of or decrease in muscle size is called _____.

3. _____ connect bone to bone.

4. _____ connect muscle to bone.

5. _____ are used as a support to hold injured bones in alignment while they are healing.

MULTIPLE CHOICE Choose the best answer for each question or statement.

1. Flexion refers to
   a. bending a part of the body.
   b. straightening a part of the body.
   c. relaxing a part of the body.
   d. All of the above.

2. Which of the following is not true about bones?
   a. There are 206 bones in the body.
   b. Bones are the framework of the body.
   c. Bones work together to provide body motion.
   d. Bones store vital minerals.

3. Which of the following is not true about muscles?
   a. Muscles provide the motion for our bodies.
   b. Muscles provide the motion for structures within our bodies.
   c. Muscles have an exceptionally rich blood supply.
   d. Muscles are joined by sutures.

4. All of the following are diseases and disorders of the musculoskeletal system *except*
   a. bursitis.
   b. dermatitis.
   c. arthritis.
   d. osteoporosis.

5. Care for the total hip replacement patient may include all of the following *except*
   a. keeping a wedge-shaped pillow between the legs.
   b. turning the patient to the back and to the unoperated side.
   c. the patient will bear full weight on the operative leg.
   d. the patient cannot bend more than 60 degrees for 10 days after surgery.

TIME-OUT

TIPS FOR TIME MANAGEMENT

Answer call lights as quickly as possible. This will save time by preventing possible accidents or injuries when patients grow tired of waiting for help and attempt to get up alone. Remember that all call lights must be answered, whether or not the particular room is assigned to you.

THE NURSING ASSISTANT IN ACTION

You are assigned to care for a frail, elderly woman who has difficulty walking. She has stooped posture and osteoporosis. The slippers she is wearing do not seem to be staying on her feet very well. You are concerned she may trip or fall as she is making her way to the dining room to eat. You offer her your arm and say, "Let me escort you to your table, Ms. Sanford." She refuses your help and tells you she is perfectly capable of walking on her own. Your coworker overhears her remark and comments that if she falls it is her own fault.

What Is Your Response/Action?

CRITICAL THINKING

CUSTOMER SERVICE Many patients find it difficult to do anything when they are in pain. If you have patients who have arthritis, do not attempt to get them to the bathroom for a shower if they are complaining of stiffness or pain. It is better to wait until after they have taken their medication to reduce pain or swelling, and they are feeling less discomfort. Some patients find the warm shower makes them feel better. Remember that many patients feel worse when exposed to cold and dampness, so avoid chilling patients as you give them a bed bath.

CULTURAL CARE Male patients in some cultures consider complaining of pain or asking for assistance a sign of weakness. Pay attention to signs of pain like grimacing or gritting of the teeth if you are moving patients or assisting them. Reassure patients that you are there to help as needed and you will allow them to do as much as they can for themselves.

COOPERATION WITHIN THE TEAM You may be the first person who notices that there is a problem with a patient's cast or that he may have an infection. Be sure to report any of the following to your supervisor: pain, swelling, blue finger beds or toenails, numbness, foul odor or drainage, or any signs of fever. The patient may be more likely to ask you a question about any of these things to see if it is a problem.

EXPLORE MediaLink

Additional interactive resources for this chapter can be found on the Companion Website at www.prenhall.com/wolgin. Click on Chapter 16 and "Begin" to select the activities for this chapter.

For chapter-related NCLEX-style questions and an audio glossary, access the accompanying CD-ROM in this book.

OBJECTIVES

When you have completed this chapter, you will be able to:

- Describe the functions of the skin, including how heat is conserved and dispersed.
- List the conditions to take note of or report when examining a person's skin.
- Describe the common disorders of the skin.
- Describe age-related changes in the skin.
- Describe pressure ulcers and list the factors that contribute to their development.
- Discuss how to prevent pressure ulcers.
- Discuss guidelines for foot care.
- Describe the equipment and devices that reduce pressure on the skin.
- Describe the procedure for safe skin cleansing and moisturizing.

MediaLink

www.prenhall.com/wolgin

Use the address above to access the free, interactive Companion Website created for this textbook. Get hints, instant feedback, and textbook references to chapter-related NCLEX-style questions. Link to other interesting sites.

AUDIO GLOSSARY:

Use the Companion Website, or the CD-ROM disk enclosed with your textbook, to hear the pronunciation of key terms in the chapter.

KEY TERMS

atrophic skin
bony prominences
dermis
epidermis
friction injuries
incontinent
integumentary system
lesion
obese
perineum
pressure ulcers
shear injuries

INTRODUCTION

Nursing assistants often care for patients who are elderly or who have disabilities. These patients are at high risk for skin injuries. This chapter provides you with the knowledge and skills needed to provide care that promotes comfort, protects the skin, and prevents injury to the skin. This includes assessing skin conditions, safe skin cleansing and moisturizing, and the careful planning of daily activities to include time to complete skin care.

The Skin (Integumentary System)

ALERT

For all patient contact, adhere to Standard Precautions (⊕ Chapter 5, pages 83–85). Wear protective equipment as indicated.

integumentary system The body system that includes the skin, hair, nails, and sweat and oil glands, that provides the first line of defense against infection, maintains body temperature, provides fluids, and eliminates wastes

The components of the **integumentary system** include the skin, hair, nails, and sweat and oil glands. The skin provides the first line of defense against infection, the maintenance of body temperature, the balance of body fluids, and the elimination of wastes. Skin covers and protects underlying structures from injury or bacterial invasion. Skin also contains nerve endings from the nervous system. A cross section of the skin is shown in Figure 17–1◆.

The skin helps regulate the body temperature by controlling the loss of heat from the body. To promote heat loss, the blood vessels near the skin dilate, and the increased blood flow brings more heat to the skin's surface. Then the skin temperature rises and more heat is lost from the hot skin to the cooler environment. Even more important in heat loss is the evaporation of sweat (perspiration) that carries heat away from the skin.

Perspiration is released from the body through *sweat glands,* which are distributed over the entire skin surface. The glands open through ducts or pores. The body also disposes of certain waste products through perspiration.

Conversely, when the body must conserve heat, sweating stops and blood vessels constrict. This prevents the blood from carrying heat to the skin. The skin temperature falls, decreasing heat loss. In this way, the body temperature is kept almost constant.

Oil glands below the skin's surface secrete a thick, oily substance through the ducts that lead to the skin surface. In this way, the skin is lubricated and kept soft and pliable. The oil also provides a protective film for the skin, which limits the absorption and evaporation of water from the surface. During the aging process, these oil glands sometimes fail to function properly, and the skin becomes dry, scaly, and delicate.

FIGURE 17–1 ◆

A cross section of the skin

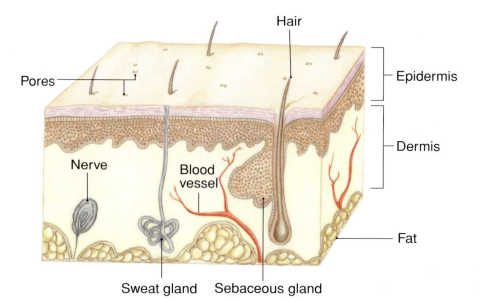

Appendages of the Skin

In addition to the skin and the sweat and oil glands, other parts of the integumentary system include the hair and the nails. Each hair has a root embedded in the skin into which the oil glands of the skin open. Fingernails and toenails grow from the nail bed at the base underneath. If the nail bed is destroyed, the nail stops growing.

The skin covers the entire body. The outer layer of the skin (the layer you can see) is called the **epidermis**. Cells are constantly flaking off or being rubbed off this outer layer of skin. Beneath the epidermis is the **dermis**. In this layer of skin are the new cells that will replace the cells that are lost from the epidermis. *Pigment* is found in the epidermis and is responsible for the color of the skin. In sunlight, through a chemical reaction, the amount of pigment increases and a suntan results. Fair-skinned people have less pigment and are more easily sunburned.

Moisture on the skin can pick up dust and dirt from the air. This moisture can also mix with the skin particles being flaked off the epidermis. This process causes a condition that promotes the growth and spread of bacteria, which is the main reason for keeping the skin clean. The skin is where the battle against infection begins.

epidermis The outer layer or surface of the skin

dermis The inner layer of skin

Primary Functions of the Skin

The primary functions of the skin are to:

- Cover and protect underlying body structures from injury and invasion by micro-organisms
- Help regulate body temperature by controlling loss of heat from the body
- Provide a first line of defense against infection
- Store energy in the form of fat and vitamins
- Eliminate wastes through perspiration
- Allow sensory perception, that is, the sense of touch (the nerves in the skin can sense heat, cold, pain, and pressure)

Inspecting the Skin

KEY IDEA

Patients who are totally immobile, are incontinent, and have limited sensation are at greatest risk for skin breakdown.

Caregivers are often the first to notice subtle changes in a patient's skin or appearance which may signal serious health problems. When examining a person's skin, be sure to note the following:

- Skin color
- Skin temperature
- Excessive moisture or dryness
- Darkened or reddened areas, especially over bony prominences
- Rashes
- Swelling
- Bruising
- Skin tears
- Wounds/ulcers
- Other abnormalities

Common Disorders of the Skin

The common disorders of the skin are:

lesion An abnormality, either benign or cancerous, of the tissues of the body, such as a wound, sore, rash, boil, tumor, or growth

- **Skin lesions:** a **lesion** is an abnormality of body tissues, either benign or cancerous, such as a wound, sore, rash, boil, tumor (lumps), or growth
- **Scales:** layers of dead skin found on the skin surface
- **Excoriations:** reddened, scratched, or broken areas caused by the wearing away of the skin's surface
- **Pressure ulcer:** area of tissue destruction or a lesion resulting from prolonged, unrelieved, pressure

pressure ulcers Also called bedsores; areas of the skin that become broken and painful; caused by continuous pressure on a body part and usually occur when a patient is kept in one position for a long period of time

- **Vascular ulcer:** area of skin breakdown related to abnormalities of the vascular system
- **Diabetic ulcer:** an ulcer that occurs in people with diabetes resulting from dysfunction of the nerve
- **Furuncle:** acute inflammation that starts in a hair follicle
- **Impetigo:** superficial infection caused by streptococci staphylococci, or other bacteria
- **Fungus:** caused by plantlike organisms, which includes athlete's foot
- **Infestations:**
  - Pediculosis capitus (scabies/head lice)
  - Pediculosis corporis (body lice)
  - Pediculosis pubis (crab lice)
- **Herpes zoster (shingles):** inflammatory condition caused by the chicken pox virus that produces painful eruptions
- **Dermatitis:** reaction to irritating or allergenic materials
- **Psoriasis:** chronic condition of crusty circular patches for which the cause is unknown
- **Burns:** excessive exposure to heat or fire
- **Maceration:** skin breakdown (reddened area) caused by excessive moisture usually in skin folds of perineum of incontinent patients

atrophic skin Thin, fragile, less elastic skin frequently associated with aging

friction injuries Injuries resulting from the patient sliding against hard surfaces

shear injuries Result from the skin remaining in place on top of a surface while the underlying structures, such as the bone, slide downward

- **Atrophic skin:** fragile, thin skin, often associated with aging
- **Friction injuries:** result from the patient sliding against hard surfaces
- **Shear injuries:** result from skin remaining in place on top of a surface and the underlying structures, such as the bone, sliding downward without the skin moving

 AGE-SPECIFIC CONSIDERATIONS

Changes in the Skin

As people age, they develop atrophic skin, which can become thin, fragile, and less elastic (like tissue paper). Atrophic skin can be injured more easily. Elderly people need gentle cleansing and moisturizing (applying lotion) to keep their skin as healthy as possible and prevent skin tears and scrapes, which can lead to infection.

An elderly person's skin may also develop brown spots, particularly on the hands and arms. Fingernails and toenails may thicken and become abnormally shaped.

Always report any changes in skin condition to your immediate supervisor, particularly:

- Redness of skin (*erythema*), which can mean increased body temperature, prolonged pressure, infection, or injury

- A blue or gray color (*cyanosis*), which can mean decreased circulation, a life-threatening condition

- A black or "scablike" skin area (*eschar*), which can disguise a more serious skin problem underneath. A scab does not necessarily mean that a wound is healing well

- A very pale or white color can mean circulatory problems related to anemia, impaired circulation to body parts, or shock

KEY IDEA

An elderly person usually experiences loss of fat under the skin, which makes sitting or lying on hard surfaces even more uncomfortable. In addition, loss of fat makes a person feel cold even when room temperatures feel warm to others. For this reason, it is important to keep elderly patients dressed warmly or well covered in bed or when you are giving nursing care.

Care of the Patient with Potential Skin Problems

Pressure Ulcers

Pressure ulcers, also called decubitus ulcers or bedsores, are areas where the skin has broken down because of prolonged underlying pressure (Figure 17–2◆). Injury to the skin comes from pressure on a part of the body where there is loss of circulation (blood flow), which destroys tissues. The pressure cuts off circulation and nourishment to skin areas over the **bony prominences**. These are places where bones are close to the surface of the skin. The pressure can come from the weight of the body lying in one position for too long or from splints, casts, or bandages. If pressure ulcers are not treated, they quickly get larger and become very painful. Even wrinkles in the bed linen can be a cause of pressure sores.

bony prominences Places where bones are close to the surface of the skin

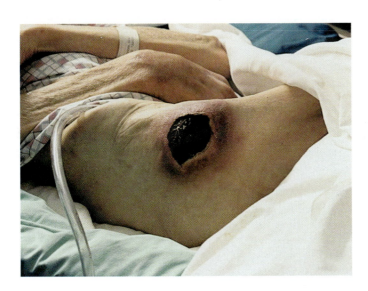

FIGURE 17–2 ◆

Pressure ulcers are broken areas of the skin caused by the loss of circulation to that area; ulcers are the result of continual pressure when a patient remains in the same position too long

Injury to the skin comes from pressure on a part of the body where there is loss of circulation (blood flow), which destroys tissues.

Pressure ulcers are often made worse by continued pressure, moisture, and lack of cleanliness. Irritating substances on the skin such as perspiration, urine, feces, material from wound discharges, or soap that has been left on the skin after a bath all tend to make skin conditions worse.

Risk Factors for Pressure Ulcer Development

Certain conditions are associated with pressure ulcer breakdown. Patients with even one of these risk factors are at risk for skin breakdown. The patient with more than one risk factor is at even greater risk. These patients need considerable assistance from the nurses to prevent pressure ulcers. The conditions for risk include:

- *Loss of Sensory Perception:* patients who are unresponsive and have a limited ability to feel pain over large parts of their bodies
- *Moist Skin:* skin that is almost constantly moist from perspiration, urine, or loose stools can break down
- *Limited Activity:* patients who are bedfast and chairfast
- *Immobility:* patients who do not move on their own while in bed or in the chair
- *Friction and Shear:* frequent sliding down and pulling up in bed can cause the patient to slide over the sheets
- *Poor Nutrition or Poor Hydration:* patients who do not eat all their food and are not on tube feedings can be vulnerable to skin breakdown

Notify your supervisor if a patient starts to decrease activity and stops eating regular meals and snacks. Early small areas of skin breakdown also need to be reported immediately. They can signal much larger problems.

Signs of a Pressure Ulcer

The signs of a pressure ulcer on the skin are heat, redness, tenderness, discomfort, and a feeling of burning. When there is a darkened or reddened area that doesn't fade after 20 minutes, a pressure ulcer has formed (Figure 17–3◆). If pressure is not relieved, the skin may break open. Specific treatments for pressure sores are prescribed by a doctor or

FIGURE 17–3 ◆

Tissue under pressure; the ulcer visible on the surface is often much smaller than the skin damage below the skin surface

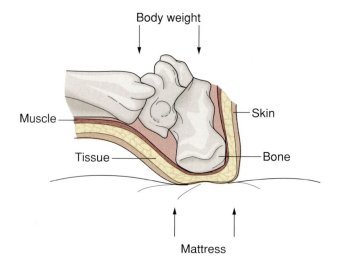

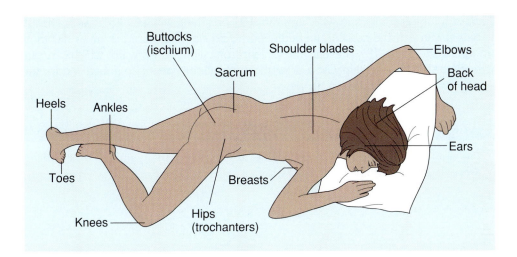

FIGURE 17–4 ◆

Check for signs of pressure ulcers over bony prominences

nurse specialist. The wound must be kept clean. As you have already learned, the skin is the body's first line of defense against infection.

KEY IDEA

Bony prominences are the areas where pressure sores are most likely to occur when patients lie or sit on them continually.

Places to check on the body for signs of pressure are the bony areas (prominences) (Figure 17–4◆). These include the shoulder blades, elbows, knees, heels, hips, sides of ankles, back of the head, above the ears, and the lower tip of the spine (sacrum). Sitting in any type of chair for too long can cause pressure over the bones in the buttocks (ischium). Usually these areas are covered only by a thin layer of skin.

Preventing Pressure Ulcers

Once a mild ulcer has formed, it can be very hard to cure. It is critical that nursing assistants report the first sign of a pressure sore to their immediate supervisor so that steps can be taken to prevent further damage.

KEY IDEA

Preventing pressure ulcers is the responsibility of the entire health care team. We now know that nearly all pressure sores *can* be prevented.

Immobile patients and bedridden patients are at risk for developing friction and shear injury from sliding over rough surfaces. When the head of the bed is elevated too high, the patient slides down in bed causing a *friction/shear injury*. Position the head of the bed below 30 degrees (Figure 17–5◆) unless there is a medical reason to have it elevated.

FIGURE 17–5 ◆

Example of head of bed raised 30 degrees; heels are raised off the bed

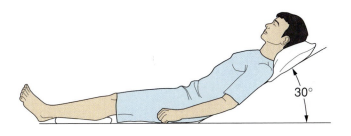

Patients on tube feedings and who have difficulty breathing will need to have the head of the bed elevated. If the head of the bed needs to be elevated, raise the knees slightly before raising the head. This prevents the patient from sliding downward, which can cause friction and shear on the skin. Use a draw sheet to pull the patient up in bed and for turning to prevent friction and shear injuries.

KEY IDEA

The nursing assistant can group activities together and plan work so that patients are assisted into different positions within a safe time frame.

obese Very overweight

GUIDELINES — OBRA

PREVENTING PRESSURE ULCERS

The nursing assistant can help to prevent bedsores by doing the following:

- Change the patient's position every 2 hours. A turning schedule at the bedside is helpful when there are multiple caregivers (Figure 17–6◆).

- Be careful when using bedpans. Pressure from sitting on the rim and friction when moving the patient on and off the bedpan can create or worsen ulcers. Never leave the patient on the bedpan longer than necessary. Use care when removing the bedpan to avoid spilling urine on the skin. Urine is irritating to the skin and can cause further damage to a reddened or tender area. Powdering the rim of the bedpan can minimize friction when removed.

- Keep the patient's body as clean and dry as possible. Change the patient's gown or clothing if it is damp. Wash the patient's skin with mild soap or use special incontinent cleansers to remove urine or feces. Rinse well with clean warm water. Use moisture barriers on the skin to prevent contact with discharged materials from wounds, which can cause irritation.

- If a part of the patient's body shows signs of developing a pressure ulcer, notify the skin care nurse or health care provider and do not position the patient on that area until the redness or ulcer has disappeared. Position the patient on the turning surfaces that do not have ulcers.

- Use powder or corn starch sparingly where skin surfaces come together and form creases. Examples are under the breasts of women patients, between buttocks, and in the folds of skin on the abdomen or groin. Do not apply powder in areas of open sores or surgical incisions. When bathing the patient, be sure to wash the powder or corn starch off completely. This is especially important in caring for obese patients. Corn starch is less caking when in contact with moisture and is preferred over powders. To help prevent caking, the corn starch or powder should be rubbed into the skin, much like when applying lotion.

- **Obese** (very overweight) patients tend to develop sores where body

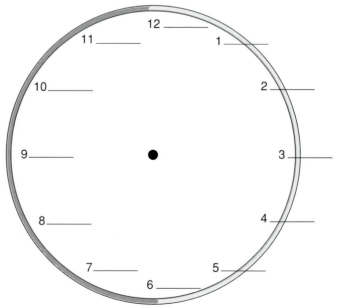

Turning schedule: Indicate position change on the lines above.
R = right side; L = left side; B = back; S = stomach; C = chair.

FIGURE 17–6 ◆

A sample turning schedule

GUIDELINES *(continued)*

parts rub against each other, causing friction. Places to check on obese patients are the folds of the body where skin touches skin, such as under the breasts, between the folds of the buttocks, and between the thighs. Pillows are used to provide support, separate skin surfaces, and prevent skin breakdown. It is necessary to avoid all skin-to-skin contact. Use pillows between the knees.

- Keep linens wrinkle free and dry at all times.

- Remove crumbs, hair pins, and any other hard objects from the bed promptly.

- If the patient is **incontinent** (unable to control urine or feces), use incontinent pads. These can be disposable or reusable. Never use more than two layers of incontinent pads. If more than two layers of incontinent pads are used, the patient will be at greater risk of pressure sore develop-

ment. To be sure that plastic never touches the patient's skin, place a sheet between the patient and the plastic disposable pads (Figure 17-7◆). Change the incontinent pads immediately when they become wet.

- Disposable plastic diapers can be used when the incontinent patient is

out of bed. However, they must be removed when the patient is returned to bed. The closed, wet plastic environment can result in maceration of the skin and skin breakdown.

- For pressure ulcer staying and treatment see Table 17-1.

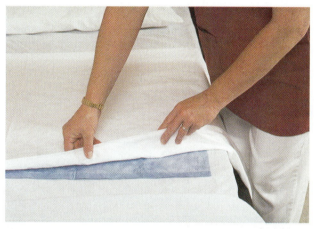

FIGURE 17-7 ◆
Place a sheet between disposable plastic incontinent pads and the patient

Foot Care

Preventing pressure ulcers on the feet requires special attention and knowledge.

incontinent Unable to control urine or feces

KEY IDEA

Pressure sores on the feet can be serious, sometimes leading to amputation and even death.

GUIDELINES   **OBRA**

FOOT CARE

- Never soak a patient's feet without a doctor's order.

- Wash a patient's feet daily with mild soap and water.

- Rinse well and dry the feet thoroughly. Do not pull towels through toes as this can cut the skin.

- Apply lotion to the feet except for the area between toes.

- Notify the nurse or podiatrist for nail care. Do not attempt to trim a patient's nails unless you have been trained to do so.

- Use pillows to dangle heels (Figure 17-8◆). Place each pillow lengthwise under the calf and tuck in to prevent heel from touching.

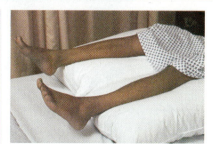

FIGURE 17-8 ◆
Use pillows to dangle the heels to prevent pressure areas

TABLE 17–1

Pressure Ulcer Staging and Treatment*

STAGE†	TREATMENT PROTOCOL FOR PRESSURE ULCER STAGES
Stage I: Nonblanchable erythema of Intact skin, the heralding lesion of skin ulceration.	*Stage I:* Apply an adhesive film dressing over the red area. These dressings are semipermeable to oxygen and prevent bacterial invasion. Healing can occur in 24 hours.
Stage II: Partial-thickness skin loss involving epidermis or dermis. The ulcer is superficial and presents clinically as an abrasion, blister, or shallow crater.	*Stage II:* Apply a transparent adhesive film dressing if ulcer is not draining. If wound is draining irrigate with normal saline and apply a hydrocolloid dressing. These occlusive dressings remain in place for 5–7 days, creating a moist environment that promotes epithelializatiod and restoration of the epidermis.
Stage III: Full-thickness skin loss involving damage or necrosis of subcucaneous tissue that may extend down to, but not through, underlying fascla. The ulcer presents clinically as a deep crater with or without the undermining of adjacent tissue.	*Stage III:* Irrigate with normal saline, cover with a hydrocolloid dressing. With excessively draining wounds, absorptive products are placed in the wound for absorption, and then the dressing is applied.
Stage IV: Full-thickness skin loss with extensive destruction, tissue necrosis, or damage to muscle, bone, or supporting structures (tendon or joint capsule are examples). Undermining and sinus tracts may be associated with this stage ulcer.	*Stage IV:* Chemical debridement, autolysis, or surgery are required for treatment of this stage. Wet-to-damp or wet-to-tacky dressing changes are used for small wounds; surgical interventions are used for larger wounds.

*SOURCE: Pressure Ulcers in Adults: Prediction and Prevention. Rockvile. MO: U.S. Department of Health and Human Services, Public Health Service, Agency for Health Care Policy and Research.

†Pressure ulcers are classified in stages by the degree of tissue damage observed.

Accurate staging of pressure ulcers is not possible until eschar has sloughed or wound is debrided.

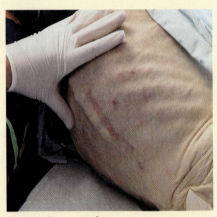

Stage I Pressure ulcer.

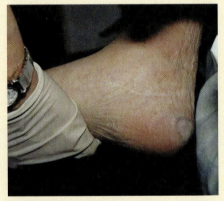

Stage II Pressure ulcer.

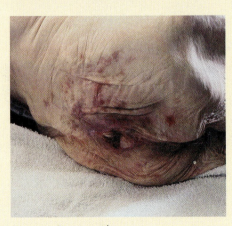

Stage III Pressure ulcer.

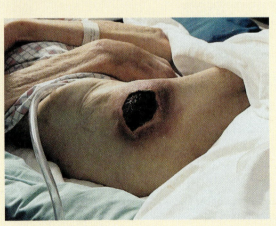

Stage IV Pressure ulcer.

Equipment and Devices That Reduce Pressure on the Skin

Special equipment may be ordered to reduce the pressure on the skin. Devices are available to protect patients while they are in bed or sitting in chairs. Bed and chair cushions are made from a variety of materials. Foam mattresses and overlays can be used for patients at low risk. Air and gel mattresses provide greater pressure reduction for people at high risk for breakdown.

Mattresses, Overlays, and Beds

Foam Mattresses

- ***Purpose:*** A softer mattress prevents pressure ulcers.
- ***Precautions:*** Turn patients every 2 hours and elevate the heels of immobile patients. Ask if your institution has this type of mattress.

Four-Inch High-Density Foam

- ***Purpose:*** An overlay for assisting in the prevention of pressure ulcers.
- ***Precautions:*** Place foam in plastic covering to prevent soiling. Use for one patient only, then discard.

Static Air Mattress

- ***Purpose:*** An overlay for preventing pressure ulcers.
- ***Precautions:*** Follow the manufacturer's operating instructions. Do not puncture. Turn the patient every 2 hours and elevate the heels of immobile patients. Use for one patient only, then discard (Figure 17–9a◆).

Alternating Air Mattress

- ***Purpose:*** Redistributes the pressure on a timed, automatic basis.
- ***Precautions:*** Be sure the motor and mattress are working correctly. Do not puncture. Use only one loosely applied sheet between the patient and the mattress.

Eggcrate Mattress

- ***Purpose:*** Provides comfort.
- ***Precautions:*** These mattresses do not protect patient from pressure ulcers (Figure 17–9b◆).

Specialty Bed

- ***Purpose:*** Provides pressure relief over most of the body and is an excellent device to promote wound healing.
- ***Precautions:*** Patients still need to be turned while on a specialty bed and their heels and the back of the head still need to be elevated off the bed surface while the patient is immobile. Use the manufacturer's recommended incontinent pads (Figure 17–10◆).

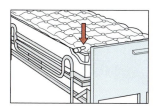
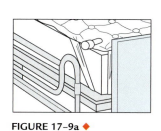

FIGURE 17–9a ◆

Static air mattress overlay

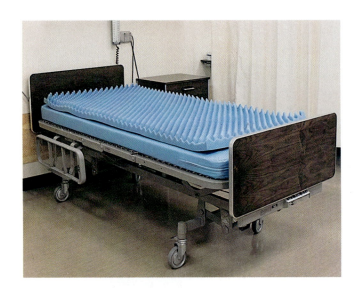
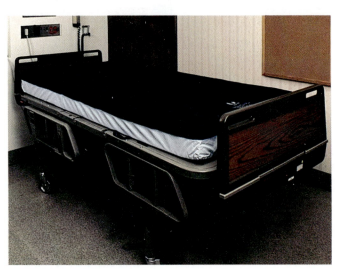

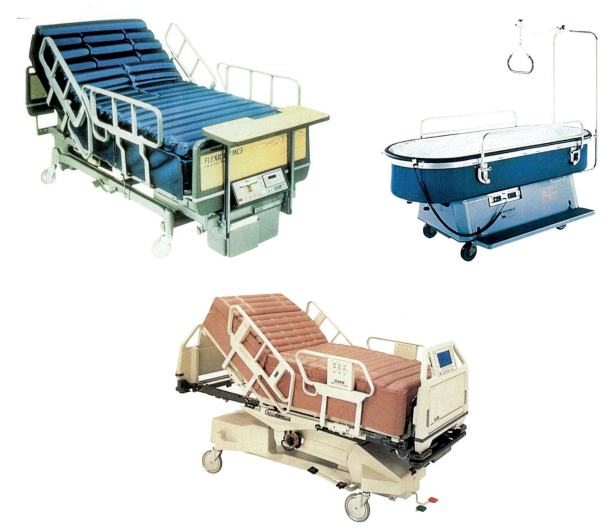

FIGURE 17–9b ◆

Eggcrate and special gel nonpressure mattresses reduce skin breakdown

FIGURE 17–10 ◆

An air fluidized mattress is one type of specialty bed used for patients at risk for skin breakdown

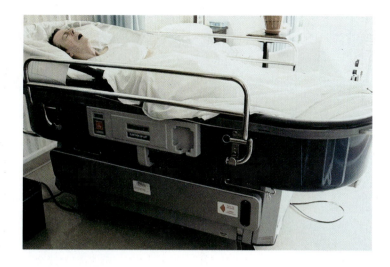

Chair Cushions

Special pressure reduction devices can be used in chairs. Patients at risk for pressure ulcers need therapeutic foam (4-inch, high-density foam, gel pads or air pads) in their chairs (Figure 17–11◆). Do not allow patients to sit on *round doughnuts* without a doctor's order as this can cause poor circulation.

Wheelchair cushions conform to the body when a patient is sitting. Place the cushion properly in the chair and cover with a cloth.

Extremities: Foot, Heel, Arms

A pillow placed lengthwise under the calf with the heel dangling is the best device for protecting the heels. Many other products do not stay in place or the straps for attachment cause pressure ulcers.

Protective Boots

- **Purpose:** To reduce pressure. These come in multiple shapes and styles, but the most effective styles have scooped-out heels to relieve pressure completely.
- **Precautions:** If the boot contains any plastic, do not allow contact with the other, unprotected foot.
- **Alternative example:** High-top style athletic shoes can be used as an alternative orthotic device to prevent foot drop. These are worn by the patient in bed 2 hours on and 2 hours off.

Orthotic Devices

- **Purpose:** To prevent foot drop and keep covers off the patient's feet.
- **Precautions:** Effective device when patient is lying on the back. Observe for pressure on the buttocks and turn patient while device is off to relieve pressure (Figure 17–12a◆ and 17–12b◆).

Foot Elevators ("Donuts")

- **Purpose:** To elevate an extremity off the bed. Very effective for immobile patients.
- **Precautions:** Must be removed for daily washing of feet and for inspection of the skin. Must be properly applied. Check skin for rubbing (Figure 17–13◆).

FIGURE 17–11 ◆

Foam cushion in wheelchair

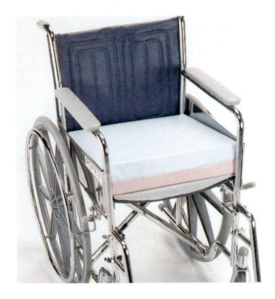

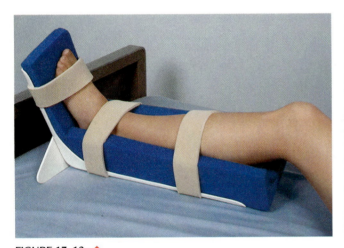

FIGURE 17–12a ◆

Footdrop splint (Photo courtesy of Posey Company, Arcadia, CA)

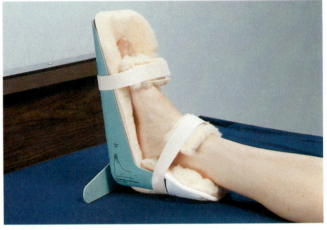

FIGURE 17–12b ◆

Footguard (Photo courtesy of Posey Company, Arcadia, CA)

FIGURE 17–13 ◆

Foot elevator (Photo courtesy of
Posey Company, Arcadia, CA)

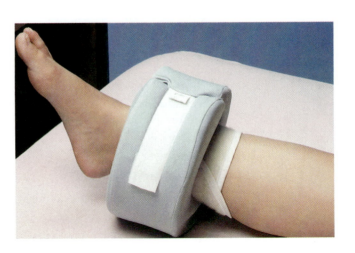

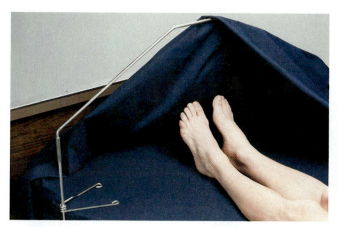

FIGURE 17–14 ◆

Bed cradle (Photo courtesy of Posey Company, Arcadia, CA)

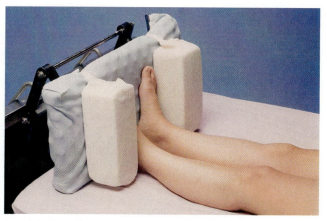

FIGURE 17–15 ◆

Adjustable footboard (Photo courtesy of Posey Company, Arcadia, CA)

Foot Cradle

- *Purpose:* To keep bed coverings off the legs and feet.
- *Precautions:* Patient may feel cold, requiring extra blankets to provide additional warmth. Be sure the bed covering is off legs (Figure 17–14◆).

Footboard

- *Purpose:* Helps prevent footdrop by keeping the foot in an upright position, as well as keeping the covers off the patient's feet.
- *Precautions:* Effective device when the patient is lying on the back. Turn the patient every 2 hours and elevate heels (Figure 17–15◆).

Sheepskin Pad

- *Purpose:* Reduces friction or rubbing against sheets.
- *Precautions:* Does not eliminate pressure (Figure 17–16◆).

Heel or Elbow Protectors

- *Purpose:* Reduces friction or rubbing against sheets. Decreases friction or rubbing against bed linens.

FIGURE 17–16 ◆

Sheepskin pad

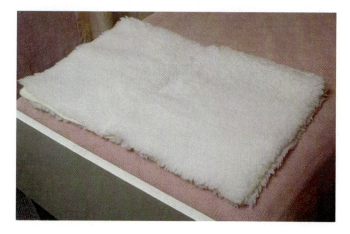

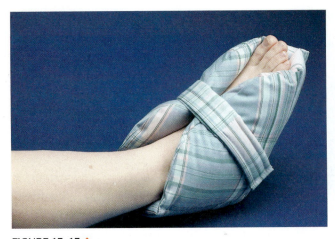

FIGURE 17–17 ◆

Heel pillow (Photo courtesy of Posey Company, Arcadia, CA)

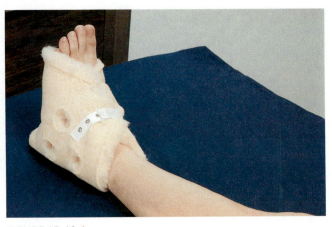

FIGURE 17–18 ◆

Heel protector (Photo courtesy of Posey Company, Arcadia, CA)

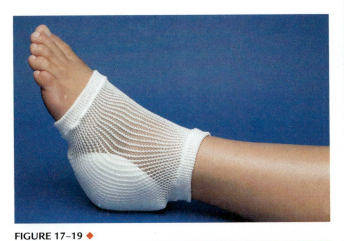

FIGURE 17–19 ◆

Elastic mesh heel protector (Photo courtesy of Posey Company, Arcadia, CA)

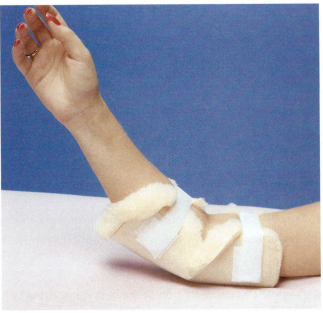

FIGURE 17–20 ◆

Elbow protector (Photo courtesy of Posey Company, Arcadia, CA)

■ **Precautions:** Make sure that these are applied properly and that they remain in place, especially when under the covers where they cannot be seen. May cause pressure ulcers if not worn properly. They do not prevent pressure ulcers (Figures 17–17◆, 17–18◆, 17–19◆, and 17–20◆).

Other Devices

Foam rings can be used to reduce the pressure on the back of the head. Unconscious patients need to have the head position changed every 2 hours even when a foam ring is used.

SAFE SKIN CLEANSING FOR THE INCONTINENT PATIENT

PROCEDURE

OBRA

RATIONALE: Keeping skin clean and protected from breakdown is a priority with incontinent patients.

PREPARATION

1. Assemble your equipment:

   a. disposable gloves

   b. tissues or disposable washcloths

   c. bedpan

   d. incontinent spray or soap

   e. towel

   f. moisture lotion or barrier

   g. corn starch or powder

   h. incontinent pad

   i. bed sheet

2. Wash your hands.

3. Identify the patient by checking the identification bracelet.

4. Ask visitors to step out of the room, if this is your hospital's policy.

5. Tell the patient that you are going to wash him.

6. Provide privacy for the patient.

7. Raise the bed to a comfortable working position.

8. Raise the side rail on the far side of the bed.

STEPS

9. Put on the disposable gloves.

10. Using tissue or disposable washcloths, wipe away as much feces and urine as possible. Then wash the area that has urine or feces on it very well, removing all waste material from the skin. Place soiled tissue into the bedpan. Use the incontinent sprays to cleanse the skin if available. These are convenient, help to eliminate odors, and the spray can be directed to specific areas.

11. If there is soap on the skin, rinse well with clean water, changing the water frequently. Many incontinent sprays do not require rinsing, thus saving time and trauma to the skin. Special cleansing foams do not run and cause less discomfort than cold sprays.

12. Pat the skin dry to prevent injury or pain from rubbing. If the skin is red and macerated, use soft tissues to blot the skin dry.

13. Apply a moisture lotion or barrier to the **perineum** (area between and around rectum and urinary opening) of any patient with incontinence.

14. Apply corn starch or powder only where skin surfaces touch other skin surfaces (creases and skin folds). Dust lightly and close to the skin surface to prevent excessive dust particles from floating into the air. The corn starch or powder should be gently rubbed into the skin. Do not apply powder in areas of open sores or surgical incisions.

15. Do not put disposable plastic diapers on the patient while still in bed. This holds moisture next to the skin and can cause skin maceration and skin infections.

16. Place an incontinent pad under the patient. Do not place patient directly on top of a plastic disposable pad. Put a sheet over the disposable plastic pad, between the pad and the patient. Do not use more than two layers of pads under the patient at a time.

17. Position, cover, and make the patient comfortable.

18. Lower the bed to a position of safety for the patient.

19. Replace the side rails to the proper position.

20. Discard disposable equipment.

21. Place soiled linen in the laundry bag, and then place the bag into the dirty linen hamper in the utility room.

22. Remove and discard gloves, then wash your hands.

FOLLOW-UP

23. Check for incontinent episodes every 2 hours. Remake the bed as necessary.

24. Report to your immediate supervisor:

   - That the patient was incontinent of urine and/or feces.

   - That the patient was washed and the skin is now clean and dry.

   - That the patient's position was changed every 2 hours, and the time of each position change.

   - Any signs of skin breakdown.

   - The color, amount, and consistency of the feces and urine you cleaned.

   - How the patient tolerated the procedure.

   - Your observations of anything unusual.

CHARTING EXAMPLE: 10/04/04 3pm Mrs. Kidd incontinent of urine. Perineal care performed and barrier cream applied to her perineum. Skin intact, no signs of breakdown. M. Worth, CNA

perineum The body area between the thighs (external genitalia and rectal area)

SUMMARY

Much of your time as a nursing assistant is spent providing routine skin care and preventing skin breakdown. Turning and repositioning the patient, eliminating friction and shear, and keeping the patient clean and dry are the keys to providing excellent care.

NOTES

CHAPTER REVIEW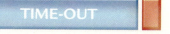

FILL IN THE BLANK Read each sentence and fill in the blank line with a word that completes the sentence.

1. _____ is the outer layer or surface of the skin.

2. _____ is the inner layer of skin.

3. A _____ _____ is an area of tissue destruction or lesion resulting
   from prolonged, unrelieved pressure.

4. When the head of the bed is elevated too high, and the patient slides down in bed, it can result in a
   _____ or _____ injury.

5. Pressure sores on the feet can be serious, sometimes leading to _____ and even death.

MULTIPLE CHOICE Choose the best answer for each question or statement.

1. Which of the following is not a function of the integumentary system?
   a. The skin is the first line of defense against infection.
   b. The skin maintains body temperature.
   c. The skin covers and protects underlying structures from injury.
   d. The skin provides movement for the body.

2. Which of the following is not an observation about skin?
   a. Color
   b. Pressure
   c. Rashes
   d. Reddened, darkened areas

3. Which of the following is not a common disorder of the skin?
   a. Arthritis
   b. Excoriations
   c. Impetigo
   d. Herpes zoster

4. As patients age, their skin may experience all of these changes *except*
   a. thinning of skin.
   b. atrophy of skin.
   c. development of brown spots.
   d. reddening of skin.

5. Which of these following conditions should you report to the nurse?
   a. Reddening of skin
   b. Cyanosis
   c. A black "scablike" skin (eschar)
   d. All of the above.

TIME-OUT

TIPS FOR TIME MANAGEMENT

Before you begin a procedure, anticipate what the patient might need during the procedure. Plan
time for as many of these needs as possible. Offer assistance to the bathroom before you begin.
Plan rest periods during the procedure if the patient is weak or short of breath.

THE NURSING ASSISTANT IN ACTION

You are caring for an elderly woman who is diabetic. The skin on both of her swollen legs is red. You see she has new sores on both legs. Ms. Francis tells you that the skin on her legs feels like it is burning. She applied some lotion on them and that only made it worse.

What Is Your Response/Action?

CRITICAL THINKING

CUSTOMER SERVICE Many frail or obese patients are unable to care for their skin as much as necessary to keep it clean and healthy. Offer to help them soak their feet or perform a back rub. The patient will usually feel better and you will have the opportunity to observe their skin at the same time.

CULTURAL CARE There are wide variations in skin color and texture. Pale thin skin can be easily damaged. You need to look carefully when examining patients with dark skin tones for signs of redness or bruising.

COOPERATION WITHIN THE TEAM Keeping skin intact and clean requires teamwork. When caring for adult patients who need to be lifted, be sure to have help from a coworker or use back-saving devices when available in the facility. Check that areas over bony prominences are protected. You are often the first person who notices skin breakdown or problems. The sooner that treatment begins, the easier it is to return the patient's skin to its usual condition. Nurses and physicians depend on your observations.

EXPLORE MediaLink

Additional interactive resources for this chapter can be found on the Companion Website at www.prenhall.com/wolgin. Click on Chapter 17 and "Begin" to select the activities for this chapter.

For chapter-related NCLEX-style questions and an audio glossary, access the accompanying CD-ROM in this book.

OBJECTIVES

When you have completed this chapter, you will be able to:

- Describe the functions of the heart and blood.
- Label a diagram with the organs of the circulatory and respiratory systems.
- Describe the functions of the respiratory system.
- Summarize how the circulatory and respiratory systems change with age.
- Identify common diseases and disorders of the respiratory and circulatory systems.
- List important precautions for patients with tuberculosis.
- List important precautions for patients receiving oxygen therapy.

MediaLink
www.prenhall.com/wolgin

Use the address above to access the free, interactive Companion Website created for this textbook. Get hints, instant feedback, and textbook references to chapter-related NCLEX-style questions. Link to other interesting sites.

AUDIO GLOSSARY:
Use the Companion Website, or the CD-ROM disk enclosed with your textbook, to hear the pronunciation of key terms in the chapter.

KEY TERMS

anemia
artery
blood pressure
cardiac
circulation
circulatory system
heart
plasma
pulmonary
respiratory system
tuberculosis (TB)
vein

INTRODUCTION

The circulatory system is responsible for getting all the necessary nutrients to a cell for its metabolism. It also carries away the cell's by-products and waste material. The circulatory system works closely with the respiratory system. Any problems in one system can affect the other system very quickly. This chapter describes the major components of each system and how each works. You will also learn about problems that may develop in the circulatory and respiratory systems, including special precautions for patients with tuberculosis, low blood pressure from inactivity, and other conditions.

The Circulatory System: Anatomy and Physiology

ALERT

For all patient contact, adhere to Standard Precautions (Chapter 5, pages 83–85). Wear protective equipment as indicated.

circulatory system The heart, blood vessels, blood, and all organs that pump and carry blood and other fluids throughout the body

The **circulatory system** (Figure 18–1♦) is made up of the heart, the blood, and the blood vessels (arteries, veins, and capillaries). Its purpose is to transport oxygen and nutrients to organs and tissues throughout the body and carry away waste products. Its functions include increasing the flow of blood to meet energy demands during exercise,

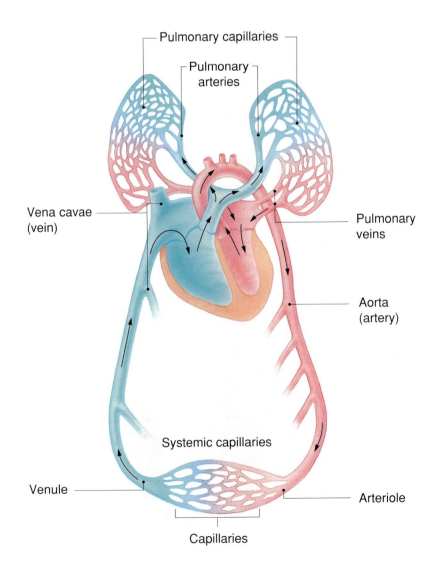

FIGURE 18–1 ♦

The circulatory system

regulate body temperature, and aid the body's immune system by transporting white blood cells and antibodies to the areas under attack by disease.

In the case of injury or bleeding, the circulatory system sends clotting cells and proteins to the injured site to stop bleeding and promote healing.

The circulatory system works closely with the respiratory system, which aids in the exchange of oxygen and carbon dioxide. Any problems in one system can quickly affect the other system.

The **heart** acts as a pump for the blood, which carries the nutrients, oxygen, and other elements needed by the cells. The blood vessels are the pathways through which the blood travels.

The Heart

The **heart** (Figure 18–2◆) is a muscular organ about the size of a fist that lies between the lungs in the chest cavity pointing slightly to the left. It is a pump that circulates blood through the lungs, where it picks up oxygen, and throughout the rest of the body.

The heart is made up of four chambers: the right atrium, the right ventricle, the left atrium, and the left ventricle.

heart A four-chambered, hollow, muscular organ that lies in the chest cavity and pumps the blood through the lungs and into all parts of the body

1. The *right atrium* receives unoxygenated blood from the body via the superior and inferior vena cava. The blood then flows through the tricuspid valve into the right ventricle.

2. The *right ventricle* pumps blood into the lungs via the pulmonary artery.

3. The *left atrium* receives oxygenated blood from the lungs via the four **pulmonary** veins. The blood flows through the bicuspid valve into the left ventricle.

pulmonary Pertaining to the lungs

4. The *left ventricle*, the heart's largest and strongest chamber, pumps the oxygenated blood into the systemic circulation of the body via the aorta.

KEY IDEA

The ventricles have thick walls of muscle. When they contract, the left ventricle pushes the blood through the largest blood vessel, the aorta, to all parts of the body.

The walls of the heart chambers are made up of *myocardial* muscle that contracts and relaxes continuously to pump the blood automatically. The pumping action occurs in two

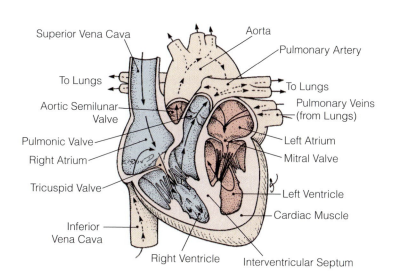

Superior Vena Cava
Aorta
Pulmonary Artery
To Lungs
To Lungs
Aortic Semilunar Valve
Pulmonary Veins (from Lungs)
Pulmonic Valve
Left Atrium
Right Atrium
Mitral Valve
Tricuspid Valve
Left Ventricle
Inferior Vena Cava
Cardiac Muscle
Right Ventricle
Interventricular Septum

FIGURE 18–2 ◆

The heart

stages for each heart beat: *systolic,* when the heart contracts to pump deoxygenated blood to the lungs and oxygenated blood to the body, and *diastolic,* when the heart is at rest.

Blood pressure is a measurement of the heart contracting and relaxing. The highest measurement (number) is the systolic pressure, which is measured when the heart is contracting, and the lower number is the diastolic measurement, which is taken when the heart is relaxing.

During each heartbeat, about 60 to 90 mL (about 2 to 3 oz.) of blood is pumped out of the heart. If the heart stops pumping, death usually occurs within 4 to 5 minutes.

blood pressure The force of the blood pushing against the walls of the blood vessels

The Blood

The blood is a kind of transportation system that transports needed elements to the cells of the body and removes waste products.

- The blood carries oxygen from the lungs to the cells.
- The blood carries carbon dioxide from the cells to the lungs.
- The blood absorbs (picks up) nutrients from the duodenum (small intestine) and carries them to the cells.
- The blood carries waste products from the cells to the kidneys to be eliminated in urine.

To carry out these functions, the blood must move continuously throughout the body. This continuous movement is called **circulation**.

The blood and blood vessels perform other functions as well:

circulation The continuous movement of blood through the heart and blood vessels to all parts of the body

- The blood transports hormones from the endocrine glands.
- The blood vessels help regulate body temperatures through dilation (enlargement) and constriction (narrowing). To bring more blood and warm up a body part, the blood vessels dilate. Constriction reduces the blood supply and lowers body temperature.
- The blood helps maintain the fluid balance of the body by helping to move sodium and potassium into and out of body cells. These elements affect how much water the body will either retain or excrete.
- The white cells of the blood defend the body against disease. They do so by destroying microorganisms they identify as a threat to the body. The white cells are sent into the blood and carried to the site of infection. There they engulf the microorganisms, and the blood carries them away to be excreted out of the body.

plasma The liquid portion of the blood

The liquid portion of the blood is called **plasma**. It contains red blood cells, white blood cells, and platelets. Platelets help to stop bleeding when the body is injured by forming clots at the site of the injury.

The red blood cells carry oxygen. People who have too few red blood cells have a type of **anemia**.

anemia A shortage of red blood cells

The white blood cells fight infection. People who have too few white blood cells have a lowered resistance to disease. An increase in white blood cells in the blood can mean that an infection is present somewhere in the body. If a patient has an inflammation in some area of the body, a physician often prescribes warm, moist compresses. These are applied to dilate the blood vessels in the area and to bring more of the important white blood cells to the place of infection to help fight it.

KEY IDEA

The blood carries oxygen and nutrients to the cells of the body. It carries away carbon dioxide (to be eliminated through the lungs) and waste products (to be eliminated through the kidneys).

The Blood Vessels

Three types of blood vessels form a complex network of tubes throughout the body. *Arteries* carry oxygenated blood away from the heart and *veins* carry blood to the heart. *Capillaries* are the tiny links between the arteries and veins where oxygen and nutrients diffuse to body tissues.

The blood vessels carrying blood that is oxygenated (having a lot of oxygen) are called **arteries**. An exception is the pulmonary artery, which carries the blood to the lungs. Arteries branch into a vast network throughout the body (Figure 18–3◆). As they branch out, the blood vessels become smaller and smaller until finally they are so thin they become capillaries.

artery Blood vessel that carries oxygenated blood away from the heart

FIGURE 18–3 ◆

The system of arteries

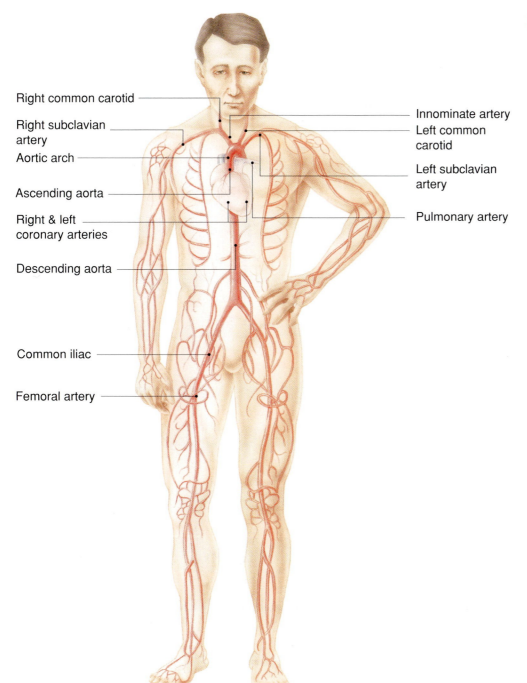

Right common carotid

Right subclavian artery

Aortic arch

Ascending aorta

Right & left coronary arteries

Descending aorta

Common iliac

Femoral artery

Innominate artery

Left common carotid

Left subclavian artery

Pulmonary artery

The walls of the capillaries are only one cell layer thick. Through these walls, gases, nutrients, waste products, and other substances are exchanged among the blood in the capillaries, the tissue fluid, and the individual cell.

After the RBCs in the blood have given up their oxygen, it returns to the heart through the **veins** (Figure 18–4◆).

The heart muscle must be supplied with blood carrying oxygen. The first branches of the aorta, the coronary arteries, come from the heart's left ventricle. These arteries surround the heart and carry needed oxygen to **cardiac** (heart muscle) tissue. If one of these coronary branches is blocked by a blood clot (thrombus), the patient has a heart attack, which can result in the death of some heart tissue. The event is called a *myocardial infarction* (MI).

vein Blood vessel that carries blood from parts of the body back to the heart

cardiac Pertaining to the heart

FIGURE 18–4 ◆

The system of veins

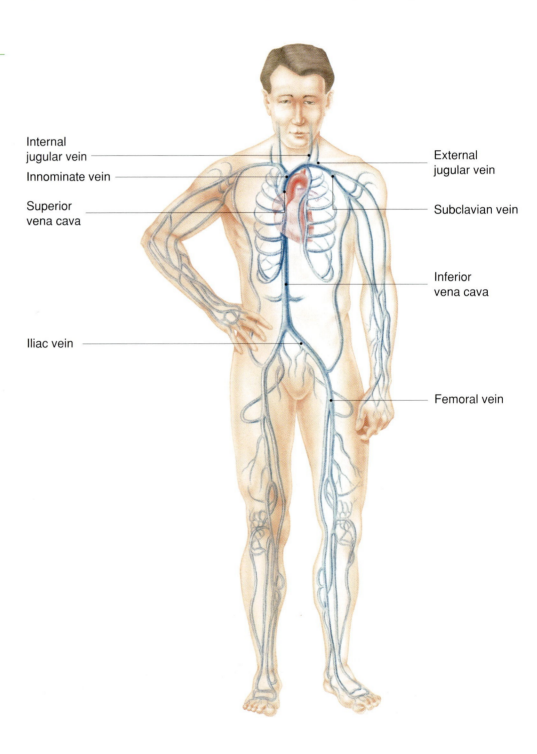

Internal jugular vein

Innominate vein

Superior vena cava

Iliac vein

External jugular vein

Subclavian vein

Inferior vena cava

Femoral vein

KEY IDEA

The following points summarize the basic differences between the arteries and veins:

- All arteries carry blood away from the heart.
- All veins carry blood back to the heart.
- All arteries (except the pulmonary artery) carry oxygenated blood.
- All veins (except the four pulmonary veins) carry deoxygenated blood.

Inactivity and Blood Circulation

When a patient is inactive, the blood circulation tends to slow down. The patient may also have a lower blood pressure (force of the blood pushing against the walls of the blood vessels). Sometimes this can cause the blood to form clots. Blood clots are dangerous. Sometimes a clot flows with the blood and becomes lodged in the blood vessels of the lungs. This condition, called a *pulmonary embolism*, is life threatening.

If you have orders to help a patient out of bed for the first time after an illness or after surgery, remember that the patient's circulation is slower and the blood pressure may be lower. Therefore, be sure the patient moves carefully and slowly. Allow the patient to sit at the edge of the bed and dangle the legs until the circulation stabilizes (comes back to normal). Then carefully help the patient to a standing position.

Sometimes this procedure will cause the blood to leave the brain suddenly, and the patient may be dizzy or feel faint. You may need more than one person to help you with the patient. Be sure to check the patient's activity restrictions with your supervisor.

The Circulatory System and the Normal Aging Process

As a person grows older, the movement of blood through the body tends to slow down. The heart muscle weakens, so the heart pumps with less force. It must work harder to keep the blood moving, yet it works less effectively. Thus, the blood flow decreases. The reduced output of the heart is one reason older people tend to tire more easily and have less reserve energy than younger people.

The heart may change in size. If it works harder to circulate the blood through the vessels, the greater work causes this muscle to grow larger. (In general, muscles get larger when they perform more work.) When some people age, they drastically reduce their physical activity. For such people, the heart may become smaller because it does not work as hard.

The blood vessels change as well. With age, they may harden and lose their ability to stretch. This causes them to become narrow. Fatty deposits and other substances may clog these narrowed vessels. Such changes further diminish blood flow and increase blood pressure. They also increase the risk of a blood vessel rupturing or becoming blocked. Thus, changes in the blood vessels can bring about physical and mental problems.

Common Diseases and Disorders of the Circulatory System

Among the diseases and disorders that most often affect the circulatory system are the following:

- ***Arteriosclerosis:*** The walls of the arteries become thicker with fatty deposits and less elastic than they should be for the normal regulation of blood flow and blood pressure.
- ***Angina pectoris:*** Heart pain that results from insufficient blood flow and oxygen to the heart muscle.

PROVIDING CARE FOR PATIENTS WITH PERIPHERAL VASCULAR DISEASE

GUIDELINES

OBRA

- Carefully inspect the feet when bathing the patient's feet or in response to patient complaint of foot discomfort. Report broken or cracked skin, color changes to red, white, black, or blue; swelling, pain,

- loss of function; corns or calluses, or loss of function.
- After washing, thoroughly dry the feet and between the toes, then apply lotion if the skin is dry.
- Avoid cutting toenails unless instructed to do so by a nurse or doctor.
- Elevate feet when patient is sitting up in a chair for more than a few

- minutes or support them with a footstool.
- Discourage habits that hinder circulation (wearing tight garters or socks, crossing legs at the knees, smoking).
- Avoid heating pads and unprotected exposure to heat or cold, because sensation is reduced.

- **Myocardial infarction (MI):** Obstruction of a blood vessel in the heart muscle results in death of heart tissue due to lack of oxygen.
- **Endocarditis:** The inner lining of the heart becomes inflamed.
- **Rheumatic heart disease:** The organism that causes rheumatic fever damages the valves of the heart.
- **Congestive heart failure:** The heart is unable to pump enough blood, and fluid builds up in the lungs.
- **Hypertension:** The blood pressure in the arteries is elevated (high).
- **Leukemia:** This is the term for cancer of the blood.
- **Anemia:** The quantity and quality of red blood cells decreases.
- **Cerebrovascular accident (CVA):** A blockage in or rupturing of arteries in the brain causes a stroke (death of brain tissue).
- **Peripheral vascular disease:** Condition resulting from restricted or poor functioning of the valves in the veins.

PROVIDING CARE FOR PATIENTS WITH HYPERTENSIVE DISEASE

GUIDELINES

- Treatment usually includes drugs that lower the blood pressure, a low-sodium diet, and encouragement of

- regular exercise. Encourage patients to follow their treatment and continue to take their medications even when they are feeling they do not need to do so.
- Encourage patients to avoid, decrease, or quit smoking.

- Observe and report the following signs and symptoms: flushed face, dizziness, nosebleeds, sudden headaches, changes in speech patterns, or blurred vision.

The Respiratory System: Anatomy and Physiology

respiratory system The group of body organs that carries on the body function of respiration; the system brings oxygen into the body and eliminates carbon dioxide

The **respiratory system** (Figure 18–5◆) provides a route or pathway for oxygen to get from the air into the lungs, where it can be picked up by the blood. The organs that make up this system include the nose and mouth, pharynx (throat), trachea (windpipe), larynx (voice box), lungs, and bronchi.

FIGURE 18–5 ◆
The respiratory system

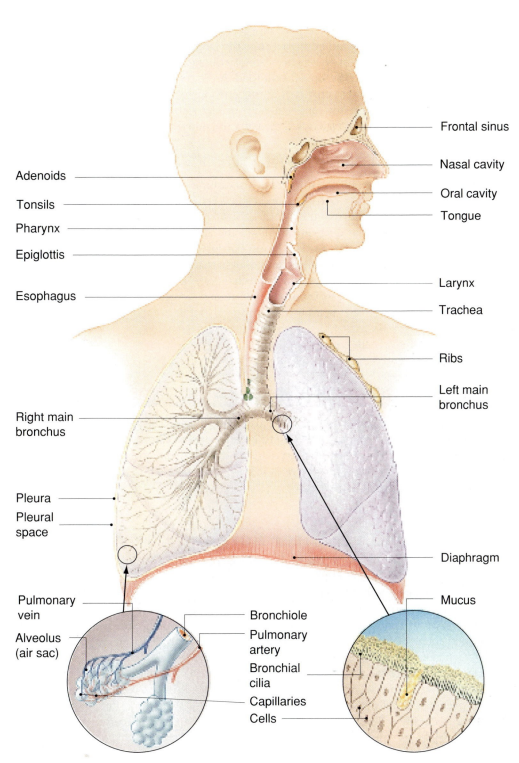

Frontal sinus

Nasal cavity

Oral cavity

Tongue

Adenoids

Tonsils

Pharynx

Epiglottis

Larynx

Trachea

Esophagus

Ribs

Left main bronchus

Right main bronchus

Pleura

Pleural space

Diaphragm

Mucus

Pulmonary vein

Bronchiole

Alveolus (air sac)

Pulmonary artery

Bronchial cilia

Capillaries

Cells

Because we must have oxygen to live, it is necessary to keep this pathway open. The structures themselves help to do this. The trachea and bronchi are kept open by incomplete cartilage rings.

On the top of the trachea, opening from the pharynx (the throat), is a structure known as the *larynx*. In addition to being the opening to the trachea, it also contains the vocal cords, which make it possible for us to talk.

An important piece of cartilage, the epiglottis, covers the opening to the trachea when food is swallowed, preventing the food from going into the lungs. A very weak patient or one who is having trouble breathing must be watched carefully during feeding so that food does not get into the trachea. This is known as aspiration of food. An unconscious patient who vomits may also be in danger of aspirating vomitus. If an unconscious patient vomits, turn the patient's head to one side immediately. You must watch the patient with great care, because if the pathway for oxygen is blocked, the patient will die without immediate treatment.

Oxygen and Carbon Dioxide Exchange

As in the body's other systems, the important work of the respiratory system is done at the level of the cell. The exchange of oxygen and carbon dioxide occurs in an area of the lungs that is so small you would have to use a microscope to see it. At the end of the last branch of the bronchus—the alveolar duct—is a small sac, the alveolus. Many oxygen molecules fill this sac after the body breathes in. The blood has less oxygen, so it can pick up a large amount of oxygen from the alveolar sac and release the carbon dioxide it is carrying. The blood is then returned to the heart to transport the oxygen around the body.

The respiratory system then is responsible for getting oxygen to the blood. Internal respiration occurs when cells that need the oxygen receive it in exchange for carbon dioxide, which is the cells' gas waste product. Both functions—the exchanges of oxygen in the lungs and at the cellular level—are equally important.

Breathing is regulated in the medulla, a part of the brain.

KEY IDEA

The circulatory and respiratory systems are tightly linked. The respiratory system delivers oxygen from the air to the blood to be transported through the circulatory system. The circulatory system delivers carbon dioxide from the body to the lungs, where the respiratory system removes it from the body. Thus, neither system can complete its work without the other.

Respiratory Care after Surgery

Often, especially after surgery, a patient must be encouraged to breathe deeply in order to keep all the air sacs open and inflated. Sometimes a nursing assistant is asked to encourage the patient to cough, especially if there is inflammation of the lung tissue. In many of the larger health care institutions, the Pulmonary Medicine Department (Respiratory Therapy) will, by a doctor's order, institute a treatment that will encourage the patient to breathe deeply and cough. An incentive spirometer is used postoperatively for this in most hospitals.

After a patient has had some kind of abdominal surgery, he may, fearing pain, resist coughing. One way to make the patient more comfortable is to place a pillow over the patient's abdomen and instruct the patient to hold it firmly against the abdomen when he coughs.

The patient is usually instructed to breathe in and out slowly and deeply twice. After breathing in deeply a third time, the patient should cough twice instead of letting the air out slowly. Make sure he covers his mouth with a tissue and turns his head away from you.

The Respiratory System and the Normal Aging Process

As adults age, the elasticity of the lung tissue can decrease. Also, the airways can become obstructed due to repeated infections or irritants, such as smoking or air pollution. This is known as chronic obstructive pulmonary disease (COPD), which refers to a group of disorders, such as bronchitis, asthma, and emphysema.

As the body ages, the circulatory system becomes less responsive. Cardiac output decreases and the structures of the heart become more rigid. The respiratory system ages as well. Geriatric adults often have less muscular strength, less lung capacity, and a weaker cough.

Infants and small children have little ability to maintain a reserve of energy and are more apt to become severely ill quickly. Crying can elevate vital signs. The intercostal muscles of infants are not fully developed and therefore may have a difficult time clearing secretions.

Common Diseases and Disorders of the Respiratory System

The following diseases and disorders are among the most common ones affecting the respiratory system:

- **Infection of the Upper Respiratory Tract:** the common cold
- **Sinusitis:** Inflammation of the sinuses
- **Pharyngitis:** inflammation of the throat
- **Cancer of the Larynx (Voice Box):** the growth of cancer in the larynx
- **Pneumonia:** infection of the lung
- **Lung Cancer:** the growth of cancer in the lungs
- **Chest Trauma:** injury to the chest
- **Tuberculosis (TB):** infection caused by a microorganism that is easily transmitted from one person to another through the air
- **Chronic obstructive pulmonary disease (COPD):** obstruction of the airways caused by repeated infections or exposure to irritants
- **Bronchitis:** inflammation of the bronchi
- **Emphysema:** obstruction of airflow in the lungs
- **Asthma:** allergy with wheezing and dyspnea (difficulty breathing)

tuberculosis (TB) A highly infectious disease that usually affects the lungs

Tuberculosis

Tuberculosis (TB) is an infection caused by bacteria known as *Mycobacterium tuberculosis.* TB primarily affects the respiratory system and destroys parts of the lung tissue. Tiny droplets containing the TB bacteria are easily transmitted from one person to another through the air by coughing, sneezing, or speaking. Depending on the environment, TB particles can remain in the air for several hours. The rate of individuals contracting TB has increased during the early 2000s.

Symptoms of TB of the lungs include a productive, persistent cough, chest pain, and/or coughing up blood. Systemic signs include fever, chills, night sweats, loss of appetite and weight, and fatigue. Sputum cultures to confirm TB can take weeks to be completed, so patients suspected of having TB are placed in isolation and begin treatment with medications immediately.

Persons who are infected but do not have the TB disease *cannot* spread the infection to other people. This is known as *latent* TB infection. A person with latent TB infection will have a positive TB skin test but not active disease. Persons at highest risk of becoming infected with TB are usually close contacts who spend a lot of time in a confined area such as family members, roommates, or coworkers.

Due to higher exposure to patients who may have TB, health care workers should receive TB tests yearly and as needed depending on exposure. A health care worker who is

FIGURE 18–6 ◆

A patient with COPD requiring oxygen

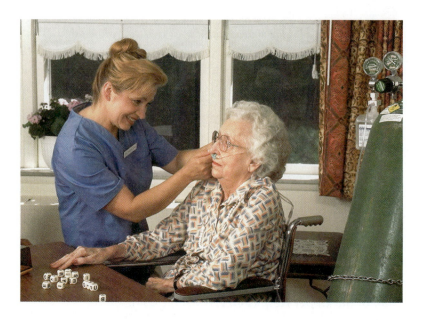

exposed to active TB unexpectedly or who develops symptoms of TB disease should be evaluated promptly.

To prevent infection, suspected patients should be placed in an isolation room with negative pressure immediately. The door to the room must be kept closed with the bathroom door open to the patient's room. Adhere to Standard Precautions at all times and wear a particulate respirator (N-95 or duckbill mask) while in the patient's room. Particulate respirators filter the air before the person wearing the respirator inhales it. Surgical masks are designed to prevent the respiratory secretions of the person wearing the mask from entering the air. The health care worker *must* wear the particulate respirator. A surgical mask will *not* provide needed protection. The patient should wear a surgical mask when being transported.

Chronic Obstructive Pulmonary Disease

A patient with chronic obstructive pulmonary disease (COPD) has several needs. She will find it difficult to breathe and will get short of breath with common activities like walking. She has a great deal of fear that she will not be able to breathe and may have a reduced appetite. Mouth care becomes very important because this patient will often breathe deeply through the mouth. Mouth breathing dries up the saliva normally present in the mouth. Saliva provides moisture that assists in cleansing the mouth. The patient may be receiving oxygen therapy (Figure 18–6◆). It is very important to permit a COPD patient to do as much as she comfortably can for herself. This helps to maintain her sense of independence and ability to function. Expect that frequent rest periods may be needed for the patient to perform the routine activities of daily living.

Indications a Patient May Require
Supplemental Oxygen

When caring for a patient there are signs that the patient may need extra or supplemental oxygen. Consider the following questions and report if you observe any to be occurring:

- Are the patient's respirations labored?
- Has the respiration rate increased?

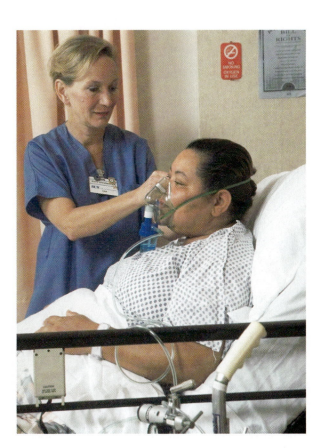

FIGURE 18–7 ◆

Patients with respiratory disease often require treatments that involve the use of oxygen

- Does the patient report feeling short of breath?
- Is the patient using accessory muscles (neck or intercostal muscles) to assist with ventilation?
- Is the patient wheezing?
- Are there signs of cyanosis—bluish nail beds or bluish hue—to the lips or mucous membranes?

Therapies Related to Respiratory Disease

A patient who has a respiratory disease may be receiving oxygen or special breathing treatments (Figure 18–7◆). A patient using oxygen must never smoke or come near an open flame because the oxygen will burn or explode. When a patient is receiving a breathing treatment, oxygen may also be used, so remember to avoid any situation involving smoking or being around an open flame. It may be important to remind visitors or family members of these precautions (Figure 18–8◆).

The oxygen orders must be followed carefully. Some patients must keep the oxygen on at all times. A patient who is receiving breathing treatments will have them ordered to be done at specific times. Check with the supervisor for specific instructions for the patient.

Try to give patient care at times that fit well with the ordered treatments. For example, after a breathing treatment, a patient generally feels better and can breathe more easily. Giving a bath or ambulating a patient after receiving treatment will enable the patient to be more active and less likely to tire.

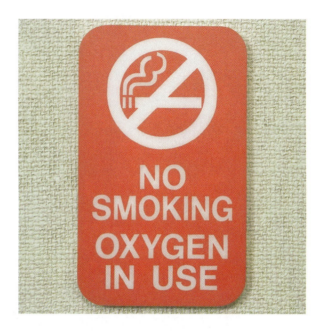

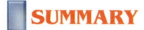

AGE-SPECIFIC CONSIDERATIONS

The use of nasal cannulas can cause irritation to the skin of the ears in the geriatric population. The nasal cannula is looped over the ears and tightened under the chin. This constant pressure of the tubing on the ears is the source of irritation and can be relieved by placing cotton or other soft material between the skin and the tubing.

Many patients, both young and old, feel claustrophobic wearing a face mask. It is often difficult to convince these patients to wear such a device and other alternatives to oxygen delivery must be considered. Another important consideration is the elderly patient with sensitive skin. If the mask is used for an extended period of time, skin breakdown may be a problem. For this reason it is important to clean the area under the mask where the skin and mask come in contact. Secondly, do not overtighten the mask straps. A secure fit to the face is desired, but not so tight as to impede circulation.

KEY IDEA

The chronic obstructive pulmonary diseases (COPD) and tuberculosis (TB) are two of many conditions that require special instructions for care and safety. Be sure to check with the supervisor to determine what the doctor's current orders are.

SUMMARY

The circulatory and respiratory systems affect the flow of blood and the exchange of oxygen between the blood and the cells of the body. The primary exchange takes place in the lungs in the alveoli. A secondary exchange is at the cellular level. The circulatory and respiratory systems work closely together. A condition that affects one system may affect the other. Patients with conditions affecting either or both systems will be limited in their activities of daily living.

NOTES

CHAPTER REVIEW

FILL IN THE BLANK Read each sentence and fill in the blank line with a word that completes the sentence.

1. The _____ is a four-chambered, hollow, muscular organ that lies in the chest cavity and pumps blood through the lungs and into all parts of the body.

2. _____ is the liquid portion of the blood.

3. The structures that carry oxygenated blood from the heart are called _____.

4. If food gets into the trachea of the lungs, it is known as _____.

5. _____ _____ disease results from restricted or poor functioning of the valves of the veins.

MULTIPLE CHOICE Choose the best answer for each question or statement.

1. Functions of the blood include all of the following *except*
   a. carries oxygen from the lungs to the cells.
   b. protects underlying structures.
   c. carries carbon dioxide from the cells to the lungs.
   d. carries waste products from the cells to the kidneys.

2. Which of the following is not true about the heart?
   a. It acts as a pump for the body.
   b. It is made up of four chambers.
   c. It is a muscular organ.
   d. It is the primary defense against infection for the body.

3. Blood pressure is
   a. the force of the blood pushing against the walls of the blood vessels.
   b. the force of the blood pushing against the valves of the heart.

   c. the force of the blood pushing against the lungs.
   d. the ability of the heart to pump blood.

4. Common diseases and disorders of the circulatory system include all of the following *except*
   a. arteriosclerosis.
   b. psoriasis.
   c. myocardial infarction.
   d. congestive heart failure.

5. Common diseases and disorders of the respiratory system include all of the following *except*
   a. sinusitis.
   b. pneumonia.
   c. anemia.
   d. bronchitis.

TIME-OUT

TIPS FOR TIME MANAGEMENT

Always have a backup plan when dealing with mechanical equipment. If the electronic thermometer is not working correctly, use a glass thermometer. If the electric bed won't raise up, use the crank. Do the best you can without wasting time waiting for someone to repair the equipment.

THE NURSING ASSISTANT IN ACTION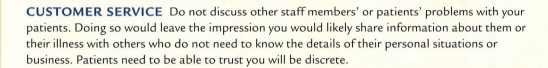

You are caring for a 57-year-old patient who has chronic emphysema and COPD. He was smoking two to three packs of cigarettes a day before being admitted to the hospital. He has difficulty breathing, coughs, and spits up lots of thick secretions. He is asking for you to give him his cigarettes. He is too sick to leave his room to go smoke outside. Your facility has a no smoking policy. You think maybe some nicotine patches might be helpful, but are unsure if his doctor would order these.

What Is Your Response/Action?

CRITICAL THINKING

CUSTOMER SERVICE Do not discuss other staff members' or patients' problems with your patients. Doing so would leave the impression you would likely share information about them or their illness with others who do not need to know the details of their personal situations or business. Patients need to be able to trust you will be discrete.

CULTURAL CARE Patients in isolation can easily feel alone or forgotten. Check on them more frequently. It can be particularly difficult to be from a different culture or unable to communicate well while in isolation for TB or another respiratory disease. The protective masks and isolation precautions need to be explained by a translator to enable the patient to better understand what is happening.

COOPERATION WITHIN THE TEAM Anticipate and plan for what your patients need before the change of shift or a scheduled class or staff meeting. This effort will be appreciated by your colleagues and help reduce the number of requests your assigned patients will have in your absence.

EXPLORE MediaLink

Additional interactive resources for this chapter can be found on the Companion Website at www.prenhall.com/wolgin. Click on Chapter 18 and "Begin" to select the activities for this chapter.

For chapter-related NCLEX-style questions and an audio glossary, access the accompanying CD-ROM in this book.

19 Measuring Vital Signs

KEY TERMS

abdominal respiration
aneroid sphygmomanometer
apical pulse
apnea
axillary
blood pressure
bradycardia
centigrade
Cheyne-Stokes respiration
diastolic blood pressure
dyspnea
exhaling
Fahrenheit
force
hypertension
hypotension
inhaling
irregular respiration
labored respiration
mercury sphygmomanometer
oral
pulse
pulse deficit
radial pulse
rate
rectal
rhythm
shallow respiration
sphygmomanometer
stertorous respiration
stethoscope
systolic blood pressure
tachycardia
thermometer
vital signs

OBJECTIVES

When you have completed this chapter, you will be able to:

- List and describe the different types of thermometers.
- Read a Fahrenheit and centigrade (Celsius) thermometer accurately.
- Demonstrate the procedure for measuring oral temperatures.
- Demonstrate the procedure for measuring rectal temperatures.
- Demonstrate the procedure for measuring axillary temperatures.
- Demonstrate the proper use of a battery-operated electronic thermometer.
- Count the radial and apical pulse.
- Report the rate and rhythm of the pulse accurately.
- Count a patient's respirations accurately.
- Determine if the patient's breathing is labored or abnormal.
- Explain systolic pressure.
- Explain diastolic pressure.
- Demonstrate the use of aneroid and mercury types of blood pressure equipment accurately and efficiently.
- Demonstrate how to use a stethoscope.
- Measure a patient's blood pressure accurately.
- Use a pain measurement scale to evaluate the intensity of a patient's pain.

MediaLink
www.prenhall.com/wolgin

Use the address above to access the free, interactive Companion Website created for this textbook. Get hints, instant feedback, and textbook references to chapter-related NCLEX-style questions. Link to other interesting sites.

AUDIO GLOSSARY:
Use the Companion Website, or the CD-ROM disk enclosed with your textbook, to hear the pronunciation of key terms in the chapter.

By measuring or "taking" a person's vital signs, you are recording measurements that reflect the physical well-being of a person. Everyone has a normal vital sign range. The vital signs are often the first key indicators that something adverse (wrong or abnormal) is going on with the patient. Vital signs which are routinely measured on every patient include temperature, respirations, blood pressure, and pulse rate. Pain intensity is commonly referred to as the "fifth vital sign."

Vital Signs

Vital signs are measurements reflecting the patient's physical well-being and condition. Vital signs include body temperature, pulse, and respirations. Blood pressure and pain intensity are two other measurements routinely ordered to evaluate and monitor patients. Increasingly you will encounter pain measurement scales that are used by patients to rate their pain intensity. This measurement is documented to help evaluate the effectiveness of pain relief measures and pain medications.

Vital signs are taken:

- Upon admission to a hospital or facility
- When ordered by an MD or as outlined on a care plan
- Any time there is an unusual situation, incident, or patient fall
- As part of a physical examination or checkup
- When a patient complains of pain
- When monitoring the patient's response to a new medication

Be aware that vital signs are influenced by the following factors:

- Changes in weather temperature
- Caffeine
- Medications
- Emotions, especially fear and anxiety
- Exercise
- Age

vital signs Measurements reflecting the patient's physical well-being and condition

Body Temperature

Body temperature is a measurement of the amount of heat in the body. The body creates heat in the process of changing food into energy. The body can also lose heat through perspiration (sweating), respiration (breathing), and excretion. The balance between the heat produced and the heat lost is the body temperature. The normal adult body temperature is 98.6° **Fahrenheit (F)** or 37° **centigrade** or **Celsius (C)**. There is a normal range in which a person's body temperature may vary and still be considered normal.

Types of Thermometers

The body temperature is measured with an instrument called a **thermometer**. There are several different types of thermometers:

- Glass
  - Oral
  - Rectal
  - Security

Fahrenheit A system for measuring temperature. In the Fahrenheit system, the temperature of water at boiling is 212°. At freezing, it is 32°. These temperatures are usually written 212°F and 32°F.

centigrade A system for measurement of temperature using a scale divided into 100 units or degrees; in this system, the freezing temperature of water is 0°C and water boils at 100°C; often referred to as *Celsius*

thermometer An instrument used for measuring temperature

- Battery-operated electronic
- Chemically treated
- Plastic single use

The *glass thermometer* is a delicate, hollow glass tube with a liquid metal called mercury, an element that is very sensitive to temperature, sealed inside it. Mercury expands (gets larger) when the temperature goes up and contracts (gets smaller) when the temperature goes down. Even if the temperature rises only slightly, the mercury will expand and travel up the tube, reflecting the change. Because mercury is toxic, mercury thermometers will eventually be replaced with thermometers containing a nontoxic substance. To reduce accidental exposure to mercury, most institutions are replacing their mercury thermometers and blood pressure equipment.

The outside of the glass thermometer is marked with lines, or calibrations, and numbers. These markings help us measure exactly the temperature readings displayed by the level of the mercury. There are three types of glass thermometers (Figure 19–1◆):

- **Oral** thermometers are used to measure the patient's temperature by mouth and also by the **axillary** method.
- **Rectal** thermometers are used to measure temperature by inserting the thermometer into the patient's rectum.
- Security thermometers are used for taking an infant's rectal temperature. Many institutions use the security or stubby type with a red knob at the stem for rectal temperatures and those with a green or blue knob at the stem for oral temperatures. Follow your institution's policy.

Battery-operated electronic thermometers eliminate human error and variations that can occur in reading a glass thermometer. An electronic thermometer is used with a disposable sheath (plastic cover) over the probe. The sheath is discarded after each use. The ear (aural) thermometer is an electronic thermometer that measures the temperature by inserting the probe gently in the ear canal. This device is capable of converting and displaying the temperature as an oral or rectal temperature. Be sure to indicate whether your thermometer converts to an oral or rectal temperature. Figure 19–2◆ is an example of an electronic thermometer that measures the temperature of the tympanic membrane or eardrum.

The *latest electronic thermometers* instantly calculate the body temperature when a sheath-covered probe is inserted into the opening of the outer ear canal. This type of thermometer is available for industrial and home use.

Chemically treated paper or plastic thermometers are now used by some health care institutions. These change color to indicate the patient's temperature.

oral Anything to do with the mouth; examples are eating and speaking

axillary The area under the arms; the armpits

rectal Pertaining to the rectum

ALERT

Mercury-filled thermometers are seen in home care settings; if one breaks:

- Increase ventilation
- Pick up mercury with an eyedropper or
- Scoop up with heavy paper
- Place mercury and glass in a plastic zipper bag
- Enclose bag in 2 more plastic bags

FIGURE 19–1 ◆

Types of glass thermometers

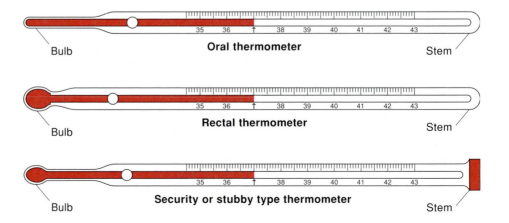

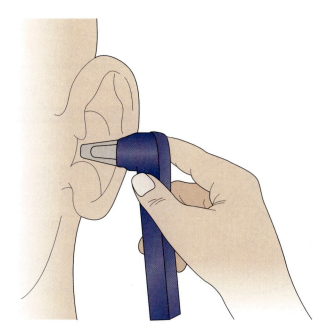

FIGURE 19–2 ◆

A type of electronic thermometer that measures the temperature by inserting the probe in the ear canal

---

| CARE OF GLASS THERMOMETERS | GUIDELINES | OBRA |

- Because glass thermometers break and shatter easily, they must be handled with care. Be especially careful to avoid breaking a thermometer while it is in a patient's mouth or rectum.

- The liquid metal, mercury, inside the thermometer is a poison; that is, it may be harmful if it is ingested (taken into the body by mouth) or if it has contact with the skin for a prolonged period of time. Adverse effects chiefly result from vapor inhalation, however. If there is a mercury spill, do not use household cleansers, a vacuum, or a broom. (See the Alert on page 384).

- Check the containers in which the thermometers are kept. Follow your instructions for cleaning these containers.

- Never clean a glass thermometer with hot water because it will cause the mercury to expand so much that the thermometer will break.

| SHAKING DOWN THE GLASS THERMOMETER | PROCEDURE | OBRA |

RATIONALE: Shaking down a glass thermometer aids in accurate measurement.

PREPARATION

1. Assemble your equipment on the bedside table:

   Thermometer in container

2. Wash your hands.

3. Before using the thermometer, check to make sure that it is not cracked or that the bulb is not chipped. The bulb is the end that is inserted into the patient's body. Never touch the bulb end of the thermometer.

STEPS

4. Hold the thermometer firmly between your fingers and your thumb at the stem, farthest from the bulb.

PROCEDURE (continued)

5. Stand clear of any hard surfaces such as counters and tables to avoid striking and breaking the thermometer while you are shaking it. For practice, you might stand with your arm over a pillow or mattress in case you accidentally drop the thermometer.

6. When you are sure that you have a good hold on the thermometer, shake your hand loosely at the wrist. Do it as if you were shaking water from your fingers (Figure 19–3◆). *Note:* Shake the mercury down to the lowest point below the numbers and lines.

7. Snap your wrist again and again. This will shake down the mercury to the lowest possible point,

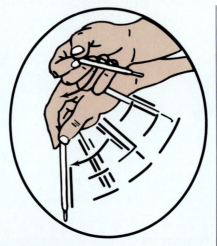

FIGURE 19–3◆
Shake down a glass thermometer by holding the thermometer stem firmly between your thumb and index finger as you snap your wrist

below the numbers and lines (calibrations).

FOLLOW-UP

8. Always shake down the mercury before and after using a glass thermometer.

| READING A FAHRENHEIT THERMOMETER | PROCEDURE | OBRA |

RATIONALE: Carefully reading a glass thermometer aids in accurate measurement.

STEPS

1. With your thumb and first two fingers, hold the thermometer at the stem. Never touch the bulb end.

2. Hold the thermometer at eye level. Turn the thermometer back and forth between your fingers until you can clearly see the column of mercury.

3. Notice the scale or calibrations. Each long line stands for 1 degree.

4. There are 4 short lines between each of the long lines. Each short line stands for two-tenths (or 0.2) of a degree.

5. Between the long lines that represent 98° and 99°, look for a longer line with an arrow directly beneath it. This special line points out normal body temperature (98.6°F).

6. Look at the end of the mercury. Notice the first line or number where the mercury ends (Figure 19–4◆). If it is one of the short lines, notice the previous longer line toward the silver tip that goes into the patient's mouth. The tem-

perature reading is the degree marked by that long line plus 2, 4, 6, or 8 tenths of a degree. For example, if the mercury ends after the 99 line, but on the second short line, the temperature is 99.4°F. If the mercury ends between the two lines, take the line it is closer to.

Note: Accuracy is extremely important. Look at the mercury carefully when reading a thermometer.

7. Write down the patient's temperature right away. If you are using a vital sign book, check to find the right column next to the patient's name and the right time of day. Write the patient's temperature using the figure you read on the thermometer. Some institutions

PROCEDURE *(continued)*

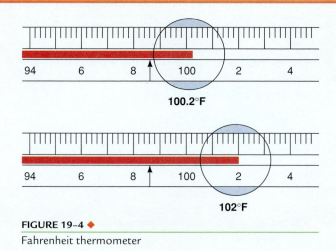

100.2°F

102°F

FIGURE 19–4 ◆
Fahrenheit thermometer

will write 99.4°F. Others will write 99⁴. Follow the method used in your institution.

CHARTING EXAMPLE: 11/01/04 12:19pm Oral T = 102°F. Notified N. Lowther, RN, that Ms. Mills is shivering and complaining of nausea. K. Fine, CNA

READING A CENTIGRADE (CELSIUS) THERMOMETER

PROCEDURE

OBRA

RATIONALE: Carefully reading a glass thermometer aids in accurate measurement.

STEPS

1. With your thumb and first two fingers, hold the thermometer at the stem.

2. Hold the thermometer at eye level. Turn the thermometer back and forth between your fingers until you can clearly see the column of mercury.

3. Notice the scale or calibrations. Each long line shows 1 degree.

4. There are 9 short lines between each number. These short lines are 1, 2, 3, 4, 5, 6, 7, 8, and 9 tenths of a degree. If the mercury ended after the 36 and on the third short line, the temperature would read 36.3°C (Figure 19–5◆). If the mercury

ended after the long line 37 and on the eighth short line, the temperature would read 37.8°C. If the mercury ends after line 37 on the fifth short line, the temperature would be referred to as 37.5°C.

Note: Accuracy is extremely important. Look at the mercury carefully when reading a thermometer.

5. Write down the patient's temperature right away. If you are using a vital sign book, check to find the right column next to the patient's

name and the right time of day. Write the patient's temperature using the figure you read on the thermometer. Some hospitals write 37°C. Others will write 37. Follow the method used in your hospital.

CHARTING EXAMPLE: 11/01/04 1:30pm Oral T = 39.5°C. Notified N. Lowther, RN, that Ms. Mills is shivering and complaining of nausea. K. Fine, CNA

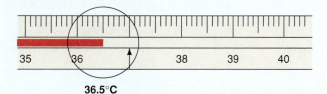

36.5°C

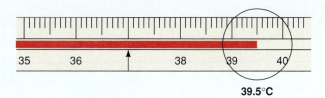

39.5°C

FIGURE 19–5 ◆
Centigrade thermometer

Recording the Patient's Temperature

For recording the patient's temperature, three symbols are used:

$°$ = degrees   F = Fahrenheit   C = Centigrade or Celsius

You will record the patient's temperatures according to the method used in your institution (Figures 19–6◆ and 19–7◆).

Fahrenheit temperature can be written in two ways:

98.6°F or 98^4 F

FIGURE 19–6 ◆

The two major scales used in the United States for measuring temperature

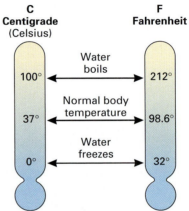

FIGURE 19–7 ◆

Temperature conversion

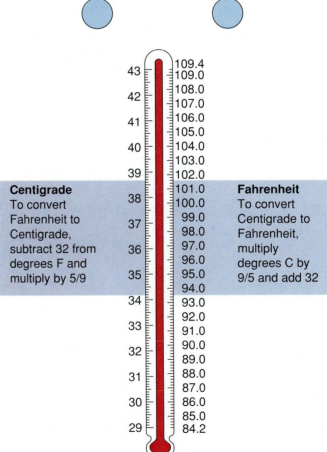

Centigrade
To convert Fahrenheit to Centigrade, subtract 32 from degrees F and multiply by 5/9

Fahrenheit
To convert Centigrade to Fahrenheit, multiply degrees C by 9/5 and add 32

TABLE 19–1

Normal Temperature Readings

METHOD	CENTIGRADE	FAHRENHEIT
Oral	37.0	98.6
Axillary	36.4	97.6
Rectal	37.5	99.6

If you are using a centigrade (Celsius) thermometer, the temperature would be written

$$37°C \quad \text{or} \quad 37.3°C \quad \text{or} \quad 37\tfrac{3}{}°C$$

Write an R in front of the temperature reading if a rectal temperature was taken. Write an A if an axillary temperature was taken. Write an O if an oral temperature was taken. See Table 19–1◆ for normal temperature readings.

MEASURING AN ORAL TEMPERATURE	PROCEDURE	OBRA

RATIONALE: Carefully using and reading a glass thermometer aids in accurate measurement.

PREPARATION

1. Assemble your equipment:
   a. Oral thermometer (Figure 19–8◆)
   b. Tissue or paper towel
   c. Vital sign form used in your institution
   d. Pen or pencil
2. Identify the patient by checking the identification bracelet.
3. Wash your hands.
4. Tell the patient you are going to take his temperature.
5. Ask the patient if he has recently had hot or cold fluids or been smoking. If the answer is yes, wait 10 minutes before taking an oral temperature.
6. Provide privacy for the patient.

7. The patient should be in bed or sitting in a chair.
8. Take the thermometer out of its container. Dry with a paper towel.
9. Shake the mercury down.

STEPS

10. Gently put the bulb end in the patient's mouth under the tongue (Figure 19–9◆).

a. Insert the thermometer gently into the patient's mouth under the tongue.
b. Position the thermometer to the side of the mouth.
c. Instruct the patient to keep the thermometer under the tongue by gently closing the lips around the thermometer. Ask him to keep his mouth and lips closed around the thermometer.

Mercury / Calibrations / Stem / Bulb

94 6 8 100 2 4 6 8 110

6 8 100

Normal body temperature is 98.6 degress Fahrenheit and is written 98.6°F.

Mercury / Stem / Bulb

35 36 38 39 40 41 42 43

36 38

Normal body temperature is 37 degrees centigrade (Celsius) and is written 37°C.

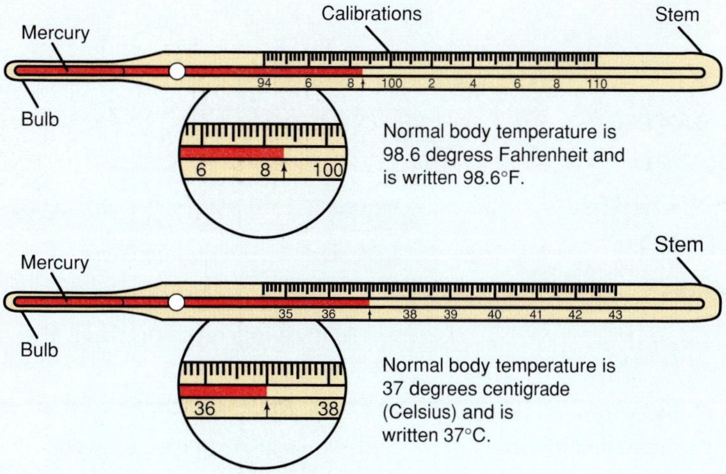

FIGURE 19–8 ◆

Normal body temperatures

PROCEDURE *(continued)*

11. Leave the thermometer in the patient's mouth for 8 minutes.

    (*Note:* The latest research states that oral temperature is more accurate when the oral thermometer remains in the mouth for 8 minutes. However, if in your institution the policy is for 3 to 5 minutes, follow the procedure of your institution.)

12. Take the thermometer out of the patient's mouth. Hold the stem end and wipe the thermometer with a tissue. Wipe the stem of the thermometer toward the bulb end.

13. Read the thermometer.

14. Record the temperature according to your institution's policy.

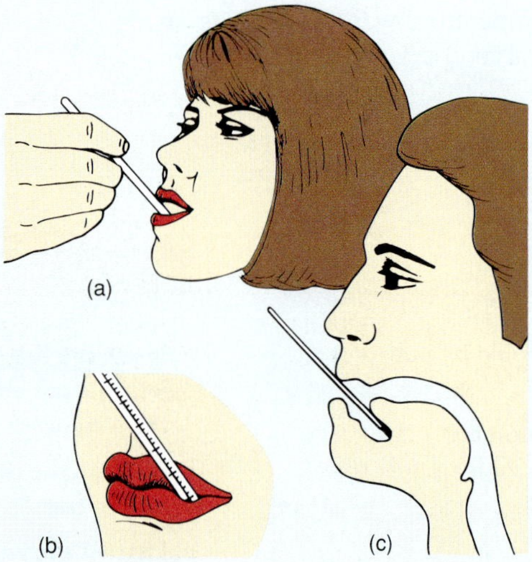

FIGURE 19–9 ◆
Gently place bulb end into patient's mouth under the tongue

FOLLOW-UP

15. Shake the mercury down. Rinse in cold water. Wipe with alcohol and replace the thermometer in its container.

16. Make the patient comfortable and replace the call light.

17. Lower the bed to a position of safety.

18. Raise the side rails when ordered or appropriate for patient safety.

19. Wash your hands.

20. Report to your immediate supervisor:

    ■ If the oral temperature was above 100°F or 37.5°C or below 97°F.

    ■ Your observations of anything unusual.

CHARTING EXAMPLE: 11/01/04 12:19pm Oral T = 102°F. Notified N. Lowther, RN, that Ms. Mills is shivering and complaining of nausea. K. Fine, CNA

USING A BATTERY-OPERATED ELECTRONIC ORAL THERMOMETER

RATIONALE: Carefully using and reading a battery-operated thermometer aids in accurate measurement.

PROCEDURE

OBRA

PREPARATION

1. Assemble your equipment:

    a. Disposable plastic probe cover

    b. Battery-operated electronic thermometer

    c. Oral (blue) attachment

    d. Vital sign form used in your institution

    e. Pen or pencil

2. Identify the patient by checking the identification bracelet.

3. Tell the patient you are going to take his temperature.

4. Wash your hands.

5. Provide privacy for the patient.

6. Check to be sure that the oral (blue top) probe connector is properly placed in its receptacle on the base of the unit.

PROCEDURE *(continued)*

STEPS

7. Remove the probe from its stored position. Insert it into a sheath or probe cover.

8. Insert the covered probe into the patient's mouth slowly until the metal tip is at the base under the tongue to the back of the patient's mouth.

9. Hold the probe in the patient's mouth. It is much heavier than a glass thermometer and some patients are unable to hold it. (Figure 19–10◆).

10. Wait about 15 seconds for the buzzer to ring for a computed temperature reading, then remove the probe from the patient's mouth.

11. Record the temperature on the vital sign form used in your institution. This is very important

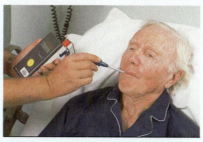

FIGURE 19–10 ◆
Hold the probe in the patient's mouth

because when you return the probe to its stored position the reading automatically returns to zero.

12. Without touching it, discard the used probe cover (sheath) immediately into a waste receptacle.

FOLLOW-UP

13. Return the probe to its stored position in the face of the thermometer.

14. Store the thermometer in its charging stand whenever it is not in use.

15. Make the patient comfortable and replace the call light.

16. Lower the bed to a position of safety.

17. Raise the side rails when ordered or appropriate for patient safety.

18. Wash your hands.

19. Report to your immediate supervisor:

   ▪ If the oral temperature was over 100°F; 37.5°C or below 97°F.

   ▪ Your observations of anything unusual.

CHARTING EXAMPLE: Record on Mr. Gunn's flow sheet 11/01/04 2:19pm Oral T = 99°F. K. Fine, CNA

> **USING A BATTERY-OPERATED ELECTRONIC TYMPANIC OR AURAL (EAR) THERMOMETER**

PROCEDURE

OBRA

RATIONALE: Carefully using and reading a battery-operated tympanic thermometer aids in accurate measurement.

PREPARATION

1. Assemble your equipment:

   a. Disposable plastic probe cover

   b. Battery-operated electronic thermometer

   c. Vital sign form used in your institution

   d. Pen or pencil

2. Identify the patient by checking the identification bracelet.

3. Tell the patient you are going to take her temperature.

4. Wash your hands.

5. Provide privacy for the patient.

STEPS

6. Make sure the probe is connected to the unit.

7. Remove the probe from its stored position. Insert the cone-shaped end of the thermometer into a

probe cover or attach a disposable probe.

8. Position the patient's head so one ear is directly in front of you.

9. For an adult or child, pull the outer ear up and back to open the ear canal. For an infant, pull the ear straight back.

10. Gently insert the covered probe into the patient's ear; slowly use a slight rocking motion if needed to insert the probe as far as possible and seal the ear canal (Figure 19–11◆).

11. Watch and wait for about 10–15 seconds for a flashing light or buzzer to ring indicating a

PROCEDURE *(continued)*

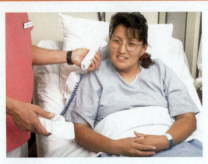

FIGURE 19–11 ◆

Gently insert covered probe into patient's ear

computed temperature reading, then remove the probe from the patient's ear.

12. Read and record the digitally displayed temperature on the vital sign form used in your institution.

This is very important because when you return the probe to its stored position the reading automatically returns to zero. Some units have built in convertors so the temperature may be displayed as an equivalent oral or rectal value in centigrade or Fahrenheit.

13. Without touching it, eject and discard the used probe cover (sheath) immediately into a waste receptacle.

FOLLOW-UP

14. Return the probe to its stored position in the face of the thermometer.

15. Store the thermometer in its charging stand whenever it is not in use.

16. Make the patient comfortable and replace the call light.

17. Lower the bed to a position of safety.

18. Raise the side rails when ordered or appropriate for patient safety.

19. Wash your hands.

20. Report to your immediate supervisor:

   ■ If the tympanic temperature was over 100°F; 37.5°C.

   ■ Your observations of anything unusual.

CHARTING EXAMPLE: Record on Ms. Sunbird's flow sheet 1/01/04 2:19pm T = 98.8°F. K. Fine, CNA

Measuring Rectal Temperature

Remember that you will always use a rectal thermometer for taking rectal temperatures. Notice that the glass rectal thermometer has a small round bulb on one end. This bulb prevents the thermometer from injuring the sensitive lining of the patient's rectum. Under the following conditions you might take a rectal temperature. Ask your supervisor for verification.

   ■ When the patient is an infant or child; follow the policies of your health care institution for pediatric patients

   ■ When the patient is having warm or cold applications on the face or neck

   ■ When the patient cannot keep her mouth closed around the thermometer

   ■ When the patient finds it hard to breathe through the nose

   ■ When the patient has sneezing or coughing spells

   ■ When the patient's mouth is dry or inflamed (red)

   ■ When the patient is restless, delirious, unconscious, or confused

   ■ When the patient is getting oxygen by cannula, catheter, face mask, or oxygen tent

   ■ When the patient has a nasogastric tube (Levine's tube, NG tube) in place

   ■ When the patient has had major surgery in the area of the face or neck

   ■ When the patient's face is partially paralyzed, as from a stroke

MEASURING RECTAL TEMPERATURE USING A GLASS THERMOMETER

PROCEDURE

OBRA

RATIONALE: Carefully using and reading an ordered rectal thermometer aids in accurate measurement.

PREPARATION

1. Assemble your equipment:
   a. Rectal thermometer
   b. Tissue or paper towel
   c. Lubricating jelly
   d. Vital sign form used in your institution
   e. Disposable gloves

2. Identify the patient by checking the identification bracelet.

3. Tell the patient that you are going to take her temperature by rectum.

4. Provide privacy for the patient.

5. Lower the head of the bed, if allowed.

6. Wash your hands and put on gloves.

7. Take the thermometer out of its container. Hold the thermometer only by the stem.

8. Inspect the bulb of the thermometer carefully for cracks or chipped places. A broken thermometer could seriously injure the patient's rectum. Do not use a chipped, cracked, or broken thermometer.

STEPS

9. Hold the thermometer at the stem end. Shake it down until the mercury is below the numbers and lines.

10. Put a small amount of lubricating jelly on a piece of tissue. Then lubricate the bulb of the ther-mometer with the lubricated tissue. This makes insertion easier and also makes it more comfortable for the patient.

11. Ask the patient to turn on her side. Assist or turn patient, if necessary. Turn back the top covers just enough so that you can see the patient's buttocks. Avoid overexposing the patient.

12. With one hand, raise the upper buttock until you can see the anus, the opening to the rectum. With the other hand gently insert the bulb 1 inch through the anus into the rectum (Figure 19–12◆). Some older patients may have external hemorrhoids, which make viewing the anus more difficult. They may be moved slightly to give a clearer view. Never use force to insert the thermometer.

13. If the patient is an infant, remove the diaper. Lay the baby on her abdomen and place your hand on her back or buttocks to support the infant. Insert the thermometer with the other hand one-half inch into the rectum. Always hold the thermometer while it is in the infant's rectum.

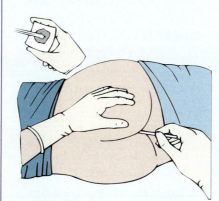

FIGURE 19–12 ◆
Insert the bulb 1 inch into the rectum through the anus

14. Hold the thermometer in place for 3 minutes. Do not leave any patient with a rectal thermometer in place, no matter what her condition.

15. Remove the thermometer from the patient's rectum. Holding the stem end of the thermometer, wipe it with a tissue from stem to bulb to remove particles of feces (Figure 19–13◆).

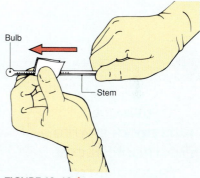

FIGURE 19–13 ◆
Hold the stem as you wipe the rectal thermometer with a tissue

16. Read the thermometer.

17. Record the temperature right away on the vital sign form used in your institution. Note that this is a rectal temperature by writing an R in front of the figure. This is necessary because an average rectal temperature is slightly higher than an oral one.

18. Shake the mercury down until it is below the numbers and lines.

19. Clean with alcohol and replace the thermometer in its container.

FOLLOW-UP

20. Dispose of gloves and wash your hands.

21. Make the patient comfortable and replace the call light.

PROCEDURE *(continued)*

22. Lower the bed to a position of safety.

23. Raise the side rails when ordered or appropriate for patient safety.

24. Report to your immediate supervisor:

   ■ If the rectal temperature is higher than 101°F or 38.3°C.

(Many institutions report the rectal temperature 101°F or 38.3°C by circling the figure in red on the vital sign form used in the institution.)

■ Your observations of anything unusual.

CHARTING EXAMPLE: Record on Ms. Snowbird's flow sheet 11/01/04 3:19pm T = 99.8°F (circle in red or mark with an "R" for rectal). K. Fine, CNA

USING A BATTERY-OPERATED ELECTRONIC RECTAL THERMOMETER

PROCEDURE   OBRA

RATIONALE: Carefully using and reading an ordered rectal thermometer aids in accurate measurement.

PREPARATION

1. Assemble your equipment:
   a. Plastic disposable probe cover (sheath)
   b. Battery-operated electronic thermometer
   c. Rectal (red) attachment
   d. Vital sign form used in your institution
   e. Pen or pencil

2. Identify the patient by checking the identification bracelet.

3. Tell the patient you are going to take his temperature.

4. Wash your hands.

5. Provide privacy for the patient.

6. Check to be sure that the rectal (red top) probe connector is seated properly in its receptacle on the base of the thermometer. Put on gloves.

STEPS

7. Remove the probe from its stored position and insert it into a probe cover (sheath). Lubricate tip of sheath.

8. Insert the covered probe slowly through the patient's anus into the rectum one-half inch.

9. Hold the probe in the patient's rectum.

10. Wait for the buzzer to ring for a computed temperature reading, then remove the probe from the rectum. Remove gloves.

11. Record the temperature on the vital sign form used in your institution. This is very important, because when you return the probe to its stored position the reading automatically returns to zero.

12. Without touching it, discard the used probe cover immediately in a waste receptacle.

13. Return the probe to its stored position in the face of the thermometer.

FOLLOW-UP

14. Store the thermometer in its charging stand whenever it is not in use.

15. Make the patient comfortable and replace the call light.

16. Lower the bed to a position of safety.

17. Raise the side rails when ordered or appropriate for patient safety.

18. Wash your hands.

19. Report to your immediate supervisor:

   ■ If the rectal temperature was over 101°F; 38.3°C.

   ■ Your observations of anything unusual.

CHARTING EXAMPLE: Record on Ms. Snowbird's flow sheet 11/01/05 3:19pm T = R (101.1°F) (circled in red). K. Fine, CNA

MEASURING AXILLARY TEMPERATURE USING A GLASS THERMOMETER

PROCEDURE   OBRA

RATIONALE: Axillary temperatures are taken on small children or adult patients unable to hold an oral thermometer in their mouths or when no tympanic thermometer is available.

PREPARATION

1. Assemble your equipment:

   a. Oral thermometer in container with proper disinfectant solution

   b. Tissue or paper towel

   c. Vital sign form used in your institution

   d. Pen or pencil

2. Identify the patient by checking the identification bracelet.

3. Tell the patient that you are going to take his temperature.

4. Wash your hands.

5. Provide privacy for the patient.

6. Holding the stem end, remove the oral thermometer from its container.

7. Rinse the thermometer with cool tap water and dry it with tissue.

8. Inspect the bulb of the thermometer carefully for cracks or chipped places. A broken thermometer could seriously injure the patient. Do not use a chipped, cracked, or broken thermometer.

STEPS

9. Remove the patient's arm from the sleeve of the gown. If the axillary region is moist with perspiration, pat it dry with a towel.

10. Place the bulb of the oral thermometer in the center of the armpit (axilla). The thermometer should be held upright by the arm and the chest, in contact with the skin.

11. Put the patient's arm across his chest or abdomen.

12. If the patient is unconscious or is too weak to help, you will have to hold the thermometer in place.

13. Leave the thermometer in place for 10 minutes (or time identified by your institution as appropriate). Stay with the patient during this time.

14. Remove the thermometer. Wipe off with tissue from the stem to the bulb if necessary.

15. Read the thermometer.

16. Shake the mercury down until it is below the numbers and lines.

17. Clean with alcohol and replace the thermometer in its container.

18. Record the temperature right away on the vital sign form used in your institution. Note that this is an axillary temperature by writing an A in front of the figure.

19. Put the patient's arm back in the sleeve of the gown.

FOLLOW-UP

20. Make the patient comfortable and replace the call light.

21. Lower the bed to a position of safety.

22. Raise the side rails when ordered or appropriate for patient safety.

23. Wash your hands.

24. Report to your immediate supervisor:

    ■ If the axillary temperature was over 99°F; 37.2°C. Many institutions report an axillary temperature over 99°F; 37.2°C by circling the figure in red on the vital sign form used in your institution.

    ■ Your observations of anything unusual.

CHARTING EXAMPLE: Record on Ms. Howell's flow sheet 11/01/04 2pm T = 98.8°F (indicate "A" for axillary or circle per agency policy). B. Miller, CNA

USING A BATTERY-OPERATED ELECTRONIC ORAL THERMOMETER TO MEASURE AXILLARY TEMPERATURE

PROCEDURE   OBRA

RATIONALE: Axillary temperatures are taken on small children or adult patients unable to hold an oral thermometer in their mouths or when no tympanic thermometer is available.

PREPARATION ◆

1. Assemble your equipment:

   a. Plastic disposable probe cover (sheath)

   b. Battery-operated electronic thermometer (Figure 19–14◆)

   c. Oral (blue) attachment

   d. Vital sign form used in your institution

   e. Pen or pencil

2. Identify the patient by checking the identification bracelet.

3. Tell the patient you are going to take his temperature.

4. Wash your hands.

5. Provide privacy for the patient.

6. Check to be sure that the oral (blue) probe connector is properly seated in its receptacle on the base of the unit.

PROCEDURE *(continued)*

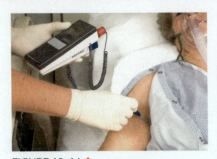

FIGURE 19–14 ◆

Taking an axillary temperature

STEPS

7. Remove the probe from its stored position. Insert it into a probe cover (sheath).

8. Put the covered probe in the center of the patient's armpit (axilla).

9. Put the patient's arm across his chest. Hold the probe in place.

10. Wait about 15 seconds for the buzzer to ring for a computed temperature reading, then remove the probe from the patient's axilla.

11. Record the temperature on the vital sign form used in your institution. This is very important, because when you return the probe to its stored position the reading automatically returns to zero.

12. Without touching it, discard the used probe cover immediately in a waste receptacle.

13. Return the probe to its stored position in the face of the thermometer.

FOLLOW-UP

14. Store the thermometer in its charging stand whenever it is not in use.

15. Make the patient comfortable and replace the call light.

16. Lower the bed to a position of safety.

17. Raise the side rails when ordered or appropriate for patient safety.

18. Wash your hands.

19. Report to your immediate supervisor:

   ■ If the axillary temperature was over 99°F; 37.2°C.

   ■ Your observations of anything unusual.

CHARTING EXAMPLE: Record on Ms. Howell's flow sheet 11/01/04 2pm T = 98.8°F (indicate "A" for axillary or circle per agency policy). A. Kwansa, CNA

Pulse

pulse The rhythmic expansion and contraction of the arteries caused by the beating of the heart; the expansion and contraction show how fast, how regular, and with what force the heart is beating

Each time the heart beats, it pumps a certain amount of blood into the arteries. This causes the arteries to expand (get bigger). Between heartbeats, the arteries contract and return to their normal size. The heart pumps the blood in a steady rhythm. The rhythmic expansion and contraction of the arteries is called the **pulse**. It is measured to show how fast the heart is beating. Measuring the pulse is a simple method of observing how the circulatory system is functioning. The pulse can be measured at a number of places on the body (pulse points) (Figure 19–15◆).

Radial Pulse

radial pulse This is the pulse felt at a person's wrist at the radial artery

rate Used to describe the number of pulse beats per minute

bradycardia Heart rate below 60

tachycardia Heart rate over 100

rhythm Used to describe the regularity of the pulse beats

force Strength or power; used to describe the beat of the pulse

At certain places on the body, the pulse can be felt easily using a person's fingers. One of the easiest and most common places to feel the pulse is at the wrist. This is called a **radial pulse** because you are feeling the radial artery (Figure 19–16◆). When taking the pulse at any pulse point, you must be able to report accurately the following:

■ **Rate:** the number of pulse beats per minute

   ■ **Bradycardia:** heart rate below 60

   ■ **Tachycardia:** heart rate over 100

■ **Rhythm:** the regularity of the pulse beats, which is whether or not the length of time between the beats is steady and regular

■ **Force** of the beat (weak, strong, or bounding)

The average normal rate of pulse for adults is from 72 to 80 beats per minute (Figure 19–17◆). Always report an adult pulse rate of under 60 and over 100 beats per minute to your supervisor.

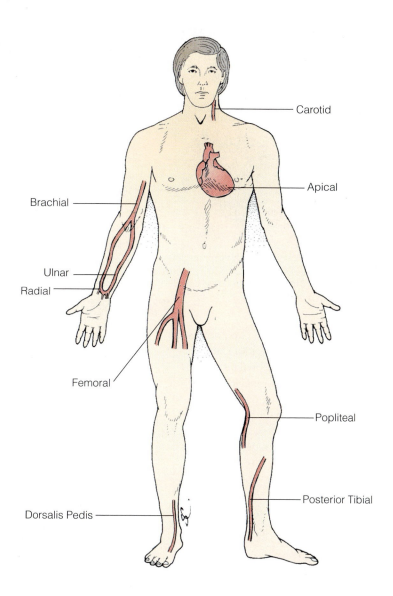

FIGURE 19–15 ◆

Points on the human body where pulse may be taken

Carotid

Apical

Brachial

Ulnar

Radial

Femoral

Popliteal

Posterior Tibial

Dorsalis Pedis

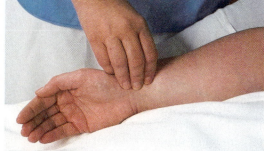

FIGURE 19–16 ◆

Measuring the radial pulse

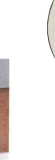

Normal pulse rates (per minute) for different age groups

- Before birth/birth 120-160
- 4 weeks to 1 year 80-160
- Childhood years 80-115
- Adult years 64-80
- Later years 60-70

FIGURE 19–17 ◆

Normal pulse rates per minute for different age groups

PROCEDURE

OBRA

MEASURING THE RADIAL PULSE

RATIONALE: The radial pulse is taken to measure the functioning of the circulatory system.

PREPARATION

1. Assemble your equipment:
   a. Watch with a second hand
   b. Vital sign form used in your institution
   c. Pen or pencil
2. Identify the patient by checking the identification bracelet.
3. Tell the patient you are going to take his pulse.
4. Wash your hands.
5. Provide privacy for the patient.
6. If the patient is standing, ask him to sit down, or have him lie in a comfortable position in bed.

STEPS

7. The patient's hand and arm should be well supported and resting comfortably.
8. Find the pulse by placing the tips of your first three fingers on the palm side of the patient's wrist in a line with her thumb directly next to the wrist bone (Figure 19–18 ◆). Press lightly until you feel the beat. If you press too hard, you may

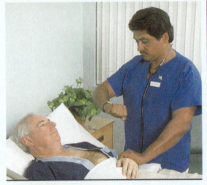

FIGURE 19–18 ◆
Press your first three fingers against the inside of the patient's wrist

stop the flow of blood and not feel the pulse. Never use your thumb. Your thumb has its own pulse and you would be counting your own pulse instead of the patient's. When you have found the pulse, notice the rhythm. Notice if the beat is steady or irregular. Notice if the force of the beat is strong, weak, or bounding.

Note: The number will be more accurate if the patient is unaware that you are counting his respirations.

9. Look at the position of the second hand on your watch. Start counting the pulse beats that you feel until the second hand comes back to the same number on the clock.
   - *Method A:* Count the pulse beats for one full minute and report the full minute. Always use this method if a patient has an irregular pulse.

   - *Method B:* Count for 30 seconds, until the second hand on the watch is opposite its position when you started. Then multiply the number of beats by 2. This is the number you record. For example, if you count 35 beats for 30 seconds, the count for one full minute is 70.
10. Record the pulse count on the vital sign form used in your institution. Be sure you write in the correct column next to the patient's name.

FOLLOW-UP

11. Make the patient comfortable and replace the call light.
12. Lower the bed to a position of safety.
13. Raise the side rails when ordered or appropriate for patient safety.
14. Wash your hands.
15. Report to your immediate supervisor:
    - If the pulse rate was under 60 or over 100 for an adult. If the pulse was irregular, circle in red the number on the vital sign form used by your institution. Sometimes "irr." is written near the number.
    - Your observations of anything unusual.

CHARTING EXAMPLE: Record on Mr. Haswell's flow sheet 11/01/04 2pm P = 78 regular. A. Kwansa, CNA

The Apical Pulse and Pulse Deficit

The pulse rate should be the same as the heart rate. However, in some patients the heartbeats are not strong enough to be transmitted along the arteries to be felt with a radial pulse. This may be due to some forms of heart disease. For these patients, an apical pulse would be taken. An **apical pulse** is a measurement of the heartbeats at the apex of the heart, located just under the left breast (Figure 19–19 ◆).

Sometimes the patient has a **pulse deficit**, a difference between the apical heartbeat and the radial pulse rate. To determine this, the apical pulse (heart rate) is counted with a stethoscope over the apex of the heart. At the same time, the pulse rate is counted at the radial

apical pulse A measurement of the heartbeats at the apex of the heart, located just under the left breast

pulse deficit A difference between the apical heartbeat and the radial pulse rate

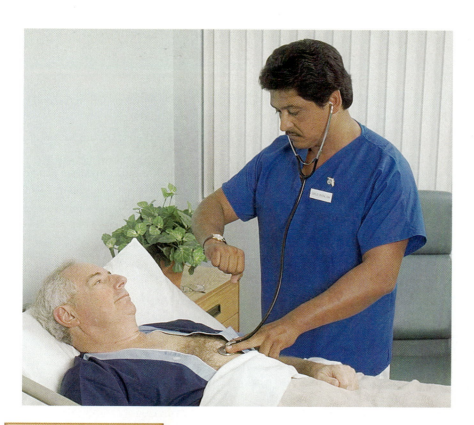

FIGURE 19–19 ◆
Measuring the apical pulse

MEASURING THE APICAL PULSE

PROCEDURE

OBRA

RATIONALE: The apical pulse is taken to directly measure the heartbeats at the apex of the heart.

PREPARATION

1. Assemble your equipment:

   a. Stethoscope and antiseptic swabs

   b. Watch with a second hand

   c. Vital sign form used in your institution (*Note:* In many institutions, this reading is reported directly to your immediate supervisor rather than writing it on the form used)

   d. Pen or pencil and note paper

2. Identify the patient by checking the identification bracelet.

3. Explain to the patient that you are going to take his apical pulse.

4. Wash your hands.

5. Provide privacy for the patient.

6. Clean the earplugs on the stethoscope with antiseptic swabs. Put the earplugs in your ears. Warm the bell or diaphragm of the stethoscope by holding it tightly for a few seconds.

STEPS

7. Uncover the left side of the patient's chest. Avoid overexposing the patient.

8. Locate the apex of the patient's heart by placing the bell or diaphragm of the stethoscope under the patient's left breast. Listen for the heart sounds.

9. Count the heart sounds for a full minute.

10. Write the full minute count on the note paper.

FOLLOW-UP

11. Cover and make the patient comfortable.

12. Replace the call light.

13. Lower the bed to a position of safety.

14. Raise the side rails when ordered or appropriate for patient safety.

15. Clean the earplugs of the stethoscope with antiseptic swabs. Return the equipment to its proper place.

16. Wash your hands.

17. Report to your immediate supervisor:

   ■ That you have taken the patient's apical pulse.

   ■ What the apical pulse rate was.

   ■ Your observations of anything unusual.

CHARTING EXAMPLE: Record on Mr. Haswell's flow sheet 11/01/04 8pm Apical P = 112 Reported to T. Ainsworth, RN. A. Kwansa, CNA

| MEASURING THE APICAL PULSE DEFICIT | PROCEDURE | OBRA |

RATIONALE: The apical pulse deficit is taken to directly measure the difference between the heartbeats at the apex of the heart and the radial pulse rate.

PREPARATION

1. Assemble your equipment:

   a. Stethoscope and antiseptic swabs

   b. Watch with a second hand

   c. Vital sign form used in your institution (*Note:* In many situations, this reading is reported directly to your immediate supervisor rather than writing it on the form used)

   d. Pen or pencil and note paper

2. Identify the patient by checking the identification bracelet.

3. Explain to the patient that you are going to take his pulse.

4. Wash your hands.

5. Provide privacy for the patient.

STEPS

6. There are two methods of taking the apical pulse deficit.

   - *Method A:* Two nursing assistants do this procedure together at the same time. One counts the radial pulse and the other counts the apical pulse for one full minute each. The difference between the two pulses is known as the apical pulse deficit. This method is used for maximum accuracy.

   - *Method B:* The nursing assistant first takes the apical pulse, and then the radial pulse. The difference between the two pulses is known as the apical pulse deficit. However, since the readings are not taken at the same time, it is not considered as accurate as the first method.

7. Count the apical pulse and the radial pulse for one full minute and record both figures.

8. Record the difference between the figures as the pulse deficit.

FOLLOW-UP

9. Make the patient comfortable and replace the call light.

10. Lower the bed to a position of safety.

11. Raise the side rails when ordered or appropriate for patient safety.

12. Clean the equipment and return it to its proper place.

13. Wash your hands.

14. Report to your immediate supervisor:

    - That you have taken the patient's apical pulse deficit.

    - The apical pulse rate.

    - The radial pulse rate.

    - The pulse deficit.

    - Your observations of anything unusual.

CHARTING EXAMPLE: Record on Mr. Haswell's flow sheet 11/01/04 8:15pm Radial P = 100 B. Miller, CNA

Apical P = 114, the apical pulse deficit is 14 A. Kwansa, CNA. Reported to T. Ainsworth, RN

pulse. The two figures are compared. The difference between the apical heartbeat and the radial pulse beat is the pulse deficit. This is called the *apical pulse deficit*. For maximum accuracy, both pulses should be taken at the same time by two nursing assistants. A different method can be used with one nursing assistant who takes the apical pulse first and then takes the radial pulse. This second method is not considered as accurate as the first method.

Respirations

The human body must have a steady supply of air. The body needs oxygen from the air in order to change food into heat and energy. When you breathe in, air is drawn into the lungs. In the lungs, oxygen is taken out of the air and absorbed into the bloodstream. The blood then carries the oxygen to the body cells. In the body cells, the oxygen is used to produce energy for the body (oxidation).

inhaling The process of breathing in air in respiration

exhaling The process of breathing out air in respiration

Respiration is the process of **inhaling** (breathing in) and **exhaling** (breathing out). One respiration includes breathing in and breathing out once. When a person breathes in, the chest gets larger (expands). When a person breathes out, the chest gets smaller

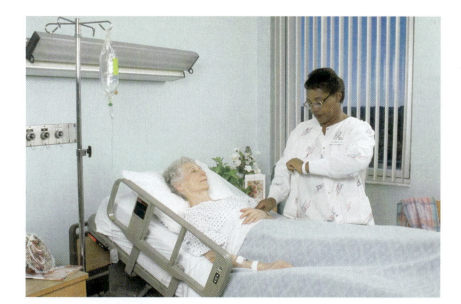

FIGURE 19–20 ◆
The patient must be unaware that you are counting respirations

(contracts). When you count respirations, the patient should be lying on his back. You watch the chest rise and fall as the patient breathes, or you feel the chest rise and fall with your hand. Either way, you should count respirations without the patient knowing it (Figure 19–20◆). If the patient thinks that breathing is being counted, he will not breathe naturally. You want to count natural breathing. Besides counting respirations, you will be noticing whether the patient seems to breathe easily or seems to be working hard to get his breath. When a person is working hard to get breath, it is called **labored respiration**. You must also notice whether the breathing is noisy.

Normally, adults breathe at a rate of from 16 to 20 times a minute. Children breathe more rapidly. The elderly breathe more slowly. Exercise, digestion, emotional stress, disease conditions, some drugs, stimulants, heat, and cold can all affect the number of times per minute that a person breathes.

Abnormal Respiration

While you are counting the patient's respirations, it is important to observe and make note of anything about his breathing that appears to be abnormal. Different types of abnormal respiration that you should be familiar with are:

1. **Stertorous respiration:** The patient makes abnormal noises like snoring or snorting sounds when breathing.

2. **Abdominal respiration:** The patient is using mostly the abdominal muscles to breathe.

3. **Shallow respiration:** Breathing with only the upper part of the lungs.

4. **Irregular respiration:** The depth of breathing changes and the rate of the rise and fall of the chest is not steady or regular.

5. **Cheyne-Stokes respiration:** One kind of irregular breathing. At first the breathing is slow and shallow; then the respiration becomes faster and deeper until it reaches a peak. The respiration then slows down and becomes shallow again. The breathing may then stop completely for 10 seconds and then begin the pattern again. This type of respiration may be caused by certain cerebral (brain), cardiac (heart), or pulmonary (chest) diseases or conditions.

labored respiration Working hard to breathe

stertorous respiration The patient makes abnormal noises like snoring sounds when breathing

abdominal respiration Breathing in which the patient is using mostly the abdominal muscles

shallow respiration Breathing with only the upper part of the lungs

irregular respiration The depth of breathing changes and the rate of the rise and fall of the chest is not steady

Cheyne-Stokes respiration One kind of irregular breathing. At first the breathing is slow and shallow; then the respiration becomes faster and deeper until it reaches a peak. The respiration then slows down and becomes shallow again. The breathing may then stop completely for 10 seconds and then begin the pattern again; this type of respiration may be caused by certain cerebral (brain), cardiac (heart), or pulmonary (lung) diseases or conditions

dyspnea Insufficient oxygenation of the blood resulting in labored or difficult breathing

apnea Periods of not breathing

6. **Dyspnea:** Insufficient oxygenation of the blood resulting in labored or difficult breathing.

7. **Apnea:** Periods of not breathing.

8. *Labored:* The patient struggles or works hard to breathe, and may make rattling, gurgling, or wheezing sounds.

MEASURING RESPIRATION

PROCEDURE   OBRA

RATIONALE: Respirations are measured to document the number of times a patient completes a cycle of inhalation and exhalation of air into the lungs.

PREPARATION

1. Assemble your equipment:
   a. Watch with a second hand
   b. Vital sign form used in your institution
   c. Pen or pencil
2. Identify the patient by checking the identification bracelet.
3. Wash your hands.
4. Provide privacy for the patient.

STEPS

5. Hold the patient's wrist just as if you were taking his pulse. This way he will not know you are watching his breathing. Count the patient's respirations, without him knowing it, immediately after counting his pulse rate.
6. If the patient is a child who has been crying or is restless, wait until he is quiet before counting respirations. If a child is asleep, count his respirations before he wakes up. Always count a child's pulse and respirations before you measure his temperature. (Most children get upset when you measure their temperature, which would abnormally elevate their pulse and respirations.)
7. One rise and one fall of the patient's chest counts as one respiration.
8. If you cannot clearly see the chest rise and fall, fold the patient's arms across his chest. You can feel his breathing as you hold his wrist.
9. Check the position of the second hand on the watch. Count "one" when you see the patient's chest rising as he breathes in. The next time his chest rises, count "two." Keep doing this for a full minute. A full minute count is required by most states as a standard of care for elderly persons. Report the number of respirations you count within that minute.
10. You may be permitted to count for 30 seconds. Count the respirations for one-half minute and then multiply the number you counted by 2. For example, if you count 8 respirations in 30 seconds (a half-minute), your number for a full minute is 16.
11. If the patient's breathing rhythm is irregular, always count for a full minute. Observe the depth of the breathing while counting the respirations.
12. Write down the number you counted immediately on the vital sign form used by your institution. Be sure you write it in the proper column, opposite the correct patient's name.
13. Note whether the respirations were noisy or labored.

FOLLOW-UP

14. Make the patient comfortable and replace the call light.
15. Lower the bed to a position of safety.
16. Raise the side rails when ordered or appropriate for patient safety.
17. Wash your hands.
18. Report to your immediate supervisor:
    - Whether the respirations were noisy or labored.
    - Whether the respirations were irregular.
    - The time they were measured.
    - If the respirations were less than 14 or more than 28 a minute.
    - Your observations of anything unusual.

CHARTING EXAMPLE: Record on Mr. Haswell's flow sheet 11/01/04 2pm R = 22 regular. A. Kwansa, CNA

Blood Pressure

Blood pressure is the force of the blood pushing against the walls of the blood vessels. When you take a patient's blood pressure, you are measuring this force of the blood flowing through the arteries.

There is always a certain amount of pressure in the arteries. This is because the heart, by pumping blood, is constantly forcing it to circulate through the body. The blood goes first into the arteries. It then circulates throughout the whole body. The amount of pressure in the arteries depends on two things:

1. The rate of heartbeat
2. How easily the blood flows through the blood vessels

The heart contracts as it pumps the blood into the arteries. When the heart is contracting, the pressure is highest. This pressure is called the **systolic pressure**. As the heart relaxes between each contraction, the pressure goes down. When the heart is most relaxed, the pressure is lowest. This pressure is called the **diastolic pressure**. When you take a patient's blood pressure, you are measuring both.

In young, healthy adults, the normal blood pressure range is between 100 and 140 millimeters (mm) mercury (Hg) for systolic pressure. Normal diastolic pressure is between 60 and 90 mm Hg. The way these figures are written is:

$$120/80 \text{ or } \frac{120 = \text{Systolic}}{80 = \text{Diastolic}}$$

When a patient's blood pressure is higher than the normal range for her age and condition, it is referred to as high blood pressure or **hypertension**. When a patient's blood pressure is lower than the normal range for her age or condition, it is referred to as low blood pressure or **hypotension**.

Instruments for Measuring Blood Pressure

When you take a patient's blood pressure, you will be using an instrument called a **sphygmomanometer**, which is a combination of three Greek words:

- *sphygmo,* meaning pulse
- *mano,* meaning pressure
- *meter,* meaning measure

This instrument, however, is usually referred to as the blood pressure cuff. The four main parts of this instrument are the manometer, valve, cuff, and bulb.

Two kinds of instruments are used for taking blood pressure. One is the **mercury** type. The other is the **aneroid (dial)** type. Both kinds have an inflatable, cloth-covered rubber bag or cuff that is wrapped around the patient's arm. Both kinds also have a rubber bulb for pumping air into the cuff. The procedure for measuring blood pressure is the same, except for measuring the reading. When you use the mercury type, you will be watching the level of a column of mercury on a measuring scale (Figure 19–21a◆). When you use the dial (aneroid) type, you will be watching a pointer on a dial (Figure 19–22◆). The newer, electronic sphygmomanometers give a digital reading (Figure 19–21b◆).

When you measure a patient's blood pressure, you will be doing two things at the same time. You will listen to the brachial pulse as it sounds in the brachial artery in the patient's arm. You also will watch an indicator (either a column of mercury or a dial) in order to take a reading.

You will use a stethoscope (Figure 19–23◆) to listen to the brachial pulse. The **stethoscope** is an instrument that makes it possible to listen to various sounds in the patient's body, such as the heartbeat or breathing sounds in the chest. The stethoscope is a

blood pressure The force of the blood exerted on the inner walls of the arteries, veins, and chambers of the heart as blood flows or circulates through the structures

systolic blood pressure The force with which blood is pumped when the heart muscle is contracting; when taking a patient's blood pressure, the systolic blood pressure is recorded as the top number

diastolic blood pressure In taking a patient's blood pressure, one records the bottom number as the reading for the diastolic pressure; this is the relaxing phase of the heartbeat

hypertension High blood pressure

hypotension Low blood pressure

sphygmomanometer An apparatus for measuring blood pressure

mercury sphygmomanometer Blood pressure equipment containing a column of mercury

aneroid sphygmomanometer Dial-type blood pressure equipment

stethoscope An instrument that allows one to listen to various sounds in the patient's body, such as the heartbeat or breathing sounds

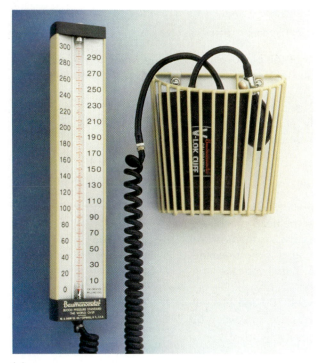

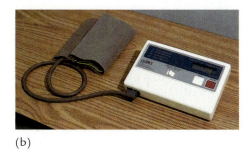

(b)

(a)

FIGURE 19–21 ◆

Two types of
sphygmomanometers:
(a) mercury, (b) electronic

tube with one end that picks up sound when it is placed against a part of the body. This end is either bell-shaped (called a bell) or it is round and flat (called a diaphragm). The other end of the tube splits into two parts. These parts have tips on the ends and fit into the listener's ears.

In many institutions, the blood pressure equipment hangs on the wall over the bed. A smaller-sized cuff must be used for children and a larger-sized for obese (overweight) patients. Do not take blood pressure on an arm that has an IV (intravenous) setup in it, or surgical site on it (example: postmastectomy), or from a patient with an AV shunt (catheter used for dialysis).

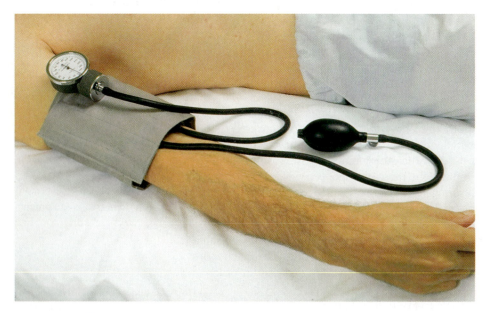

FIGURE 19–22 ◆

Aneroid sphygmomanometer

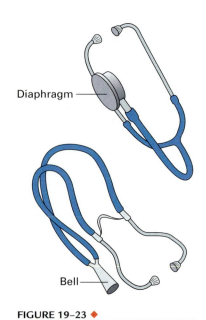

Diaphragm

Bell

FIGURE 19–23 ◆

Stethoscopes

USING A STETHOSCOPE

GUIDELINES

- Point the earplugs of the stethoscope forward before you place them in your ears. This action enables you to hear sounds through the stethoscope.

- Place the earplugs of the stethoscope in your ears.
- Use your fingertips to find the brachial pulse at the inner side of the arm above the elbow, or under the left breast to listen to the apical heartbeat.

- Hold the bell of the stethoscope in place with your fingers.
- Listen carefully for the sounds.
- Remember to clean both the earplugs and the diaphragm or bell of the stethoscope after or between each patient skin contact.

Electronic Blood Pressure Monitoring Apparatus

The latest development in the electronic blood pressure apparatus is an infrared photoelectric system in which a miniature cuff is placed around the left index finger, inflating to the correct pressure necessary to obtain a proper reading and then deflating once the measurement has been determined. Use of this type of equipment eliminates the use of a stethoscope and human error.

With an automatic digital blood pressure monitor a cuff is placed around the wrist. The arm must be at the level of the heart, and no stethoscope is needed.

NONINVASIVE BLOOD PRESSURE MONITORING (NIBP)

GUIDELINES

- Patient selection: No exclusion based on age. With appropriately sized cuffs and hoses, NIBP monitors can be used on patients of all ages.
- Do **not** use NIBP in patients with the following:
  - Highly irregular or rapid cardiac rhythms
  - Excessive body movement or excessive external movement
  - Extreme hypotension or hypertension
- Do **not** place an NIBP cuff on the following:

- The same extremity with an IV infusion line
- The same extremity where SpO_2 is being monitored
- An extremity with impaired circulation
- NIBP monitors have performance limits; in rare circumstances, they cannot determine extremes in blood pressure.
- Inflation of the cuff will impede IV flow.
- Identified patients for whom NIBP monitoring is not acceptable should be communicated to all caregivers. These include those with atrial dysrhythmias and tremors.

- Application of device and initial monitoring:
  - Upper arm is preferred site for cuff placement.
  - Forearm and ankle can also be used.
- Select proper cuff size. Cuff width should equal 40% of arm circumference. Too loose or too small a cuff will lead to falsely high readings. Too large a cuff can lead to falsely low readings.
- Obtain at least one BP reading through auscultation to use as baseline reading.

MEASURING BLOOD PRESSURE USING A SPHYGMOMANOMETER

RATIONALE: Blood pressure is measured to document the force of the patient's blood flowing through the arteries.

PREPARATION

1. Assemble your equipment:

   a. Sphygmomanometer (blood pressure cuff)

   b. Stethoscope

   c. Antiseptic swabs

   d. Vital sign form used in your institution

   e. Pen or pencil

2. Identify the patient by checking the identification bracelet.

3. Tell the patient that you are going to measure his blood pressure.

4. Wash your hands.

5. Provide privacy for the patient.

6. Wipe the earplugs of the stethoscope with antiseptic swabs.

STEPS

7. Have the patient resting quietly. He should be either lying down or sitting in a chair.

8. If you are using the mercury apparatus, the measuring scale should be level with your eyes.

9. The patient's arm should be bare up to the shoulder, or the patient's sleeve should be well above the elbow without limiting or constricting circulation.

10. The patient's arm from the elbow down should be resting fully extended on the bed. Or it might be resting on the arm of the chair or

your hip, well supported, with the palm upward.

11. Unroll the blood pressure cuff and loosen the valve on the bulb. Squeeze the compression bag to deflate it completely.

12. Snugly and smoothly, wrap the cuff around the patient's arm $\frac{1}{2}$" to 1" above the elbow. Do not wrap it so tightly that the patient is uncomfortable from the pressure. You may need to use a different-size cuff for a patient with very thin arms (a child, for example) or very large arms (Figure 19–24◆).

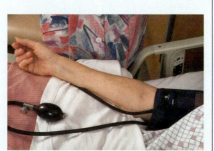

FIGURE 19–24 ◆
Placement of blood pressure cuff

13. Leave the area clear where you will place the bell or diaphragm of the stethoscope.

14. Be sure the manometer is in position so you can read the numbers easily.

15. Put the earplugs of the stethoscope into your ears.

16. With your fingertips, find the patient's brachial pulse at the inner aspect of the arm above the elbow (brachial artery) (Figure 19–25◆). This is where you will place the diaphragm or bell of the stethoscope. The diaphragm should be held firmly against the patient's skin, but it should not touch the cuff of the apparatus (Figure 19–26◆).

17. Tighten the thumbscrew of the valve to close it by turning it clockwise. Be careful not to turn it too

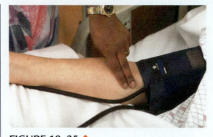

FIGURE 19–25 ◆
Checking for the brachial pulse

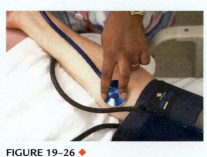

FIGURE 19–26 ◆
Place diaphragm over the brachial artery

tightly. If you do, you will have trouble opening it.

18. Hold the stethoscope in place. Inflate the cuff quickly. When the radial pulse is no longer felt, inflate the cuff an additional 30 mm Hg. (Inflating the cuff to an unnecessarily high pressure is painful to the patient.)

19. Open the valve counterclockwise. This allows the air to escape. Let it out slowly until the sound of the pulse comes back. A few seconds must go by without sounds. If you do hear pulse sounds immediately, you must stop the procedure and completely deflate the cuff. (Repeat Step 18, this time inflating the cuff slightly higher.) Again, slowly loosen the thumbscrew to let the air out. Listen for a repeated pulse sound. At the same time, watch the indicator.

20. Note the calibration (number) that the pointer passes as you hear the

first sound (Figure 19–27◆). This point indicates the systolic pressure (or the top number).

21. Continue releasing the air from the cuff. When you hear the last beat, note the calibration. This is the diastolic pressure (or bottom number).

22. Deflate the cuff completely and remove it from the patient's arm.

23. Record your reading on the vital sign form used in your institution.

24. After using the blood pressure cuff, roll it up over the manometer and replace it in the case.

25. Wipe the earplugs and diaphragm of the stethoscope again with an antiseptic swab. Put the stethoscope back in its proper place (Figure 19–28◆).

26. Make the patient comfortable and replace the call light.

27. Lower the bed to a position of safety.

28. Raise the side rails when ordered or appropriate for patient safety.

29. Wash your hands.

30. Report to your immediate supervisor:

   ■ That you have measured the patient's blood pressure.

   ■ The time that you measured the blood pressure.

   ■ Your observations of anything unusual.

CHARTING EXAMPLE: Record on Mr. Haswell's flow sheet 11/01/04 2pm BP = 148/82. A. Kwansa, CNA

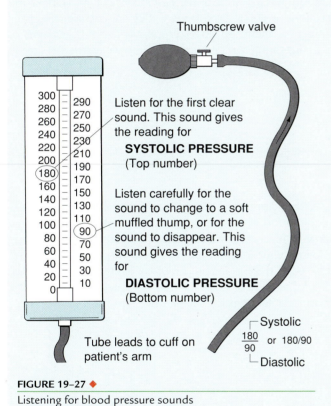

Thumbscrew valve

Listen for the first clear sound. This sound gives the reading for **SYSTOLIC PRESSURE** (Top number)

Listen carefully for the sound to change to a soft muffled thump, or for the sound to disappear. This sound gives the reading for **DIASTOLIC PRESSURE** (Bottom number)

Tube leads to cuff on patient's arm

$\begin{array}{l}\text{Systolic} \\ \frac{180}{90} \text{ or } 180/90 \\ \text{Diastolic}\end{array}$

FIGURE 19–27 ◆

Listening for blood pressure sounds

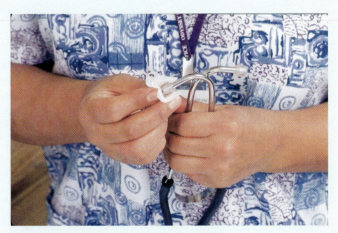

FIGURE 19–28 ◆

Wipe the ear plugs using an antiseptic wipe

Pain—The Fifth Vital Sign

Increasingly you will encounter pain measurement scales with which patients are asked to rate their pain intensity. This measurement is documented to help evaluate the effectiveness of pain relief measures and pain medications. The nursing assistant plays a valuable role in recognizing changes in the patient. Use a pain measurement scale to evaluate the intensity of a patient's pain. Document the value or number that the patient identifies as the amount of pain or discomfort he is currently experiencing.

There are many reasons a patient may experience pain and it is important that the cause be identified. Common causes of pain include:

- Infection
- Cancer
- Postsurgical
- Inflammation of joints, stiffness, or arthritis
- Skin—open wounds, tears, cuts, or decubitus
- Chronic diseases

It is important to take patients' complaints of pain seriously and document how they describe the pain. A patient may use words like *dull, achy, like a knife, throbbing, cramping, unbearable,* or *stabbing.* Observe closely patients who may not be able to communicate with words. The patient may cry, moan, groan, or yell when touched. Some caregivers find pain scales with happy and sad faces are ways to measure children's pain or that of adults when language or communication is a barrier. Some patients have chronic pain and they will usually have pain medications prescribed for them. If they are experiencing pain, the medication may not be working for them. Be sure to report patients' complaints of pain to your supervisor. When you are caring for a patient or taking vital signs, be sure to ask about the pain.

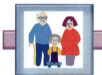

AGE-SPECIFIC CONSIDERATIONS

Vital Signs

Age-specific care for vital signs is very important. Be sure to use the appropriate size equipment for your patient. Use the appropriate size cuff and the most appropriate type of thermometer. If this is not followed, inaccurate vital signs will be obtained. When using glass thermometers, be sure to follow your institution's policy for the use of glass thermometers, especially with children. Glass thermometers can break easily, and mercury exposures are dangerous for patients of all ages. If you will care for patients in several age groups, be sure you know the "normal" vital signs for each group.

SUMMARY

In this chapter you learned how to measure the patient's vital signs—temperature, pulse, respirations, and blood pressure. You learned the normal reading or normal range for each type of measurement using the various types of equipment available or appropriate. For example, the normal reading for a temperature measured rectally is 99.6°F; 37.5°C while the reading for a normal temperature measured orally is 98.6°F; 37.0°C. There are also several different types of rectal and oral thermometers available. Procedures presented here demonstrate how to use many types of equipment and the facilities you will work in will have similar equipment. Over the years as you continue to work in the health care field, you will see the development of and will be trained to use new equipment. What is most important is that you know and understand the criteria for normal readings and that you know what equipment to use and how to use it when you are measuring a patient's vital signs. Pain is also measured, recorded, and reported. The nursing assistant plays a vital role in recognizing signs of pain and documenting changes in the patient's fifth vital sign.

NOTES

CHAPTER REVIEW

FILL IN THE BLANK Read each sentence and fill in the blank line with a word that completes the sentence.

1. Body _____ is the measurement of the amount of heat in the body.

2. _____ temperatures are measured under the armpit of the patient.

3. Glass thermometers often contain a dangerous poison called _____ .

4. One of the easiest and most common places to take a pulse is the _____ pulse.

5. The _____ pressure heard when taking a blood pressure represents the contraction of the heart.

MULTIPLE CHOICE Choose the best answer for each question or statement.

1. When using a glass thermometer, do all of the following *except*
   a. wash your hands.
   b. hold the mercury tip end and shake.
   c. stand back from any hard surfaces to avoid breaking the thermometer.
   d. shake the thermometer down after use.

2. If a patient cannot read, what type of pain measurement scale could you use?
   a. One with words
   b. One with numbers
   c. One with sad and happy faces
   d. One with birds and flowers

3. When taking a patient's pulse, it is important to note
   a. the rate.
   b. the rhythm.
   c. the force.
   d. All of the above.

4. Apnea is
   a. difficult breathing.
   b. when the patient uses his abdominal muscles to breathe.
   c. not breathing.
   d. fast breathing followed by slow, shallow breaths.

5. Do not take a blood pressure in an arm with
   a. an IV.
   b. a surgical site.
   c. an AV shunt.
   d. All of the above.

TIME-OUT

TIPS FOR TIME MANAGEMENT

Regardless of how organized you are and how well you manage your time, you can only do so much work in one shift. Realize that you cannot do everything for everyone, even if you would like to. Know your limits and do not take on more than you can perform. Rather, make constructive suggestions about the division of work among all the staff members.

THE NURSING ASSISTANT IN ACTION
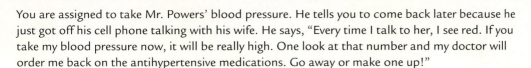

You are assigned to take Mr. Powers' blood pressure. He tells you to come back later because he just got off his cell phone talking with his wife. He says, "Every time I talk to her, I see red. If you take my blood pressure now, it will be really high. One look at that number and my doctor will order me back on the antihypertensive medications. Go away or make one up!"

What Is Your Response/Action?

CRITICAL THINKING
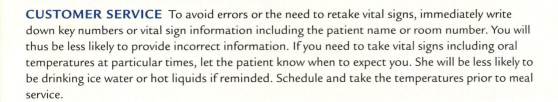

CUSTOMER SERVICE To avoid errors or the need to retake vital signs, immediately write down key numbers or vital sign information including the patient name or room number. You will thus be less likely to provide incorrect information. If you need to take vital signs including oral temperatures at particular times, let the patient know when to expect you. She will be less likely to be drinking ice water or hot liquids if reminded. Schedule and take the temperatures prior to meal service.

CULTURAL CARE You may encounter patients who are from a culture where they are raised to be stoic and bear pain without complaint. If you notice a patient grit his teeth, grimace, sweat, or look pale, inquire about pain or discomfort. Often pain medication is ordered that will enable the patient to be more comfortable and be able to rest.

COOPERATION WITHIN THE TEAM Sometimes, patients require frequent measurements of vital signs. Anticipate and plan for what your patient needs before a scheduled team or staff meeting. If you need to take a break or go to eat, try to do so after taking the vital signs rather than tell your coworker relieving you that the vital signs were due 5 minutes ago, but not done. Your coworker likely has patient care responsibilities of her own that are as important as your duties.

EXPLORE MediaLink
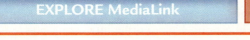

Additional interactive resources for this chapter can be found on the Companion Website at www.prenhall.com/wolgin. Click on Chapter 19 and "Begin" to select the activities for this chapter.

For chapter-related NCLEX-style questions and abn audio glossary, access the accompanying CD-ROM in this book.

Video:

- Risk Management; Vital Signs—Measuring Blood Pressure—Measuring Orthostatic Blood Pressure

20 The Gastrointestinal System and Related Care

KEY TERMS

absorption
anus
appendicitis
bile
constipation
continuous
diarrhea
digestion
duodenum
enema
evacuation
fecal impaction
flatus
gastrointestinal (GI) system
gastrostomy
gastrostomy tube (GT)
gavage
intermittent
large intestine
lavage
liver
nasogastric tube
ostomy
ostomy appliance
pancreas
peristalsis
rectal irrigation
rectum
retention
saliva
Sims's position
small intestine
sphincter
stoma
suction

OBJECTIVES

When you have completed this chapter, you will be able to:

■ Identify the major components of the gastrointestinal system and describe the digestive process.

■ Describe the age-related changes in the gastrointestinal system.

■ List the common disorders and diseases of the gastrointestinal system.

■ Define and describe two different tubes used for tube feedings.

■ Describe three ways that a nasogastric tube can be used.

■ Describe how to recognize and manage diarrhea.

■ Describe how to recognize and remove fecal impaction.

■ List the steps for administering a cleansing enema.

■ Describe what steps may be taken to help keep stool consistency soft and the bowels moving.

■ Describe the procedures for the different types of rectal treatments.

■ Describe the psychological aspects of caring for the ostomy patient.

■ Give ostomy care.

■ Define the key terms used in this chapter.

MediaLink
www.prenhall.com/wolgin

Use the address above to access the free, interactive Companion Website created for this textbook. Get hints, instant feedback, and textbook references to chapter-related NCLEX-style questions. Link to other interesting sites.

AUDIO GLOSSARY:
Use the Companion Website, or the CD-ROM disk enclosed with your textbook, to hear the pronunciation of key terms in the chapter.

Good nutrition and a functioning bowel are vital to a patient's health. This chapter provides you with an overview of the gastrointestinal system and the knowledge required for administering various procedures designed to promote gastrointestinal health, including feeding through a nasogastric tube, rectal cleansing, and ostomy care. Common disorders and diseases of the gastrointestinal system are also covered.

INTRODUCTION

ALERT

For all patient contact, adhere to Standard Precautions (Chapter 5, pages 83–85). Wear protective equipment as indicated.

The Gastrointestinal System (Digestive System)

The **gastrointestinal system** is responsible for breaking down the food that is eaten into a form that can be used by the body's cells. This action is both mechanical and chemical. The digestive tract is about 30 feet long and consists primarily of the mouth, esophagus, stomach, small intestines, and large intestines (Figure 20–1◆).

gastrointestinal (GI) system
The GI tract is about 30 feet long and consists primarily of the mouth, esophagus, stomach, small intestines, and large intestines

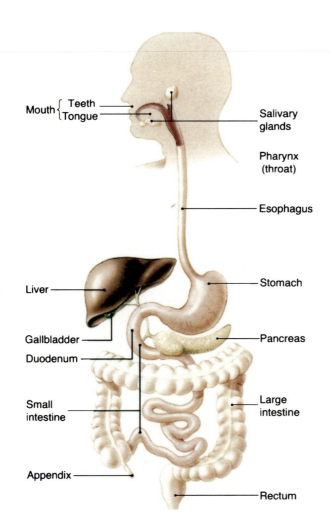

Mouth { Teeth / Tongue

Salivary glands

Pharynx (throat)

Esophagus

Liver

Stomach

Gallbladder

Pancreas

Duodenum

Small intestine

Large intestine

Appendix

Rectum

FIGURE 20–1 ◆

The gastrointestinal system

KEY IDEA

The mouth, pharynx, esophagus, stomach, small intestines, and large intestines are all important in the reduction of food to simple compounds and the absorption of nutrients.

digestion Breaking down the food that is eaten into a form that can be used by the body cells; this process is both mechanical and chemical

saliva The secretion of the salivary glands into the mouth; saliva moistens the food and helps in swallowing; it contains an enzyme (protein) that helps digest starches

duodenum The first loop of the small intestine

small intestine The first, smaller portion of the bowel, including the duodenum, where most of digestion and food breakdown occurs; also known as the small bowel

absorption Part of the digestive process in which digestive juices and enzymes break down food into usable parts

pancreas Produces digestive juices and enzymes responsible for food breakdown in the small intestines

bile Substance manufactured by the liver that helps the food breakdown process

peristalsis Rhythmic contractions of the muscle walls of the small and large intestines

large intestine Distal colon that absorbs water from stool

Digestion begins in the mouth, where food is chewed and mixed with the substance called **saliva**, which contains chemicals that begin to act on the food being chewed. During swallowing, the food moves in a moistened ball down the esophagus to the stomach. The stomach churns and mixes the food at the same time it is being broken down chemically. The most important area of digestion is the **duodenum**, the first loop of the **small intestine**, where **absorption** begins. It is here that the digestive juices and enzymes, not only from the duodenum itself but also from the **pancreas**, finish the job of breaking down food into usable parts. In addition, **bile**, a fluid that has been stored in the gallbladder after being manufactured in the liver, enters the duodenum and helps the reduction process.

A large amount of water is necessary for the chemical reduction of food into its end products. The food is moved by rhythmic contraction, called **peristalsis**, of the muscle walls of the small and large intestines. The next step is absorption.

Some of the final products of digestion are absorbed in the area of the duodenum. These end products are:

- Amino acids, the building blocks for all growth and repair of body tissue, which come from dietary proteins
- Fatty acids and glycerols from fat
- Simple sugars, such as glucose, from carbohydrates
- Water and nutrients

The lining of the duodenum is composed of thousands of tiny fingerlike projections called *villi* (singular, *villus*) (Figure 20–2◆). Each villus is capable of absorbing the end products of digestion. The products are then moved into the bloodstream, where they are carried to individual cells.

Some digestion continues to take place in other parts of the small intestine. What is left of the food moves through the **large intestine**, where water is reabsorbed into the body.

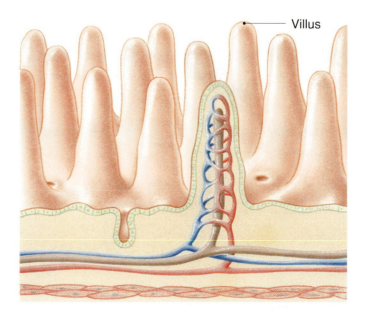

Villus

FIGURE 20–2 ◆

Small intestine

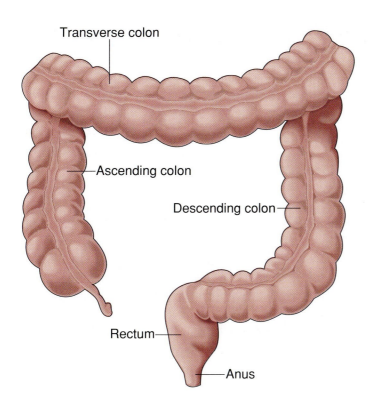

FIGURE 20–3 ◆
Large intestine

The material that cannot be used by the body is excreted from the rectum, through the anus, as feces.

The **liver** not only manufactures the bile that aids in digestion, it is also a storage area for *glucose,* a form of sugar released in large amounts when the cells need it for energy to carry on their activities. In addition, the liver is the place where *toxins,* or poisons, are removed from the blood. Damage to the liver can be caused by drinking alcoholic beverages or taking drugs that are harmful to its tissues.

The appendix is located at the lower right side of the abdomen, between the small intestine and the large intestine. *Inflammation* (swelling and irritation) and *infection* of the appendix is known as **appendicitis**. Surgery to remove an inflamed appendix, called an appendectomy, is usually performed to correct this condition.

The lowest portion of the large intestine curves in an S-shape into the **rectum** (Figure 20–3◆). The rectum is made of very delicate tissue. It has an internal sphincter muscle and an external sphincter muscle. A **sphincter** is a ring-shaped muscle that surrounds and controls a natural opening in the body, such as the anus. Sometimes blood vessels that supply this area become enlarged and filled with blood clots, causing hemorrhoids.

liver Responsible for manufacturing bile and is a storage area for glucose; the liver also is the place where toxins, or poisons, are removed from the blood

appendicitis Inflammation (swelling and irritation) and infection of the appendix, typically with pain in the right lower quadrant; surgery called an appendectomy is usually performed to remove the appendix

rectum The lowest portion of the large intestine, which curves in an S-shape and stores fecal material

sphincter Ring-shaped muscle that surrounds and controls a natural opening in the body, such as the anus

AGE-SPECIFIC CONSIDERATIONS

Age-Related Changes in the Gastrointestinal System

As a person ages, changes occur in the gastrointestinal system that cause the process of digestion to be less efficient. The flow of saliva decreases, as does the number of taste buds, so a person's appetite is likely to decrease as well. In addition, an older person may experience difficulty chewing and swallowing. A weakened gag reflex means an increased risk of choking. Reduced digestive juices make food more difficult to digest, and the absorption of vitamins and minerals is also reduced.

Due to the changes in the gastrointestinal system as a patient ages, care needs of the elderly patient need to be adapted. Decreases in saliva as well as an increased difficulty with chewing and swallowing may result in the need for longer mealtimes for the elderly. They benefit from sitting up while eating to aid digestion and prevent choking. Due to decreases in peristalsis, the elderly may need more fiber and fluids in their diets. The muscular contractions that move food through the digestive system slow down.

Common Disorders and Diseases of the Gastrointestinal System

- *Malignancy:* cancerous tumor that can occur anywhere and in any organ of the gastrointestinal system
- *Ulcers:* gastric (stomach) ulcers, duodenal ulcers, and ulcerative colitis; lesions of mucous membrane exposed to digestive juices
- *Hernias:* occur when there is a weakness in the walls of the muscle, and the underlying tissue pushes through
- *Cholecystitis:* inflammation of the gallbladder
- *Cholelithiasis:* stones in the gallbladder
- *Constipation:* difficult, infrequent defecation with passage of unduly hard and dry fecal material
- *Diarrhea:* abnormally frequent discharge of fluid fecal material from the bowel
- *C. Diff (Clostridium Difficile):* an infectious bacterial disease that causes severe gastrointestinal discomfort and diarrhea; treated with antibiotics
- *Appendicitis:* inflammation of the appendix
- *Peritonitis:* inflammation of the peritoneal cavity
- *Intestinal obstruction:* interruption in the normal flow of intestinal contents along the gastrointestinal tract
- *Hemorrhoids:* varicose veins of the anal canal or outside the external sphincter of the rectum and anus
- *Hepatitis:* inflammation of the liver caused by viruses
- *Hepatic cirrhosis:* chronic disease of the liver caused by viruses
- *Jaundice:* abnormally high concentration of bilirubin in the blood causing a yellow discoloration of the skin and sclerae of the eyes
- *Polyps:* growths on the lining of the intestines that can become cancerous if not treated

Tube Feedings

Oftentimes nursing assistants care for patients who have tubes in the body for the purpose of putting food into the body (or for draining fluids from the body). Frequently, a patient cannot eat or drink because of an illness, surgery, or an injury. In these cases, other methods are used to meet the patient's food and fluid needs. The use of feeding tubes is ordered by the doctor, and the nurse carries out the order. One of the main roles of the nursing assistant caring for a patient with a feeding tube is to protect the patient and keep the patient safe. Think about how uncomfortable it is to have tubing inserted into your body. Provide comfort for the patient and always be careful when you work around feeding tubes. Remember to check and follow the policy of your particular institution or agency regarding your role in caring for a patient with a feeding tube.

Nasogastric Tubes

A **nasogastric tube** (NG tube) is inserted by a skilled nurse or a physician through one of the patient's nostrils, down the back of the throat, and through the esophagus into the patient's stomach. These tubes are used for suctioning the stomach and short-term tube feedings. In such feedings, a nutrition formula is given to a patient through the tube at regular times. Nasogastric feeding is also called **gavage** (Figure 20–4◆).

Fluids are removed from the patient's body through tubes by gravity or **suction**. When fluids are removed by gravity, the collecting container is placed near the patient at a level that is lower than the patient's body. The fluid drips into the container. Suction is used to remove thick secretions that cannot be drawn out easily by gravity. Low-level or intermittent suction is most often used. A suction canister will be connected to a suction machine (Figure 20–5a◆) or to a wall-mounted suction unit (Figure 20–5b◆).

The nasogastric tube can be used to withdraw a specimen of the stomach contents for testing. When a nasogastric tube is being used to drain substances out of the stomach or to collect a specimen, the patient is given nothing by mouth (NPO). The food would only be drawn back out through the tube. Another procedure called a **lavage** refers to the washing out of the stomach through a nasogastric tube, usually with normal saline.

nasogastric tube A tube placed through one of the patient's nostrils (naso-), down the back of the throat, and through the esophagus into the patient's stomach (-gastric)

gavage Feeding through a nasogastric tube

suction Using negative pressure to remove material, usually fluid

lavage The washing out of the stomach through a nasogastric tube, usually with normal saline

KEY IDEA

When a nasogastric tube is used to drain substances from the stomach or to collect a specimen, the patient is given nothing by mouth (NPO).

CARING FOR THE PATIENT WITH A NASOGASTRIC TUBE (NG)

GUIDELINES

- Before giving any fluid through an NG tube, be sure to check to see that the tube is in the stomach by inserting air through a syringe while listening with a stethoscope over the stomach

- Confirm that a doctor has checked the x-ray and approved use of the tube.

- Never pull on the tube when moving the patient or changing the patient's position.

- Remember to fasten the connecting tubing to the patient's clean gown after you have finished bathing the patient. This eases the strain on the tube and prevents accidental withdrawal. The NG tube may be taped to the bridge of the patient's nose. Notify the nurse if tape becomes loose.

- Keep the tube clean and free from mucous deposits at the entrance to the nostril.

- Observe the patient's nostrils for any signs of pressure damage from the tube and report them to the nurse for retaping of the tube.

- If the patient begins to gag or vomit while the tube is in place, report this immediately.

- Report immediately to your supervisor if you see what appears to be leakage from the tube or suction system. Never open the collecting containers to empty the drainage without instructions to do so.

- Report if the level of fluid in the container stops rising. The tubing may be blocked or drainage may be complete.

- The drainage collected through the tube is measured at regular intervals. Note the color, kind, and amount of material and record on the output side of the intake and output sheet.

- If a specimen of the drainage is needed, collect the amount at the time specified.

- If there is a rapid increase in the amount of material being drained or any change in the material itself, report to your supervisor.

FIGURE 20–4 ◆

Nasogastric tubes (stomach tubes)

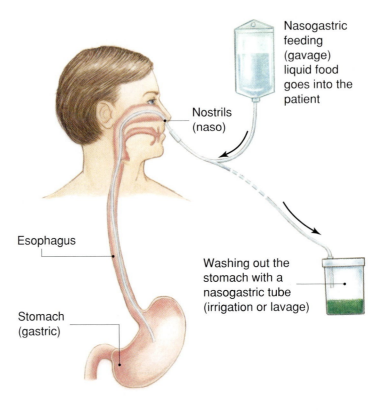

Nasogastric feeding (gavage) liquid food goes into the patient

Nostrils (naso)

Esophagus

Washing out the stomach with a nasogastric tube (irrigation or lavage)

Stomach (gastric)

FIGURE 20–5a ◆

Patient with portable suction (vacuum) apparatus with a nasogastric tube

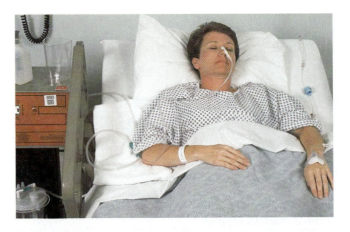

FIGURE 20–5b ◆

Patient connected to wall-mounted suction unit

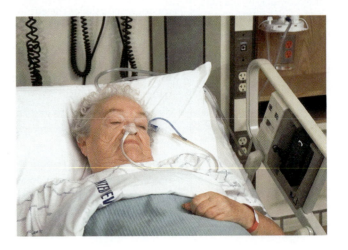

Gastrostomy Tubes

A **gastrostomy** is an opening made through the abdomen to the stomach for the purpose of feeding (Figure 20–6◆). Children and adults who are unable to eat by mouth (typically with disorders of the gastrointestinal or central nervous system) are likely to have a gastrostomy. There are three main types of gastrostomy tubes: a long-term surgical gastrostomy tube; a percutaneous endoscopic gastrostomy (PEG) tube; and a percutaneous endoscopic gastrostomy with a jejunal extension (PEG-J) tube. A surgical gastrostomy, in which a **gastrostomy tube (GT)** is inserted into the stomach, is done in an operating room with the patient under general anesthesia. After a surgical gastrostomy, patients are usually fitted with a "replacement tube" made of silicone. The PEG technique is simple to perform and safer than the standard surgical procedure for elderly or weak patients. A PEG-J is used to feed patients who are at risk for aspiration. The tube has an extension that feeds into the jejunum (Figures 20–7◆).

gastrostomy An opening made through the abdomen to the stomach for the purpose of feeding

gastrostomy tube (GT) Tube inserted into the abdomen for the introduction of fluids

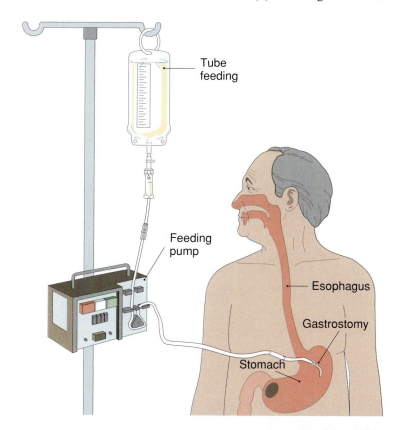

Tube feeding

Feeding pump

Esophagus

Gastrostomy

Stomach

FIGURE 20–6 ◆

Art of gastrostomy tube feeding

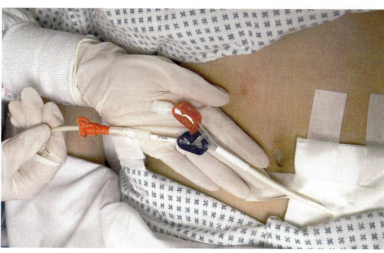

FIGURE 20–7 ◆

Patient with a jejunostomy gastrostomy tube

The tubes usually have a balloon to keep the tube in the stomach and a retainer device to keep the tube stabilized at its exit site. It is very important that the tube site is cleaned each day and that the fit of the tube is checked. A tube retainer that is too tight can cause a pressure sore inside the stomach or on the abdominal wall. Silicone gastrostomy tubes can last for many months. Be sure to check the policy of the health care agency where you work. Report to your supervisor any tubes that are cracked, plugged, or not working properly.

KEY IDEA

Be sure to clean the tube site each day and to check the fit of the tube.

GUIDELINES

GASTROSTOMY TUBE (GT, PEG, OR PEG-J) DAILY CARE

- Cleanse around the gastrostomy site with mild soap and water; pat dry.
- Give tube a twist to ensure that the tube is not too tight against the abdominal wall.

- If the tube does not twist easily, loosen the tube retainer device so that there is 1/8-inch distance between the skin and the retainer disc or triangle.
- Once the gastrostomy site has healed (usually 2 to 3 weeks after surgery) NO DRESSINGS are needed at the site.

- Watch for any signs of irritation or leakage at the gastrostomy site and report these immediately to a supervisor.
- When a patient puts tension on a G-tube, the tube should be stabilized with a mesh netting or wrap to prevent dislocation of the tube or tissue breakdown.

Enteral Feedings (Tube Feedings)

Tube feedings are done only on the order of a physician. The registered dietitian is responsible for assessing the patient's nutritional status and providing recommendations to meet the identified needs. Each institution establishes its own policy for starting the tube feeding. Usually, the policy states that a nasogastric feeding is to be started by the registered nurse or the licensed practical nurse. The nursing assistant watches the level of the feeding and makes sure the formula is being fed slowly into the patient's stomach.

KEY IDEA

Although nasogastric feeding is customarily started by a registered nurse or licensed practical nurse, the nursing assistant is responsible for watching the level of the feeding and making sure the formula is being fed slowly into the patient's stomach.

Commercial formulas are bought ready to use or may require mixing/diluting by the nurse. The formulas contain all the nutrients required for a well-balanced diet, including vitamins and minerals.

The formula is administered at room temperature. A tube feeding container is connected to the stomach by a tube. The rate is controlled by a pump or a special valve so the formula is fed into the patient's stomach very slowly. For adults, the tube must be flushed with 40cc of water before and after the feeding or every 8 hours. This flushing serves two purposes:

- To provide extra fluid intake for the patient
- To maintain tube patency (open tubes)

continuous Uninterrupted, without a stop

intermittent Alternating; stopping and beginning again

TUBE FEEDINGS — GUIDELINES

- Tube feedings are done by gravity and/or by pump. They may be **continuous** or **intermittent** feedings.

- Force from a syringe is never used during the feeding as it may cause abdominal distress in the patient.

- Never use formula taken directly from a refrigerator without warming it to room temperature before feeding the patient.

- Before starting feedings, check the placement of the tube.

- Elevate the head of the bed 30 degrees or higher or have the patient sit up in a chair or wheelchair during the tube feeding to prevent aspiration into the lungs. Stop or hold tube feedings when directed. Refer to your institution's policy and procedure manual or check with your supervisor if you are in doubt.

- Be sure to give the correct amount of formula and water.

- If the tube feeding appears obstructed, stop the feeding and report to your immediate supervisor.

- Report to your immediate supervisor:
  - The time the feeding was started and completed.
  - If continuous feeding, the amount infused.
  - The amount of water flushed before and after.
  - How the patient tolerated the procedure.
  - Your observations of anything unusual.

Patients who do not have a functioning GI tract may be able to receive a venous feeding called *total parenteral nutrition (TPN)*. TPN is infused via a central or peripheral vein. Many complications are associated with TPN, such as gut degradation and infection. This therapy is also very expensive and should only be used when the gut is not functioning.

Diarrhea and Constipation

The care of patients with diarrhea and constipation is an important part of the nursing assistant's role. **Diarrhea** is characterized by frequent, watery stools. This problem may be temporary, due to an infection or a particular food. Diarrhea can often be seen in the patient who gets gastrostomy tube feedings. Whatever the cause, diarrhea is unhealthy and can result in severe illness and dehydration. Be sure to note the amount of urine output a patient has because this is an indication of dehydration. Whenever diarrhea is observed, it must be reported immediately.

diarrhea Abnormally frequent discharge of fluid fecal material from the bowel

Diarrhea is always unhealthy and may result in severe illness and dehydration. Always report diarrhea immediately to your supervisor.

A dietary remedy for diarrhea is the *BRAT* diet. *BRAT* stands for bananas, rice, applesauce, and tea. The foods help to thicken the stool and the tea is helpful for replacing lost fluid.

When a person has diarrhea, she needs frequent skin care (every 1 to 2 hours) to prevent the skin around the anus and buttocks from becoming sore and irritated. Protective ointments such as A&D ointment can help to prevent breakdown. Nurses may choose to use a fecal collection pouch for a patient who is unaware of her incontinence. Fecal pouches may be used by nursing assistants who have been instructed in application technique.

Constipation

constipation Difficult, infrequent defecation with passage of unduly hard and dry fecal material

Constipation is difficult, infrequent defecation with passage of unduly hard and dry fecal material. The most common cause of constipation is lack of adequate fluid intake. The average adult needs eight to ten 8-ounce glasses of fluid each day to stay well hydrated.

The most common cause of constipation is lack of adequate fluid intake, so it is important to see that the patient gets enough fluids each day. In addition, bulk-forming foods and physical activity help combat constipation.

To help the patient avoid constipation it is important to be sure that the patient takes enough fluids every day. Bulk-forming foods such as grains, fruits, and vegetables will help the bowel to stay stimulated and moving. If enough bulk is not available in the diet, then fiber supplements such as Metamucil® can be given. Be sure to assist the patient to take all of the bulk supplements and drink plenty of fluid.

Physical activity also helps to keep the bowels moving. Patients who can walk should be encouraged to do so. For patients who do not walk, wheelchair or bed exercises can be very helpful.

Fecal Impaction

fecal impaction Hard, puttylike fecal material resulting from prolonged retention of stool in the rectum

Prolonged unrelieved constipation leads to **fecal impaction**. The stool becomes hard, puttylike, and very difficult to expel from the rectum. The patient may try to have a bowel movement several times a day. Only small amounts of watery liquid feces may be passed through the anus. The patient will usually feel or complain of rectal pain, discomfort, and cramping. The mass is felt by inserting the digital finger of a gloved hand into the patient's rectum. It often becomes necessary to digitally remove the fecal impaction using lubricant. A physician's order is required to perform this procedure. In many states, this procedure can be performed by the CNA. Before performing this procedure, be sure to check first with your supervisor.

CHECKING FOR A FECAL IMPACTION

GUIDELINES

- Be certain your state allows you to perform this procedure.

- You supervisor should be available in case you have questions or the patient experiences problems.
- Be aware that while performing this procedure the patient can experience reduced heart rate if you stimulate the vagus nerve in the rectum.

- Do not perform this procedure if you have not received the necessary training or met agency requirements to do so.

CHECKING FOR A FECAL IMPACTION

PROCEDURE

RATIONALE: Inserting a gloved finger into the rectum is required to determine that a fecal impaction is present.

PREPARATION

1. Assemble equipment:
   a. Lubricant
   b. Gloves, two pair
   c. Basin of warm water
   d. Soap
   e. Protective underpad
   f. Bedpan and tissue
   g. Bath blanket
   h. Towel
2. Identify the patient by checking the identification bracelet.
3. Explain the procedure to the patient, emphasizing the need to relax as much as possible.

4. Ask about any allergies, including iodine-based antiseptics, latex, and adhesive tape.
5. Ask about any history of slow heart rate or dizziness.
6. Provide privacy for the patient.
7. Wash your hands.

STEPS

8. Place the protective pad under the patient's buttocks.
9. Position the patient in the left side-lying, or Sims's, position.
10. Drape the patient with the bath blanket so that only the buttocks are exposed.
11. Put on gloves.
12. Liberally lubricate your digital finger.
13. With your nondominant hand, separate the buttocks to expose the anus position.
14. Ask the patient take a deep breath through the mouth. While they are taking the breath, insert your lubricated finger into the anus.

15. Check for a hard fecal mass then withdraw your finger. Observe for any signs of rectal bleeding. Discard and put on clean gloves.
16. Offer the bedpan if needed.
17. Wash the patient's anal area with soap and water and towel dry.

FOLLOW-UP

18. Remove underpad. Return bedpan to proper place.
19. Remove and discard gloves and all disposable items used.
20. Wash your hands.
21. Document and report the results to your supervisor.

CHARTING EXAMPLE: 11/20/04 4pm Checked Mrs. Hayes for fecal impaction. Hard mass felt in lower rectum. Tolerated the procedure well, no bleeding or change in heart rate noted. Mrs. Hayes was able to pass a small amount of stool following the procedure. She is still very uncomfortable and complaining of rectal pain. G. Davis, CNA

PROCEDURE

REMOVING A FECAL IMPACTION

The facility's practices and policy will reflect the standard or rule in your state on allowing nursing assistants to perform this procedure.

RATIONALE: Inserting a lubricated, gloved finger into the rectum is required to dislodge and remove fecal impaction when present.

PREPARATION

1. Assemble equipment:
   a. Lubricant
   b. Gloves, two pair
   c. Basin of warm water
   d. Soap
   e. Protective underpad
   f. Bedpan and tissue
   g. Bath blanket
   h. Towel
2. Identify the patient by checking the identification bracelet.
3. Explain the procedure to the patient, emphasizing the need to relax as much as possible.
4. Ask about any allergies, including iodine-based antiseptics, latex, and adhesive tape.
5. Ask about any history of slow heart rate or dizziness.

6. Provide privacy for the patient.
7. Wash your hands.

STEPS

8. Place the protective pad under the patient's buttocks.
9. Position the patient in the left side-lying, or Sims's, position.
10. Drape the patient with the bath blanket so that only the buttocks are exposed.
11. Put on gloves. Check and record the patient's pulse and rhythm.
12. Liberally lubricate your middle index finger.
13. With your nondominant hand, separate the buttocks to expose the anus position.
14. Ask the patient to take a deep breath through the mouth. While they are taking the breath, insert your lubricated finger into the anus.
15. Check for a hard fecal mass, then hook your finger around a portion of feces then withdraw your finger.
16. Drop the feces in the bedpan and observe for any signs of rectal bleeding.
17. Clean your finger with toilet tissue, lubricate it again and repeat Steps 13 through 16 until you no longer feel any feces to remove.

18. Stop and check the patient's pulse and note how they are tolerating the procedure after each one to two times you repeat Steps 13 through 16. If the patient experiences a slowed pulse rate or a change in heart rhythm, call your supervisor or RN to check the patient. Discard and put on clean gloves.
19. Offer the bedpan if needed.
20. Wash the patient's anal area with soap and water and towel dry.

FOLLOW-UP

21. Remove underpad. Return bedpan to proper place.
22. Remove and discard gloves and all disposable items used.
23. Wash your hands.
24. Document and report the results to your supervisor.

CHARTING EXAMPLE: 11/20/04 4:30pm Checked Mrs. Hayes for fecal impaction. Hard mass felt in lower rectum. Removed several large pieces of hard, dark, sticky stool. Tolerated the procedure well, no bleeding or change in heart rate noted. Pulse 76 and regular. Mrs. Hayes was able to pass a small amount of stool following the procedure. She says she is feeling less uncomfortable and has reduced rectal pain. G. Davis, CNA

Rectal Treatments

enema Procedure of evacuation or washing out of waste materials (feces or stool) from a person's lower bowel

retention The patient keeps the enema fluid (oil) in the rectum for 20 minutes

Enemas, which promote the removal of waste materials from a patient's lower bowel to relieve constipation or remove fecal impaction, are administered by nursing assistants. A *cleansing enema* washes out waste materials (feces or stool) from the person's lower bowel. An *oil retention enema* inserts oil into the rectum to soften the stool. **Retention** means that the patient keeps the fluid (oil) in the rectum for 20 minutes. Giving enemas has been made easier in recent years by the use of disposable, prepackaged enema kits and solutions. These plastic enema kits contain an enema bag, tubing, and a clamp and are for single patient use. Prepackaged solutions with nozzles for administering to the patient may also be prescribed.

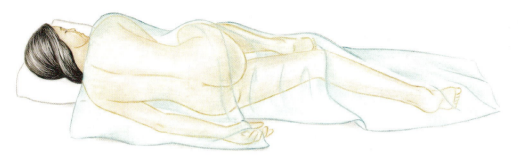

FIGURE 20–8 ◆

Patient lying on left side (left Sims's position)

> **KEY IDEA**
>
> If the patient has any complaints before you start giving the enema, report this to your immediate supervisor. Do not proceed with the enema until you are told to do so.

Occasionally, a patient may complain of a cramplike pain after the enema has started. If this happens, stop the flow of solution until the pain goes away. If you stop the flow and then start again when the pain is gone, the full prescribed amount of solution can usually be given without causing the patient very much discomfort.

Positioning the Patient for the Enema

When the patient is on the left side with the right knee bent toward the chest, it is called left **Sims's position** (Figure 20–8◆). This is also called the *enema position* because most patients are given enemas in the left Sims's position.

Sims's position Patient positioned on the left side with the right knee bent toward the chest, often called the enema position

The Cleansing Enema

The cleansing enema is given only when it has been ordered by the patient's physician (Figure 20–9◆). This enema is used most often to promote evacuation of the lower bowel when this does not happen naturally. **Evacuation** means discharge of the contents of the lower bowel through the rectum and **anus**.

evacuation Discharge of the contents of the lower bowel through the rectum and anus

anus Muscular opening that controls elimination of stool from the rectum

> **KEY IDEA**
>
> Cleansing enemas may be given in preparation for certain diagnostic tests. They are frequently used in preparing a patient for procedures or surgery.

The solution used in the cleansing enema will vary. It may be a commercial preparation, a solution of salt and water (saline), a mixture of soap and water, or plain tap water.

FIGURE 20–9 ◆

Administering a cleansing enema

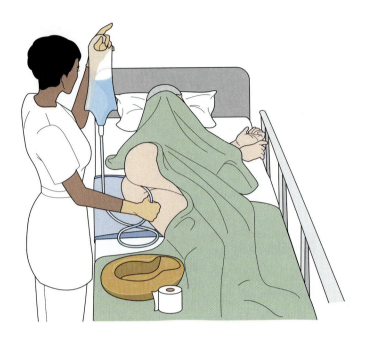

<table>
<tr><td colspan="2">**PROCEDURE**</td><td>**OBRA**</td></tr>
</table>

THE CLEANSING ENEMA

RATIONALE: Cleansing enemas are used to remove stool from the lower bowel in preparation for tests or surgery.

PREPARATION

1. Assemble your equipment:

   a. Disposable enema kit: enema container, tubing, and clamp

   b. Lubricating jelly

   c. Graduated pitcher

   d. Bath thermometer

   e. Solution as instructed by the registered nurse:

   - *Soapsuds:* 1 package of enema soap, 1000 cc of water, 105°F (40.5°C)

   - *Saline:* 2 teaspoons salt, 1000 cc of water, 105°F (40.5°C)

   - *Tap water:* 1000 cc of water, 105°F (40.5°C)

   f. Bedpan and cover/bedside commode

   g. Urinal, if necessary

   h. Emesis basin

   i. Toilet tissue

   j. Disposable bed protector

   k. Paper towel

   l. Bath blanket

   m. Disposable plastic gloves

2. Wash your hands.

3. Identify the patient by checking the identification bracelet.

4. Ask visitors to step out of the room, if this is your hospital's policy.

5. Tell the patient that you are going to give him an enema while he is in bed.

6. Provide privacy for the patient.

STEPS

7. Cover the patient with a bath blanket. Without exposing the patient, fan-fold the top sheets to the foot of the bed. Have the patient covered only with the bath blanket.

8. Place the disposable bed protector under the patient's hips and buttocks.

9. Turn the patient on the left side. Bend the right knee toward the chest. (This is the left Sims's position.)

10. Place the bedpan at the foot of the bed within easy reach.

11. Close the clamp on the enema tubing.

12. Fill the graduated pitcher with 1000 cc of water at 105°F (40.5°C).

13. Pour the water from the graduate into the enema container.

PROCEDURE (continued)

14. a. If your instructions call for a soapsuds enema, add one package of enema soap to the water in the container. Use the tip of the tubing to mix the solution gently so that no suds form.

 b. If your instructions call for a saline enema, add 2 teaspoons of salt to the water in the container.

 c. If your instructions call for a tap water enema, do not add anything to the water.

15. Open the clamp on the enema tubing. Let a little of the solution run through the tubing into the bedpan. This will eliminate any air in the tubing, warm the tube, and avoid giving the patient flatus. Then close the clamp.

16. Put the lubricating jelly on a piece of toilet tissue. Lubricate the enema tip by rubbing the jelly on it with the tissue, beginning at the end and going up the tube 2 to 4 inches. Be sure the tip is well lubricated and the opening is not plugged.

17. Expose the patient's buttocks by raising the blanket in a triangle over the anal area (Figure 20–10◆). Put on disposable gloves.

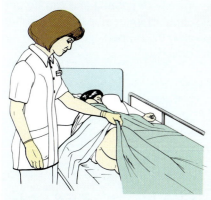

FIGURE 20–10 ◆
Raise the blanket to expose the patient's buttocks

18. Raise the upper buttocks so you can see the anal area.

19. Gently insert the enema tip 2 to 4 inches through the anus into the rectum (slow insertion prevents spasm of the sphincter) (Figure 20–11◆). If you feel resistance or if the patient complains of pain, stop and report this to your immediate supervisor.

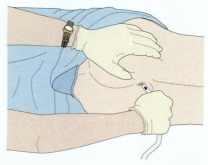

FIGURE 20–11 ◆
Insert the enema tip 2–4 inches through the anus

20. Open the clamp and hold the enema container 12 inches above the anus or 18 inches above the mattress (the higher the container, the greater the pressure exerted) (Figure 20–12◆).

21. Tell the patient to take slow, deep breaths. Explain that this will help relieve any cramps caused by the

enema. It will also help the patient to relax.

22. When most of the solution has flowed into the patient's rectum, close the clamp. Slowly withdraw the rectal tubing. Wrap it in the paper towel to avoid contamination, and place the tubing into the empty enema container. Encourage the patient to hold the solution for as long as possible.

23. Help the patient onto the bedpan or commode. If using a bedpan, raise the back of the bed, if allowed. Put the toilet tissue where the patient can reach it easily.

24. The patient may be allowed to go to the bathroom to expel the enema. If so, assist the patient to the bathroom and stay near the bathroom to assist the patient if needed. Tell the patient not to flush the toilet. This is so the results can be observed.

25. When the patient is in the bathroom or on the bedpan, make sure the signal cord is within reach. Check on the patient every few minutes.

26. Dispose of the enema equipment while the patient is on the bedpan.

27. When observing the results of an enema, look for anything that does

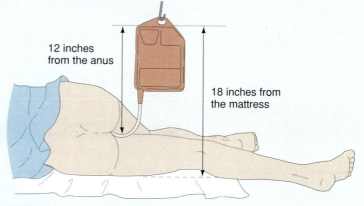

12 inches from the anus

18 inches from the mattress

FIGURE 20–12 ◆
Hang or hold the enema bag 12 inches above the anus or 18 inches above the mattress

PROCEDURE *(continued)*

not appear normal. Check color, consistency, odor, and amount.

a. Report to the registered nurse if the stool:
- Is very hard
- Is very soft
- Is large in amount
- Is small in amount
- Is accompanied by flatus (gas)

b. Collect a specimen and report to the registered nurse if the stool:
- Is black (tarlike)
- Is streaked with red, white, yellow, or gray
- Has a very bad odor
- Looks like perked coffee grounds

28. Empty the bedpan, clean it, and put it in its proper place.

29. Remove the disposable bed protector and discard.

30. Remove the bath blanket. At the same time, raise the top sheets to cover the patient.

31. Wash the patient's hands or have the patient wash his own hands.

FOLLOW-UP

32. Make the patient comfortable.

33. Lower the bed to a position of safety for the patient.

34. Raise the side rails where ordered, indicated, and appropriate for patient safety.

35. Place the call light within easy reach of the patient.

36. Wash your hands.

37. Report to your immediate supervisor:
- That you have given the patient a cleansing enema.
- The time the enema was given.

- The type of solution used.
- The results, color of stool, consistency, flatus (gas) expelled, and unusual material noted.
- Whether or not a specimen was obtained.
- How the patient tolerated the procedure.
- Your observations of anything unusual.

CHARTING EXAMPLE: 12/7/04 7pm 1000cc cleansing soapsuds enema given. Enema returned with dark brown stool. Procedure tolerated well. W. Waverly, CNA

The Prepackaged, Ready-to-Use Enema

The prepackaged, ready-to-use enema is an effective, easy-to-use enema. The physician must order this type before it can be administered. This enema is used frequently in the home as well as in the health care institution. It is completely disposable and can be purchased in any pharmacy or obtained from the central supply room in a health care institution. Many health care institutions have a policy of *warming* the prepackaged, ready-to-use enema. Follow your employing health care institution's policies.

GIVING THE READY-TO-USE CLEANSING ENEMA

PROCEDURE

OBRA

RATIONALE: These enemas provide a disposable, easy-to-use way to remove stool from the lower bowel.

PREPARATION

Note: Always read the package instructions for giving the enema.

1. Assemble your equipment:
   a. Disposable prepackaged enema
   b. Bedpan and cover/bedside commode
   c. Urinal, if necessary
   d. Disposable bed protector
   e. Toilet tissue
   f. Disposable plastic gloves

2. Wash your hands.

3. Identify the patient by checking the identification bracelet.

PROCEDURE (continued)

4. Ask visitors to step out of the room, if this is your hospital's policy.

5. Tell the patient that you are going to give her an enema while she is in bed.

6. Provide privacy for the patient. Ask patient if she needs to urinate. If so, provide equipment.

STEPS

7. Cover the patient with a bath blanket. Without exposing the patient, fan-fold the top sheets to the foot of the bed. Have the patient covered only with the bath blanket.

8. Place the disposable bed protector under the patient's hips (buttocks). Warm the enema if this is the policy of your employing health care institution.

9. Turn the patient on the left side. Bend the right knee toward the chest. (This is the left Sims's position.)

10. Place the bedpan at the foot of the bed within easy reach.

11. Open the enema package. Take out the disposable enema. Remove the cap (Figure 20–13◆). Put on disposable plastic gloves.

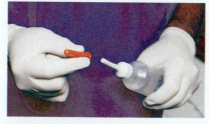

FIGURE 20–13 ◆
Remove the cap

12. Expose the patient's buttocks by raising the blanket in a triangle over the anal area.

13. Raise the upper buttocks so you can see the anal area.

14. Gently insert the enema tip, which is prelubricated, 2 inches through the anus into the rectum (Figure 20–14◆).

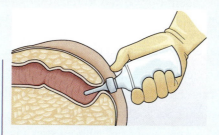

FIGURE 20–14 ◆
Insert the enema tip 2" through the anus into the rectum

15. Squeeze the plastic bottle gently until all the liquid goes into the patient's rectum.

16. Remove the tube from the patient's anus. Put the empty plastic bottle back in the box (Figure 20–15◆). You will discard it later, in the dirty utility room. Encourage the patient to hold the solution as long as possible.

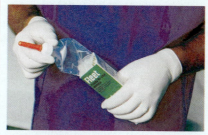

FIGURE 20–15 ◆
Return empty bottle into the box for disposal

17. Help the patient onto the bedpan. Raise the back of the bed, if allowed. Put the toilet tissue where the patient can reach it easily.

18. The patient may be allowed to use a bedside commode or go to the bathroom to expel the enema. If so, assist the patient to the bathroom and stay near the bathroom to assist the patient if needed. Tell the patient not to flush the toilet. This is so the results can be observed.

19. When the patient is in the bathroom or on the bedpan, make sure the signal cord is within reach. Check on the patient every few minutes.

20. Discard the disposable enema equipment. Return to the patient when she is finished using the bedpan. Check the contents for color of stool, consistency, amount, unusual material, or anything abnormal. If you observe anything unusual, collect a specimen.

21. Empty the bedpan. Clean it and put it in its proper place.

22. Remove the disposable bed protector and discard it.

23. Remove the bath blanket. At the same time, raise the top sheets to cover the patient.

24. Wash the patient's hands or have the patient wash her own hands.

FOLLOW-UP

25. Make the patient comfortable.

26. Lower the bed to a position of safety for the patient.

27. Raise the side rails where ordered, indicated, and appropriate for patient safety.

28. Place the call light within easy reach of the patient.

29. Wash your hands.

30. Report to your immediate supervisor:

   ■ That you have given the patient a cleansing enema.

   ■ The time the enema was given, the results, color of stool, consistency, flatus expelled, and any unusual material noted.

   ■ How the patient tolerated the procedure.

   ■ Your observations of anything unusual.

CHARTING EXAMPLE: 12/7/04 8pm Ready-to-use enema given. Mrs. Blake had a bowel movement at 8:10pm. Enema returned with dark brown stool. Procedure tolerated well. W. Waverly, CNA

The Oil Retention Enema

The procedure for giving the retention enema is different from that for the cleansing enema. The patient is expected to retain (hold in) the enema solution for 10 to 20 minutes. Sometimes a soapsuds (cleansing) enema is given 20 minutes after the oil retention enema has been expelled.

Retention enemas are given to:

- Help soften the feces and gently stimulate evacuation
- Lubricate the inside surface of the lower intestine
- Soften the stool, if necessary
- Ease the passage of feces without straining
- Provide laxative benefits when oral laxatives are not allowed
- Soften fecal impaction (hard stool retained in the lower bowel) when straining might be harmful or painful

---

PROCEDURE   OBRA

GIVING THE READY-TO-USE OIL RETENTION ENEMA

RATIONALE: These enemas provide a disposable, easy-to-use way to lubricate and remove stool from the lower bowel.

PREPARATION

Note: Always read the package instructions for giving the enema.

1. Assemble your equipment:
   a. Disposable, prepackaged, ready-to-use enema kit
   b. Bedpan and cover/bedside commode
   c. Urinal, if necessary
   d. Disposable bed protector
   e. Equipment for soapsuds enema if ordered by the physician; give 20 minutes after oil retention enema
   f. Toilet tissue
   g. Disposable gloves
2. Wash your hands.
3. Identify the patient by checking the identification bracelet.

4. Ask visitors to step out of the room, if this is your hospital's policy.
5. Tell the patient that you are going to give him an oil retention enema while he is in bed.

STEPS

6. Provide privacy for the patient.
7. Cover the patient with a bath blanket. Without exposing the patient, fan-fold the top sheets to the foot of the bed. Have the patient covered only with the bath blanket.
8. Place the disposable bed protector under the patient's hips (buttocks).
9. Turn the patient on the left side. Bend the right knee toward the chest. (This is the left Sims's position.)
10. Place the bedpan at the foot of the bed within easy reach.
11. Open the package. Take out the disposable, prepackaged, ready-to-use enema bag filled with oil. Remove the cap. Put gloves on. Warm the oil enema if this is the policy of your health care institution.
12. Expose the patient's buttocks by raising the blanket in a triangle over the anal area.

13. Raise the upper buttocks so you can see the anal area.
14. Gently insert the enema tip, which is prelubricated, 2 inches through the anus into the rectum.
15. Squeeze the plastic bottle gently until all the liquid goes into the patient's rectum.
16. Remove the tube from the patient's anus. Put the empty plastic bottle back in the box. You will discard it later.
17. Explain to the patient that it is necessary to retain (hold in) the oil for 20 minutes. Encourage the patient to stay in the Sims's position, if at all possible. Check on the patient every few minutes.
18. Your instructions may require you to give a soapsuds enema after the patient has retained the oil for 20 minutes. If so, give the soapsuds enema at that time.
19. Help the patient onto the bedpan. Raise the back of the bed, if allowed. Put the toilet tissue where the patient can reach it easily.
20. The patient may be allowed to go to the bathroom to expel the enema. If so, assist the patient to

PROCEDURE *(continued)*

the bathroom and stay near the bathroom to assist the patient if needed. Tell the patient not to flush the toilet. This is so the results can be observed.

21. When the patient is in the bathroom or on the bedpan, make sure the signal cord is within reach. Check on the patient every few minutes.

22. Discard the disposable enema equipment.

23. Return to the patient when he is finished using the bedpan or bathroom. Check the contents for color of stool, consistency, amount, unusual material, or anything abnormal. If you observe anything unusual, collect a specimen.

24. Empty the bedpan. Clean it and put it in its proper place.

25. Remove the disposable bed protector and discard it.

26. Remove the bath blanket. At the same time, raise the top sheets to cover the patient.

27. Wash the patient's hands or have the patient wash his own hands.

FOLLOW-UP

28. Make the patient comfortable.

29. Lower the bed to a position of safety for the patient.

30. Raise the side rails where ordered, indicated, and appropriate for patient safety.

31. Place the call light within easy reach of the patient.

32. Wash your hands.

33. Report to your immediate supervisor:

    ■ That you have given the patient an oil retention enema.

    ■ The time the oil retention enema was given, the results, color of stool, consistency, flatus expelled, and unusual material noted.

    ■ How the patient tolerated the procedure.

CHARTING EXAMPLE: 12/7/04 8pm Oil retention enema given and held for 15 minutes. Mr. Blake had a bowel movement at 8:20pm. Enema returned with dark brown stool. Procedure tolerated well. W. Waverly, CNA

The Harris Flush (Return-Flow Enema)

The Harris flush is an irrigation of the rectum (**rectal irrigation**). Irrigation means washing out. Clean water runs into the rectum. **Flatus** (gas) and water run out of the rectum. Again, clean water runs into the rectum. Flatus and water run out of the rectum in the return flow. The procedure is repeated for 10 minutes until the patient is relieved of excess gas.

rectal irrigation Repeated washing out of the rectum; clean water runs into the rectum, gas (flatus) and water run out of the rectum, as in the Harris flush

flatus Intestinal gas

GIVING THE HARRIS FLUSH (RETURN-FLOW ENEMA)

PROCEDURE

OBRA

RATIONALE: Return-flow enemas are used to irrigate and remove flatus from the lower bowel.

PREPARATION

Note: Always read the package instructions for giving the enema.

1. Assemble your equipment:

    a. Disposable enema bag, tubing, and clamp

    b. Lubricating jelly

    c. Graduated pitcher

    d. Bath thermometer

    e. Urinal, if necessary

    f. Disposable plastic gloves

    g. Emesis basin

    h. Toilet tissue

    i. Disposable bed protector

    j. Paper towel

    k. Bath blanket

    l. Bedpan/bedside commode

2. Wash your hands.

3. Identify the patient by checking the identification bracelet.

4. Ask visitors to step out of the room, if this is your hospital's policy.

5. Tell the patient that you are going to give her a Harris flush, which is a rectal irrigation that will relieve gas.

6. Provide privacy for the patient.

PROCEDURE (continued)

STEPS

7. Cover the patient with a bath blanket. Without exposing the patient, fan-fold the top sheets to the foot of the bed. Have the patient covered only with the bath blanket.

8. Place the disposable bed protector under the patient's hips and buttocks.

9. Turn the patient on the left side. Bend the right knee toward the chest. (This is the left Sims's position.)

10. Put the bedpan at the foot of the bed within easy reach.

11. Close the clamp on the enema tubing.

12. Fill the graduated pitcher with 500 cc of water, 105°F (40.5°C). Measure the temperature of the water with the bath thermometer.

13. Pour the water from the graduated pitcher into the enema container.

14. Open the clamp on the enema tubing to let water run through the tubing into the bedpan. This will get rid of any air that may be in the tubing to avoid giving the patient flatus and will also warm the tube. Close the clamp.

15. Put the lubricating jelly on a piece of toilet tissue. Lubricate the enema tip by rubbing the jelly on it with the tissue. Be sure the tip is well lubricated and the opening is not plugged.

16. Expose the patient's buttocks by raising the blanket in a triangle over the anal area. Put gloves on now.

17. Raise the upper buttocks so you can see the anal area.

18. Gently insert the enema tip 2 inches through the anus into the rectum.

19. Open the clamp. Hold the enema container 12 inches above the anus. Allow about 200 cc of water to enter the rectum.

20. Lower the enema bag below the bed frame. Let the water run back into the enema bag without removing the tube from the patient's rectum.

21. Hold the enema bag 12 inches above the anus. Let 200 cc of water run into the patient's rectum; then lower the bag. Allow the water to run back into the enema bag. Keep the tube in the patient's rectum.

22. Continue letting water in and out of the rectum for 10 to 20 minutes, as you are instructed.

23. Tell the patient to take slow deep breaths. Explain that this kind of breathing will help relieve the pressure and cramps caused by the enema. It will also help her to relax.

24. Observe the amounts (large or small) of flatus the patient expels as the water runs out of the patient into the enema bag.

25. Remove the tubing when the treatment is finished. Wrap the enema tip in the paper towel. This is to avoid contamination. Place it in the disposable enema container.

26. Help the patient onto the bedpan. Raise the back of the bed, if allowed. Put the toilet tissue where the patient can reach it easily. Give the patient the signal cord. Check on the patient every few minutes.

27. The patient may be allowed by the nurse to go to the bathroom to expel more flatus. If so, assist the patient to the bathroom. Tell the patient to notice the amount of flatus (large or small amounts) that is expelled.

28. Discard the disposable enema equipment while the patient is on the bedpan or in the bathroom.

29. Return to the patient when she is finished using the bedpan or bathroom. Check the contents for bowel movement, color of stool, consistency, amount, unusual

material, or anything abnormal. If you observe anything unusual, collect a specimen. Ask the patient if flatus was expelled.

30. Empty the bedpan, clean it, and put it in its proper place.

31. Remove the disposable bed protector and discard it.

32. Remove the bath blanket. At the same time, raise the top sheets to cover the patient.

33. Wash the patient's hands, or have the patient wash them.

FOLLOW-UP

34. Make the patient comfortable.

35. Lower the bed to a position of safety for the patient.

36. Raise the side rails where ordered, indicated, and appropriate for patient safety.

37. Place the call light within easy reach of the patient.

38. Wash your hands.

39. Report to your immediate supervisor:

   - That you have given the patient a Harris flush.

   - The time the Harris flush was given and how long it was continued.

   - The results, amount of flatus expelled, and unusual material noted.

   - Whether or not a specimen was obtained.

   - How the patient tolerated the procedure.

   - Your observations of anything unusual.

CHARTING EXAMPLE: 12/8/04 8pm Harris Flush enema given, bowel irrigated for 15 minutes. Mrs. Blake released flatus. Procedure tolerated well. W. Waverly, CNA

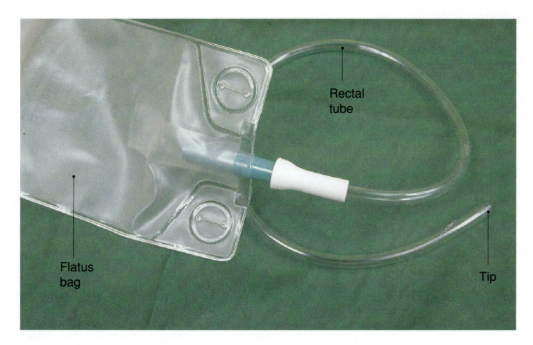

Rectal
tube

Flatus
bag

Tip

FIGURE 20–16 ◆
Disposable flatus bag and
rectal tube

Disposable Rectal Tube with Connected Flatus Bag

A rectal tube with connected bag is used to relieve intestinal gas (flatus) that often accumulates in the patient's lower bowel (Figure 20–16◆). You will use the rectal tube only once a day for 20 minutes, unless otherwise instructed. The whole kit—tube and bag—is discarded after one use.

USING THE DISPOSABLE RECTAL TUBE WITH CONNECTED FLATUS BAG

PROCEDURE   **OBRA**

RATIONALE: Flatus bags are used remove flatus from the lower bowel.

PREPARATION

1. Assemble your equipment:
   a. Disposable rectal tube with connected flatus bag
   b. Small piece of adhesive tape
   c. Tissue
   d. Lubricating jelly
   e. Disposable gloves
2. Wash your hands.

3. Identify the patient by checking the identification bracelet.
4. Ask visitors to step out of the room, if this is your hospital's policy.
5. Tell the patient that you are going to insert a rectal tube for the purpose of relieving him of gas (flatus).
6. Provide privacy for the patient.

STEPS

7. Turn the patient on the left side. Bend the right knee toward the chest. (This is the left Sims's position.)
8. Expose the patient's buttocks by raising the blanket in a triangle

over the anal area. Put on the disposable plastic gloves.
9. Lubricate the tip of the rectal tube. Do this by squeezing lubricating jelly onto the tissue and rubbing the jelly on the tip. Be sure the opening at the end of the tube is not clogged. (If the rectal tube is prelubricated, this step is not necessary.)
10. Raise the upper buttocks so you can see the anal area.
11. Gently insert the rectal tube 2 to 4 inches through the anus into the rectum.
12. Use a small piece of adhesive tape to attach the tube to the patient's buttocks in order to hold the tube in place.

PROCEDURE *(continued)*

13. Let the tube remain in place for 20 minutes. Then remove and discard the equipment. (Usually this procedure is done once in a 24-hour period.)

FOLLOW-UP

14. Make the patient comfortable.

15. Lower the bed to a position of safety for the patient.

16. Raise the side rails where ordered, indicated, and appropriate for patient safety.

17. Place the call light within easy reach of the patient.

18. Wash your hands.

19. Report to your immediate supervisor:
   - The time the rectal tube was inserted and the time it was removed.
   - The patient's comments about the amount (small or large) of flatus that was expelled through the tube.
   - How the patient tolerated the procedure.
   - Your observations of anything unusual.

CHARTING EXAMPLE: 12/8/04 8pm Flatus bag used for 20 minutes to remove flatus from the lower bowel. Mr. Blake released 1/2 filled bag of flatus. Procedure tolerated well. W. Waverly, CNA

Rectal Suppositories

Rectal suppositories are inserted into the rectum to aid in elimination, to promote healing, to relieve pain, or to re-toilet train an incontinent patient. Adults use a single or double-cone shaped suppository; children use a long, thin suppository. Simple, nonmedicinal suppositories are made of soap, glycerine, or cocoa butter, and may be administered by nursing assistants. Medicinal suppositories, which contain drugs, are not administered by nursing assistants.

ostomy A surgical procedure (operation) in which a new opening, called a stoma, is created in the abdomen, usually for the discharge of wastes (urine or feces) from the body

stoma A surgically made opening connecting the urinary or intestinal tract with the outside, such as in a urostomy or colostomy

The Ostomy

An **ostomy** is a surgical procedure in which a new opening, called a **stoma**, is created, usually in the abdomen, for the discharge of wastes (urine or feces) from the body. A stoma created surgically may be used to divert the path of the patient's feces from the rectum. This is done when the colon is diseased or injured. The ostomy is often performed to remove tumors. Sometimes the surgery is done to permit repair of bowel injuries. An ostomy may be created to treat inflammatory bowel disease (IBD) like ulcerative colitis and Crohn's disease.

KEY IDEA

An ostomy is a surgical procedure that provides the patient with an artificial opening connecting a body passage with outside, such as in a tracheotomy or colostomy. An ostomy may be temporary or permanent.

Figures 20–17◆ through 20–21◆ describe types of ostomies and show the position of the stoma in each case.

Sigmoid colostomy

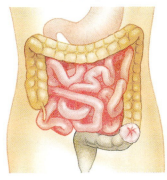

Descending colostomy

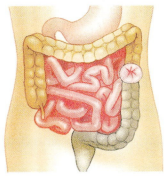

FIGURE 20–17 ◆

Following surgery, the type of discharge from a sigmoid or descending colostomy may be semiliquid until, through management of diet, the stool begins to resemble a normal bowel movement

Transverse (double barrel)

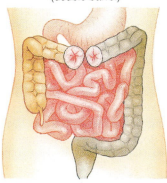

Transverse-loop colostomy

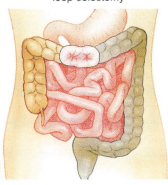

FIGURE 20–18 ◆

Frequently, the transverse double barrel and the transverse loop colostomy are temporary; common patient problems with these types of ostomies include skin irritation and leakage from the appliance

Ileal conduit

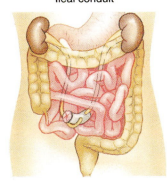

Bilateral cutaneous ureterostomy

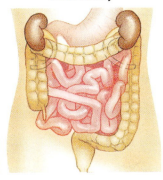

FIGURE 20–19 ◆

Urinary diversion is performed for malfunction of the urinary bladder. When the patient has a bilateral cutaneous ureterostomy or an ileal conduit, prevention of leakage and skin protection are of utmost importance

Ascending colostomy

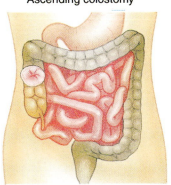

FIGURE 20–20 ◆

The ascending colostomy is essentially the same as the transverse colostomy. Common patient problems include skin irritation, leakage from the appliance, and odor control

FIGURE 20–21 ◆

The ileostomy; a common
patient problem with the
ileostomy is skin irritation

Ileostomy

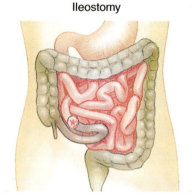

ostomy appliance Collecting
pouch usually attached to the
skin around the stoma with
adhesive

A person with a stoma must wear an **ostomy appliance** to collect waste from the stoma (Figure 20–22◆). This is a collecting pouch usually adhered to the skin around the stoma with an adhesive barrier. The stoma is red due to its abundant blood supply. It may bleed slightly during care. This is normal and is not something that should worry the patient. However, bleeding that does not stop should be reported.

As a nursing assistant, you may be taking care of a patient who has had the surgery for some time and already has been fitted with an ostomy appliance. Sometimes the patient is able and wants to care for the ostomy himself. In this case, assist the patient as he needs. Ask the patient how you can assist, as each patient develops a routine in doing self-care and will appreciate your interest and concern. A new surgical patient with a new ostomy is cared for by a registered nurse who teaches self-care and does a frequent assessment of the stoma.

Psychological Aspects of Ostomies

The psychological reaction of the patient to an ostomy will vary with each patient. Dealing with the ostomy may at first be a bit overwhelming to the patient. Faced with an altered body image, the patient may feel a keen sense of loss, become quiet and withdrawn, or very angry, hostile, noisy, and disruptive. The patient may develop mood changes, appearing very anxious or depressed. Anxiety is a natural and common response; fear is another. Either emotion can cause the patient to develop feelings of doom or panic. Family

FIGURE 20–22 ◆

Ostomy appliance in place over
the stoma

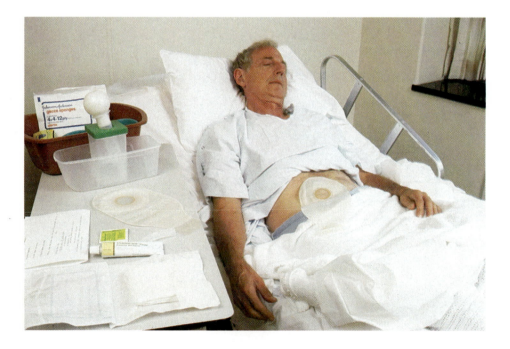

members and significant others who provide emotional support are very important. Allow the patient time to express his feelings during your contact with him.

The nurse or enterostomal therapy nurse (a nurse specializing in ostomy care) should be contacted to arrange for an *ostomy visitor* if the patient desires. An ostomy visitor is someone who has had ostomy surgery and has had special training. The shared experience of someone who has had an ostomy and is living with a stoma can help the patient see that positive adjustment is possible. As the caregiver it is important not to convey either verbally or nonverbally a negative reaction to the patient. Your patient needs encouragement and support.

Caring for an Ostomy

It is desirable for the patient to be moving toward independence in ostomy self-care prior to discharge. It is important for the patient to know and demonstrate how to empty the appliance, clean the tail, and replace the clamp prior to discharge. To get to that point, you can assist by practicing with the patient how to empty the ostomy pouch.

Shortly after surgery and until the patient is up without assistance, it is easier for the patient to have the pouch emptied while in bed. Ideally, in the future, the patient will be able to empty the pouch while sitting on the toilet, with the pouch between the legs. It is often difficult for the patient to do this during the post-op stay, but you should inform the patient that the toilet method is the best and most natural (especially away from home, for example, in a public restroom). With this method, no extra equipment (containers) is needed.

KEY IDEA

It is easier to empty the ostomy pouch when it is about 1/3 filled. Hot water destroys the pouch's odor proofing.

PROCEDURE   **OBRA**

EMPTYING THE OSTOMY POUCH

RATIONALE: Pouches provide a container to collect stool discharged from the bowel.

PREPARATION

1. Assemble your equipment:
   a. Plastic container (for contents of pouch)
   b. Toilet tissue
   c. Disposable bed protector
   d. Basin with warm water
   e. Soap
   f. Wet washcloth
   g. Hand towel
   h. Disposable gloves
   i. Container of water, if pouch is to be rinsed (optional)
2. Identify the patient by checking the identification bracelet.
3. Tell the patient you will empty the ostomy pouch. If the patient is able, assist him.
4. Provide privacy for the patient.
5. Raise the bed to a comfortable working position. Raise the head of the bed. This helps the stool settle into the bottom of the pouch and also allows the patient to see what you are doing.
6. Put on gloves.
7. Encourage the patient to watch. Ask "Would you like to empty the pouch?"

STEPS

8. Cover the patient with the bath blanket. Without exposing the patient, fan-fold the top sheet and the bedspread to the bottom of the bed.
9. Place the disposable bed protector under the patient's hips and put container and roll of toilet tissue on the bed where it is easily accessible to you.
10. Holding the bottom of the pouch up, remove the clamp from the pouch and set the clamp aside.

PROCEDURE *(continued)*

11. Drain the pouch into the container. If the stool is thick, slide fingers down the outside of the pouch, squeezing out the contents into the container.

12. After emptying the pouch, measure the contents, if necessary, and then flush.

13. *Optional:* Rinse pouch with container of water, if patient wishes. Empty rinse water in plastic container. (Some patients like to rinse out the pouch. The pouch is odor proof whether it is clean or full of stool as long as the pouch is intact.)

14. Wipe the end of the pouch off with the tissue on the outside and also on the inside of the narrow opening.

15. Wipe off the clamp with tissue and place the clamp back on the bottom of the pouch.

16. If the patient has helped, give him a wet washcloth with soap and water to wash his hands.

FOLLOW-UP

17. Cover the patient. Lower the head of the bed if required or patient's preference.

18. Make the patient comfortable and replace the call light.

19. Lower the bed to a position of safety.

20. Raise the side rails when ordered or appropriate for patient safety.

21. Clean basin with soapy water, rinse, dry, and replace in its proper place. Discard disposable equipment. Bag and dispose of soiled linen in the laundry hamper.

22. Dispose of gloves and wash your hands.

23. Report to your immediate supervisor:

    - That the ostomy pouch was emptied.

    - Record as output on I + O records.

CHARTING EXAMPLE: 12/9/04
11pm Ostomy pouch emptied of 250cc loose stool. W. Waverly, CNA

CHANGING THE OSTOMY APPLIANCE

PROCEDURE   OBRA

RATIONALE: Disposable ostomy bags provide a container to collect stool discharged from the colostomy stoma.

PREPARATION

1. Assemble your equipment:
   a. Disposable bed protector
   b. Bath blanket
   c. New pouch (may be 1 or 2 pieces)
   d. Toilet tissue
   e. Basin of warm water (115°F; 46°C)

   f. Non-cream-based soap or cleanser as ordered by your immediate supervisor
   g. Washcloth
   h. Disposable gloves
   i. Towels

2. Identify the patient by checking the identification bracelet.

3. Tell the patient that you will assist them in changing the ostomy appliance.

4. Wash your hands and put on gloves.

5. Provide privacy for the patient.

6. Raise the bed to a comfortable working position.

STEPS

7. Place a towel over the patient's abdomen, exposing only the appliance.

8. Place the disposable bed protector under the patient's hips. This is to keep the bed from getting wet or dirty.

9. Gently remove the soiled pouch. Use a push-pull method to remove barrier.

10. Dispose of the pouch in the appropriate container. Wipe the area around the ostomy with a warm wet washcloth. This is to remove any stool from the skin.

11. Rinse the entire area well. Be careful not to leave any soap on the skin. (Soap has a drying effect and may irritate the skin.)

12. Dry the area gently with a bath towel.

13. Prepare the new barrier (Figure 20–23◆). A colostomy stoma

PROCEDURE *(continued)*

needs a barrier 1/8-inch larger than the stoma measurement. It may need to be sized and cut out. For urostomy and ileostomy stomas, no skin should show between the wafer and the stoma. The opening of the wafer should fit around the stoma at the area where the skin meets the stoma. Use stoma adhesive paste if necessary. Note: There are 1- and 2-piece appliances. Become familiar with the supplies available to you.

14. Apply new wafer to skin; hold in place for 30 seconds with your hand to help adhesive stick well (Figure 20–23c◆). Apply clamp to bottom of pouch.

15. Remove the disposable bed protector. Change any damp linen. Bag and dispose of soiled linen in the laundry hamper.

FOLLOW-UP

16. Make the patient comfortable and replace the call light.

17. Lower the bed to a position of safety.

18. Raise the side rails when ordered or appropriate for patient safety.

19. Remove all used equipment.

20. Wash your hands.

21. Report to your immediate supervisor:

    - That the ostomy wafer and pouch were changed.

- The amount of drainage.
- The consistency of the stool.
- The color and appearance of the stoma and skin around stoma.
- How the patient tolerated the procedure.
- Your observations of anything unusual.

CHARTING EXAMPLE: 12/10/04 11am Disposable ostomy appliance removed and changed. Bag emptied of 100 cc loose stool. Stoma adhesive applied to hold appliance ostomy in place. Skin intact surrounding stoma. W. Waverly, CNA

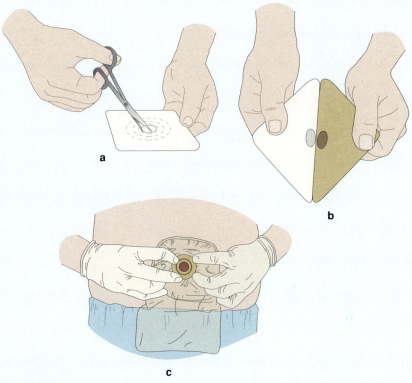

FIGURE 20–23 ◆
Replacing an ostomy appliance. (a) Use a measuring guide to size and cut opening in the barrier. (b) Remove covering if wafer is self-adhesive, or apply stoma adhesive paste. (c) Hold in place for 30 seconds.

SUMMARY

Caring for patients with digestive-related problems requires a knowledge of the gastrointestinal system itself as well as the common disorders and diseases of the system. It is also important to be familiar with the types of age-related changes that can occur in the gastrointestinal system. Tube feeding is a common procedure and it is important to understand the guidelines for care of a patient on tube feedings. Causes of diarrhea and constipation have been discussed to enable the nursing assistant to make changes to prevent and remedy problems. Learning how to recognize and manage diarrhea and constipation also contributes to a patient's comfort and health. The nursing assistant is relied upon to understand the proper technique for safe administration of the procedures given in this chapter and to have knowledge of the patient care guidelines. The nursing assistant is also responsible for reviewing and following the policies and procedures of the institution or agency where the nursing assistant is employed regarding each of these procedures and their administration and the nursing assistant's role.

NOTES

CHAPTER REVIEW

FILL IN THE BLANK   Read each sentence and fill in the blank line with a word that completes the sentence.

1. The GI tract is about _____ feet long.

2. _____ begins in the mouth, where food is chewed and mixed with saliva.

3. The rhythmic contractions of the muscle walls of the small and large intestine are called _____.

4. A feeding through a nasogastric tube is called a _____ feeding.

5. Intestinal gas is called _____.

MULTIPLE CHOICE   Choose the best answer for each question or statement.

1. All of the following are diseases and disorders of the gastrointestinal system *except*
   a. ulcers.
   b. jaundice.
   c. pericarditis.
   d. hemorrhoids.

2. When caring for a patient with a nasogastric tube, do all of the following *except*
   a. never pull on the tube when moving a patient.
   b. observe the patient's nostrils for signs of pressure.
   c. report any leakage to your supervisor immediately.
   d. remove the tube immediately if blood is noted.

3. When caring for a patient with a gastrostomy tube, do all of the following *except*
   a. cleanse around the gastrostomy site with mild soap and water, pat dry.
   b. twist the tube to ensure the tube is not adhered to the wall of the abdomen.
   c. watch for signs of irritation or leakage and report it to your supervisor immediately.
   d. be sure that feedings flow quickly when administered.

4. Diarrhea is
   a. only unhealthy in children.
   b. not something you need to report to your supervisor.
   c. unhealthy and may result in severe illness or dehydration.
   d. always a sign of eating too much spicy food.

5. Which of the following guidelines for checking for a fecal impaction is incorrect?
   a. Be certain your state allows you to perform this procedure.
   b. Your supervisor should be available in case you have questions or the patient experiences problems.
   c. Be aware that while performing this procedure the patient can experience an increased heart rate if you stimulate the vagus nerve in the rectum.
   d. Do not perform this procedure if you have not received the necessary training or met agency requirements to do so.

TIME-OUT

TIPS FOR TIME MANAGEMENT

If you must wait for a decision from a superior before performing care on a particular patient, use the time wisely. Avoid standing outside an office door for a prolonged time. Instead, tell your superior where to find you when the decision has been made; then continue your work.

THE NURSING ASSISTANT IN ACTION

Mr. Brammer has been receiving medications that cause his stools to become very hard. He tells you that he is constipated and has not had a bowel movement for several days. He is complaining of rectal pain and discomfort. He says in a frustrated voice, "I keep trying to go to the bathroom and nothing happens! Why didn't my doctor tell me about this sooner? I am afraid I will have hemorrhoids forever if this keeps up. I feel like there is a brick stuck in my rectum."

What Is Your Response/Action?

CRITICAL THINKING

CUSTOMER SERVICE Many patients find it difficult to move their bowels in your presence. Provide as much privacy for them as you can. If you need to ask them questions about their bowel movements, try to avoid doing so in front of family and visitors because it can be very embarrassing for them.

CULTURAL CARE If you need to check a patient for or remove a fecal impaction, there may be patients who would prefer for personal or cultural reasons that only the same gender nursing assistant performs this procedure on them. Many cultures would consider it inappropriate for a male to be providing this type of care to a woman. If you are unsure, ask the patient if this is a problem before you begin the procedure.

COOPERATION WITHIN THE TEAM If you are going to be performing procedures that can be time consuming (changing ostomy appliances or removing a fecal impaction), when possible try to choose a time that will not be in conflict with other scheduled patient therapies or right before a meal is to be served. The food may not keep well or the patient may not feel like eating right after these procedures. The efforts of the dietary department to prepare a good meal will be lost.

EXPLORE MediaLink

Additional interactive resources for this chapter can be found on the Companion Website at www.prenhall.com/wolgin. Click on Chapter 20 and "Begin" to select activities for this chapter.

For chapter-related NCLEX-style questions and an audio glossary, access the accompanying CD-ROM in this book.

21 Nutrition for the Patient

443

OBJECTIVES

When you have completed this chapter, you will be able to:

- Define the components and importance of a well-balanced diet using the food group pyramid. Provide examples of foods included in each group.
- Describe the six classes of nutrients.
- List the three functions of essential nutrients.
- Identify examples of when a patient may be at nutrition risk.
- List conditions when a patient may need a special diet.
- Define examples of therapeutic diets and explain the purpose of each.
- Prepare the patient for mealtime and serve the food tray.
- Observe and record information concerning meals.
- Distribute between-meal nourishment and drinking water.

MediaLink

www.prenhall.com/wolgin

Use the address above to access the free, interactive Companion Website created for this textbook. Get hints, instant feedback, and textbook references to chapter-related NCLEX-style questions. Link to other interesting sites.

AUDIO GLOSSARY:

Use the companion Website, or the CD-ROM disk enclosed with your textbook, to hear the pronunciation of key terms in the chapter.

KEY TERMS

- calorie
- calorie count
- enterally
- essential nutrient
- extra nourishment
- malnutrition
- nutrient
- nutrition status assessment
- omit
- parenteral nutrition
- registered dietitian (RD)
- regular diet
- therapeutic diet

ALERT

For all patient contact, adhere to Standard Precautions (Chapter 5, pages 83–85). Wear protective equipment as indicated.

As a nursing assistant, your role in providing good nourishment to the patient is essential. This chapter is designed to provide guidelines for evaluating your patient's nutritional needs and delivering a well-balanced diet. Many patients require alterations to their regular diet, and you will learn about special diets and when they are needed.

In addition, this chapter will provide information on preparing the patient for mealtime, feeding the patient, and delivering water and extra nourishment. Nutrition plays a vital role in the recovery and maintenance of health. Your active participation in helping your patients meet their nutritional needs is essential.

A Well-Balanced Diet

calorie Unit for measuring the energy produced when food is digested in the body

The key to a healthy, well-balanced diet is eating the correct amounts of a variety of foods. A vital function of food is to provide energy, which is measured in a unit of heat called a **calorie**. The foods that are essential for keeping the body well are divided into groups (Figure 21–1 ◆). If you eat the recommended number of portions of foods from each group on the pyramid every day, your diet will be adequate for good health. The number and size of portions will depend on the age, size, and activities of the individual. An increasing number of Americans are obese because they eat large portions of unhealthy food. At the same time the amount of calories burned or used by physical work or excercise by all age groups

FIGURE 21–1 ◆

The food guide pyramid

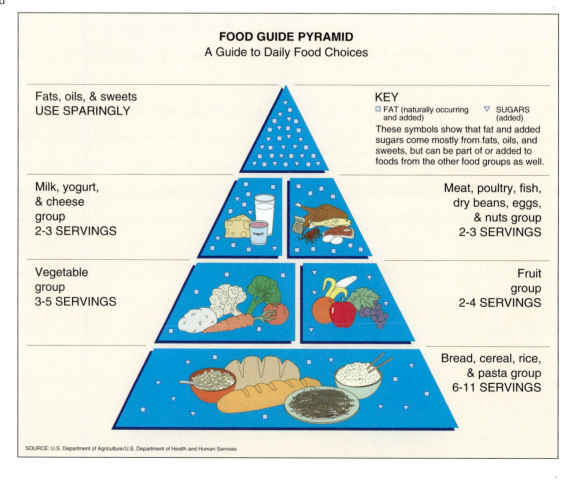

FOOD GUIDE PYRAMID
A Guide to Daily Food Choices

Fats, oils, & sweets
USE SPARINGLY

KEY
□ FAT (naturally occurring and added)   ▽ SUGARS (added)
These symbols show that fat and added sugars come mostly from fats, oils, and sweets, but can be part of or added to foods from the other food groups as well.

Milk, yogurt, & cheese group
2-3 SERVINGS

Meat, poultry, fish, dry beans, eggs, & nuts group
2-3 SERVINGS

Vegetable group
3-5 SERVINGS

Fruit group
2-4 SERVINGS

Bread, cereal, rice, & pasta group
6-11 SERVINGS

SOURCE: U.S. Department of Agriculture/U.S. Department of Health and Human Services

have decreased. The serving sizes for the food pyramid can be found on individual product labels. There are ongoing discussions about modifying the food pyramid.

The food group pyramid is divided into six categories:

- **Breads, cereals, rice, grains, and pasta** are examples of *complex carbohydrates* that provide energy. This group also contributes fiber to the diet which aids in digestion. The U.S. Department of Agriculture (USDA) recommends six to eleven servings per day from this group.

- **Vegetables** supply numerous vitamins, minerals, and fiber with virtually no fat. The benefits of eating a diet with many vegetables are quite extensive. The USDA recommends at least three to five servings per day from this group.

- **Fruits** also supply numerous vitamins, minerals, and fiber with almost no fat. The USDA recommends a minimum of two to four servings per day from this group.

- **Milk, yogurt, and cheese** provide protein, vitamins, and important minerals such as calcium. The USDA recommends two to three servings per day from this group.

- **Meat, poultry, fish, dry beans, eggs, soy, legumes, and nuts** provide protein. The USDA recommends two to three servings per day from this group.

- **Fat, oils, and sweets** should be eaten sparingly because this group contains fat, simple carbohydrates, and very little, if any, protein, complex carbohydrates, vitamins, or minerals. These foods include salad dressings, cream, butter, margarine, sugars, soft drinks, candies, sweet desserts, and alcoholic beverages.

What Are Nutrients?

Nutrients are chemical substances found in food. Over 50 nutrients are needed for the human body to function and must be consumed in your diet every day. These are called **essential nutrients**. There are six classes of essential nutrients:

1. **Carbohydrates** are divided into complex and simple carbohydrates. Examples of complex carbohydrates include bread, cereal, rice, grain, pasta, nuts, fruits, and vegetables. Examples of simple carbohydrates include juice, soda, sugar, and syrup.

2. **Protein** is divided into complete (essential) and incomplete (nonessential) amino acids. Complete protein examples include meat, fish, poultry, and cheese. Incomplete protein examples include beans, legumes, nuts, and peas.

3. **Fat** found in food may be saturated, monounsaturated, or polyunsaturated. Examples of fat sources include oil, butter, and margarine. Other foods that may contain fat are meat, peanut butter, cheese, nuts, and cream.

    The optimal distribution of calories includes:

   - 55 percent from complex carbohydrates

   - 15 percent from protein

   - 30 percent or less from fat

     When reading labels, it is necessary to know that:

   - Carbohydrates have 4 calories per gram

   - Protein has 4 calories per gram

   - Fat has 9 calories per gram

4. **Water** has no caloric value. The primary sources of water include drinking water, other beverages, soups, fruits, and vegetables.

5. **Vitamins** are divided into water-soluble and fat-soluble forms. Some examples of water-soluble vitamins include vitamin C, biotin, pantothenic acid, pyridoxine,

nutrient Chemical substances found in foods

essential nutrient Nutrients needed for the human body to function; they must be consumed in the diet every day

folacin, vitamin B$_{12}$, niacin, thiamin, and riboflavin. Examples of fat-soluble vitamins include vitamins A, D, E, and K. Vitamins contribute little caloric value.

6. ***Minerals*** are divided into macro and trace minerals. There are over 22 essential minerals. Some examples include calcium, phosphorus, sulfur, potassium, sodium, chloride, magnesium, chromium, fluoride, zinc, iodine, copper, and selenium. Minerals also deliver minimal caloric value.

Essential nutrients have three functions in the body:

1. To form and maintain body cell functions
2. To provide energy
3. To regulate body processes

After food is ingested, it enters the digestive tract where the nutrients are changed into simple forms. These simple forms are then carried by the blood to the body cells, where the special functions of each are carried out.

Regular and Special Diets

regular diet A basic, or well-balanced, diet containing appropriate amounts of foods from each of the food groups

therapeutic diet Any special diet

registered dietitian (RD) Person responsible for the preparation of well-balanced regular and therapeutic (special) diets to meet patients' nutritional needs

Eating a well-balanced diet is very important when you are healthy and feeling well. Good nourishment is even more important when a person is ill. The nutrition department in your institution will be preparing a well-balanced diet of nourishing meals for many different patients. This basic balanced diet is often called a **regular diet**. This regular diet is often modified to meet a patient's special nutritional needs. This diet is known as a **therapeutic (special) diet**. A **registered dietitian (RD)** assesses a patient's nutritional status and ensures that appropriate therapeutic diets are implemented.

Patient requests for special diets due to religious or cultural practices should be directed to your supervisor who will arrange for the patient to speak with someone from the nutrition department.

Alterations to a regular diet may be needed for various reasons. A few examples include:

■ Changing the consistency of the food, as in pureed or soft

■ Increasing or decreasing the caloric content

■ Changing the amounts of one or more nutrients, as in high protein, low potassium, low phosphorus, and fluid restriction

■ Omitting foods the patient is allergic to, such as lactose

■ Increasing the frequency of meals, such as six small meals a day

■ Altering the menu because of cultural or religious requirements

A complete description of each therapeutic diet can be found in the diet manual at your institution. Table 21–1 ◆ is *not* comprehensive and details only the most common diet orders.

Note: Additional information on special diets can be obtained from the American Dietetic Association.

enterally Delivery of a nutrition formula through a tube for patients with a functional GI tract who are unable to take in adequate calories or food by mouth

Patients who are unable to eat by mouth can be fed **enterally** through the use of a tube feeding. Enteral tube feedings are indicated if a patient has a functioning gastrointestinal (GI) tract. For patients with a nonfunctioning GI tract such as gastric obstructions, total parenteral nutrition may be indicated. Total **parenteral nutrition** is the infusion of dextrose, amino acids, and lipids into the venous system. Refer to Chapter 20 for more information on these modalities.

parenteral nutrition Nutrition therapy delivered by an IV catheter for patients with a nonfunctioning GI tract

Nutrition Status Assessment

Registered nurses (RNs) or registered dietitians (RDs) routinely assess each patient's nutritional status. However, it is important to communicate any noted problems with a patient's nutritional intake. As a nursing assistant, you will be able to observe any problems a patient may

TABLE 21–1

Examples of Different Types of Patient Diets

TYPE OF DIET	DESCRIPTION	COMMON PURPOSE
Regular	Provides a well-balanced variety of complete nutrition. This diet must be tailored for age.	To maintain or attain optimal nutrition status in patients who do not require a special diet.
Clear liquid	Clear broth and juices, ginger ale, gelatin, popsicles, clear coffee, and tea.	To provide calories and fluid in a form that requires minimal digestion. Commonly ordered after surgery.
Full liquid	Strained soups/cereals, coffee, fruit and vegetable juices, ginger ale, gelatin, custard, ice cream, sherbet, pudding, tea.	For those unable to chew or swallow solid food. Used as a transitional diet between clear liquids and solid foods.
Soft	Foods soft in consistency; no strongly flavored foods that could cause distress.	Used for patients who are unable to chew or swallow hard or coarse foods.
Mechanical soft	Same food included in a soft diet except food is ground or strained.	For patients with difficulty chewing or swallowing soft food.
Bland	Foods mild in flavor; omits spicy food, caffeine, and alcohol.	Omits food that may cause excessive gastric acid secretion (ulcers).
Low residue	Food low in fiber and bulk, also omits all foods that contain seeds.	Used for patients with acute colitis, enteritis, and diverticulitis.
High residue/fiber	Food high in fiber such as whole grains, cereals, fruit, vegetables, and legumes.	Used for bowel regulation, high cholesterol, and high glucose; protects against colon cancer and diverticulosis.
Low calorie	Low in calorically dense food such as fat.	For patients who need to lose weight.
Diabetic	Precise balance of carbohydrates, protein, and fats, devised according to the needs of the individual patient.	For diabetic patients; matches food intake with the insulin requirements.
High protein	Meals supplemented with high-protein foods such as meat, fish, cheese, milk, and eggs and oral supplements.	Assists in the repair of tissues wasted by disease. Used for increased protein needs (wound healing).
Low fat; low cholesterol	Limited amounts of butter, cream, oil, and margarine. Limited fried food, high fat meat, and dairy.	For patients who have difficulty digesting fat. Examples include pancreatitis, cholestasis, and heart and hepatic disease.
Lactose free or low lactose	Excludes or limits food that contains lactose (milk products).	Used to prevent cramping and diarrhea in patients with a lactose deficiency.
Low sodium (low salt)	Limited amounts of foods containing sodium; no salt packet on tray. This diet may be restricted in protein, sodium, phosphorus, fluid, and potassium.	May be needed for patients with liver, cardiac, and renal disease. Used for patients with acute or chronic renal failure.
Gluten restricted	Restricts gluten containing foods such as wheat, rye, barley, and oats.	Used for patients with gluten-sensitive enteropathy.

have eating. This will allow you to report any concerns about the patient's nutrition status to your supervisor or the registered dietitian. The **nutrition status assessment** may include:

- How well the patient eats and drinks (record what the patient eats or drinks for a **calorie count**)
- Chewing or swallowing problems
- Complaints of nausea, vomiting, constipation, or diarrhea
- Reports of recent weight changes

nutrition status assessment Assessment by an RN or RD as to what a patient eats and how the body uses it; determination of any special nutritional needs

calorie count Counting or adding up a total of all calories consumed in a 24-hour period

malnutrition Poor
nutrition status

The prevalence of malnutrition in the hospital is very high. **Malnutrition** means poor nutrition status. Patients with a poor appetite need encouragement to meet their nutritional needs. The patient's surroundings should be cheerful and attractive. The sight and aroma of food should be as appetizing as possible. You often can increase patients' appetites by showing them what they will be eating and providing some positive comments about the food. Obtaining patients' food preferences is one important way you may be able to increase their intake. In some settings, it is possible for patients to eat with others. The companionship and socialization can also encourage or promote the desire to eat—thereby improving the patient's appetite.

Assisting Patients with Foods

Mealtime is a break in the often boring hospital routine and gives the patient something to look forward to. Many patients also enjoy making food selections from the menu. This is a time when you can encourage the patient to select a well-balanced meal.

When the food tray is delivered, do everything you can to make the patient's meal as pleasant and comfortable as possible. Make sure the room is clean, quiet, free of unpleasant odors, and not too warm or cold. Take away things that might spoil the patient's appetite—items such as an emesis basin, urinal, or bedpan.

AGE-SPECIFIC CONSIDERATIONS

Patients of all ages enjoy social contact while eating. Children have food preferences just like adults. Encourage children to eat, but do not force them. Offer small amounts frequently. For adolescents, try to obtain foods that are familiar, and favorites too. Emphasize healthy choices, but in a way that is typical for the age group, i.e., pizza. For the elderly, perform and encourage oral care prior to meals to improve the preceptor of taste and the flavor of food. Encourage the patient to sit up in the chair for meals and to wait 30 to 60 minutes after meals for food to digest.

| PREPARING THE PATIENT FOR A MEAL | PROCEDURE | OBRA |

RATIONALE: Efforts to enable a patient to eat comfortably will improve her appetite.

PREPARATION

1. Assemble your equipment:
   a. Bedpan or urinal
   b. Basin of warm water (115°F; 46.1°C)
   c. Washcloth
   d. Towel
   e. Robe and slippers
2. Identify the patient by checking the identification bracelet.
3. Wash your hands.

STEPS

4. Tell the patient you are getting her ready for her next meal.
5. Provide privacy for the patient.
6. Offer the bedpan or urinal or assist the patient to the bathroom.
7. Have the patient wash her hands or offer the patient assistance.
8. Raise the backrest so the patient is in a sitting position, if this is allowed. If not, you might prop up her head by using several pillows.
9. Clear the over-bed table. Put it in a convenient position for the patient's meal.
10. If the patient wants to sit in a chair to eat and this is allowed, assist her with her robe and slippers. Help the patient out of bed and to the chair.

PROCEDURE *(continued)*

FOLLOW-UP

11. Make the patient comfortable and replace the call light.

12. Check that the telephone is still within reach.

13. Lower the bed to a position of safety for the patient.

14. Raise the side rails when ordered or appropriate for patient safety.

15. Wash your hands.

16. Report the following to your immediate supervisor:

    ■ The patient is ready for the next meal.

    ■ How the patient tolerated the procedure.

    ■ Your observations of anything unusual.

CHARTING EXAMPLE: 12/01/04 11:55am Assisted Mrs. Chow to the bathroom and to bedside chair for her lunch. S. Goode, CNA

SERVING THE FOOD

PROCEDURE   OBRA

RATIONALE: Patients unable to prepare their tray will not be able to eat their prescribed diet.

PREPARATION

1. Wash your hands.

2. Check the tray before you give it to the patient. Make sure the tray looks appetizing and nothing is missing (including silverware). Make sure nothing has spilled. Correct anything that is wrong.

3. Be sure you are giving the right tray to the right patient. Check the menu card, which will have the patient's name on it, against the patient's identification band to be sure they match (Figure 21–2◆).

STEPS

4. Put the tray on the over-bed table. Adjust it to a height comfortable for the patient.

5. Arrange the dishes and silverware so the patient can reach everything easily. Be sure drinking water is handy.

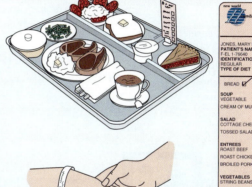

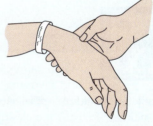

FIGURE 21–2 ◆

Check to be sure the name on the menu card matches the patient's identification band

6. Help any patient who needs it (Figure 21–3◆). For example, if a patient seems to be weak or asks for help, you might offer to spread the napkin on his lap or tuck it under his chin. Spread butter on the bread. Cut up whatever needs cutting. Pour tea or coffee. Do not give any more help than is really needed. The more a patient can do for himself, the better.

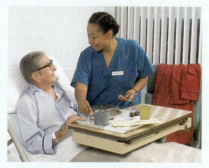

FIGURE 21–3 ◆

Help any patient requiring assistance to eat

PROCEDURE *(continued)*

7. A patient may discover that he cannot eat when the food is served. Report this to your supervisor. If permitted, you may take the tray away and keep the hot food warm until the patient wants to eat.

8. When you are sure the patient can go on with his meal by himself, leave the room.

9. Go back for the food tray when the patient has finished eating.

10. Note how much the patient has eaten and how much he has had to drink.

11. Record the intake for those patients who are on calorie counts or intake and output records.

12. Record how the patient has eaten his meal on the daily activity flow sheet. Record this information separately for breakfast, lunch, and supper:

   a. Did the patient eat all the food served?

   b. Did the patient eat about half the food served?

   c. Did the patient eat very little food?

   d. Did the patient decline to eat anything?

13. Take the tray away and put it in its proper place.

14. If the patient ate sitting in a chair, help him back into bed.

15. Put personal articles back where the patient wants them.

16. If the patient ate in bed, brush crumbs from the bed, smooth out the sheets, and straighten the bedding.

17. Assist the patient with oral care as needed.

FOLLOW-UP

18. Make the patient comfortable and replace the call light.

19. Lower the bed to a position of safety for the patient.

20. Raise the side rails when ordered or appropriate for patient safety.

21. Wash your hands.

22. Report the following to your immediate supervisor:

- That you have served the patient his food.

- The amount of food eaten (all, half, or refused to eat).

- Your observations of anything unusual.

CHARTING EXAMPLE: 12/02/04 12.30pm Helped Mr. Cohen to eat his lunch. He ate all his food. S. Goode, CNA

AGE-SPECIFIC CONSIDERATIONS

When caring for patients of all ages, try to find out food preferences and favorites. When possible, give them some choice in when and what they eat. Children appreciate what is familiar, therefore encourage family to assist with mealtimes. To assist the elderly, make sure there is adequate lighting so that they can see the food. Have them wear their glasses as well.

Patients Requiring Assistance to Eat

Some patients are incapable of feeding themselves and, therefore, will have to be fed. The reasons include the following:

- The patient cannot use his hands.

- The doctor wants the patient to save his strength and to be on "complete bed rest."

- The patient may be too weak to feed himself.

- The patient may have difficulties with swallowing (for example, due to a stroke or cleft palate) and may need assistance.

- The patient may have dysphasia, which is difficulty in chewing or swallowing due to damage to the nerves and muscles involved in swallowing (from head and neck cancer, multiple sclerosis, Parkinson's or Alzheimer's disease).

Usually, it is hard for adults to accept the idea of not being able to eat independently. Because he may be physically challenged or handicapped, the patient may experience feelings of resentment or even depression. Be friendly and natural. Encourage the patient to do as much as he can for himself. Also, remember that because of medical reasons a patient may not always be allowed to help. You will learn how to judge the amount of help the patient can give you when he is being fed. For example, if the patient is strong enough, you might let him hold his own bread.

When feeding a challenged patient, the most important thing is not to rush him through his meal. The time it takes to chew food, for example, may seem long to you, but the patient is probably very weak; otherwise, he would be able to eat without your help.

Remember that you should not bring the food tray or have it delivered until you have prepared the patient for the meal and are ready to feed him. Again, make sure you are serving the correct tray to the patient. Preparations before mealtime are the same for the challenged patient who cannot feed himself. Be observant throughout. Watch for signs of choking, coughing, or anything unusual.

Signs and symptoms of dysphasia include pocketing of food in the mouth, drooling, coughing, especially following sips of liquids, choking on food, frequent clearing of the throat, and speaking in a wet, gargly voice.

GUIDELINES

FEEDING A PATIENT WITH DYSPHASIA

- Positioning the patient with a 90° flexion of hips and a 45° neck flexion is recommended. Pillows can be used behind the back and neck if needed to maintain this position. If the patient is in bed, the knees can be cranked up to prevent the patient from slipping down.
- Feeding liquids can be easier using a cut-out cup and reminding the patient to keep his head down, suck in a small amount of liquid, swallow, then rest.
- Place solid food on the tongue with a spoon. Wait and be sure the mouth is empty before offering more food. Very cold foods or Italian ices between every five or six bites can make it easier for some patients to eat. Avoid offering dry foods, for example, bread, waffles, and pancakes. Extra honey, syrup, butter, or applesauce can help make these foods easier to swallow for patients who desire them.
- Encourage the patient to swallow twice after each bite.
- Present food from the midline and below.
- Be patient and offer verbal cues as needed.
- Check that the mouth is empty after the feeding and have the patient remain sitting up for 30 minutes.

PROCEDURE   OBRA

FEEDING THE PHYSICALLY CHALLENGED PATIENT OR THE PATIENT WHO IS UNABLE TO FEED HIMSELF

RATIONALE: Patients unable to prepare their tray and feed themselves will not be able to eat their prescribed diets.

PREPARATION

1. Assemble your equipment on the over-bed table:
   Patient's tray
2. Check the name on the card on the tray against the patient's identification bracelet.
3. Tell the patient you are going to feed him or assist with the meal.

STEPS

4. Wash your hands.
5. If allowed the patient should be in high Fowler's position.
6. If you plan to be seated while you feed the patient, bring a chair to a convenient position beside the bed.

PROCEDURE (continued)

7. Check the tray to make sure everything is there. If anything is missing, have it brought in or get it yourself.

8. Tuck a napkin under the patient's chin.

9. Season the food the way the patient likes it. However, do this only if his request agrees with the prescribed diet.

10. For most patients unable to feed themselves you will use a spoon. Fill the spoon only half-full. Give the food to the patient from the tip of the spoon, not the side. Put the food in one side of the patient's mouth so he can chew it more easily. If a patient is paralyzed on one side of his body, make sure you feed him on the side of his mouth that is not paralyzed.

11. If the patient cannot see the tray, name each mouthful of food as you offer it. Offer the different foods in a logical order, for example, soup or juice before the main course. Alternate between liquids and solid foods throughout the meal. Feed the patient as you yourself would want to eat. Or follow the patient's suggestions about how he wants to alternate between various kinds of foods and a beverage.

12. If the patient is unable to see and would like to feed himself, you can describe the position of the food on the tray. For example, cold liquids are in the left corner, hot liquids in the right corner. Describe the food on the plate in terms of a clock face (Figure 21–4♦). For example, "Baked potato at 2 o'clock, peas at 4 o'clock, carrots at 5 o'clock, roast beef at 8 o'clock, and bread at 11 o'clock."

13. Try to maintain the patient's independence as much as possible.

14. Warn the patient if you are offering something hot. Never offer extremely hot liquids; allow them

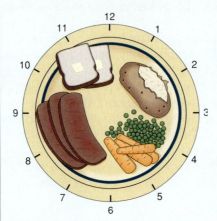

FIGURE 21–4 ♦
Describe the food on the plate and its placement in terms of a clock face

to cool. Use a straw for giving liquids (Figure 21–5♦). Use a new straw for each beverage.

15. Feed the patient slowly. Remember that he may chew and swallow very slowly. Allow plenty of time between mouthfuls.

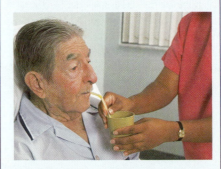

FIGURE 21–5 ♦
Use a straw when offering liquids

16. Encourage the patient to finish the meal, but do not use force.

17. When the patient has finished eating, help him to wipe his mouth with the napkin, or do this for the patient.

18. Note how much the patient has eaten and how much he has had to drink.

19. Record fluid intake on the intake and output sheet or as directed by

your supervisor, when the patient is on intake and output.

20. Record how the patient has eaten his meal on the daily activity sheet or as directed by your supervisor. Record this information separately for breakfast, lunch, and supper:

    a. Did the patient eat all the food served?

    b. Did the patient eat about one-half the food served?

    c. Did the patient eat very little food?

    d. Did the patient refuse to eat anything?

21. As soon as you are sure the patient is finished with the tray, take it away. Put it in its proper place.

FOLLOW-UP

22. Adjust the backrest of the bed to make the patient comfortable, if this is allowed.

23. Brush crumbs from the bed, smooth the sheets, and straighten the bedding.

24. Assist the patient with oral care or provide oral care as needed.

25. Make the patient comfortable and replace the call light.

26. Lower the bed to a position of safety for the patient.

27. Raise the side rails when ordered or appropriate for patient safety.

28. Wash your hands.

29. Report the following to your immediate supervisor:

    ■ That you have fed the patient.

    ■ Your observations of anything unusual.

CHARTING EXAMPLE: 12/02/04 12:30pm Assisted Mr. Cohen to eat his lunch. He ate all his food except the jello. S. Goode, CNA

Between-Meal Nourishment

Extra nourishment in the form of food or drink is offered to patients during the day. This is a hospital "snack" given to patients to provide energy or to break the routine. Patients are often given extra nourishment as part of their medical care. Examples of snacks are crackers and cheese, fruit and milk, and oral supplements such as a milkshake. In some institutions, extra nourishment is passed out to patients by workers from the food service department. However, you may be assigned this responsibility. If you are, your immediate supervisor will give you a list of which patients can have an extra nourishment and which have special restrictions. It is important to deliver the nourishment at the scheduled time that is ordered for patients on a special diet.

extra nourishment Snacks

KEY IDEA

The nourishment or snacks provided must be acceptable within the therapeutic or special diet and will be included in the diet order.

PROCEDURE

SERVING BETWEEN-MEAL NOURISHMENT

RATIONALE: Patients are offered snacks as part of their prescribed diets or to provide additional nourishment for patients with poor appetites.

PREPARATION

1. Wash your hands.
2. Assemble your equipment on a tray or a cart:
   a. Nourishment
   b. Cup, dish, and a spoon or straw
   c. Napkin

STEPS

3. Identify the patient by checking the identification bracelet.

4. If the patient has a choice of items, ask what the patient prefers.
5. Prepare the nourishment.
6. Take the nourishment to the patient on a tray or cart.
7. Encourage the patient to take the nourishment, assisting as needed. Offer a straw if this is more convenient.
8. After the patient has finished, collect the tray.
9. Discard the disposable equipment.
10. Record the intake for those patients who are on intake and output records or calorie counts. (See *Procedure: Determining the Amounts Consumed* in Chapter 22.)

FOLLOW-UP

11. Make the patient comfortable and replace the call light.

12. Lower the bed to a position of safety for the patient.
13. Raise the side rails when ordered or appropriate for patient safety.
14. Wash your hands.
15. Report the following to your immediate supervisor:
    - That you have served the between-meal nourishment.
    - Your observations of anything unusual.

CHARTING EXAMPLE: 12/05/04 8:30pm Assisted Mr. Cohen to eat all his evening snack. S. Goode, CNA

Passing Drinking Water

Part of your job as a nursing assistant will be to see that the patients you are caring for have plenty of fresh water at their bedsides, unless a doctor orders otherwise. Some patients are not allowed to have more than a certain amount of water. Some, for brief periods, may not have water at all.

Fresh ice water is passed to patients at regular intervals during the day. Your supervisor will tell you the schedule of your institution. Disposable pitchers and cups are used everywhere. Most patients like ice water. Others want water without ice, straight from the tap. You will be told which patients are allowed to have a choice. If a patient is not allowed to have ice, his water pitcher will be tagged "**Omit** Ice." Some patients are allowed ice chips only.

omit Leave out

PROCEDURE

PASSING DRINKING WATER

RATIONALE: Patients are offered drinking water to maintain body functions or provide additional fluids to consume when thirsty.

PREPARATION

1. Assemble your equipment:
   a. Moving table (cart) with small ice chest and cover or disposable water pitcher liners
   b. Ice cubes
   c. Scoop
   d. Paper or disposable cups
   e. Disposable water pitchers
   f. Straws
   g. Paper towels
2. Wash your hands.

STEPS

3. Fill the disposable water pitcher liners or ice chest with ice cubes and cover it.
4. Put all the equipment on the table.

5. Before you pass drinking water, be sure you know:
   a. Which patients are NPO (nothing by mouth)
   b. Which patients are on restricted fluids and get only a measured amount of water
   c. Which patients get only tap water (**omit** ice)
   d. Which patients may have ice water
   e. Which patients may not have a straw
6. Roll the moving table into the hall outside the patient's room.
7. Go into the room and pick up one patient's water pitcher/container. Record the patient's intake. Empty it in the sink in the room.
8. Remove and discard the disposable liner.
9. Walk to the water table in the hall. Insert a new water pitcher liner into the pitcher/container. Fill it half full with tap water.
10. Fill the pitcher to the brim with ice cubes, *being sure the scoop does not touch the water pitcher.*
11. Replace the water pitcher on the same patient's table from which it was taken. If the pitcher is labeled

with the patient's name, check it against the identification bracelet.
12. Throw away used paper cups.
13. Wipe the table with a clean paper towel. Discard the towel.
14. Place several clean paper cups next to the water pitcher.
15. Place several straws next to the water pitcher.
16. Be sure the patient can reach the water pitcher easily.
17. Offer to pour a fresh glass of water for the patient.

FOLLOW-UP

18. Wash your hands.
19. Report the following to your immediate supervisor:
    - That you have passed fresh drinking water to the patient.
    - Your observations of anything unusual.

CHARTING EXAMPLE: 12/05/04 11:30pm (Usually not documented but mentioned in verbal report to the oncoming shift CNA) Passed fresh drinking water to all patients except those ordered NPO. S. Goode, CNA

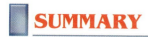

SUMMARY

Good nutrition is key to the recovery of many patients. Your role in providing that support includes observing the patient's needs, delivering food, water, and extra nourishment according to the order, and identifying any special circumstances that you encounter. Special diets are quite common and this chapter has provided an overview of many examples. A well-balanced diet containing the essential nutrients is important for all patients. Your knowledge of the food group pyramid can assist patients with their menu selections. As a nursing assistant, your role in providing good nutrition to the patient and identifying any patient nutrition problems is extremely important.

NOTES

CHAPTER REVIEW

FILL IN THE BLANK Read each sentence and fill in the blank line with a word that completes the sentence.

1. The process of counting or adding up all of the calories consumed in a 24-hour period is called a _____ _____.

2. The food group guide to a well-balanced diet that is divided into six categories is the _____ _____.

3. Difficulty swallowing or chewing is called _____.

4. When feeding patients, it is important not to _____ them while they eat.

5. A _____ or snack is given to patients to provide energy or as part of their medical care.

MULTIPLE CHOICE Choose the best answer for each question or statement.

1. How many servings of breads, cereals, and pastas are recommended on the food pyramid?
   a. 2–3
   b. 3–5
   c. 5–6
   d. 6–11

2. How many servings of vegetables are recommended on the food pyramid?
   a. 2–3
   b. 3–5
   c. 5–6
   d. 6–11

3. Which of the following is generally not allowed on a clear liquid diet?
   a. apple juice
   b. jello
   c. tomato juice
   d. tea

4. When feeding a patient who has dysphasia, do all of the following *except*
   a. position the patient with his head up 90 degrees.
   b. offer dry foods such as crackers.
   c. encourage the patient to swallow twice after each bite.
   d. be patient and offer verbal cues.

5. Obesity is an increasing problem because
   a. the fast-food industry encourages ordering the "Biggie Size."
   b. people are more physically active.
   c. parents cannot control their children's diets.
   d. many people are eating more food calories than they burn.

TIME-OUT

TIPS FOR TIME MANAGEMENT

Occasionally you may finish your work early and have time to spare. Avoid spending this extra time in the breakroom reading a magazine. Instead, use the time to restock supplies and talk with patients. Go back to the room of a patient who likes to chat or is lonely and sit with him or her. Visit a patient who does not have visitors very often.

THE NURSING ASSISTANT IN ACTION
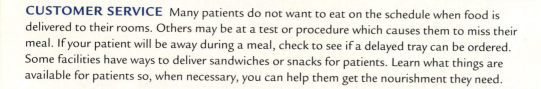

Mrs. Smith has been hospitalized to control her diabetes and high blood pressure. She is ordered on a low-sodium, diabetic diet. After her family visits, you come to deliver her bedtime snack and find Mrs. Smith eating a hamburger, french fries, and drinking a large soda. This meal contains a great deal of sodium and sugar. She says to you, "You know how I cannot eat the food you all serve me here. Let me just enjoy this one little meal and pretend you didn't see me eating just now."

What Is Your Response/Action?

CRITICAL THINKING

CUSTOMER SERVICE Many patients do not want to eat on the schedule when food is delivered to their rooms. Others may be at a test or procedure which causes them to miss their meal. If your patient will be away during a meal, check to see if a delayed tray can be ordered. Some facilities have ways to deliver sandwiches or snacks for patients. Learn what things are available for patients so, when necessary, you can help them get the nourishment they need.

CULTURAL CARE Many patients will have food choices or preferences that are different from what is offered to them. If you notice a patient is not eating, ask if there is something else she would like or a reason he does not want to eat. Sometimes family members can bring in seasonings and spices that would make the food taste better to the patient. As long as it does not conflict with the diet ordered, there is no reason not to accommodate a patient's taste.

COOPERATION WITHIN THE TEAM You may be better able to anticipate some patients' dietary needs than other members of the team, especially if you are more familiar with a patient's culture or language. If you see this is the case, offer to help the dietician or other team members communicate with the patient or family or share important cultural food considerations they may not know about.

EXPLORE MediaLink
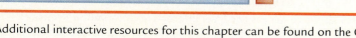

Additional interactive resources for this chapter can be found on the Companion Website at www.prenhall.com/wolgin. Click on Chapter 21 and "Begin" to select activities for this chapter.

For chapter-related NCLEX-style questions and an audio glossary, access the accompanying CD-ROM in this book.

22 The Urinary System and Related Care

KEY TERMS

absorb
anuria
balance of fluids
bladder distention
calibrated
catheter
convert
cubic centimeter
cystitis
dehydration
discharge
dysuria
edema
eliminate
evaporate
fluid
fluid balance
fluid imbalance
fluid intake
fluid output
force fluids
graduate
homeostasis
incontinent
indwelling urinary catheter
insensible fluid loss
nothing by mouth (NPO)
parenteral intake
peristaltic waves
perspiration
residual
restrict fluids
retain
tissue fluid
urethra
urinary system (excretory system)
urinate
urine
void

OBJECTIVES

When you have completed this chapter, you will be able to:

- State the main function of the urinary system.
- Label the four components of the urinary system and explain the function of each.
- Describe three processes by which urine is formed.
- Differentiate normal and abnormal urine.
- List common diseases and disorders of the urinary system.
- Explain fluid balance and imbalance.
- List the reasons for recording accurate measures of fluid intake and output.
- Accurately measure fluids using the metric system.
- Measure the capacity of serving containers.
- List ways to encourage a patient to increase fluid intake.
- Explain ways to restrict the patient's intake of fluid.
- List the ways in which the body loses fluid.
- Explain the function of urinary catheters and demonstrate their daily care.
- Apply a condom catheter.
- Discontinue an indwelling catheter.

MediaLink
www.prenhall.com/wolgin

Use the address above to access the free, interactive Companion Website created for this textbook. Get hints, instant feedback, and textbook references to chapter-related NCLEX-style questions. Link to other interesting sites.

AUDIO GLOSSARY:
Use the companion Website, or the CD-ROM disk enclosed with your textbook, to hear the pronunciation of key terms in the chapter.

Several body systems participate in the elimination of waste products from the body. One such system is the urinary system. This vital body system plays a major role in maintaining homeostasis, the body's ability to maintain a steady state. Other systems that remove waste include the integumentary, respiratory, and digestive systems. Major organs of these systems include skin, lungs, and intestines, respectively. This chapter focuses on the four components of the urinary system—left and right kidneys, left and right ureters, bladder, and urethra—and the specific functions of these organs. The major function of this system is the formation and excretion of urine. The processes involved in the formation of urine and the significance of fluid balance in maintaining homeostasis are explained. A discussion of metric units of measurement required for monitoring and recording fluid intake and output are presented along with the concepts of force fluids, restrict fluids, and nothing by mouth (NPO). Your role is key in monitoring and recording fluid intake and output. Catheter care and catheterization procedures are included.

INTRODUCTION

ALERT

For all patient contact, adhere to Standard Precautions (⚭ Chapter 5, pages 83–85). Wear protective equipment as indicated.

Anatomy and Physiology of the Urinary System

As nursing assistants you will have a major responsibility in helping other members of the health care team monitor the patient's urinary system function. The physician may order strict measurement of some patient's fluid intake and output. Since the **urinary system** is the system for excreting a large volume of fluid (urine), it is important that you understand some of the basic anatomy and physiology of the system (Figure 22–1 ◆). Descriptions of the four components that make up this system and the related function of each component follow.

urinary system (excretory system) The group of body components including the kidneys, ureters, bladder, and urethra that removes wastes from the blood and produces and eliminates urine

FIGURE 22–1 ◆

The urinary system

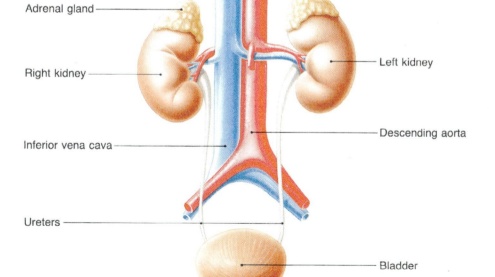

- Adrenal gland
- Right kidney
- Inferior vena cava
- Ureters
- Left kidney
- Descending aorta
- Bladder
- Urethra

FIGURE 22–2 ◆

The nephron unit

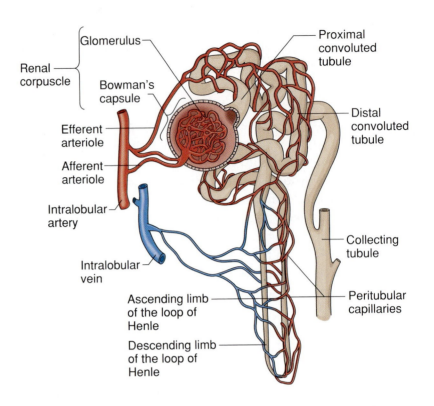

Kidneys

The two kidneys are identical structures that look like lima beans. Fat and connective tissue surround the kidneys to provide support and help maintain the kidneys in normal position. The functional unit of the kidneys is called a *nephron*. Each kidney has more than 1 million nephrons. A nephron consists of a glomerulus, Bowman's capsule, and a tubular system. The glomerulus is a cluster of capillaries. This network of capillaries lies within a cupping of a tube known as Bowman's capsule. Extending from each Bowman's capsule is a renal tubule consisting of several sections. These different sections form the tubular system that consists of the proximal convoluted tubule, the descending limb of the loop of Henle, the ascending limb, the distal convoluted tubule, and a collecting tubule (see Figure 22–2◆).

Formation of Urine

The main functions of the urinary system occur in the structural units (glomerulus, Bowman's capsule, and tubular system) of the nephrons. The three functions—glomerular filtration, tubular reabsorption, and tubular secretion—are the complex processes by which **urine** is formed and excreted by the kidney. Urine is the fluid secreted by the kidneys, stored in the bladder, and excreted through the urethra.

Step 1: Glomerular Filtration   Urine formation starts in the glomerulus with filtration of blood. The semipermeable membrane of the glomerulus allows free passage of water and certain solutes. This fluid is called glomerulus filtrate, and it flows into the Bowman's capsule. Glomerulus filtrate contains both essential and nonessential material.

Step 2: Tubular Reabsorption   Tubular reabsorption is the taking back of water and certain solutes—essential minerals dissolved in the water that the body needs. The process involves the movement of substances out of the filtrate into the blood. About 97 to 99 percent of the filtrate is reabsorbed by the tissues thereby restoring essential materials to the body.

urine The fluid secreted by the kidneys, stored in the bladder, and excreted through the urethra

Step 3: Tubular Secretion   Tubular secretion is the final step in the process of urine formation. It involves the movement of substances out of the blood into the filtrate for excretion thereby removing nonessential materials from the body.

KEY IDEA

Urine formation is the complex process that cleans blood plasma of unnecessary substances while selectively reabsorbing other essential materials. Specifically, waste products are removed and fluids, electrolytes, blood pressure, and pH are regulated to help the body maintain a normal state.

Ureters

Once urine is formed, it drips from the kidney into the ureter. The two ureters are tubes that help to form the renal pelvis at the end that connects to the kidney (see Figure 22–1). These tubes are about 10 to 12 inches in length. The primary function of the ureters is to collect urine (in renal pelvis) and drain urine to the bladder. Urine flow through the ureters is aided by **peristaltic waves**, or involuntary contractions, similar to those of the digestive tract. Once urine drains from the ureters into the bladder, there are valves around the openings to prevent the backflow of urine when the bladder contracts. The urinary tract is sterile.

peristaltic waves Waves of involuntary contractions

Bladder

The bladder is the third component in the urinary system, and it serves as a reservoir for urine before it leaves the body. This collapsible organ is key to the excretion of urine. The muscular wall of the bladder contains stretch receptors. When these receptors are stimulated by as little as 300 cc to a completely full bladder, messages are sent to the brain that cause the person to urinate, or **void** (discharge urine from the body).

void To urinate, pass water

Urethra

The **urethra**, a small tube leading from the bladder floor to the external environment, serves to empty the bladder of collected urine. Because the urethra is open to the outside of the body, it may also provide a passageway for disease-causing organisms. The normal flow of urine will generally flush bacteria out. When organisms enter the bladder, a bladder infection (cystitis) may occur. The infection may also spread through the ureters to the kidney, causing a kidney infection (nephritis). Cystitis and nephritis are often called urinary-tract infections. Long-term nephritis may lead to kidney damage.

Women have shorter urethras than men. Therefore, women are at greater risk to acquire urinary tract infections.

urethra A small tube that serves to empty urine from the bladder to the external environment

Diseases and Disorders of the Urinary System

In a healthy person, fresh voided urine is a clear, straw color that turns cloudy upon standing. Painful urination, discoloration of urine, or failure to void are abnormal conditions that should be reported to appropriate members of the patient care team. Table 22–1◆ lists some common diseases and disorders of the urinary system and the causes, results, or symptoms associated with the disease or disorder.

TABLE 22–1

Diseases and Disorders of the Urinary System

DISEASE OR DISORDER	CAUSE, RESULT, OR SYMPTOM
Acute renal failure	Loss of kidney function
Anuria	No urine
Cancer of the urinary bladder	Malignant tumor
Chronic renal failure	Progressive deterioration of kidney function
Cystitis	Inflammation of the urinary bladder
Dysuria	Painful voiding
Hematuria	Blood in the urine
Hydronephrosis	Distention of the pelvis of one or both kidneys (urine is being made but cannot be excreted due to urinary backup)
Injury to the bladder	Due to trauma
Nocturia	Frequent urination at night
Oliguria	Very small amount of urine in 24 hours (usually less then 500 cc in 24 hours)
Polyuria	Unusually large volume of urine in 24 hours
Pyelonephritis	Infection of the kidney (acute or chronic)
Pyuria	Pus in the urine, an infection
Renal colic	Sharp, severe pain in lower back over kidney that accompanies forcible dilation of a ureter due to a stone or urinary calculus
Tuberculosis of the kidney	Caused by *Mycobacterium tuberculosis* in the kidney
Tumors of the kidney	Considered malignant until proven otherwise
Urethral stricture	Narrowing of the urethra caused by infection or instrumentation; results in frequent voiding, dysuria, and hematuria (blood in the urine)
Urethritis	Inflammation of the urethra, often by sexually transmitted diseases such as chlamydia or gonorrhea
Urinary retention	Inability to urinate
Urinary tract infection (UTI)	Presence of pathogenic microorganisms in the urinary tract
Urolithiasis (renal calculi)	Presence of stones in the urinary (excretory) system

anuria Inability to urinate, no urine output

cystitis Inflammation of the urinary bladder

dysuria Painful voiding

homeostasis Stability of all body functions at normal levels

tissue fluid A watery environment around each cell that acts as a place of exchange for gases, food, and waste products between the cells and the blood

urinate To discharge urine from the body; other words for this function are void, micturate, and pass water

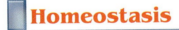

Homeostasis

Homeostasis is the body's attempt to keep its internal environment stable or in balance. Examples of the body's ability to maintain homeostasis include these:

- The body temperature stays constant.
- The blood pressure stays within specific limits.
- The chemistry of the blood stays within certain normal limits.

The urinary system is perhaps the most important system for maintaining homeostasis. This is because, as described above, the urinary system determines the content (water and chemical) of the blood. The blood content, in turn, determines the content of the **tissue fluid**, which is the immediate environment of the cells. Many changes in kidney function, some normal, can be found in urine samples. Diagnostic studies of the urinary system include urinalysis, creatinine clearance, urine culture, residual urine, protein determination, and glucose testing. You may be directly involved in collecting urine samples and performing certain tests (see Chapter 23). Changes in kidney function are also revealed in accurate measurement of intake and output. Sometimes in illness, especially after surgery, the patient is unable to void (**urinate**).

Fluid Balance and Fluid Imbalance

Fluid balance means that the body eliminates just about the same amount that it takes in. An **imbalance of fluid** occurs when the body keeps, or **retains**, too much **fluid** or when the body loses too much fluid (Figure 22–3◆). In some medical conditions, fluid may be held in the body tissues and cause them to swell. This is called **edema**. When a patient experiences a fluid loss, or decrease in the amount of fluids in tissues, it is called **dehydration**. Inadequate fluid intake may be caused by vomiting, bleeding, wound drainage, severe diarrhea, or excessive sweating (**perspiration**). When a patient's body loses more fluid than is taken in or when the body retains fluid (puts out less fluid than it has taken in) the doctor can treat the condition in various ways. A specific method is prescribed to meet the needs of the individual patient. The only way a doctor can know when a patient's **balance of fluids** is not right is by knowing the patient's measurable intake and output.

fluid balance The same amount of fluid that is taken in by the body is given out by the body

fluid imbalance When too much fluid is kept in the body or when too much fluid is lost

retain To keep or hold in

fluid Applies to liquid substances

KEY IDEA

A starving person can lose half of his body protein and almost half his body weight and still live, but losing only one-fifth of the body's fluid will result in death. This is why it is very important for the doctor to know the patient's balance of fluid.

Water is essential to human life (Figure 22–4◆). Next to oxygen, water is the most important thing for the body. About 50 to 60 percent of the adult human body is water. In an infant 70 to 80 percent of the body composition is water; this places infants at high risk when fluid is lost. On the other hand, older adults are also at risk because of a decrease in the body's water content to about 45 to 50 percent.

edema Abnormal swelling of a part of the body caused by fluid collecting in that area; usually the swelling is in the ankles, legs, hands, or abdomen

dehydration A decrease in the amount of water in the tissues occurring when fluid output exceeds input or intake

FIGURE 22–3 ◆
Fluid intake and output

perspiration Sweat

balance of fluids See *fluid imbalance*

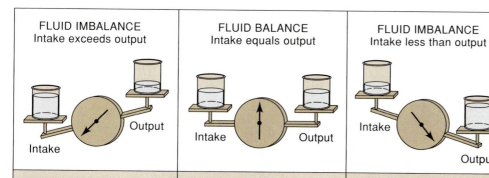

FLUID IMBALANCE Intake exceeds output	FLUID BALANCE Intake equals output	FLUID IMBALANCE Intake less than output
Results from: Excessive intake . . . large amounts of • Liquids • Food or Restricted output . . . limited amounts of • Urine • Perspiration	**Results from:** Normal intake of • Liquids • Food • Breathing (inhaling) or Normal output • Breathing (exhaling) • Perspiration • Urine • Feces	**Results from:** Restricted intake . . . limited amounts of • Liquids • Food or Excessive output . . . large amounts of • Urine • Vomitus • Blood • Drainage • Perspiration • Stool (diarrhea)

FIGURE 22–4 ◆

Water is essential to human life

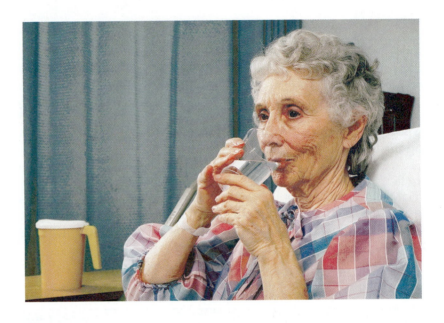

FIGURE 22–4 ◆

Water is essential to human life

Fluid Intake

Through eating and drinking, the average healthy adult will take in about 3 quarts (3,312 cc) of fluid every day. This is his **fluid intake**. Although solid foods also contain some liquid, most of the fluids in the body are taken in when a person drinks liquids. Therefore, a patient's *fluid intake* includes everything the patient drinks: water, milk, milk drinks, fruit juices, soup, tea, coffee, or anything liquid. Ice cream and gelatin also are counted as liquids (Figure 22–5◆). Fluids taken in through an intravenous tube and/or nasogastrointestinal tube are also included in the patient's total fluid intake. Fluids and nutrients taken intravenously are referred to as **parenteral intake**. Fluid intake needs increase with high temperatures (weather), exercise, fever, illness, and excessive fluid loss.

fluid intake The fluid taken into the body, from whatever source

parenteral intake Fluids taken in intravenously

FIGURE 22–5 ◆

Although solid foods also contain some liquid, most of the fluids in the body are taken in when a person drinks liquids

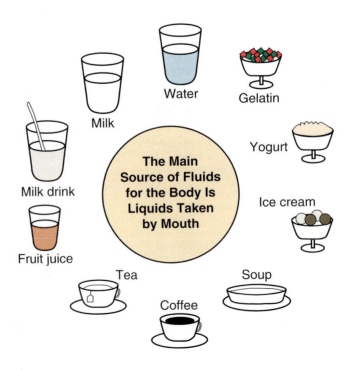

The Main Source of Fluids for the Body Is Liquids Taken by Mouth

Water — Gelatin — Yogurt — Ice cream — Soup — Coffee — Tea — Fruit juice — Milk drink — Milk

Fluid Output

Fluid output is the sum total of liquids that come out of the body. Most adults will eliminate the same amount of fluid taken in. Therefore, the adult above also will **eliminate** about 3 quarts (3,312 cc) of fluid every day. Fluid is discharged from the body of a healthy person in several ways:

- Most of the fluid passes through the kidneys and is discharged as urine.
- Some of the fluid is lost from the body through perspiration.
- Some fluid is **evaporated** from the lungs in breathing.
- The rest is **absorbed** and **discharged** through the intestinal system.

To urinate means to discharge urine from the body. Other terms for this body function are void and pass water. Fluid that is lost by breathing and perspiration is called **insensible fluid loss**. Approximately 100 to 200 cc of fluid is discharged from the body in feces. Output also includes emesis (vomitus), drainage from a wound or from the stomach, loss of blood, and diarrhea.

fluid output The fluid passed or excreted out of the body; for example urine, vomit, diarrhea

eliminate To rid the body of waste products, to excrete, expel, remove, put out

evaporate To pass off as vapor, as water evaporating into the air

absorb To take or soak in, up, or through

KEY IDEA

It is difficult to measure accurately the amount of fluid discharged through evaporation and breathing. Therefore, a person may seem to have a greater fluid intake than output. There is, however, a fluid balance in the normally functioning body.

discharge Flowing out of material (secretion or excretion) from any part of the body such as pus, feces, urine, or drainage from a wound

insensible fluid loss Fluid that is lost from the body without being noticed, such as in perspiration or air breathed out

---

Many times the health care team will help with maintaining fluid balance by increasing or decreasing a patient's fluid intake or providing medical interventions to aid in the elimination of fluid. Therefore, it is very important for members of the nursing staff to keep accurate records of fluid intake and output. The record of the patient's intake and output is kept for a full 24-hour period. These records may be kept for any period of time (shift, days, or weeks) as prescribed by the physician. With some patients, the doctor is only interested in knowing the 24-hour totals. However, in sicker patients and patients with acute renal failure, he may want to know the fluid balance on an hour-by-hour basis. In some cases, the fluid balance may be monitored less frequently than every hour. The most important thing for you to remember is that the **records must be accurate**.

Unit of Measurement

The metric system of measurement is used in many countries of the world. In the United States, we normally use one system for measuring liquids (ounces, pints, quarts) and a different system for measuring lengths (inches, feet, yards, miles). You probably have already noticed that many quantities used in the health care field are measured in cubic centimeters or milliliters. Because most institutions use these terms for measuring intake and output, you should understand what they mean.

KEY IDEA

Scientists, engineers, and many health care institution personnel use the metric system for measuring liquids, lengths, and weight. The basic metric unit of measurement of length is the meter, which is a little longer than a yard. A centimeter [one one-hundredth (1/100) of a meter] is about four-tenths (4/10) of an inch.

FIGURE 22–6 ◆

Proportionate size of cubic inch and cubic centimeter

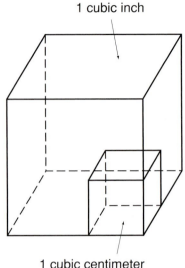

1 cubic inch

1 cubic centimeter

Cubic Centimeters

cubic centimeter Having a volume equal to a cube whose edges are 1 centimeter long

The term *cc* is an abbreviation for **cubic centimeter**, a unit of measurement in the metric system. A cubic centimeter can be thought of as a square block with each edge of the block 1 centimeter long (Figure 22–6◆). If we filled this block with water, we would have 1 cubic centimeter (1 cc) of water.

The liter is the basic unit of liquid measure in the metric system. It is approximately the same as a quart. A milliliter (1/1000 liter) is the amount that would fill a cubic centimeter. Therefore the two units are often used interchangeably. The patient's liquid intake is measured in cubic centimeters (cc) or milliliters (ml).

graduate A measuring cup marked along its side to show various amounts so that the material placed in the cup can be measured accurately; the marks are called *calibrations*

Graduate Containers

A container called a **graduate** (Figure 22–7◆) or a measuring cup is used to measure intake and output (I&O). The side of the graduate is marked (**calibrated**) with a row of short lines and numbers. These show the amount of liquid in both milliliters and ounces

calibrated Marked with lines and numbers for measuring

FIGURE 22–7 ◆

Examples of calibrated containers

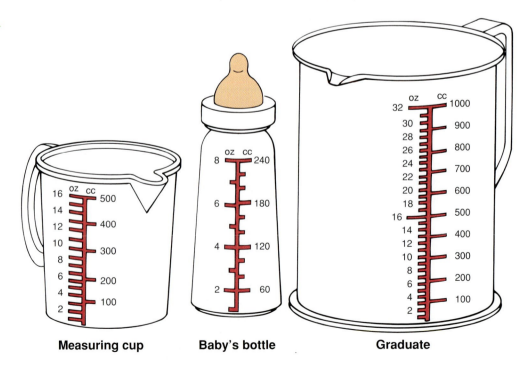

Measuring cup   Baby's bottle   Graduate

TABLE 22–2

U.S. Customary Liquid Measure with Approximate Equivalent Apothecary and Metric Measurements

cc = cubic centimeter	150 cc = 5 oz
ml = milliliter	180 cc = 6 oz
oz = ounce	210 cc = 7 oz
1cc = 1 ml	240 cc = 8 oz
1/4 teaspoon = 1 cc	270 cc = 9 oz
1 teaspoon = 4 cc	300 cc = 10 oz
30 cc = 1 oz	500 cc = 1 pint
60 cc = 2 oz	1000 cc = 1 quart
90 cc = 3 oz	4000 cc = 1 gallon
120 cc = 4 oz	

(see Table 22–2♦). This graduate is like the measuring cup you use at home to measure ingredients for cooking, only larger. Another calibrated graduate used in the home is a baby's milk bottle. This, too, is marked with a row of short lines and numbers. They show the amount of milk in both ounces and milliliters. When full, most baby bottles contain 8 ounces, or 240 cubic centimeters (cc). To give the baby 4 ounces of milk, or 120 cc, you would fill it half-full or to the 4-ounce line.

Some things to remember about graduate containers are as follows:

- They are all calibrated.
- They are made of metal, glass, cardboard, or plastic.
- They are used for measuring liquids in cubic centimeters (cc).
- They are used for measuring liquids in ounces (oz).
- The measuring cup is used to measure liquids in the home.
- The baby's bottle is used to measure liquids in the home.
- The calibrated graduate is used to measure fluid.

It is very important that you observe the exact amounts of fluids taken in by the patient and that you record them accurately. You will have to measure the amount of liquid contained in each serving container, bowl, glass, or cup used by the patient. If your institution does not have a list of the amounts contained in each container, bowl, glass, or cup, you will find it helpful to make such a list yourself (see Table 22–3♦).

TABLE 22–3

Capacities of Serving Containers

4-oz juice cup	120 cc
6-oz cup	180 cc
8-oz cup	240 cc
12-oz cup	360 cc
1-cup milk carton	240 cc
4-oz ice cream cup	120 cc
6-oz Jell-O cup	180 cc
6-oz coffee cup	180 cc
1-qt water pitcher	1000 cc

Measuring And Recording Fluid Intake

Tell the patient that her fluid intake is being measured and recorded. Encourage her to help you, if she is not too ill, by asking her to keep track of how much liquid she drinks. This is your responsibility, however, not the patient's. Also, inform family members and visitors that patient's fluid intake is being recorded.

Fluids taken in by patients intravenously are recorded by the registered nurse. This record may also be kept on the intake and output sheet in a special column headed Parenteral Intake.

KEY IDEA

> Regardless of how fluids are consumed, the important thing is that the doctor know as accurately as possible how much fluid the patient has taken in. *This is your responsibility, not the patient's.* You must monitor what your patients have on their meal trays and any fluids taken between meals.

The proper time for the nursing assistant to record the patient's fluids on the intake and output sheet is as soon as the patient has consumed the fluids. Before the end of each shift, the complete amount of intake should be totaled (added). Your task will be to remember to record all fluid taken each time the patient eats or drinks. Think about fluid intake every time you remove a tray, water pitcher, glass, or cup from a patient's bedside. Remember especially to check the water pitcher.

When measuring fluid intake, you will have to note the difference between the amount the patient actually drinks and the amount he leaves in the serving container. You will be required to **convert** (change) amounts such as a bowl of soup, glass of orange juice, or cup of tea into cc (cubic centimeters) when recording them.

convert Change

PROCEDURE

MEASURING THE CAPACITY OF SERVING CONTAINERS

OBRA

RATIONALE: Glasses and dishes vary in size. Having a list of those used by the patient will be a time-saving measure.

PREPARATION

1. Assemble your equipment in the utility room:

   a. Complete set of dishes, bowls, cups, and glasses used by the patients

   b. Graduate (measuring cup)

   c. Water

   d. Pen and paper

STEPS

2. Fill the first container with water.

3. Pour this water into the graduate.

4. Place the graduate on a flat surface for accuracy in measurement.

5. At eye level, carefully look at the level of the water and determine the amount in cc (cubic centimeters).

6. Write this information on the paper. For example, one carton of milk = 240 cc.

7. Repeat these steps for each dish, glass, bowl, or cup used by the patient.

FOLLOW-UP

8. You will have a complete list to use when measuring intake.

CHARTING EXAMPLE: Write the list and keep it in the area where you will be measuring the fluids.

**DETERMINING
THE AMOUNTS
CONSUMED**

PROCEDURE

OBRA

RATIONALE: Measuring is more accurate than guessing the amount consumed.

PREPARATION

1. Assemble your equipment on the bedside table:

   a. Graduate

   b. Pen and paper

   c. Leftover liquids in their serving containers

STEPS

2. Pour the leftover liquid into the graduate.

3. Look at the level and determine the amount in cc.

4. From your list (see preceding procedure), determine the amount in the full serving container.

5. Subtract the leftover amount from the full-container amount. This figure is the amount the patient actually drank.

6. Immediately record this amount on the intake side of the intake and output sheet.

EXAMPLE

1. Assemble equipment.

2. Pour the leftover orange juice into the graduate.

3. Look at the level of the juice. There are 60 cc in the graduate (Figure 22–8◆).

4. Look at the list. A full glass of juice = 240 cc.

5. Subtract:

$$
\begin{array}{rl}
240\ cc = & \text{full glass} \\
-60\ cc = & \text{amount left over} \\
\hline
180\ cc = & \text{amount the patient} \\
& \text{actually drank}
\end{array}
$$

6. Record: 180 cc on the intake side of the I&O sheet.

CHARTING EXAMPLE: 10/24/04 9am Mark 180cc on the intake flow sheet. J. Jones, CNA

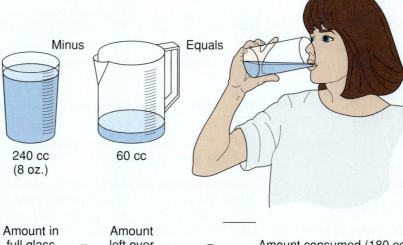

Minus   Equals

240 cc   60 cc
(8 oz.)

Amount in   Amount   Amount consumed (180 cc)
full glass   –   left over   =
240 cc   60 cc

FIGURE 22–8 ◆
Measuring intake

Force Fluids, Restrict Fluids, and NPO

Force Fluids (FF)

Patients who need to have more fluids added to their normal intake are put on **force fluids** and often need encouragement to drink more (Figure 22–9◆). FF is the abbreviation for force fluids. Patients may also be placed on FF when they fail to take in the normal amount of fluid that the body needs. A list of ways you can persuade the patient to drink more fluids and guidelines for patients on force fluids follow:

- Offer fluids in small quantities.

- As permitted by the patient's therapeutic diet, provide different kinds of fluids, especially drinks, the patient prefers; examples are hot tea, gelatin, soda, ice cream, milk, juice, broth, coffee, custard, and water.

force fluids Extra fluids to be taken in by a patient according to the doctor's orders (FF)

FIGURE 22-9 ◆

Sign placed on door or bed of patient who is on forced fluids

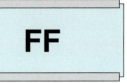

FF

- Offer liquids without being asked.
- Remind patient of the importance of fluids in getting better.

FORCE FLUIDS — GUIDELINES

- Verify that patient is on force fluids.
- Place a sign stating *force fluids* on the bed or door.
- Encourage the patient to drink the amount of fluids required. For

example, 800 cc every 8 hours means the patient would have to drink 100 cc every hour. At the end of the 8-hour shift, the patient would have taken in 800 cc of fluids.

- Record the amount taken in by the patient in ccs on the intake side of the intake and output sheet.

Restrict Fluids

For some patients, the doctor writes orders to restrict fluids (Figure 22–10◆). This means that fluids may be limited to certain amounts. When you are caring for a patient on **restrict fluids**, it is important to follow orders exactly and to measure accurately. Your calm and reassuring attitude can make a big difference in how the patient feels and reacts. Usually, the water pitcher is removed from the bedside. Frequent oral hygiene is often necessary as it helps keep the mucous membranes of the mouth moist.

restrict fluids Fluids that are limited to certain amounts

FIGURE 22-10 ◆

Sign placed on door or bed of patient who is on restricted fluids

RESTRICT FLUIDS

RESTRICT FLUIDS — GUIDELINES

- Verify the patient is on restrict fluids.
- Patient must stay within the fluid-intake limits stated by your immediate supervisor.

- Place a sign stating *restrict fluids* on the bed or door.
- Remind patient that fluids are restricted.

- Record the amount on the intake side of the intake and output sheet.
- Schedule the patient intake so that it covers 24 hours.

Nothing by Mouth

For some patients, the doctor writes orders that the patient is to have **nothing by mouth (NPO)**. This means that the patient cannot eat or drink anything at all. You may be asked to take away the patient's water pitcher and glass at midnight. You will post a sign saying NPO (Figure 22–11◆). NPO is taken from the Latin *nils per os,* which means nothing by mouth. Persons are usually NPO before and after surgery and before some lab tests or certain x-ray procedures. An NPO sign is put at the foot or the head of the bed or on the door of the patient's room. Some institutions do not allow a patient on NPO to have oral hygiene. Patients often become very irritable when they are not allowed to have anything to eat or drink. They may, therefore, be hard for you to deal with. Calm and reassuring behavior on your part can help the patient get through a very uncomfortable period. A smile and a few kind words will go a long way here.

nothing by mouth (NPO)
Cannot eat or drink anything at all

NPO

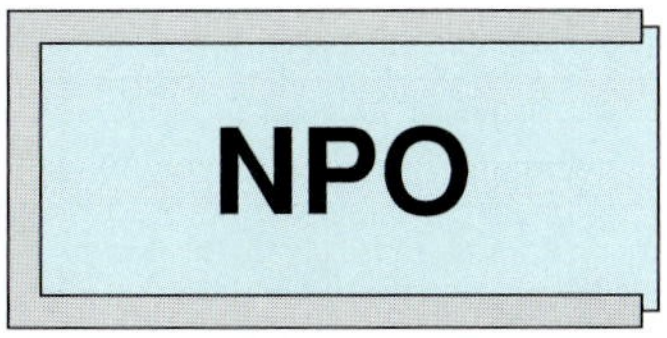

FIGURE 22–11 ◆

Sign placed on door or bed of patient who is on nothing by mouth restriction

GUIDELINES

NOTHING BY MOUTH

- Verify the patient is on NPO.
- Explain to patient the NPO (nothing by mouth) restriction.

- Place a sign stating *NPO* on the bed or door.
- Remove the water pitcher and anything else with which the patient could take a drink or eat.

- Do not give any liquids or food to this patient.
- Make a note on the intake side of the intake and output sheet that the patient is NPO.

Measuring and Recording Fluid Output

A patient who is on intake and output must have both measured and recorded. This means that every time the patient uses the urinal, emesis basin, or bedpan, the urine and other liquids must be measured and recorded (Figure 22–12◆).

You should tell the patient his output is being measured and ask him to cooperate. A female patient must urinate in a bedpan or specipan. The specipan is a disposable container that fits into the toilet bowl under the seat. The specipan can be placed in the patient's toilet bowl, if the patient is allowed out of bed. This pan covers only the front of the toilet, so stool can be expelled through the back of the toilet and toilet paper can be tossed. Ask the patient not to place toilet paper in the bedpan. Provide a wastepaper basket for her. Then discard tissue into the toilet or hopper. Female patients must also be asked not to let their bowels move while urinating into a bedpan. Male patients on output must be instructed to use a urinal.

KEY IDEA

Provide each patient on output with a bedpan, specipan, or urinal. Any device used for measuring a patient's output must be used for that patient only and disposed of or sterilized when the patient is discharged. Be sure to follow Standard Precautions.

FIGURE 22–12 ◆

Intake and output sheet

| CITY MEMORIAL HOSPITAL |
| DAILY INTAKE AND OUTPUT RECORD   Name _____ |

Solutions	Rate (cc/hr)	Solutions	Rate (cc/hr)
A		D	
B		E	
C		F	

Date: ____   Yesterday's Weight: _____   Today's Weight: _____

		INTAKE							OUTPUT				
HOUR	ORAL	Feeding Tube		IV		IV		IVPB		Other	Other	Urine	Emesis	Stool	Other
		Amt. Up	Amt. Abs.	Amt. Up	Amt. Abs.	Amt. Up	Amt. Abs.	Amt. Up	Amt. Abs.				
11 p.m.													
12 p.m.													
1 a.m.													
2 a.m.													
3 a.m.													
4 a.m.													
5 a.m.													
6 a.m.													
8 hr. total													
7 a.m.													
8 a.m.													
9 a.m.													
10 a.m.													
11 a.m.													
12 noon													
1 p.m.													
2 p.m.													
8 hr. total													
3 p.m.													
4 p.m.													
5 p.m.													
6 p.m.													
7 p.m.													
8 p.m.													
9 p.m.													
10 p.m.													
8 hr. total													
24 hr. total													
Combined 24 hour total		INTAKE				OUTPUT							

GUIDE FOR RECORDING I & O:
Juice Glass......................120 cc   Insulated Hot Mug........210 cc   Cereal Bowl..............180 cc   Ice Cream....................120 cc
Coffee Cup.....................210 cc   Cold Cup (small)..........120 cc   Milkshake Container......210 cc   Jello Container...........120 cc
                                        Jumbo Paper Cup........300 cc   Water Pitcher................900 cc   Milk Container..............240 cc

---

PROCEDURE   OBRA

MEASURING URINARY OUTPUT

RATIONALE: Urinary output reflects kidney functioning.

PREPARATION

1. Assemble your equipment in the patient's bathroom:

   a. Bedpan, cover, urinal, or specipan

   b. Graduate (measuring container or calibrated container)

   c. Intake and output sheet

   d. Pencil or pen

   e. Disposable gloves

2. Wash your hands and put on gloves.

STEPS

3. Pour the urine from the bedpan or urinal into a graduate.

4. Place the graduate on a flat surface for accuracy in measurement.

5. At eye level, carefully look at the level of urine in the graduate to see the number reached by the level of the urine.

6. Record this amount in cc, as well as the time, on the output side of the intake and output sheet.

FOLLOW-UP

7. Wash, rinse, and return the graduate to its proper place.

8. Wash, rinse, and return the urinal or bedpan to its proper place.

9. Dispose of gloves and wash your hands.

10. Report to your immediate supervisor:

    ■ That you have measured the output for the patient.

    ■ Your observations of anything unusual.

CHARTING EXAMPLE: 9/14/04 7pm Record urinary output in the Output column of the patient's I&O sheet: output 400 cc. M. Gonzalez, CNA

Urinary Catheters

The urinary **catheter** is the most common kind of catheter used for draining urine out of the body (Figure 22–13◆). This catheter (made of plastic or silicon) is inserted through the patient's urethra into the bladder. This catheter may also be used when a patient is unable to void (urinate) naturally, or it may be used to measure the amount of urine left in the bladder after a patient has voided naturally (**residual** urine). When a patient is unable to void, the bladder may stretch out. The bladder is distended and the patient's symptom is described as urinary retention, or a **bladder distention**.

Sometimes a urinary catheter is used for only one withdrawal of urine. Sometimes, however, it is kept in place in the bladder for a number of days or even weeks.

Sometimes the bladder-drainage catheter is used to help keep an **incontinent** patient dry. An incontinent patient is one who cannot control his urine and/or feces. An **indwelling urinary catheter** is a tube inserted through the patient's urethra into the bladder to allow for urinary drainage. It really is two tubes, one inside the other. The inside tube is connected at one end to a kind of balloon. After the catheter has been inserted, the balloon is filled with water or air so the catheter will not slip out through the urethra. Urine drains out of the bladder through the outer tube. The urine collects in a container attached to the bed frame lower than the patient's urinary bladder. This is always maintained as a closed system, which means it is never opened except when emptying the urine collecting bag. A commercially prepared condom catheter is sometimes used for external drainage of urine from a male incontinent patient (see later section).

You will empty this container, measure the urine, and record the amount. This will always be done whenever it is full and always before the end of your working shift. The measurement is not taken from the soft expandable plastic urine collection container. A hard plastic graduate is always used as it is more accurate.

Figure 22–14◆ shows a condom catheter and drainage bag used for ambulatory patients and Figure 22–15◆ shows the plastic urine container for the nonambulatory patient.

catheter A device for draining urine out of the body

residual Remaining or left over

bladder distention A stretching out of the bladder when urine produced is not excreted

incontinent Unable to control urine or feces

indwelling urinary catheter A bladder drainage tube that is allowed to remain in place within the bladder

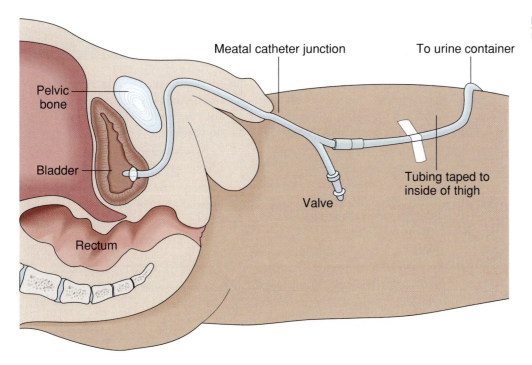

FIGURE 22–13 ◆

Urinary catheter in the male

Meatal catheter junction

To urine container

Pelvic bone

Bladder

Tubing taped to inside of thigh

Valve

Rectum

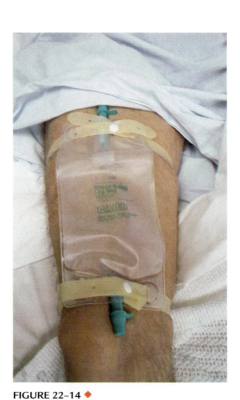

FIGURE 22–14 ◆
Leg drainage bag for ambulatory patient

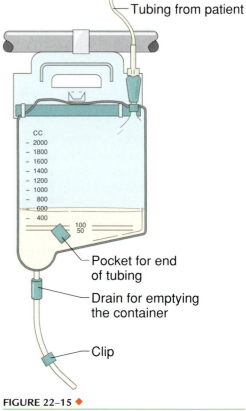

FIGURE 22–15 ◆
Plastic urine container for nonambulatory patient

GUIDELINES

INDWELLING URINARY CATHETER

- Check from time to time to make sure the level of urine has increased. If the level stays the same, report this to your immediate supervisor.

- If the patient says he feels that his bladder is full or that he needs to urinate, report this to your immediate supervisor.

- If the patient is allowed to get out of bed for short periods, the bag goes with the patient. It must be held lower than the patient's urinary bladder (below hip level) at all times to prevent the urine in the tubing and bag from draining back into the urinary bladder.

- Check to make sure there are no kinks in the catheter and tubing. Be sure the patient is not lying on the catheter or the tubing. This would stop the flow of urine.

- The catheter may be loosely taped or strapped at all times to the patient's inner thigh. This keeps it from being pulled on or being pulled out of the bladder.

- Most patients with urinary drainage through a catheter are on output. You must keep a careful record of urinary output.

- Keep tubing and drainage bag from touching the floor.

- Catheter care should be done as ordered for these patients.

- Report to your immediate supervisor any complaints the patient may have of burning, tenderness, or pain in the urethral area or any changes in the appearance of the urine.

CHECKING CATHETERS AND CONTAINERS	GUIDELINES

- Check tubing for kinks.

- Be sure patient is not lying on tubing.
- Check level in container for increase in level. If level remains the same or increases rapidly, report to your immediate supervisor.

- The plastic urine container is hung on bed frame below the level of the patient's urinary bladder.

EMPTYING URINE FROM AN INDWELLING CATHETER CONTAINER	PROCEDURE	OBRA

RATIONALE: Urine is removed to accurately measure output.

PREPARATION

1. Assemble your equipment:
   a. Calibrated graduate
   b. Alcohol swab
   c. Disposable gloves
2. Wash your hands and put on gloves.

STEPS

3. Open the drain at the bottom of the plastic urine container and let the urine run into the graduate; then close the drain, wipe with alcohol swab, and replace in the holder on the bag.
4. Measure the amount of urinary output.
5. Record the amount immediately on the output side of the intake and output sheet.

FOLLOW-UP

6. Wash and rinse the graduate and put it in its proper place.

7. Dispose of gloves and wash your hands.
8. Document or report to your immediate supervisor:
   - That you have emptied the urine container (drainage bag) and measured the amount of output.
   - That you have recorded the amount on the output side of the intake and output sheet.
   - Your observations of anything unusual.

CHARTING EXAMPLE: 12/02/04 11pm 1200 cc pale clear urine emptied from drainage bag. Recorded 1200 cc on I/O sheet. C. Keller, CNA

Daily Indwelling Catheter Care

The catheter is attached to tubing that should be strapped or taped loosely to the inner side of the patient's thigh. This is so it does not pull and irritate the bladder. This tubing leads to a plastic urine container. The container is attached to the bed frame. It is kept lower than the level of the urinary bladder so that there is a constant downhill flow from the patient caused by gravity. The urine collects in the plastic container.

This is a *closed* drainage system. The system must never be opened. If the patient is allowed to get out of bed, the container is carried at a lower level than the patient's bladder. A careful record of urinary output is kept for all patients who have indwelling catheters in place.

KEY IDEA

Daily care of patients with indwelling catheters is very important to prevent infection. Aseptic technique should be used at all times when you are handling and caring for the equipment.

AGE-SPECIFIC CONSIDERATIONS

Patients of all ages may have concerns and fears about being catheterized, after being catheterized, or while having a catheter in place. Children may fear where the tube will go inside their body. Elderly patients may fear a loss of mobility and independence. All patients may fear pain and the loss of privacy. To respond to these concerns, be certain to close the door or pull the curtain. Explain the procedure to the patient in terms that he or she can understand; use pictures if appropriate.

GIVING DAILY INDWELLING CATHETER CARE

PROCEDURE   OBRA

RATIONALE: Catheter care prevents urinary infections.

PREPARATION

1. Assemble your equipment:
   a. Disposable catheter care kit
   b. Disposable gloves
   c. Disposable bed protector
2. Identify the patient by checking the identification bracelet.
3. Wash your hands.
4. Tell the patient you are going to clean the area around his catheter tube. Make sure the patient's genital area has already been washed or that perineal care has been done.
5. Provide privacy for the patient.
6. Raise bed to a comfortable working position.
7. Make sure there is plenty of light.

STEPS

8. Cover the patient with a bath blanket. Without exposing him, fan-fold the top sheets to the foot of the bed. Have the patient covered with only the blanket.
9. Open the catheter kit. Put on the disposable gloves. Place the disposable bed protector under the patient's buttocks.
10. Observe for crusting, lesions, discharge, or anything else abnormal.
11. Take the applicators from the kit. The applicators are covered with antiseptic solution. With your gloved thumb and forefinger (index finger), gently separate the labia on female patients. If the male patient has a foreskin, gently pull it back to apply antiseptic solution to the entire area. Apply antiseptic solution on the entire area where the catheter enters the patient's body. Work from the cleanest area to the dirtiest. Gently replace the male's foreskin if you have pulled it back.
12. Check the strap or tape to be sure the tubing is taped correctly in place.

13. Remove the disposable bed protector.
14. Cover the patient with the top sheets. Remove the bath blanket.

FOLLOW-UP

15. Make the patient comfortable and replace the call light.
16. Lower the bed to a position of safety for the patient.
17. Raise the side rails when ordered or appropriate for patient safety.
18. Discard disposable equipment.
19. Remove gloves and wash your hands.
20. Report to your immediate supervisor:
    - That catheter care has been given.
    - The time it was given.
    - How the patient tolerated the procedure.
    - Your observations of anything unusual.

CHARTING EXAMPLE: 12/03/04 3pm Catheter care given. R. Martin, CNA

Many health care institutions have discontinued daily indwelling catheter care. They consider daily washing of the genital area with soap and water as sufficient to maintain cleanliness. Follow the policy of your employing health care institution and the instructions of your immediate supervisor with regard to indwelling catheter care.

In some health care institutions, the nursing assistant does not discontinue an indwelling catheter. However, if the health care institution where you are employed has a policy to this effect and it is on your job description that you are expected to discontinue indwelling catheters, follow the guidelines on page 475.

Fluid Output and the Incontinent Patient

If a patient is incontinent of urine, record this on the output side of the I&O sheet each time the patient wets the bed. Even though the urine cannot be measured, the doctor at least knows that the patient's kidneys are functioning.

DISCONTINUING AN INDWELLING CATHETER	GUIDELINES

- Note there are differences in how the indwelling catheter is discontinued. Follow the exact steps required by your employer or state.
- Place protective pad under patient as urine may leak.

- Cut the end of the indwelling catheter off with a bandage scissors (Figure 22–16◆), which will deflate the balloon inside the patient, or use a 10-cc syringe to remove contents of inflated balloon, if permitted by your employing health care institution.
- Gently pull the catheter out.

- If you meet any resistance, do *not* apply force.
- Wait a minute; then gently pull the catheter out. It should come out easily. Give perineal care.
- Dispose of used or soiled equipment appropriately using standard precautions.

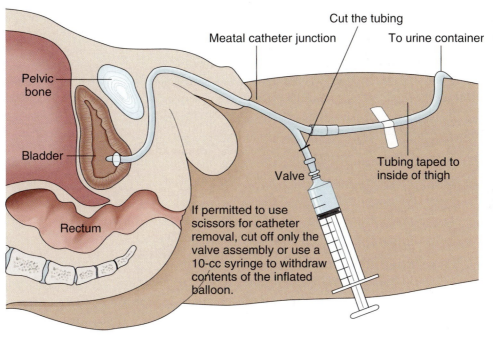

FIGURE 22–16 ◆

Deflate balloon prior to removing an indwelling catheter. Be sure to follow procedure used in your state of employment or taught by your instructor

KEY IDEA

Care must be taken to properly deflate the retention balloon while holding the catheter. A catheter accidentally can be retracted into a male's urethra if the catheter is improperly cut to deflate the balloon. Should this occur, removal from the bladder requires cystoscopic surgery or radiological interventions. Remove the catheter using a slow, steady movement to minimize the patient's pain or discomfort.

The Condom Catheter

Condom catheters or urinary sheaths are frequently used for males who have urinary incontinence. Condom Catheters are designed with a soft rubber sheath that slides over the penis and is held in place with elastic tape. Tubing connects the catheter with a drainage bag made to be worn on the leg (see Figure 22–17a◆). The advantage of the condom catheter is that it provides a way to maintain a higher quality of life and reduces the fear of having urinary accidents and wet clothing. Some patients prefer condom catheters to wearing adult diapers or pads.

The condom catheter is changed daily. It is important to thoroughly wash and dry the penis and perineal area before applying a new condom catheter. Read and follow the manufacturers' instructions. It is important to use elastic tape rather than adhesive tape as it will expand when the penis changes size and will not constrict blood flow to the penis.

APPLYING A CONDOM CATHETER ON A MALE PATIENT

PROCEDURE   **OBRA**

RATIONALE: To improve quality of life for incontinent males.

PREPARATION

1. Assemble your supplies
   a. Condom catheter kit
   b. Drainage bag or leg bag and cap
   c. Basin of warm water
   d. Soap, washcloth, and towel
   e. Gloves
   f. Bed protector
   g. Paper towels
2. Identify the patient by checking the identification bracelet.
3. Explain the procedure to the patient.
4. Ask about any allergies including latex.
5. Provide privacy for the patient.
6. Wash your hands.

STEPS

7. Cover the patient with a bath blanket. Fan-fold top bed linens to the patient's lower legs.

8. Ask the patient to raise his buttocks to enable you to slide the bed protector under him. (Turn the patient on his side to place the bed protector under his buttocks if he is unable to lift himself.)
9. Assemble the equipment making sure the drainage bag or leg bag is ready with the drain closed and cap in place.
10. Arrange the bath blanket to expose the genital area.
11. Put on gloves.
12. Remove condom catheter if patient has one in place by removing elastic tape and rolling the condom sheath off the penis. Disconnect the drainage tubing from the condom and cap the drainage tube. Discard the tape and condom.

13. Provide male perineal care (see p. 267) Check the penis for signs of skin breakdown, redness, or irritation.
14. Prepare the new condom by removing the protective backing and exposing the adhesive strip. Remove the fenestrated drape from the kit, and using your nondominant hand, place the penis through the hole in the drape. Keep dominant hand sterile.

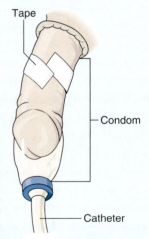

FIGURE 22–17b ◆
Tape is applied in a spiral fashion to secure the condom catheter to the penis.

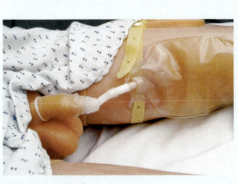

FIGURE 22–17a ◆
A condom catheter attached to a leg bag.

PROCEDURE *(continued)*

15. Firmly hold the penis as you roll the condom over the penis. Be sure to leave a 1-inch space at the end of the condom catheter (see Figure 22–17a).

16. Secure the condom with the elastic tape applied in a spiral (see Figure 22–17b). Do *not* apply the tape completely around the penis as it can prevent circulation.

17. Connect the condom with the drainage bag or attach the leg bag.

18. Remove bed protector and bath blanket. Position the patient for comfort, and replace the linens.

FOLLOW-UP

19. Measure and record the amount of urine in the bag.

20. Clean basin and return items to their proper place. Remove and discard gloves and all disposable items used.

21. Wash hands.

22. Document and report the results to your supervisor.

CHARTING EXAMPLE: 12/1/04 9am Condom catheter removed and perineal care given. No signs of skin irritation noted. New condom catheter applied and attached to leg bag. 300 cc urine emptied from drainage bag. G. Bates, CNA

Advanced Skills

Advanced skills are performed only by CNAs who have demonstrated competence to do the skill in both a facility and state that permit it.

Inserting an Indwelling Catheter

GUIDELINES

URINARY CATHETERIZATION

- Urinary catheterization generally requires a physician's order.

- Catheterization may be routine to health care providers, but it can be frightening to patients. Reduce the patient's anxiety by explaining the purpose of the procedure and providing privacy.

- Do not remove more than 800 to 1000 cc of urine at one time from adults to prevent bladder collapse and electrolyte imbalance.

- On female patients, if the catheter tip is accidentally inserted into the vagina, it is considered contaminated and must be discarded. You will need to get a new kit and start over. Your facility procedure may recommend not removing a catheter accidentally inserted into the vagina until after the new catheter has been correctly inserted in the urethral opening (the urinary meatus).

- Be aware that individuals from some cultures believe it is inappropriate for a caregiver to catheterize a patient of the opposite sex. Accommodate the patient's preferences.

KEY IDEA

Infection is the most common complication of having an indwelling urinary catheter, and the risk of infection increases with the length of time the catheter remains in place. Use of correct sterile technique will significantly reduce the patient's risk of infection.

INSERTING AN INDWELLING URINARY CATHETER IN A FEMALE PATIENT USING CORRECT STERILE TECHNIQUE

PROCEDURE

RATIONALE: Urinary catheterization is an ancient procedure. It involves inserting a hollow tube up the urethra into the bladder under sterile conditions. Common reasons for catheterization are to empty the bladder for surgery, to obtain a specimen, to instill medications, to bypass an obstruction, or to determine accurate urinary output.

PREPARATION

1. Assemble your equipment:

   a. Catheter kit (contains paper drape, urinary catheter, syringe, lubricant, antiseptic solution, cotton balls, urine collection tray, specimen cup) (see Figure 22–18◆).

   b. Sterile gloves

2. Identify the patient by checking the identification bracelet.

3. Explain the procedure to the patient emphasizing the need to maintain the sterile field. Tell the patient you will be inserting an indwelling catheter into her.

4. Ask about any allergies including iodine-based antiseptics, latex, and adhesive tape.

5. Provide privacy for the patient.

6. Wash your hands.

STEPS

7. Position the patient in the dorsal recumbent position with knees flexed, exposing the labia.

8. Drape the patient so that only the perineum is exposed.

9. Remove the full drape from the kit with your fingertips, and place, plastic side down, just under the patient's buttocks (ask her to raise her hips).

10. Put on sterile gloves.

11. Prepare the items in the kit for use during insertion, maintaining sterile technique.

12. Test the balloon for defects. Deflate the balloon, and leave the syringe

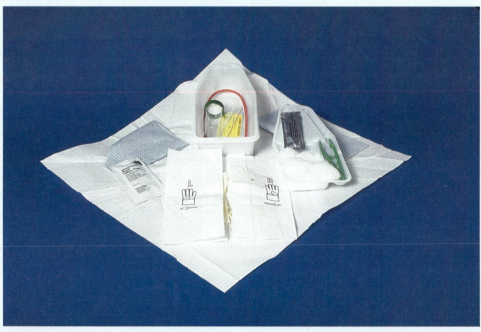

FIGURE 22–18 ◆

Catheter kit

PROCEDURE *(continued)*

on the catheter. Liberally lubricate the catheter tip.

13. With your nondominant hand, separate the labia minora, and hold this position until the catheter is inserted (see Figure 22–19◆). (*Note:* The dominant hand is the only sterile hand now; the contaminated hand continues to separate the labia.)

14. Using cotton balls, cleanse the meatus with the aseptic solution:

    a. Making one downward stroke with each cotton ball, begin at the labia on the side farthest from you, and move toward the labia nearest you.

    b. Afterward, wipe once down the center of the meatus.

    c. Wipe once with each cotton ball, and discard.

15. Insert the tip of the catheter slowly through the urethral opening 3 to 4 inches or until urine returns.

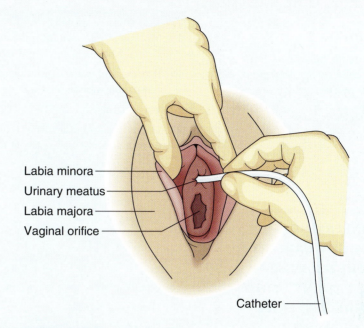

Labia minora
Urinary meatus
Labia majora
Vaginal orifice

Catheter

FIGURE 22–19 ◆
Inserting a urinary catheter into a female

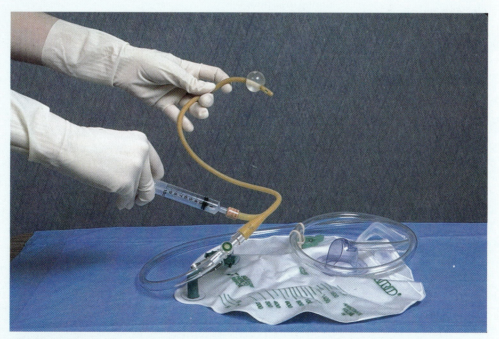

FIGURE 22–20 ◆
Testing the retention of a balloon catheter with a syringe

PROCEDURE *(continued)*

16. Advance the catheter another 0.5 to 1.0 inch.
17. Inflate the balloon with the attached syringe, and gently pull back on the catheter until it stops, or catches (see Figure 22-20♦).

FOLLOW-UP

18. Measure the amount of urine in the drainage bag container, and record.
19. Remove and discard gloves and all disposable items used.
20. Wash hands.
21. Document and report the results to your supervisor.

CHARTING EXAMPLE: 11/20/04
4pm Inserted an indwelling catheter into Mrs. Hayes. Tolerated the procedure well. 800 cc clear pale yellow urine drained into bag. Specimen collected and sent to lab for urinalysis as ordered. K. Little, CNA

INSERTING A STRAIGHT URINARY CATHETER INTO A MALE PATIENT USING CORRECT STERILE TECHNIQUE

PROCEDURE

RATIONALE: Urinary catheterization is an ancient procedure. It involves inserting a hollow tube up the urethra into the bladder under sterile conditions. Common reasons for catheterization are to empty the bladder for surgery, to obtain a specimen, to instill medications, to bypass an obstruction, or to determine accurate urinary output.

PREPARATION

1. Assemble your equipment: sterile gloves, fenestrated drape, cotton balls, iodine cleansing solution, water soluble lubricant, a size 14–16 French urinary straight catheter, urine collection basin, sterile urine cup, forceps.
2. Identify the patient by checking the identification bracelet.
3. Explain the procedure to the patient. Tell the patient you will be catheterizing him.
4. Ask about any allergies including iodine-based antiseptics, latex, and adhesive tape.

5. Provide privacy for the patient.
6. Wash your hands.

STEPS

7. Drape the patient with bed linens so that only the penis is exposed.
8. Assemble the equipment, and put on gloves.
9. Prepare the items in the kit for use during insertion.
10. Remove the fenestrated drape from the kit, and using your nondominant hand, place the penis through the hole in the drape. Keep dominant hand sterile.
11. Pull the penis up at a 90-degree angle to the patient's supine body.
12. With your nondominant hand, gently grasp the glans (tip) of the penis; retract the foreskin if uncircumcised.
13. Using cotton balls, cleanse the meatus and the glans with the iodine cleansing solution, beginning at the urethral opening and moving toward the shaft of the penis; make one complete circle around the tip of penis with each cotton ball. (The forceps may be used to hold the cotton ball.)
14. Direct the open end of the catheter into the collection container. Lubricate and insert the tip of the

catheter slowly through the urethral opening 7 to 9 inches or until urine returns (see Figure 22-21♦).
15. Allow urine to drain until it stops. Collect a sterile urine specimen if needed. Then remove the catheter.

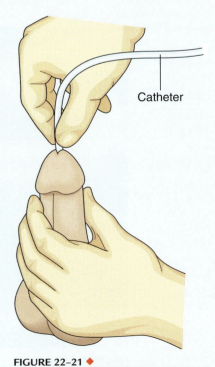
Catheter

FIGURE 22-21 ♦
Side view of male anatomy with indwelling urinary catheter in place

16. Cleanse the perineal area and replace the foreskin of the penis. Reposition the patient for comfort, and replace the linens.

FOLLOW-UP

17. Measure the amount of urine in the collection container, and record.

18. Remove and discard gloves and all disposable items used.
19. Wash hands.
20. Document and report the results to your supervisor.

CHARTING EXAMPLE: 11/20/04
4pm Inserted and removed a straight catheter into Mr. Hanes. Tolerated the procedure well. 750 cc clear pale yellow urine obtained. Urine specimen collected and sent to lab for urinalysis as ordered. K. Little, CNA

SUMMARY

The urinary system—kidneys, ureters, bladder, and urethra—is one of the systems responsible for maintaining homeostasis. Essential to this function is the formation and excretion of urine which occurs in the kidneys. The ureters collect the urine formed in the kidneys and drain it into the bladder. The bladder, a collapsible organ, acts as a reservoir. When the bladder receptors are stretched, muscle receptors in the wall of the bladder send messages to the brain causing a person to urinate. The urethra serves to empty the bladder of urine. Because of its exposure to the external environment, disease-causing organisms can enter the body through the urethra. Understanding the urinary system, including the nature and formation of urine and the diseases and disorders associated with the system, provides a sound basis to fulfill your responsibilities monitoring and recording fluid intake and output and providing indwelling catheter care.

The enthusiasm and caring support that you bring to the care of your patients is often helpful in improving the patients' attitudes toward their own progress. For example, patients on force fluids, restrict fluids, nothing by mouth, and even incontinent patients may feel stressed by their present circumstances. Your encouraging words or thoughtful manner may ease the situation for them and allow them to be more cooperative.

NOTES

CHAPTER REVIEW

FILL IN THE BLANK Read each sentence and fill in each blank line with a word that completes the sentence.

1. A patient may be _____ if there is a decrease in the amount of water in her tissues.

2. _____ _____ is the sum total of liquids that come out of the body.

3. Patients who need to increase their fluid intake may need to _____ _____.

4. Patients are often NPO before and after _____.

5. When a patient is incontinent, it means she is unable to control either her _____ or _____.

MULTIPLE CHOICE Choose the best answer for each question or statement.

1. Which of the following is not a structure of the urinary system?
   a. Ureters
   b. Valves
   c. Bladder
   d. Urethra

2. The following are all diseases and disorders of the urinary system *except* for
   a. hematuria.
   b. acute renal failure.
   c. bursitis.
   d. renal colic.

3. All of the following may result in dehydration *except*
   a. vomiting.
   b. diarrhea.
   c. sweating.
   d. hypertension.

4. The unit of measurement health care providers use to measure intake and output is
   a. cc.
   b. oz.
   c. mm/hg.
   d. lbs.

5. When measuring the capacity of a container, you should do all of the following except
   a. place container on a flat surface.
   b. view the container at eye level.
   c. swirl the fluid to get the best reading.
   d. carefully record your reading on paper.

TIME-OUT

TIPS FOR TIME MANAGEMENT

Take the time you need to do the task correctly. When you attempt to cut corners, you compromise the patient's safety and well-being. Rushing through tasks increases stress for you and for the patient. When you are stressed, you are more likely to make mistakes. You will not save any time by rushing through a job.

THE NURSING ASSISTANT IN ACTION

You are a student doing a clinical day working in a nursing care facility. Another student requests your help assisting Ms. Clark, a resident, to the bathroom. Before you get her positioned on the toilet, she has urinated and released some diarrhea on your uniform pant leg.

What Is Your Response/Reaction?

CRITICAL THINKING

CUSTOMER SERVICE Residents may have less control over their bladders and bowels or take longer to use the bathroom than you think necessary. They will notice your comments, actions, and impatience if you keep trying to hurry them. Avoid expressing your frustration and feelings to the residents as they are likely to feel more anxious or upset.

CULTURAL CARE Be aware that individuals from some cultures believe it is inappropriate for a caregiver to provide perineal care or catheterize a patient of the opposite sex. Whenever possible, accommodate the patient's preferences. If there is a caregiver of the same sex as the patient qualified to perform the procedure, that person should be assigned to assist with that patient care procedure. A notation should be made on the care plan alerting staff of this preference. Your supervisor can assist you in problem solving when you encounter patient preferences that you are unsure how to handle.

COOPERATION WITHIN THE TEAM There are times when male caregivers will be requested to perform several procedures like catheter care or catheterization on male patients who are assigned to female coworkers. When their workloads are, or appear to be uneven, pitch in and help with other care required by patients or residents assigned to your coworkers. Patient personal comfort and preferences are more important than who has what assigned to them on any given day.

EXPLORE MediaLink

Additional interactive resources for this chapter can be found on the Companion Website at www.prenhall.com/wolgin. Click on Chapter 22 and "Begin" to select the activities for this chapter.

For chapter-related NCLEX-style questions and an audio glossary, access the accompanying CD-ROM in this book.

23 Specimen Collection

KEY TERMS

asepsis
clean catch
expectorate
feces
genital
medical asepsis
midstream
saliva
specimen
sputum
stool

OBJECTIVES

When you have completed this chapter, you will be able to:

- List the types of specimens nursing assistants are expected to collect.
- Label specimens properly.
- Explain the need for accuracy in specimen collection.
- Explain the need for asepsis in specimen collection.
- Collect a routine urine specimen.
- Collect a routine urine specimen from an infant.
- Collect a midstream, clean-catch urine specimen.
- Collect a 24-hour urine specimen.
- Strain the urine.
- Collect a sputum specimen.
- Collect a stool specimen.
- Prepare a Hemoccult slide.

MediaLink
www.prenhall.com/wolgin

Use the address above to access the free, interactive Companion Website created for this textbook. Get hints, instant feedback, and textbook references to chapter-related NCLEX-style questions. Link to other interesting sites.

AUDIO GLOSSARY:
Use the Companion Website, or the CD-ROM disk enclosed with your textbook, to hear the pronunciation of key terms in the chapter.

Specimen collection is a vital part of the duties and responsibilities of a nursing assistant. The physician often utilizes the results of tests that are performed on specimens that you will collect to diagnose or order treatment for a patient. Accuracy and proper technique are, therefore, essential to proper specimen collection. The information in this chapter will help you understand the need for asepsis and the correct method for obtaining the ordered specimens.

 INTRODUCTION

Specimen Collection

As one of its natural living functions, the human body regularly gets rid of various waste materials. Most of the body's waste materials are discharged in the urine and feces. The body also gets rid of wastes in the material coughed up and spit out of the mouth (**expectorated**). This material is called sputum.

These body waste materials, when tested in the laboratory, often show changes in the sick person's body. By examining the results of laboratory tests, doctors get information that can help them make their diagnosis and decide on appropriate treatment for the patient.

For these reasons, the doctor will sometimes need **specimens** (samples) of these waste products: urine, feces, and sputum. Members of the health care institution nursing staff are responsible for collecting such specimens.

When you are collecting specimens, you must be very accurate in following the procedure and labeling the specimen. You have to collect the specimen at the exact time that is indicated. You must look at the patient's identification bracelet for the correct name, identification number, and room number when filling out the cover or label on the specimen container (Figure 23–1◆). The time and date the specimen was obtained should be printed on the label. The label must be printed clearly so that it can be read easily. It must be attached to the container immediately after the specimen has been collected. Unlabeled specimens should be thrown away so that mistakes will not be made. For example, misdiagnosis, incorrect treatment, or delays in discharge can occur if there are labeling errors.

ALERT

For all patient contact, adhere to Standard Precautions (⚭ Chapter 5, pages 83–85). Wear protective equipment as indicated.

expectorate To cough up matter from the lungs, trachea, or bronchial tubes and spit it out

specimen A sample of material taken from the patient's body; examples are urine specimens, feces specimens, and sputum specimens

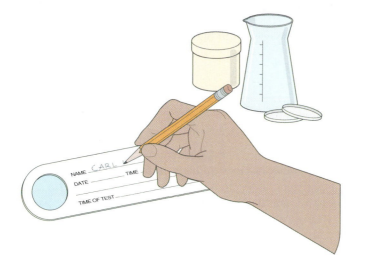

FIGURE 23–1◆

Be accurate when filling out the specimen label

SPECIMEN COLLECTION ACCURACY	GUIDELINES	OBRA
Be sure you follow all the "rules" listed here: ■ Right patient—from whom the specimen is to be collected. ■ Right specimen—as ordered by the doctor.	■ Right time—when the specimen is to be collected. ■ Right amount—measured exactly for each specimen. ■ Right container—the cup that is correct for each specimen. ■ Right label—filled out properly from the patient's identification bracelet. ■ Right requisition or laboratory slip—lists the kind of laboratory examination or test to be done.	■ Right method—procedure by which you collect the specimen. ■ Right asepsis—washing your hands before and after collecting the specimen. ■ Right attitude—how you approach and speak to the patient.

KEY IDEA

When you are collecting specimens, you must be very accurate in following the procedure and labeling the specimen. You have to collect the specimen at the exact time that is indicated.

Asepsis in Specimen Collection

asepsis Free of disease-causing organisms

As you learned from the chapter on infection control, **asepsis** means free of disease-causing organisms. When collecting specimens, it is very important to use good asepsis technique. You must wash your hands very carefully before and after collecting each specimen to prevent spreading bacteria (Figure 23–2◆).

medical asepsis Special practices and procedures for preventing the conditions that allow disease-producing bacteria to live, multiply, and spread

Medical asepsis means preventing the conditions that allow disease-producing bacteria to live, multiply, and spread. As a nursing assistant, you will share the responsibility for preventing the spread of disease and infection by using aseptic technique.

KEY IDEA

Remember especially to wash your hands before and after collecting specimens.

AGE-SPECIFIC CONSIDERATIONS

Specimen Collection

Give very easy-to-follow directions and explanations to young children or any older adult who has difficulty remembering steps to follow. It may be necessary to stay with them and talk them through the steps to obtain the desired specimen.

Teenagers and many adults are uncomfortable or embarrassed when giving urine or stool specimens. Respect their privacy when requesting or receiving the specimen from them, especially if this occurs in an outpatient office or area where other patients may overhear you.

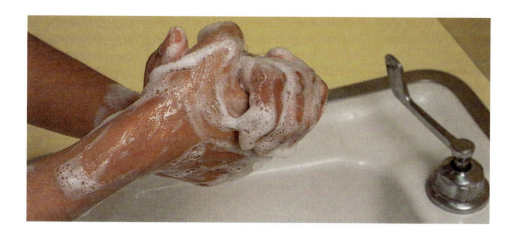

 # Urine Specimens

Urine specimens are collected at different times for different reasons. For example, urine specimens may be ordered as part of a series of tests required at the time of admission or before surgery. In addition to the routine urine specimen collection, there are the midstream, clean-catch, and the 24-hour specimen collections. Procedures for each type of specimen collection and for straining urine follow.

Routine Urine Specimen

The usual single urine specimen collected is called the routine urine specimen. This is the specimen that is taken routinely on admission, daily, or preoperatively by the nursing assistant and sent to the laboratory. Urine may be examined for blood or bacteria (urinary tract infection).

COLLECTING A ROUTINE URINE SPECIMEN	PROCEDURE	OBRA

RATIONALE: Urine samples are collected to test for bacteria, infection, drug screens, sugar, or ketones.

PREPARATION

1. Assemble your equipment:

   a. Patient's bedpan and cover, or urinal, or specipan

   b. Graduate used for measuring output

   c. Urine specimen container and lid

   d. Label, if your institution's procedure is not to write on the lid

   e. Laboratory requisition or request slip, which should be filled out by the head nurse or team leader.

   f. Disposable gloves

2. Identify the patient by checking the identification bracelet.

3. Tell the patient a urine specimen is needed.

4. Wash your hands.

5. Prepare the label by copying all necessary information from the patient's identification bracelet or using the addressograph. Record the time and date.

STEPS

6. Provide privacy for the patient.

7. Explain the procedure to the patient and if he is able, have the patient collect the specimen himself.

8. Put on gloves prior to handling the bedpan or urinal.

9. Have the patient urinate into a clean bedpan, urinal, or specipan, or directly into a specimen cup.

10. Ask the patient not to put toilet tissue into the bedpan or specipan,

PROCEDURE *(continued)*

but to use the plastic-lined waste-basket temporarily. You will then discard the tissue in the toilet or hopper.

11. Take the bedpan or urinal to the patient's bathroom or to the dirty utility room.

12. Pour the urine into a *clean graduated container* that is used for that patient only.

13. If the patient is on output, note the amount of the urine and record it on the intake and output sheet.

14. Pour urine from the graduate into a specimen container and fill it three-fourths full, if possible (Figure 23–3a◆).

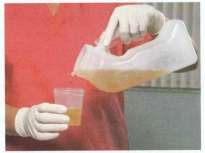

FIGURE 23–3a ◆
Pour urine from the clean graduated container into the specimen container

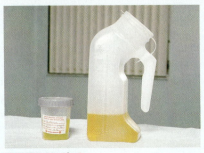

FIGURE 23–3b ◆
Place the correct label on the container with the correct patient name

15. Put the lid on the specimen container. Place the correct label on the container for the correct patient (Figure 23–3b◆). Place specimen in a plastic bag if this is the practice in your institution.

16. Pour the leftover urine into the toilet or hopper.

17. Clean and rinse out the graduate. Put it in its proper place in the patient's bathroom.

18. Clean the bedpan or urinal and put it in its proper place.

19. Dispose of gloves and wash your hands.

FOLLOW-UP

20. Make the patient comfortable and replace the call light. (If patient collected the specimen, allow him to wash his hands.)

21. Lower the bed to a position of safety.

22. Raise the side rails when ordered or appropriate for patient safety.

23. Send or take the labeled specimen container to the laboratory with a requisition or laboratory request slip.

24. Report to your immediate supervisor:

   ■ That a routine urine specimen has been obtained.

   ■ That the specimen has been sent to the laboratory.

   ■ The date and time of collection.

   ■ Your observations of anything unusual.

CHARTING EXAMPLE: 12/12/04 8pm Urine sample obtained from Mr. Chang and sent to lab for analysis as ordered. He is resting comfortably in bed. S. Fowler, CNA

COLLECTING A ROUTINE URINE SPECIMEN FROM AN INFANT

RATIONALE: Specimen collectors are applied on infants when needed to collect urine samples.

PROCEDURE

PREPARATION

1. Assemble your equipment on the bedside table:

   a. Urine specimen bottle or container

   b. Plastic disposable urine collector

   c. Label, if your institution's procedure is not to write on the lid

   d. Laboratory request slip, which should be filled out by the head nurse, or team leader.

   e. Disposable gloves

2. Wash your hands.

3. Identify the patient by checking the identification bracelet.

4. Ask all visitors except parents or guardian to step out of the room.

PROCEDURE (continued)

STEPS

5. Tell the parents or guardian and the patient that you want to collect a urine specimen. (Children who are not yet toilet trained can understand language and are more likely to cooperate if told.)

6. Pull the curtains around the bed (even a 2-year-old may be shy about having his pants pulled down in front of the strangers who may be visiting the child in the next bed).

7. Put on disposable gloves.

8. Take off the child's diaper.

9. Make sure the child's skin is clean and dry in the **genital** area. This is where you are going to apply the urine collector, which is a small plastic bag.

10. Remove the outside piece that surrounds the opening of the plastic urine collector. This leaves a sticky area, which is placed around the baby boy's penis or the baby girl's vulva (Figure 23–4◆). Do not cover the baby's rectum.

11. Put the child's diaper on as usual.

12. Dispose of gloves and wash your hands.

13. Return and check every half hour to see if the infant has voided. You cannot feel the diaper to find out. You must put on gloves, open the diaper, and look at the urine collector.

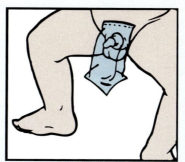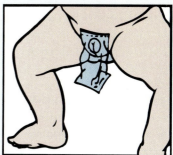

FIGURE 23–4 ◆

Placement of urine specimen collectors on boy and girl infants

14. When the infant has voided, carefully remove the plastic urine collector. It comes off easily. Wash off any sticky residue, rinse, and pat dry.

15. Replace the child's diaper.

16. Put the specimen in the specimen container and cover it immediately.

17. Label the container properly by checking the patient's identification bracelet.

18. Dispose of gloves and wash your hands.

19. The labeled specimen container must be sent or taken to the laboratory with the requisition or laboratory request slip.

FOLLOW-UP

20. Make the baby comfortable.

21. Lower the crib to a position of safety.

22. Pull the curtains back to the open position.

23. Raise the crib side rails to assure patient safety.

24. Report to your immediate supervisor:

   ■ That a routine urine specimen has been obtained.

   ■ That the specimen has been sent to the laboratory.

   ■ The date and time of collection.

   ■ Your observations of anything unusual.

CHARTING EXAMPLE: 12/12/04 8pm Urine sample obtained from Baby Channel and sent to lab for analysis as ordered. C. Taylor, CNA

genital Refers to the external reproductive organs

Midstream, Clean-Catch Urine Specimen

A special method is used to collect a patient's urine when the specimen must be free from contamination. This special kind of specimen is called a midstream, clean-catch urine specimen. In some health care facilities, a disposable midstream, clean-catch package can be obtained from the central supply room. All the equipment and supplies necessary for this specimen are in the kit.

    Midstream means catching the urine specimen between the time the patient begins to void and the time he stops. **Clean catch** means the urine is not contaminated by anything outside the patient's body. The procedure requires careful washing of the genital area.

midstream Catching the urine specimen between the time the patient begins to void and the time he stops

clean catch Means the urine for this specimen is not contaminated by anything outside the patient's body

COLLECTING A MIDSTREAM CLEAN-CATCH URINE SPECIMEN

PROCEDURE   OBRA

RATIONALE: Clean-catch urine samples are collected after cleansing the perineal area or penis to remove external bacteria prior to obtaining the urine sample to test.

PREPARATION

1. Assemble your equipment:

   a. Obtain a requisition slip from your supervisor for a disposable collection kit for this specimen, or go to the CSR exchange cart, if used in your institution, and get the kit. If your institution does not use disposable equipment, CSR will supply the cotton balls and solution to be used for the cleansing process according to your institution's policy.

   b. Label and container

   c. Disposable gloves

   d. Laboratory request slip, which should be filled out by the nurse, team leader, or ward clerk

   e. Patient's bedpan or urinal, if the patient is unable to go to the bathroom

2. Identify the patient by checking the identification bracelet.

3. Tell the patient you need a midstream, clean-catch urine specimen.

4. Wash your hands.

5. Provide privacy for the patient.

STEPS

6. Explain the procedure. If the patient is able, he may collect this specimen on his own in his bathroom.

7. If the patient is not able to collect the specimen himself, help him with the procedure.

8. Open the disposable kit.

9. Remove the towelettes and the urine specimen container from the kit.

10. For female patients:

    a. Put on the disposable gloves.

    b. Use all three towelettes to clean the perineal area.

    c. Separate the folds of the labia (lips) and wipe with one towelette from the front to the back (anterior to posterior) on one side. Then throw away the towelette.

    d. Wipe the other side with a second towelette, again from front to back. Discard the towelette.

    e. Wipe down the middle from front to back, using the third towelette, and discard it.

11. For male patients:

    a. Put on the disposable gloves.

    b. If the patient is not circumcised, pull the foreskin back (retract foreskin) on the penis to clean, and hold it back during urination.

    c. Use a circular motion to clean the head of the penis. Discard each towelette after each use.

12. Explain to the patient that he is to start to urinate into the bedpan, urinal, or toilet. After the flow of urine has started, he is to stop urinating. The specimen container is then placed under the patient and he is to start urinating again, directly into the urine specimen container. After obtaining the specimen, remove the container before the flow of urine stops. This procedure catches the urine that is passed in the middle of the void. If the patient cannot stop urinating, once having started, move the container into the stream of urine to collect the middle of the stream specimen directly into the urine specimen container.

13. If a funnel type of container is used, remove the funnel and discard it.

14. Cover the urine container immediately with the lid from the kit. Be careful not to touch the inside of the container or the inside of the lid.

15. Label the container right away. Copy all needed information from the patient's identification bracelet. Record the date and time of collection.

16. Clean the bedpan or urinal. Put it in its proper place.

17. Discard all used disposable equipment.

18. Dispose of gloves and wash your hands.

FOLLOW-UP

19. Make the patient comfortable and replace the call light.

20. Lower the bed to a position of safety.

21. Raise the side rails when ordered or appropriate for patient safety.

22. The labeled specimen container must be sent or taken to the laboratory with a requisition or laboratory request slip, which is usually filled out by the head nurse, team leader, or ward clerk.

23. Report to your immediate supervisor:

    ■ That a midstream, clean-catch urine specimen has been obtained.

    ■ That it has been sent or taken to the laboratory.

    ■ The date and time of collection.

    ■ Your observations of anything unusual.

CHARTING EXAMPLE: 12/12/04 9pm Clean–catch urine sample obtained from Mr. Chang and sent to lab for analysis as ordered. He is resting comfortably in bed. S. Fowler, CNA

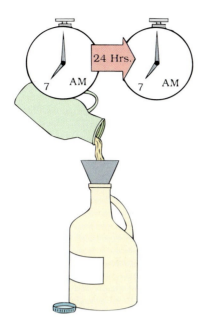

FIGURE 23–5 ◆
Write down the 24-hour period in which the urine is collected

KEY IDEA

Clean catch means the urine is not contaminated by anything outside the patient's body. The procedure requires careful washing of the genital area.

24-Hour Urine Specimen

A 24-hour urine specimen is a collection of all urine voided by a patient over a 24-hour period. All the urine is collected for 24 hours (Figure 23–5◆). An example would be to measure the kidney functioning of a diabetic patient.

When you are to obtain a 24-hour urine specimen, it is necessary to ask the patient to void and discard the first voided urine in the morning. This is because this urine has remained in the bladder an unknown length of time. The test should begin with the bladder empty. For the next 24 hours, save all the urine voided by the patient. On the following day at the same time, ask the patient to void and add this specimen to the previous collection. In this way the doctor can be sure that all the urine for the test came from the urinary bladder during the 24 hours of the test period.

COLLECTING A 24-HOUR URINE SPECIMEN	PROCEDURE	OBRA

RATIONALE: 24-hour urine samples are collected to measure kidney functioning over a 24-hour period.

PREPARATION

1. Assemble your equipment:

   a. Large container, usually a 1-gallon plastic disposable bottle

   b. Funnel, if the neck of the bottle is small

   c. Graduate, used for measuring output, if the patient is on intake and output

   d. Patient's bedpan, urinal, or specipan

   e. Label for the container

   f. Laboratory request slip, which should be filled out by the nurse, or team leader.

   g. Sign, to be placed over or on the patient's bed and in the patient's bathroom, to indicate

PROCEDURE *(continued)*

that a 24-hour urine specimen is being collected

h. Disposable gloves

2. Identify the patient by checking the identification bracelet.

STEPS

3. Tell the patient that a 24-hour urine specimen is needed.

4. Explain the procedure. Tell the patient you will be placing the large container in her bathroom.

5. Wash your hands.

6. Fill in the label for the large container. Copy all needed information from the patient's identification bracelet. Record the date and time of the first collection. Attach the label to the urine specimen container (the large, 1-gallon, plastic disposable bottle). Place the container in the patient's bathroom. In many institutions specimens are refrigerated or kept on ice to control odor and the growth of bacteria.

7. Post the sign over or on the patient's bed and in the patient's bathroom. This is so all personnel will be aware that a 24-hour specimen is being collected.

8. Provide privacy each time the patient voids if she uses a bedpan or urinal at bedside rather than a specipan or urinal in the bathroom. Ask the patient to avoid placing tissue in the bedpan with the specimen, as tissue absorbs urine needed for testing. Provide the patient with a plastic-lined

wastepaper basket to temporarily dispose of the toilet tissue. Then discard it in the toilet or hopper.

9. If the patient is on intake and output, measure all the urine each time the patient voids. Write the amount on the intake and output sheet.

10. When the collection starts, have the patient void. Throw away (discard) this first amount of urine. This is to be sure that the bladder is completely empty. This first voiding should not be included in the specimen. This is usually done in early A.M. per institutional policy. The test will continue until the same time the next day.

11. You may be instructed to refrigerate the urine or put it on ice. If so, fill a large bucket with ice cubes. Keep the large urine container in the ice in the patient's bathroom. All nursing assistants caring for this patient for the next 24 hours will be responsible for keeping the bucket filled with ice.

12. For the next 24 hours, save all urine voided by the patient. Pour the urine from each voiding into the large container.

13. At the end of the 24-hour period, have the patient void at the same time the test was started the day before. Add this to the collection of urine in the large container. This will be the last time you will collect the urine for this test.

14. The large labeled container with the 24-hour collection of urine is taken to the laboratory with a requisition or laboratory request slip that is made out by the head nurse, or team leader.

15. Clean the equipment and put it in its proper place. Discard disposable equipment.

16. Remove the 24-hour specimen sign from the patient's bed.

FOLLOW-UP

17. Make the patient comfortable and replace the call light.

18. Lower the bed to a position of safety.

19. Raise the side rails when ordered or appropriate for patient safety.

20. Wash your hands.

21. Report to your immediate supervisor:

- That a 24-hour urine specimen has been obtained.

- That the specimen has been sent to the laboratory.

- The date and time of collection.

- Your observations of anything unusual.

CHARTING EXAMPLE: 12/12/04 7am 24-hour urine sample collected from Mr. Chang. Jug labeled and sent to lab for analysis as ordered. M. White, CNA

Straining the Urine

The urine is strained to determine if a patient has passed stones (calculi) or other matter from the kidneys. The doctor may order that all urine passed by the patient is to be strained.

The labeled specimen container must be taken to the laboratory with a requisition or laboratory request slip at the nurse's request.

PROCEDURE

STRAINING THE URINE

OBRA

RATIONALE: Urine samples are collected and strained to determine if a patient has passed a kidney stone or calculi.

PREPARATION

1. Assemble your equipment in the patient's bathroom:

   a. Disposable paper strainers or gauze squares

   b. Specimen container with cover or a small plastic bag to be used as a specimen container

   c. Label, if your institution's procedure is not to write on the cover

   d. Patient's bedpan and cover, urinal, or specipan

   e. Laboratory request slip, which should be filled out by the nurse, or team leader.

   f. Sign to be placed over or on the patient's bed indicating that all urine must be strained

   g. Disposable gloves

2. Identify the patient by checking the identification bracelet.

STEPS

3. Tell the patient that each time she urinates it must be into a urinal, bedpan, or specipan, as all urine must be strained. Caution the patient not to put any tissue into the container. Provide the patient with a plastic-lined wastepaper basket to temporarily dispose of the toilet tissue. Then discard it in the toilet or hopper.

4. Provide privacy whenever the patient voids.

5. Wash your hands and put on gloves.

6. When the patient voids, take the bedpan or urinal to the patient's bathroom. Pour the urine through the strainer or gauze into the measuring container (Figure 23–6◆).

7. If any particles show up on the gauze or the paper strainer, place the gauze or paper strainer with particles in a plastic bag or specimen container. Do not attempt to remove the particles because they may be lost or damaged.

8. Label the specimen container immediately. Copy all needed information from the patient's

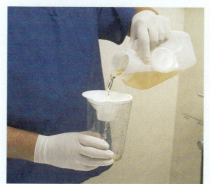

FIGURE 23–6 ◆
Pour urine through gauze or strainer into measuring container

identification bracelet. Record the date and time of collection.

9. Measure the amount of the voiding and record it on the intake and output sheet, if the patient is on intake and output.

10. Discard the urine.

11. Clean and rinse the bedpan and graduate and put them in their proper places.

12. Dispose of gloves and wash your hands.

FOLLOW-UP

13. Make the patient comfortable and replace the call light.

14. Lower the bed to a position of safety.

15. Raise the side rails when ordered or appropriate for patient safety.

16. Report at once to your immediate supervisor:

    ■ That, in straining the urine, particles were obtained.

    ■ That a specimen was collected.

    ■ The date and time of collection.

    ■ Your observations of anything unusual.

CHARTING EXAMPLE: 12/12/04 7am Urine sample collected from Mr. Sullivan and strained as ordered. No particles were seen or collected. He continues to be experiencing a great deal of pain even after receiving pain medication. M. White, CNA

Sputum Specimen

Sputum is a substance collected from a patient's lungs that contains saliva, mucus, and sometimes pus or blood. It is thicker than ordinary **saliva** (spit). Most of it is coughed up from the lungs and bronchial tubes. In some health care facilities, this procedure is carried out by the Respiratory Therapy Department (Pulmonary Medicine). Sputum specimens are studied to determine if a patient has pneumonia or tuberculosis.

Usually, early morning is the best time to obtain this specimen.

sputum Waste material coughed up from the lungs or trachea

saliva The secretion of the salivary glands into the mouth; saliva moistens food and helps in swallowing

PROCEDURE

COLLECTING A SPUTUM SPECIMEN

RATIONALE: Sputum samples are collected to test for evidence of infection, bacteria, or to diagnose pulmonary diseases such as TB or pneumonia.

PREPARATION

1. Assemble your equipment:

   a. Sputum container with cover and tissues

   b. Label, if your institution's procedure is not to write on the cover

   c. Laboratory request slip, which should be filled out by the nurse, or team leader.

   d. Disposable gloves

2. Identify the patient by checking the identification bracelet.

STEPS

3. Tell the patient that a sputum specimen is needed.

4. Wash your hands and put on gloves.

5. If the patient has eaten recently, have her rinse out her mouth with water. If she wants to have oral hygiene at this time, help her as necessary.

6. Give the patient a sputum container (Figure 23–7a ◆). Ask her to take three consecutive deep breaths and on the third exhalation to cough deep from within the lungs to bring up the thick sputum. Explain that saliva (spit) and nose secretions are not adequate for this test.

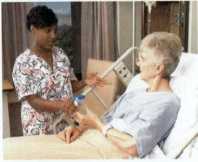

FIGURE 23–7a ◆
Tell patient to cough deep within the lungs to bring up sputum for the specimen

7. The patient may have to cough several times to bring up enough sputum for the specimen. One to two tablespoons is usually the required amount (Figure 23–7b ◆).

8. Cover the container immediately. Be careful not to touch the inside of either the container or the cover to avoid contamination.

9. Label the container right away. Copy all needed information from the patient's identification bracelet. Record the time of collection and the date.

10. The labeled specimen container must be sent or taken immediately to the laboratory with a requisition or laboratory request slip. This should be filled out by the nurse or ward clerk. The test must be done in the laboratory before the sputum begins to dry.

FOLLOW-UP

11. Make the patient comfortable and replace the call light.

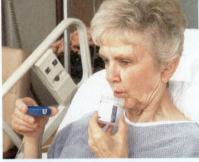

FIGURE 23–7b ◆
Patient brings up sputum for the specimen

12. Lower the bed to a position of safety.

13. Raise the side rails when ordered or appropriate for patient safety.

14. Dispose of gloves and wash your hands.

15. Report at once to your immediate supervisor:

    ■ That a sputum specimen has been obtained.

    ■ The color, amount, odor, and consistency of the specimen.

    ■ That the specimen has been sent to the laboratory.

    ■ The date and time of collection.

    ■ How the patient tolerated the procedure.

    ■ Your observations of anything unusual.

CHARTING EXAMPLE: 12/12/04
8am Sputum sample obtained from Ms. Smoke. Sample labeled and sent to lab as ordered. D. Free, CNA

---

feces Solid waste material discharged from the body through the rectum and anus; other names include stool, excreta, excrement, bowel movement, and fecal matter

stool See *feces*

Stool Specimen

Feces, **stool**, b.m., bowel movement, and fecal matter all mean the same thing—the solid waste from a patient's body. The doctor sometimes orders a stool specimen to help in the diagnosis of a patient's illness where blood or parasites are present in the patient's stool.

Sometimes a warm specimen is ordered. This means that the specimen must be tested in the laboratory while the specimen is still warm from the patient's body. You will be told whether the specimen is to be warm.

In some institutions, you may be requested to prepare Hemoccult slides. The correct procedure follows.

PROCEDURE

COLLECTING A STOOL SPECIMEN

OBRA

RATIONALE: Stool specimens or samples are collected to determine if parasites or blood are present in the stool.

PREPARATION

1. Assemble your equipment (Figure 23–8◆):

   a. Patient's bedpan and cover

   b. Stool specimen container

   c. Wooden tongue depressor

   d. Label, if your institution's procedure is not to write on the cover

   e. Laboratory request slip, which should be filled out by the nurse, or team leader.

   f. Plastic bag for warm specimen, if used by your institution

   g. Disposable gloves

2. Identify the patient by checking the identification bracelet.

3. Wash your hands.

STEPS

4. Tell the patient that a stool specimen is needed. Explain that whenever he can move his bowels he is to call you so the specimen can be collected.

5. Provide privacy for the patient.

6. Have the patient move his bowels into the bedpan or into a specipan placed in the back half of the toilet.

7. Ask the patient *not to urinate into the bedpan* and not to put toilet tissue in the bedpan. Provide the patient

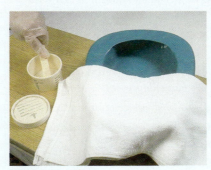

FIGURE 23–8 ◆
Equipment for collecting stool specimen

with a plastic-lined wastepaper basket to temporarily dispose of the toilet tissue. Then discard it in the toilet or hopper.

8. Prepare the label immediately by copying all needed information from the patient's identification bracelet. Record the time of collection and the date.

9. Put on gloves.

10. After the patient has had a bowel movement, take the covered bedpan to the patient's bathroom or to the dirty utility room.

11. Using the wooden tongue depressor, take about 1 to 2 tablespoons of feces from different areas of the stool in the bedpan and place them in the stool specimen container. Label the specimen container.

12. Cover the container immediately. Be careful not to touch the inside of either the container or the cover to avoid contamination.

13. Wrap the tongue depressor in a paper towel and discard it.

14. Empty the remaining feces into the toilet or hopper.

15. Clean the bedpan and return it to its proper place.

16. Dispose of gloves and wash your hands.

17. If the nurse has told you this is a warm specimen, it must be taken to the laboratory for examination while it is still warm from the patient's body. Place the stool specimen container, fully labeled, in the plastic bag (if used by your institution). Attach the laboratory request slip to the bag. Carry it immediately to the laboratory.

FOLLOW-UP

18. Make the patient comfortable and replace the call light.

19. Lower the bed to a position of safety.

20. Raise the side rails when ordered or appropriate for patient safety.

21. Wash your hands.

22. Report at once to your immediate supervisor:

    ■ That a stool specimen has been obtained.

    ■ That the specimen has been sent to the laboratory.

    ■ The date and time of collection.

    ■ Your observations of anything unusual.

CHARTING EXAMPLE: 12/12/04
8am Stool sample obtained from Mr. Black. Sample labeled and sent to lab for analysis as ordered.
N. Bugs, CNA

PREPARING A HEMOCCULT SLIDE

PROCEDURE

RATIONALE: Stool specimens are collected and examined to determine if blood is present in the stool.

Note: Some states require that Hemoccult slides be collected by a nurse.

STEPS

1. Ask the patient to move her bowels into a bedpan or specipan, whenever this is possible.

2. Wash your hands and put on gloves.

3. Check the patient's identification bracelet.

4. Label the outside of the Hemoccult slide with the patient's name, address, hospital number, and the date this specimen is collected.

5. Collect a small amount of stool on a tongue depressor.

6. Apply small amount in box A on Hemoccult slide.

7. Open side 1.

8. From a different area of the stool, collect a small amount of stool on tongue depressor.

9. Apply small amount in box B.

10. Close cover of slide card and secure.

11. Check information with patient identification bracelet.

12. Dispose of gloves and wash your hands.

FOLLOW-UP

13. Send to the laboratory or give collected sample to the nurse if it is your institution's policy to check Hemoccult specimens on the unit.

14. Report to your immediate supervisor:

   ■ That the Hemoccult specimen has been collected.

   ■ The time and date it was collected.

   ■ Your observations of anything unusual.

CHARTING EXAMPLE: 12/15/04 8am Stool sample obtained from Mr. Black. Sample sent to lab for testing. Y. Reed, CNA

◼ SUMMARY

In collecting specimens for testing, it is important to remember to always explain to the patient what you are going to do before proceeding with the collection. This step helps to gain the patient's confidence and elicits cooperation in the procedure. Standard Precautions must be maintained while collecting specimens. Care must be taken to be accurate in all information related to obtaining and labeling the required specimens.

NOTES

CHAPTER REVIEW

FILL IN THE BLANK Read each sentence and fill in the blank line with a word that completes the sentence.

1. When you ask a patient to cough up matter from the lungs, trachea, or bronchial tubes and spit it out, you are asking them to _____.

2. By testing _____, physicians can get information to assist them in making a diagnosis and deciding on care for the patient.

3. When collecting specimens, you need to be very _____.

4. Always wear _____ when collecting a specimen.

5. After collecting the specimen, make sure you _____ it, to avoid mixups.

MULTIPLE CHOICE Choose the best answer for each question or statement.

1. All of the following are important when collecting specimens *except*
   a. identifying the correct patient.
   b. accurately collecting the specimen.
   c. placing the correct label on the specimen.
   d. placing the specimens in alphabetical order.

2. Inaccurate or mislabeled specimens can lead to
   a. mistakes in diagnosis.
   b. delayed or unnecessary treatment.
   c. needing to repeat the procedure.
   d. All of the above.

3. Using medical asepsis to collect specimens includes
   a. washing your hands before collecting the specimen.
   b. wearing gloves.
   c. sterilizing the specimen.
   d. washing your hands after collecting the specimen.

4. A clean-catch urine specimen means that the urine has
   a. not been contaminated by anything outside the patient's body.
   b. been obtained without dropping the sample.
   c. been collected while the patient was wearing gloves.
   d. been obtained with a catheter.

5. When collecting a 24-hour urine, do all of the following *except*
   a. throw out the first urine when collection begins.
   b. provide the patient with two times as much fluid to drink.
   c. post a sign indicating the patient is on a 24-hour urine collection.
   d. correctly label and date the container(s).

TIME-OUT

TIPS FOR TAKING CARE OF YOURSELF

To prioritize means to rank in order of importance. If you are told to do several tasks by two different superiors, you may feel unsure about which tasks have the highest priority. Explain the situation to each superior and ask for help in establishing which tasks have first priority.

THE NURSING ASSISTANT IN ACTION

You need to obtain a patient's urine sample to use in an analysis for illegal drug use. Your facility requires that you watch the patient while the specimen is voided. The patient offers you a bag with a bottle of urine in it. He tells you, "I brought you in a sample that you can test. Just use that one. How do you expect me to pee with you standing there watching me?"

What Is Your Response/Action?

CRITICAL THINKING

CUSTOMER SERVICE If you and a coworker are caring for a patient together, avoid personal conversations and try to include the patient in anything you do talk about. Do not discuss other staff members or patient problems with your patient. Doing so would leave the impression you would likely share information about them or their illness with others who do not need to know the details of their personal situation or business. Patients need to be able to trust you will be discreet.

CULTURAL CONSIDERATIONS Patients have a right to privacy. Remember to knock before entering their room or bathroom if the door is closed. Some patients may not understand exactly what you want them to do when you are trying to obtain specimens from them. Have an interpreter explain or use pictures if you see the patient does not understand your directions. Doing so may help you avoid having to repeat procedures or unnecessarily frustrate the patient.

COOPERATION WITHIN THE TEAM If a visitor or staff from another department appears to be having trouble finding what he needs, approach him and ask if you can be of assistance. If someone calling your unit has the wrong number, transfer the call to the operator or offer to check for the correct number if you have a phone directory nearby. Your attempt to help, rather than ignore his need, will demonstrate cooperation and convey your concern.

EXPLORE MediaLink

Additional interactive resources for this chapter can be found on the Companion Website at www.prenhall.com/wolgin. Click on Chapter 23 and "Begin" to select the activities for this chapter.

For chapter-related NCLEX-style questions and an audio glossary, access the accompanying CD-ROM in this book.

Video:

- Risk Management; Specimen Collection—Collecting a Urine Specimen for Culture

24 The Endocrine System and Related Care of Diabetics

OBJECTIVES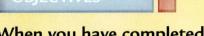

When you have completed this chapter, you will be able to:

- Label a diagram of the body showing the endocrine glands.
- Describe the function(s) of each gland.
- List the common diseases and disorders of the endocrine system.
- Recognize the signs and symptoms of diabetes mellitus, insulin shock, and diabetic coma.
- Teach the patient with diabetes how to avoid pressure points and skin problems.
- Test a patient's blood glucose level via a finger stick using a blood glucose meter.

MediaLink

www.prenhall.com/wolgin

Use the address above to access the free, interactive Companion Website created for this textbook. Get hints, instant feedback, and textbook references to chapter-related NCLEX-style questions. Link to other interesting sites.

AUDIO GLOSSARY:

Use the Companion Website, or the CD-ROM disk enclosed with your textbook, to hear the pronunciation of key terms in the chapter.

KEY TERMS

carbohydrate
diabetes mellitus
diabetic coma
endocrine glands
endocrine system
exocrine glands
gland
glucose
hormones
hyperglycemia
hypoglycemia
insulin
insulin shock
metabolism
secrete

The body depends on a well-functioning endocrine system for good health and the ability to carry out normal daily activities. When the glands of the endocrine system secrete the proper type and amount of hormones, the other systems of the body also function well. In contrast, when hormones are secreted in the wrong amount, the result is illness, of which the most common is diabetes. This chapter describes how the endocrine system works and problems that can arise from improper endocrine functioning. In particular, it addresses the nursing assistant's role in providing care to patients with diabetes.

Anatomy and Physiology of the Endocrine System

endocrine system System composed of endocrine glands; regulates body function by secreting hormones

gland An organ that is able to manufacture and discharge a chemical that will be used elsewhere in the body

secrete Produce and release into the body; glands secrete hormones

hormones Protein substances secreted by endocrine glands directly into the blood to stimulate increased activity

endocrine glands Ductless glands that produce hormones and secrete them directly into the blood or lymph

exocrine glands Glands that produce hormones and secrete them either directly or through a duct to epithelial tissue, such as a body cavity or the skin surface

The **endocrine system** consists of several **glands** that **secrete** (produce and release) liquids called **hormones**. Through these hormones, the endocrine system helps the nervous system organize and direct the activities of the body. Figure 24–1◆ shows the locations of the **endocrine glands**. The endocrine glands secrete hormones directly into the bloodstream. In contrast, **exocrine glands**, such as the salivary glands, deliver their products through ducts into a body cavity or to the skin surface, as from sweat glands.

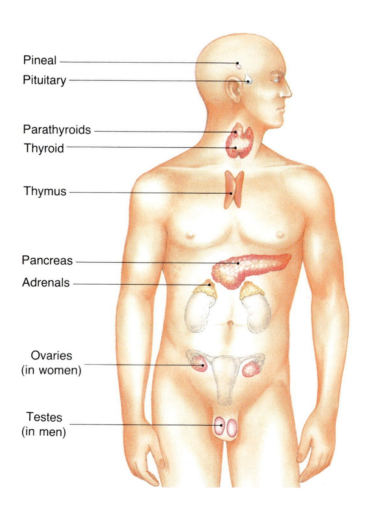

Pineal
Pituitary

Parathyroids
Thyroid

Thymus

Pancreas
Adrenals

Ovaries
(in women)

Testes
(in men)

FIGURE 24–1 ◆

Endocrine glands

The pituitary gland is the master gland. Its hormones directly affect the other endocrine glands, stimulating them to produce their hormones. Hormones from the anterior and posterior portions of the pituitary gland regulate the metabolism of the body's billions of cells. The anterior portion manufactures and releases seven hormones. The pituitary hormones are especially important in reproduction and in all functions leading to puberty (the time at which a child takes on the physical characteristics of an adult man or woman). Hormones from the pituitary gland regulate the menstrual cycle in the female and sperm production in the male. Without these hormones, humans would be unable to reproduce.

The pituitary gland and its hormones are under the direct control of the hypothalamus, a tiny piece of tissue lying near the base of the brain. This structure seems to be the link between our thinking, our emotions, and our body functions.

The thyroid gland produces a hormone that regulates growth and general metabolism. The hormones secreted by the thyroid gland influence a person's energy level, skeletal growth, sexual development, skin texture, and hair luster.

The thymus gets smaller after puberty, but it plays an important part in the body's immune system. The immune system prevents us from getting many diseases.

The parathyroids are located within the capsule of the thyroid. They produce a hormone that, along with one of the hormones in the thyroid gland, regulates the level of calcium and potassium in the blood. Calcium is important for many functions of the body, such as muscle contraction and conduction of nerve impulses.

The pancreas is both an endocrine gland and an exocrine gland (a gland that has a duct). Its endocrine portion produces the hormone insulin. **Insulin** regulates the sugar content of the blood. If the body does not have enough insulin, the person develops hyperglycemia (high blood sugar) and becomes diabetic. The diabetic patient must be treated by reducing her carbohydrate or sugar intake and by regulating the balance between insulin and **glucose** (blood sugar).

The adrenal glands lie on top of the kidneys. They are very important in helping the body adapt to stress conditions by stimulating the autonomic nervous system. In an emergency, they produce adrenalin, which enables the body to quickly produce great amounts of energy.

In the female, the ovaries are responsible for secreting the hormones estrogen and progesterone. The rise and fall of the levels of these hormones in the blood determine the menstrual cycle. The hormones are also important in causing an ovum, or egg, to develop and in maintaining a pregnancy.

In the male, the testes produce testosterone, the primary sex hormone of the male. Testosterone is responsible for the masculine physical characteristics and causes the production of sperm.

insulin Hormone that regulates the sugar content of the blood

glucose A sugar formed during metabolism of carbohydrates; blood sugar

The Endocrine System and the Normal Aging Process

With age, some endocrine glands decrease their production of hormones. For example, secretion of thyroid, parathyroid, and adrenal hormones gradually diminishes. The production of estrogen and progesterone decreases as well.

Some hormones become less effective as the body ages. An example of such a hormone is insulin.

Together, changes in hormone levels and effectiveness decrease the endocrine system's ability to regulate activities of the body. In general, however, few age-related disorders are directly related to problems with the endocrine glands. Disorders of the endocrine system may occur at any age.

Diabetes is one of the most common endocrine diseases. It affects patients of all ages and has a major impact on patient's lives. For children, establish trust by being honest and answering questions truthfully. Use fantasy play or puppets to let children express how they feel. For adolescents, try to allow them options or choices in as many aspects of their care as possible. Take time to explain things, but do not argue. Teens need information as well as emotional support to make good decisions. Adults also need information to help them make lifestyle changes.

Common Diseases and Disorders of the Endocrine System

Diseases and disorders of the endocrine system generally involve production of too much or too little of some hormone. The most common diseases and disorders are as follows:

- *Hypothyroidism:* too little hormone secreted by the thyroid gland
- *Hyperthyroidism:* too much hormone secreted by the thyroid gland
- *Hyperparathyroidism:* overactivity of the parathyroid glands
- *Hypoparathyroidism:* absence of activity of the parathyroid glands
- *Diabetes Mellitus:* abnormality of the insulin secretion of the pancreas, resulting in metabolic abnormalities
- *Cushing's Syndrome:* hyperactivity of the adrenal glands
- *Addison's Disease:* hypo-(less) function of the adrenal glands
- *Hyperpituitarism:* secretion of excessive amounts of growth hormone by the pituitary gland
- *Hypopituitarism:* pituitary insufficiency; secretion of too little hormone by the pituitary gland
- *Pituitary Tumors:* cancer that causes changes in normal growth

Diabetes Mellitus

diabetes mellitus Disorder of carbohydrate metabolism caused by inability to convert sugar into energy because of inadequate production or utilization of insulin

carbohydrate Basic food element used by the body; composed of carbon, hydrogen, and oxygen; includes sugars and starches

metabolism The process through which food elements are converted into energy for use in the human body

The most common disorder arising from problems with the endocrine system is the chronic disease known as **diabetes mellitus**. Diabetes is a disturbance of carbohydrate metabolism. In other words, the body cannot change **carbohydrate** (starches and sugar) into energy and cannot store them, called **metabolism**, because of an imbalance of the hormone insulin.

Obesity and diabetes escalated during 2001. The Centers for Disease Control and Prevention (CDC) reported that obesity climbed from 19.8 percent of American adults to 20.9 percent of American adults between 2000 and 2001, and diagnosed diabetes increased from 7.3 to 7.9 percent during the same year. The increases were evident regardless of sex, age, race, and educational status. CDC said more than 44 million Americans are considered obese, reflecting an increase of 74 percent since 1991. During the same time frame, diabetes increased by 61 percent, with an estimated 17 million people having diabetes in the United States.

There also has been an increase in the number of obese children diagnosed with diabetes. Diets high in carbohydrates and sugar combined with the decrease in children's exercise put them at higher risk to develop Type II diabetes. Changes in diet and increased exercise can eliminate or reduce the need for insulin or various prescription medications used to treat diabetes.

There are two types of diabetes:

- *Insulin-dependent diabetes mellitus (IDDM), also known as Type I or juvenile-onset diabetes:* The body produces little or no insulin, so it must be given by injection.
- *Non–insulin-dependent diabetes mellitus (NIDDM), also known as Type II or adult-onset diabetes:* The body *may* produce a normal amount of insulin but cannot use it. Type II diabetes may be controlled with diet and exercise alone, or the patient may also need oral medication or insulin.

Most diabetics have Type II (NIDDM) diabetes.

Terms Often Used with Diabetes Mellitus

Many of the patients cared for by a nursing assistant have diabetes. Therefore, it is important to recognize terms often used in connection with this condition:

- *FBS:* fasting blood sugar; a type of test to measure the amount of glucose in the patient's blood after the patient has not eaten for a given amount of time
- *GTT:* glucose tolerance test; a type of test that measures the amount of glucose in the patient's blood after the patient has consumed a specified amount of glucose
- **Hypoglycemia:** abnormally low blood sugar
- **Hyperglycemia:** abnormally high blood sugar
- *Gangrene:* necrosis (death) of a body part caused by lack of blood circulating to that part
- *Pancreas:* endocrine gland that produces insulin
- *Islets of Langerhans:* part of the pancreas that produces insulin
- *PPBS:* postprandial blood sugar; a type of test that measures the amount of glucose in the patient's blood after the patient has eaten

hypoglycemia Abnormally low blood sugar

hyperglycemia Abnormally high blood sugar

Signs and Symptoms of Diabetes Mellitus

The ability to recognize the signs and symptoms of diabetes also is very important. Although the nursing assistant does not diagnose illnesses, you can support the health care team by reporting any of the following signs to your supervisor:

- Fatigue, tiredness
- Loss of weight; hunger
- Vaginitis: inflammation of the vagina
- Skin erosions (lesions); sores healing poorly and slowly (a late sign)
- Hyperglycemia
- Glycosuria: sugar in the urine
- Polyuria: frequent and large amounts of urine
- Polydipsia: excessive thirst
- Poor vision: eyesight affected

Signs and Symptoms of Insulin Shock

One of the most common and serious complications related to diabetes is **insulin shock**, also called diabetic shock or insulin reaction. This condition occurs in patients with diabetes when they receive too much insulin, miss a meal, or have too much physical activity.

insulin shock Serious complication related to diabetes; occurs when the diabetic receives too much insulin, misses a meal, or has too much physical activity

Too much glucose leaves the blood, resulting in hypoglycemia (low blood sugar). Insulin shock has a sudden onset. The following signs and symptoms indicate that a patient may be experiencing insulin shock:

- Excessive sweating, perspiration
- Faintness, dizziness, weakness
- Hunger (polyphagia)
- Irritability, personality change, nervousness, anxious
- Numbness of tongue and lips
- Inability to awaken, coma, unconsciousness, stupor
- Headache
- Tremors, trembling
- Blurred or impaired vision
- Upon examination: low blood sugar
- Blood sugar below 70 mg/dL

Signs and Symptoms of Diabetic Coma

diabetic coma A coma (abnormal deep stupor) that can occur in a diabetic patient from lack of insulin

If the diabetic patient does not receive enough insulin to metabolize carbohydrates or when there is increased stress or infection, the patient may experience hyperglycemia (high blood sugar), resulting in **diabetic coma**, also called diabetic acidosis. A diabetic coma may have a gradual onset, but it can be life threatening. Therefore, knowledge of its signs and symptoms is crucial:

- Air hunger, heavy labored breathing, increased respirations
- Loss of appetite
- Nausea and/or vomiting
- Weakness
- Abdominal pain or discomfort
- Generalized aches
- Increased thirst and parched tongue
- Sweet or fruity odor of the breath
- Flushed skin
- Dry skin
- Increased urination
- Dulled senses
- Loss of consciousness
- Upon examination: high blood sugar
- Blood sugar above 250 mg/dL

Caring for the Diabetic Patient:
Reducing Pressure Points

Two conditions related to diabetes make pressure points a particular concern for the diabetic. First, a person with diabetes is more susceptible to arteriosclerosis, which involves narrowing of the arteries. Arteriosclerosis results in less blood flowing to the extremities, especially the legs and feet. Second, changes may occur in the nerves of the feet, causing less nerve sensation, a condition called neuropathy. When a person with diabetes has neuropathy, he is not aware when a pressure point is causing skin irritation. One extreme complication of such skin irritations is gangrene (no blood passes to a toe or to the foot). The body part with gangrene dies and must be surgically amputated.

To avoid skin irritation and its consequences, all patients with diabetes must reduce pressure points. Teaching the following guidelines will help patients do this.

CARE OF THE FEET AND SKIN FOR DIABETICS	GUIDELINES	OBRA

- Avoid standing or lying in one position for a long period of time. Change from sitting to walking or from lying to sitting and walking.
- Never walk barefoot or in stocking feet. Always wear shoes for protection because a cut will have difficulty healing.
- Never cross knees. Never wear rubber or elastic bands for garters, and never

roll stockings or socks. This stops circulation in the lower extremities.
- Bathe every day, washing the feet very well.
- Never use very hot water for a shower or bath, as a burn will not heal readily.
- When drying the body after a shower or bath, do not rub hard; pat dry, especially between the toes.
- Use skin cream to prevent hard, dry skin areas.
- Follow the physician's instructions for cutting toenails.

- Do not use any nonprescription drugs, internally or externally, without the physician's permission.
- Tell every physician, dentist, eye doctor, and podiatrist who examines you that you have diabetes.
- Wear shoes and stockings that fit so that they do not cause pressure points by restricting movement in the toes.
- If you see any open skin, red area, scratched skin, sores, blisters, or any area of skin that looks other than normal, call and report this to your physician.

Testing of Blood Glucose

When a patient has diabetes, certain changes or adjustments in lifestyle are important. Some patients also need to use medication to keep their diabetes under control. The amounts of medication and food a diabetic needs are related to how high or low the blood sugar is. The symptoms listed previously can occur if the blood sugar is not at a desirable level. Testing procedures that can identify high or low blood sugar are therefore key in determining the correct amounts of medication and food.

In hospitals and nursing homes today, the most common method of testing the level of blood sugar is to use a blood glucose meter. In the past, urine testing was used to help monitor the diabetic's glucose levels. (Excess sugar in the blood is excreted in the urine.) However, doctors have found that routine urine testing is less accurate than testing blood samples with a blood glucose meter. Testing the blood reveals high or low blood sugar sooner than waiting until excess sugar has reached the urine.

Self-monitoring of blood glucose using meters can greatly improve the home patient's quality of life. It allows the patient to know whether the patient's diet, exercise, and medication protocol are working. Home testing of blood glucose enables the patient to have some control of the diabetes, rather than feeling that diabetes is controlling the patient's life.

There are many types of meters, each with different features. These meters are available at local pharmacies and medical supply stores. There are many manufacturers of battery-operated blood glucose meters (Figure 24–2◆). One new device allows the diabetic patient to obtain the blood sample from the forearm. This method is less painful than finger sticks. In addition, scientists are currently developing noninvasive methods of monitoring blood glucose. You may encounter patients who wear a watch-like device that measures their blood glucose level. As technology advances and the cost of these devices becomes more affordable, it will be easier for diabetics to maintain awareness of their glucose levels.

FIGURE 24–2 ◆

This Accu Check meter measures the level of glucose in a blood sample

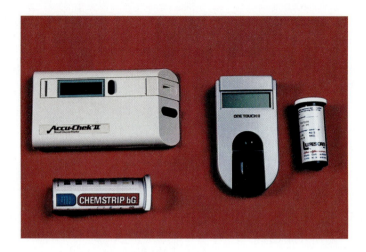

TESTING FOR GLUCOSE USING THE ONE-TOUCH PROFILE DIABETES TRACKING SYSTEM

PROCEDURE

RATIONALE: Measuring glucose levels can help diabetics control their disease.

PREPARATION

1. Wash your hands.

2. Explain to the patient that you are going to test his blood sugar.

3. Make the patient comfortable and wash his hands with soap and water.

4. Assemble your equipment:

   a. One-Touch Profile meter

   b. Test strips

   c. Penlet and lancet

   d. Disposable pipet

   e. Disposable gloves

   f. Bandage

STEPS

5. Match the code on the test strips to the number on the meter. Check the expiration date on the test strips. Discard them if they have expired. The code number may have to be reset. Follow the manufacturer's instructions. (Figure 24–3(a)◆)

6. Remove test strip from container. Close the container. Do not touch the white area of the strip.

7. Press Power and insert the strip into the meter (Figure 24–3(b)◆).

8. Put on disposable gloves.

9. Insert the lancet into the Penlet according to the manufacturer's directions. (Figure 24–3(c)◆).

10. Place the end of the lancet firmly against the side of a fingertip of the patient.

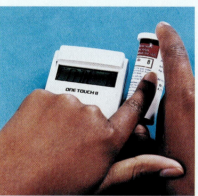

(a)

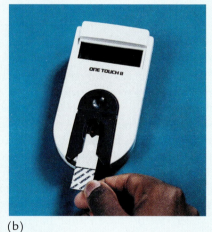

(b)

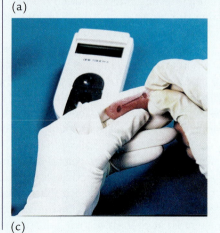

(c)

FIGURE 24–3 ◆

Press power and insert the strip into the meter (Photo Courtesy of Johnson & Johnson)

PROCEDURE *(continued)*

11. Press the button on top of the Penlet.

12. Squeeze the finger gently to obtain a large drop of blood.

13. Using a disposable pipet, slowly draw up the drop of blood and apply the sample to the test strip. This method prevents contamination of the patient and is preferred in a hospital or nursing home setting where several different patients use the same blood glucose meter. An alternative method for individual use (at home, for example) is to apply the blood sample directly to the strip (Figure 24-4◆).

14. Wait a short time for the results to appear on the blood glucose meter (Figure 24-5◆).

15. Apply a bandage to the patient's finger.

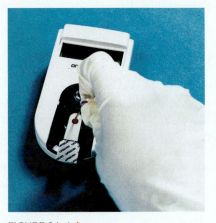

FIGURE 24-4 ◆

Apply the blood sample directly to the strip.

FOLLOW-UP

16. Remove disposable gloves and wash your hands.

17. Record the results. Notify the supervisor if the results are above or below normal.

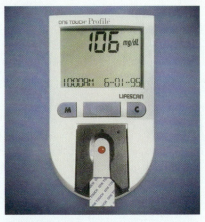

FIGURE 24-5 ◆

The results appear on the blood glucose meter. (Photo courtesy of Johnson & Johnson)

CHARTING EXAMPLE: 12/30/04
11:55am Blood sugar 106
R. Alvarez, CNA

Urine Testing for Acetone

Very rarely, the nursing assistant may be asked to test a patient's urine. A fresh urine sample may be tested with test strips to measure for acetone, which can appear in the urine as a result of abnormal blood glucose levels (Figure 24-6◆). Follow your institution's guidelines.

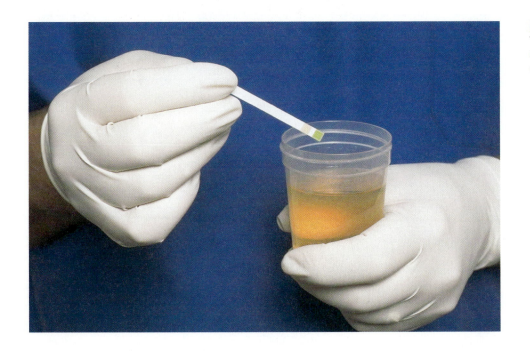

FIGURE 24-6 ◆

Test strips may be used to measure the acetone level in a urine sample

Each bottle of test strips has pictures and instructions for using the specific product. Check the expiration date, and do not use any test strips past that date. Anytime you perform a urine test for acetone, use a fresh urine sample, wash your hands before and after the test, and wear disposable gloves (see Chapter 23).

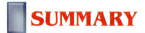

SUMMARY

Understanding how the endocrine system regulates normal body metabolism is important for the caregiver. In particular, a nursing assistant can help correct problems and even save lives by identifying quickly any symptoms that indicate a patient's level of blood sugar is abnormal. The most common method of glucose monitoring for patients is the use of a blood glucose meter. This method can help the patient and the caregiver monitor the patient's blood glucose levels. At-home use of a blood glucose meter by the patient gives more independence and the ability to control daily activities and medication.

NOTES

CHAPTER REVIEW

FILL IN THE BLANK Read each sentence and fill in the blank line with a word that completes the sentence.

1. The hormone that regulates the sugar content of the blood is called _____.

2. The process through which food elements are converted into energy for use in the body is called _____.

3. Abnormally low blood sugar is called _____.

4. Abnormally high blood sugar is called _____.

5. The most common way to test blood glucose is with a _____ _____ _____.

MULTIPLE CHOICE Choose the best answer for each question or statement.

1. The endocrine system consists of several glands that secrete liquids called
   a. hormones.
   b. urine.
   c. insulin.
   d. glucose.

2. The master gland of the endocrine system is the
   a. pancreas.
   b. pituitary.
   c. ovaries.
   d. thyroid.

3. Which of the following is not a disease or disorder of the endocrine system?
   a. Diabetes mellitus
   b. Hyperthyroidism

   c. Crohn's disease
   d. Addison's disease

4. The most common disorder of the endocrine system is
   a. cancer.
   b. hypoglycemia.
   c. impotence.
   d. diabetes mellitus.

5. Insulin shock occurs when the body has
   a. too much insulin.
   b. too little insulin.
   c. too much cholesterol.
   d. too little cholesterol.

TIME-OUT

TIPS FOR TAKING CARE OF YOURSELF

Take responsibility for your own actions. "I made a mistake" are difficult words to say.
Take responsibility for an error and take appropriate steps to correct it.

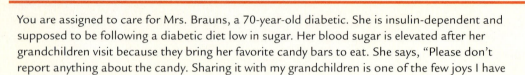

THE NURSING ASSISTANT IN ACTION

You are assigned to care for Mrs. Brauns, a 70-year-old diabetic. She is insulin-dependent and supposed to be following a diabetic diet low in sugar. Her blood sugar is elevated after her grandchildren visit because they bring her favorite candy bars to eat. She says, "Please don't report anything about the candy. Sharing it with my grandchildren is one of the few joys I have since my husband died."

What Is Your Response/Action?

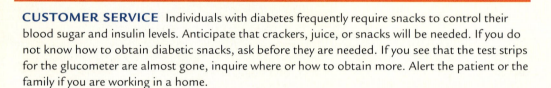

CRITICAL THINKING

CUSTOMER SERVICE Individuals with diabetes frequently require snacks to control their blood sugar and insulin levels. Anticipate that crackers, juice, or snacks will be needed. If you do not know how to obtain diabetic snacks, ask before they are needed. If you see that the test strips for the glucometer are almost gone, inquire where or how to obtain more. Alert the patient or the family if you are working in a home.

CULTURAL CARE Type II or adult-onset diabetes is increasingly seen and diagnosed in obese children. Individuals at highest risk include anyone with a diabetic parent or grandparent. African American, Hispanic, Latino, and American Indian cultures have higher numbers of diabetics.

COOPERATION WITHIN THE TEAM Many special procedures require extra time to perform and should be completed once started. If you will be applying anti-embolism stockings and anticipate that another patient will require your assistance during the time you need to apply the stockings, first attempt to take care of the need in advance. You can ask a coworker to watch for the light while you are busy, but respect that they have patients to care for as well.

EXPLORE MediaLink

Additional interactive resources for this chapter can be found on the Companion Website at www.prenhall.com/wolgin. Click on Chapter 24 and "Begin" to select activities for this chapter.

For chapter-related NCLEX-style questions and an audio glossary, access the accompanying CD-ROM in this book.

Video:

- Risk Management; Specimen Collection—Perform a Blood Glucose Evaluation.

25

The Reproductive System and Related Care

OBJECTIVES

When you have completed this chapter, you will be able to:

- Label a diagram with the female organs of the reproductive system and explain how each organ helps in the process of reproduction.
- Label a diagram with the male organs of the reproductive system and explain how each organ helps in the process of reproduction.
- Explain the meaning of sexuality and how the nursing assistant can appropriately respect the sexuality of patients.
- List the common disorders of the reproductive system.
- List the common sexually transmitted diseases (STDs).
- Explain HIV/AIDS precautions to all patients.
- Describe how to prepare a patient for a pelvic exam.
- Give a vaginal irrigation (douche).
- Identify important aspects of postpartum care.

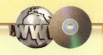

MediaLink
www.prenhall.com/wolgin

Use the address above to access the free, interactive Companion Website created for this textbook. Get hints, instant feedback, and textbook references to chapter-related NCLEX-style questions. Link to other interesting sites.

AUDIO GLOSSARY:
Use the Companion Website, or the CD-ROM disk enclosed with your textbook, to hear the pronunciation of key terms in the chapter.

KEY TERMS

AIDS
estrogen
fertile
fertilization
gynecological (GYN) patient
HIV
menopause
menstruation
ova/ovum
ovulation
pelvic inflammatory disease (PID)
perineal area
reproductive system
sexually transmitted diseases (STDs)
sperm
testosterone
vagina (vaginal canal)
vaginal irrigation (douche)

INTRODUCTION

ALERT

For all patient contact, adhere to Standard Precautions (⊂⊃ Chapter 5, pages 83–85). Wear protective equipment as indicated.

To meet the needs of patients, the nursing assistant must have an understanding of the female and male reproductive systems. Because of misinformation or cultural values, patients may be sensitive to care they receive for this area of their bodies. Even if their own cultural identity differs from that of their patients, caregivers must maintain a compassionate and professional approach to patient care. This chapter provides guidance by discussing the male and female reproductive systems, sexuality, and patient care related to the reproductive system.

The Reproductive System

reproductive system The group of body organs that makes possible the creation of a new human life

ova/ovum The female reproductive cell(s) produced in the ovaries which is capable of uniting with a sperm cell and developing into a new organism

estrogen A female hormone that causes a buildup of the lining of the uterus to prepare it for possible pregnancy; also responsible for the development of secondary sexual characteristics

perineal area The area of the body between the thighs; includes the area of the anus and the external genital organs

The **reproductive system** is the group of body organs that makes possible the creation of a new human life. In the process of reproduction (creation of new life), the male and female each have an essential role.

Female Reproductive System

In the female, the primary reproductive organs are the two ovaries (Figure 25–1♦). The main task of the ovaries is the production of **ova** (eggs)/**ovum** (egg) and female hormones. The ovaries are the major sites of production of **estrogen** and progesterone in the amounts required for normal female growth, development, and function. The **perineal area** (the external genitalia and rectal area) has three openings:

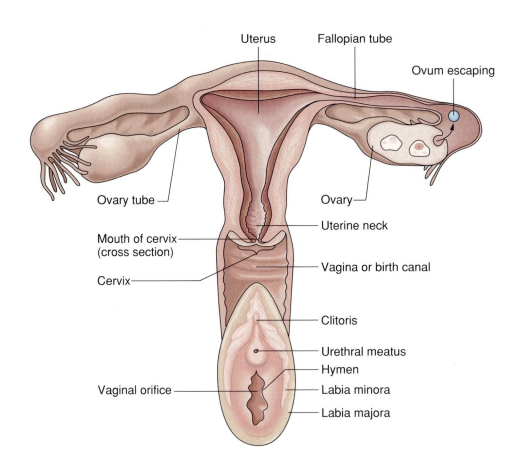

FIGURE 25–1 ♦

Female reproductive organs

1. The external urinary meatus, the end of the urethra

2. The **vagina** or **vaginal canal**, which serves as the organ for intercourse and the birth canal

3. The anus, the last portion of the gastrointestinal tract

The reproductive process begins with **ovulation**. During ovulation, an ovum is released from one ovary into the opening of the fallopian tube, through which it travels to the uterus (womb). Ovulation usually occurs once each month, and a woman normally is **fertile** (able to become pregnant) during this time. Also, estrogen is released, causing a buildup of the lining of the uterus (endometrium), preparing it for a possible pregnancy. The process of ovulation is controlled by hormones from the pituitary gland, under the control of the hypothalamus. These hormones are involved in the development of the ovum and in maintaining pregnancy.

Fertilization occurs at this stage if an ovum unites with a **sperm** cell released from the male during intercourse. Artificial insemination is a process sometimes used to fertilize the ovum. After the egg is fertilized, it normally grows and develops in the uterus over a period of 40 weeks (Figure 25–2◆). Then the baby is born when the uterus contracts, gradually pushing the baby through the vagina (birth canal). In some cases, the baby is surgically removed from the uterus in an operation called a cesarean birth.

If the woman does not become pregnant, the next menstrual period begins about 14 days after ovulation. **Menstruation** is the periodic (monthly) loss of some blood and a small part of the lining of the uterus (Figure 25–3◆). The discharge flows out of the vagina for 4 to 7 days. As the woman reaches age 45 to 55, menstruation gradually becomes less frequent, leading to the normal cessation of menstrual cycles, or **menopause**.

vagina (vaginal canal) The canal leading from the cervix to the outside of the female body; serves as the organ for intercourse and the birth canal

ovulation Process whereby an ovum is released from one ovary into the opening of the fallopian tube and moves to the uterus

fertile Able to become pregnant; capable of reproduction

fertilization Joining of a sperm and ovum to form a new cell

sperm The male reproductive cell produced in the testes, which is released from the male during intercourse

menstruation Periodic (monthly) loss of some blood and a small part of the lining of the uterus when a woman is not pregnant

menopause Time during which menstruation stops, resulting in decreased hormone production and an end of fertility

---

KEY IDEA

The reproductive cycle of a fertile woman begins with ovulation, during which the ovaries release an egg. The egg may be fertilized (joined by a sperm) so that it can develop into a fetus, or the egg may pass out of the body during menstruation.

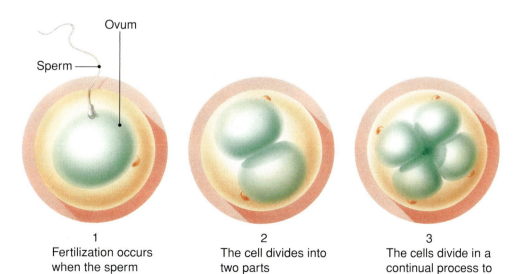

1
Fertilization occurs when the sperm and ovum join to form a single cell

2
The cell divides into two parts

3
The cells divide in a continual process to form a living being

FIGURE 25–2 ◆

Fertilization and cell division

FIGURE 25–3 ◆

The menstrual flow cycle, a physiological process in women of childbearing age

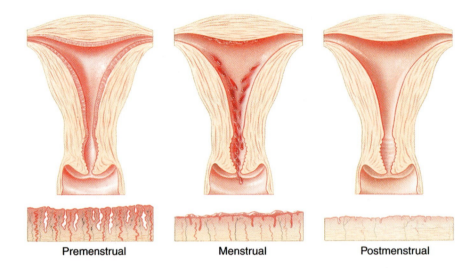

Premenstrual   Menstrual   Postmenstrual

Male Reproductive System

In the male, the primary reproductive organs are the testes (testicles), which produce sperm (Figure 25–4◆). The testes are paired glands that lie in a sac called the scrotum. The scrotum is located outside the body, posterior to the penis, which is the primary male sex organ.

The penis has three columns of spongy or cavernous tissue. During sexual excitement, blood rushes in through the penile artery and the veins constrict, trapping the blood so it fills these spaces. Then the penis becomes erect. This activity occurs under the influence of **testosterone**, the primary male sex hormone, which is also manufactured in the testes. It is secreted into the blood through the influence of the hormones from the anterior pituitary, which is under the control of the hypothalamus.

testosterone The primary male sex hormone; manufactured in the testes

FIGURE 25–4 ◆

Male reproductive organs

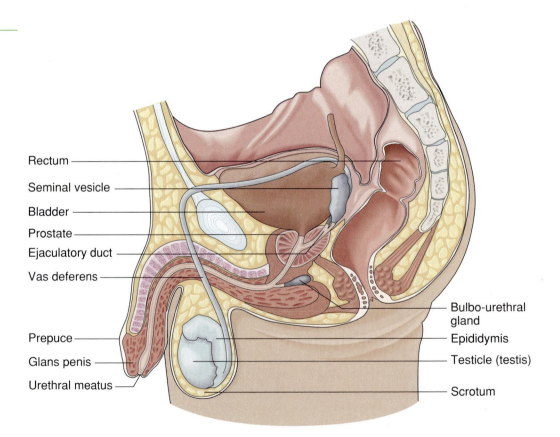

Rectum

Seminal vesicle

Bladder

Prostate

Ejaculatory duct

Vas deferens

Prepuce

Glans penis

Urethral meatus

Bulbo-urethral gland

Epididymis

Testicle (testis)

Scrotum

During intercourse, sperm travel up the vas deferens, or sperm duct, to the urethra. The sperm enter the urethra with secretions from other glands in the male reproductive system. These glands—the seminal vesicles, the prostate gland, and the bulbo-urethral gland (Cowper's gland)—contribute water, nutrients, and vitamins. Together, these secretions plus the sperm make up the semen. When the male has an orgasm, the semen is ejaculated (expelled) so that the sperm can travel up his partner's vagina, enabling a sperm to join with an ovum.

The penis has only one duct. It is used for the flow of urine and for the ejaculation of sperm in the semen. During intercourse, the internal sphincter of the male's urinary bladder closes tightly, so urine does not become mixed with the semen.

KEY IDEA

The male participates in the reproductive process by producing sperm in the testes. When a male ejaculates during intercourse, the semen carries many sperm up the vagina, where one sperm may fertilize an ovum.

Sexuality

A person's reproductive system is just one part of that person's sexuality. Sexuality means the group of characteristics that identify the differences between male and female. During all the stages of growth and development, people are sexual beings. Their sexuality arises from their emotions, thoughts, and experiences related to warm, loving, and caring feelings shared between people, whether associated with the sex organs or not. Also, inherited sexual characteristics influence individual behavior patterns.

Because sexuality is a part of each person, the nursing assistant needs to care for patients in ways that respect their sexuality appropriately. Appropriate care is considerate of the patient's need for privacy. The nursing assistant should close doors and privacy curtains when providing patient care and should not talk in front of others about conditions the patient may find embarrassing. Also, the nursing assistant can show respect for the patient's sexuality by helping the patient look attractive. As needed, the nursing assistant can help the patient choose attractive clothing, care for the hair, and apply makeup, as appropriate.

The nursing assistant should expect that patients will have different views about sexuality and their reproductive systems. For example, cultural values may make some patients extremely concerned about privacy and reluctant to discuss problems related to sexual function or reproductive organs. Occasionally a patient may express his sexuality inappropriately by grabbing or touching the nursing assistant or other staff member. If this occurs, the nursing assistant should tell the patient calmly, "That is not appropriate behavior." If this response does not end the behavior, the nursing assistant should discuss the problem with her supervisor.

KEY IDEA

Sexuality describes a person's maleness or femaleness. It includes differences in male and female bodies, as well as the contrasting ways men and women learn to behave and their feelings about being a man or woman. Therefore, sexual behavior includes not only intercourse, but also many ways of touching and showing affection or attraction.

The Reproductive System and the Normal Aging Process

As a person ages, changes occur in hormone levels and in some parts of the reproductive system. Certain age-related problems are common in women, others in men.

AGE-SPECIFIC CONSIDERATIONS

When caring for adolescents, keep in mind that they are beginning to develop sexual maturity. They may have a wide range of knowledge about their bodies and varying levels of comfort with their emerging sexuality. When caring for these patients, keep privacy concerns in mind as well as issues of confidentiality. Adolescents may or may not want to be examined and cared for with their parents present.

Aging of the Female Reproductive System

A notable age-related change in the reproductive system of a woman is menopause, which typically occurs between ages 45 and 55. Besides the end of menstruation and fertility, menopause brings a decrease in the production of estrogen. The decline in estrogen production is thought to contribute to other age-related changes. Loss of elasticity of the vaginal tissues, decreased vaginal secretions, and other changes make the woman more susceptible to irritation and infection of the vulva and vagina. The decline in estrogen also can lead to a loss of calcium, causing the bones to become brittle. Many women use estrogen replacement therapy or any number of natural products available at health food or nutrition stores. Research is ongoing to study the benefits versus the risks of using estrogen replacement to relieve symptoms of menopause. Many women use it to relieve sleeplessness, excessive vaginal bleeding, irritability, hot flashes, or night sweats. The doctor will consider the risks and take the woman's family history before prescribing medication. The number of months or years the medication is taken will vary with each woman.

As a woman ages, the pelvic muscles which support the structures in the perineal area can become weak. This can lead to stress incontinence; that is, involuntary urination when lifting, sneezing, or coughing. Exercise to strengthen the pelvic muscles helps to relieve this condition. Surgery is another option.

Aging of the Male Reproductive System

When men grow older, their hormone levels also change, and the production of sperm decreases. Older men generally need more time to achieve an erection, and the erection is usually less firm but lasts longer. Perhaps the most significant age-related change affecting the male reproductive system is enlargement of the prostate gland. This firm, muscular gland encircles the urethra like a doughnut. When it expands, it squeezes the urethra and causes painful urination, decreased force of the urinary stream, and more frequent urination. If the condition remains untreated, it may lead to poor urinary control, dribbling, bleeding, obstruction, and kidney damage.

Among the most common treatments for an enlarged prostate is surgery to remove the prostate tissue surrounding the urethra. Many men fear surgery on their prostate gland (prostatectomy), because they believe it will end their sex life. The amount of semen ejaculated will be less, but, otherwise, 70 percent of the men who have had a prostatectomy are often capable of having the same sexual relations as before surgery. Some men, however, will experience a diminished ability to perform sexually after this surgery.

There have been recent advances yielding new prescription drugs to take orally (for example, Viagara), by injection, or directly applied to the penis that offer men experiencing impotence for a variety of reasons the ability to achieve erections. Urologists have the most experience treating sexual problems. Cardiac workups are advised and usually required for men at risk. There can be complications or in rare cases deaths of men who take these drugs and exert themselves. It is a common belief among men in various cultures that special teas or products containing animal, fish, or snake oils or extracts will enhance their potency.

KEY IDEA

Aging alone does not cause an end of sexual desire. As people grow older, sexual desire may change, but sexuality and sexual needs continue.

Common Diseases and Disorders of the Reproductive System

A number of disorders may affect the female reproductive system:

- **Dysmenorrhea:** painful menstruation
- **Amenorrhea:** absence of menstruation
- **Menorrhagia:** excessive bleeding during menstruation
- **Pelvic inflammatory disease (PID):** infection that spreads to all structures in the pelvic cavity
- **Vaginitis:** inflammation of the vagina
- **Cystocele:** downward protrusion of the urinary bladder into the vagina
- **Rectocele:** protrusion of the rectum into the vagina
- **Cancer of the uterus:** malignancy of the uterus
- **Fibroids:** benign tumors of the uterus
- **Tumors of the breast:** new cell growth that may be benign or malignant

Male reproductive system disorders include the following:

- **Benign prostatic hyperplasia (BPH):** enlarged prostate gland
- **Cancer of the prostate gland:** malignant tumor
- **Prostatitis:** inflammation of the prostate gland
- **Hydrocele:** abnormal accumulation of fluid within the scrotum
- **Impotence:** inability to achieve or sustain an erection
- **Varicocele:** enlargement of the veins within the scrotum
- **Tumors of the testicle:** new cell growth that may be benign or malignant
- **Tumors of the breast:** new cell growth that may be benign or malignant

Sexually Transmitted Diseases

Diseases acquired as a result of sexual intercourse with a person who is infected are called **sexually transmitted diseases (STDs)**. Some of the most common STDs are as follows:

- **Chlamydia:** infection by Chlamydia bacteria (a type of rickettsia), whose incidence is on the rise. It can cause pelvic inflammatory disease (PID) with a whitish-yellow discharge. Infertility can result from not treating the disease.

pelvic inflammatory disease (PID) Infection that spreads to all structures in the pelvic cavity

sexually transmitted diseases (STDs) Diseases acquired as a result of sexual intercourse with an infected person

- **Gonorrhea:** contagious infection caused by gonococcus bacteria. Females may have no symptoms, yet can spread the disease. Males notice a greenish-yellow discharge from the penis and have a burning sensation within 2 to 5 days of contracting the disease.

- **AIDS (acquired immune deficiency syndrome):** group of signs and symptoms that characterizes a lethal disorder in T-cell immunity associated with either Karposi's sarcoma or opportunistic infections that impair immune function; caused by infection with a virus called **HIV**, which attacks white blood cells and impairs their response to infection.

- **Syphilis:** an infectious, chronic, venereal disease characterized by lesions that may involve any organ or tissue; caused by *Treponema pallidum*, a spirochete. Early symptoms include sores followed by a rash, a sore throat, and a mild fever.

- **Genital herpes simplex (HSV):** a viral disease that may be recurrent and has no cure; open sores may be present in the genital area or inside the vagina, but most patients will not have visible signs of the disease; the sores do not need to be visible for the infection to be transmitted to another individual.

- **Human papillomavirus (HPV) infection (genital warts):** genital and anal warts caused by infection with HPV; some forms can be cancerous; there is no cure or way to get rid of the virus (HPV), and treatment usually is aimed at treating the wart itself with medication. Males may be unaware they have this disease and spread it to their partners.

HIV Human immunodeficiency virus; the microorganism that causes AIDS

KEY IDEA

STDs can be prevented by sexual abstinence. Most STDs can be prevented by using barriers such as male or female condoms during intercourse, or using other methods of practicing safe sex.

Caring for Patients with AIDS

Measures to prevent HIV infection are especially important, according to current HIV/AIDS research. One reason is that AIDS frequently is a fatal syndrome. Many promising new drugs on the market can lessen the effect of HIV/AIDS, but no cure is available as of this writing. Currently, a combination of three drugs has been most useful to treat patients. Researchers are uncertain how effective this treatment will be as the AIDS virus mutates and may not continue to respond to the drugs. New cases continue as it is not always possible to know who may transmit the disease and because a person can carry the virus (HIV) for many years before developing AIDS.

Tests are available that indicate exposure to HIV, but these tests do not confirm a diagnosis of AIDS. To be diagnosed with **AIDS**, the patient must not only test positive for HIV but also meet at least one of the criteria set by the Centers for Disease Control and Prevention (CDC). The CDC criteria include development of certain infections, cancers, wasting of the body, and dementia. A person infected with HIV can transmit the virus whether or not he has AIDS.

Both heterosexuals and homosexuals can be afflicted by HIV/AIDS. The following groups are most at risk for HIV/AIDS: IV drug users, people who engage in homosexual acts, people who have received contaminated blood, and anyone who has sexual intercourse with a person in these groups. At this time, the fastest growing numbers of new HIV infections are in the heterosexual group.

AIDS Viral infection characterized by decreased immunity to opportunistic infections

HIV/AIDS can be transmitted by blood and other body fluids or secretions that may contain blood. Gloves and protective eye gear are mandatory to protect the nursing assistant from exposure due to splashing when handling *any* patient's body fluids, such as blood, urine, feces, or saliva. If you as a nursing assistant come upon a needle and syringe, or any sharp object, you should immediately dispose of it in a puncture-proof container. Needles should never be bent, broken, or recapped.

The AIDS patient, too, requires protection. Because the immune system is suppressed, the patient needs to be protected from such normally routine illnesses as colds. The patient's privacy also may need to be protected, in compliance with HIPPA's patient confidentiality rules, because many people are afraid of AIDS or have negative feelings about members of some major risk groups (homosexuals and IV drug users). Therefore, the nursing assistant should maintain confidentiality and follow the institution's policy and should not disclose that a patient has AIDS. However, a patient's condition needs to be known to the patient's caregivers.

The nursing assistant can also support the emotional well-being of the patient with AIDS. Having a terminal illness is distressing for any patient. And because this disease is widely feared, the patient's family and friends may be reluctant to touch or spend time with him. The nursing assistant can help by being sensitive and nonjudgmental with the patient. Also, when the nursing assistant works with the AIDS patient and touches him appropriately, her behavior can serve as a model to family members, helping them view the risks more realistically.

KEY IDEA

HIV is not spread by casual contact like hugging, coughing, or sharing a bathroom. The Standard Precautions (see Chapter 5, pages 83–85) provide protection against AIDS as well as other blood-borne diseases.

Care of the Gynecological Patient

A female patient receiving care of the reproductive system (including the breasts) is known as a **gynecological (GYN) patient** (Figure 25–5◆). Care of the gynecological patient often includes pelvic exams. Occasionally, the nursing assistant may also give a vaginal irrigation (also called a douche).

gynecological (GYN) patient Patient being treated for diseases or conditions of the female reproductive organs, including the breasts

FIGURE 25–5 ◆
Many gynecological patients appreciate support and reassurance

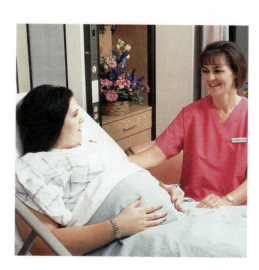

Preparing the Patient for a Pelvic Exam

A pelvic examination is very important for assessing the condition of the female reproductive organs. However, patients often find the exam embarrassing or uncomfortable, so the nursing assistant should be especially careful to maintain privacy and comfort.

PREPARING THE PATIENT FOR A PELVIC EXAM

PROCEDURE

RATIONALE: Performed to allow the doctor or nurse midwife to assess a female's reproductive organs or to collect specimen cultures.

PREPARATION

1. Assemble the equipment (Figure 25-6◆):
   a. Disposable gloves
   b. Microscope slides
   c. Cotton applicators
   d. Cotton balls
   e. Pap smear fixative
   f. Vaginal speculum
   g. Uterine dressing forceps
   h. Lubricant
   i. Wooden tongue blade

2. Wash your hands and put on disposable gloves.

3. Provide privacy for the patient.

4. Tell the patient you are going to prepare her for a pelvic exam.

STEPS

5. Have the patient empty her bladder in the bathroom or assist with a bedpan.

6. Help the patient undress while providing coverage with a blanket.

7. Position the patient on her back with her knees separated and legs flexed (Figure 25-7◆). Stirrups may be used to position the legs and feet. An additional drape may be used to cover the legs.

8. If you leave the room before the exam, place the call light within easy reach of the patient. However, you may be asked to remain during the exam.

9. After the exam, assist the patient to dress or put on a gown.

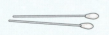
Cotton applicators

Wooden tongue blade

Microscope slides

Pap smear fixative

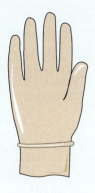
Glove

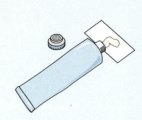
Lubricant

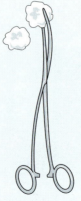
Uterine dressing forceps

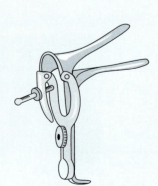
Vaginal speculum

FIGURE 25–6 ◆
Assemble equipment for the pelvic exam

PROCEDURE *(continued)*

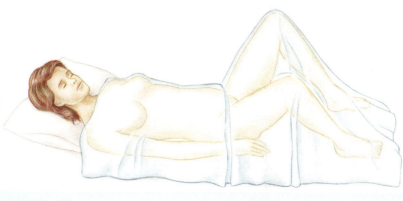

FIGURE 25–7 ◆

Position patient on her back with knees separated and legs flexed

FOLLOW-UP

10. Make sure the patient is comfortable.
11. Care for the equipment according to the institution's policy.
12. Remove your gloves and wash your hands.

13. Report to the supervisor:
  ■ That the exam was performed.
  ■ What time the exam was performed.

CHARTING EXAMPLE: 1/15/04, 2pm Pelvic exam performed by Dr. Smith. Pap smear labeled and sent to the lab. C. Smith, CNA

KEY IDEA

When providing any type of gynecological care, the nursing assistant must be especially careful to protect the patient's privacy and to respect her ideas of modesty.

Vaginal Douche or Nonsterile Irrigation

The introduction of a solution into the vagina with an immediate return of the solution by gravity is called a **vaginal irrigation** or **douche**. This type of irrigation is usually used for cleansing the vaginal canal or relieving inflammation of the vaginal tract. A doctor may order this treatment to cleanse before surgery or an examination, in cases of severe discharge, to treat an inflammation, or to neutralize secretions in the vaginal canal.

When used to excess, vaginal irrigation can wash away normal protective secretions. This is one reason why such a procedure should never be done without a physician's order.

In carrying out a vaginal irrigation, follow the rules of medical asepsis. In some institutions this procedure is done while the patient is on the toilet. Follow the instructions of your immediate supervisor.

vaginal irrigation (douche)
The introduction of a solution into the vagina with an immediate return of the solution by gravity; usually used for cleansing the vaginal canal or relieving inflammation of the vaginal tract

NONSTERILE VAGINAL IRRIGATION (DOUCHE)

PROCEDURE

RATIONALE: Purpose is to cleanse the vaginal canal or relieve irritation.

PREPARATION

1. Assemble your equipment:
   a. Disposable douche
   b. Bedpan and cover (towel)
   c. Bath blanket
   d. Disposable waterproof bed protector
   e. Disposable gloves
2. Wash your hands and put on disposable gloves.
3. Identify the patient by checking the identification bracelet.
4. Ask visitors to step out of the room.
5. Tell the patient you are going to give her a vaginal douche.
6. Provide privacy for the patient.

STEPS

7. Offer the patient the bedpan, explaining that her bladder must be empty to ensure the desired results from the douche.
8. Remove the bedpan. Measure output if the patient is on intake and output. Record on the I&O sheet. Empty the contents of the bedpan; wash it and place it on a chair nearby.
9. Remove gloves and wash your hands. Put on clean gloves.
10. Wash the patient's hands.

11. Place the patient into the dorsal recumbent position. The head of the bed should be flat. Drape the patient with a small sheet.
12. Cover the patient with a bath blanket. Without exposing her, fan-fold the top sheets to the foot of the bed. The patient holds the bath blanket while you do this. Leave the patient covered with only the bath blanket.
13. Place the disposable bed protector under the patient's hips (buttocks).
14. Raise the bed to a comfortable working position.
15. Open the douche kit.
16. Cleanse the perineum with soap and water, using a washcloth.
17. Place the bedpan under the patient's hips (buttocks).
18. With solution flowing, insert the douche nozzle tip into the vagina from 2 to 3 inches with an upward and then downward and backward gentle movement.
19. Allow the solution to flow.
20. Help the patient to sit up on the bedpan by raising the back of the bed, if allowed (Fowler's position). This will help the solution to drain from the vagina.
21. Dry the perineum with toilet tissue and discard into the bedpan.
22. Remove the bedpan and cover with towel.
23. Help the patient to turn on her side and dry the buttocks with toilet tissue.
24. Replace the bed protector with a dry one if wet.
25. Lower the bed to its lowest horizontal position.

26. Change any linen that has become damp.
27. Raise the top sheets over the bath blanket and then remove the bath blanket from under the top sheets.

FOLLOW-UP

28. Make the patient comfortable.
29. Lower the bed to a position of safety for the patient.
30. Raise the side rails where ordered, indicated, and appropriate for patient safety.
31. Place the call light within easy reach of the patient.
32. Observe the contents of the bedpan. Collect a specimen to show to your immediate supervisor if the returned solution is not as clear as when it was inserted.
33. Discard disposable supplies.
34. Clean the bedpan and return to its proper place.
35. Remove disposable gloves and wash your hands.
36. Report to your immediate supervisor:
    - That the vaginal irrigation was done.
    - The time the vaginal irrigation was done.
    - Whether a specimen was collected, and why.
    - How the patient tolerated the procedure.

CHARTING EXAMPLE: 2/24/04, 3:30pm Vaginal irrigation performed; tolerated well. V. Juarez, CNA

Postpartum Care

During vaginal delivery of a baby, the vaginal canal stretches and sometimes tears through the perineal muscles. This can cause postpartum edema and tenderness. Sometimes during the birth the doctor will make a small cut (episiotomy) in the vagina to make the opening larger and to prevent tearing. This episiotomy will require stitches and will also be tender. Postpartum perineal care (cleansing of the perineum) promotes healing, cleanses, and gives comfort to that area.

Perineal care must be performed by the patient or caregiver after each elimination of urine or feces. It is generally performed by the patient on the toilet. The following procedure is for postpartum perineal care given in bed.

POSTPARTUM PERINEAL CARE

PROCEDURE

RATIONALE: Used to promote healing, cleanse, or relieve discomfort in the perineal area.

PREPARATION

1. Assemble your equipment:
   a. Disposable bed protector
   b. Bedpan and cover
   c. Squirt bottle (peri bottle)
   d. Toilet paper
   e. Disposable gloves
2. Wash your hands.
3. Identify the patient by checking the identification bracelet.
4. Ask visitors to leave the room, if this is your hospital's policy.
5. Tell the patient you are going to clean the genital area.
6. Provide privacy for the patient.
7. Be sure there is plenty of light. Raise the bed to a comfortable working position.

STEPS

8. Cover the patient with a bath blanket. Without exposing her, fan-fold the top sheets to the foot of the bed. Have the patient covered only with the blanket. Put on gloves.
9. Fill the squirt bottle with warm water at 100°F (37.7°C) or use the solution provided in your institution.
10. Place the disposable bed protector under the patient's hips (buttocks).
11. Help the patient to get on the bedpan.
12. Put on disposable gloves.
13. Spray the perineum with solution, working from anterior to posterior.
14. Dry the patient gently with the toilet paper. Remove and discard the disposable gloves.
15. Remove the bedpan and disposable bed protector. Place them on a chair.
16. Cover the patient with the top sheets. Remove the bath blanket.

FOLLOW-UP

17. Make the patient comfortable.
18. Lower the bed to a position of safety for the patient.
19. Raise the side rails where ordered, indicated, and appropriate for patient safety.
20. Place the call light within easy reach of the patient.
21. Discard disposable equipment.
22. Empty, rinse, and put the equipment back where it belongs.
23. Remove your gloves and wash your hands.
24. Report to your immediate supervisor:
    - That postpartum perineal care was given.
    - Your observations of anything unusual.
    - How the patient tolerated the procedure.

CHARTING EXAMPLE: 11/14/04, 10:15am Pericare given to Mrs. Hanks who says she is feeling pain when her clean perineal pad was applied. Request for pain medication relayed to Ms. Jacobs, RN. T. Suggs, CNA

Another important function of postpartum care is observation of the amount of blood that has accumulated on the perineal pads worn by the patient. Some institutions count the number of pads, and others also want a description of the amount of blood on the pad. In addition, the nursing assistant should observe the urine for blood clots (from the vagina) the first 24 hours after birth.

KEY IDEA

Never hand a baby to a mother who is sleepy and then leave her alone. You may need to put the side rails up for safety or remain with the mother while she feeds the baby. Follow the instructions of your immediate supervisor.

Another aspect of care for the postpartum patient is help with ambulation. The type of delivery—a vaginal or a cesarean birth—may influence her ability to ambulate without discomfort. It is very important that the patient have good feeling in her legs before attempting to walk. The legs may be numb from anesthesia she received for the birth. Some types of anesthesia require the patient to lie flat for several hours after birth until the anesthesia wears off to prevent developing a severe headache. Check with your supervisor if you are uncertain about the patient's ambulation orders or ability.

Finally, if the patient has had a cesarean section birth, she will require additional care. Follow the instructions in Chapter 28 for coughing and deep breathing and use of the incentive spirometer for patients who have had surgery.

SUMMARY

The different reproductive structures in the female and male greatly influence the care provided by the nursing assistant. A basic understanding of the human reproductive anatomy and the common diseases and disorders is essential. Also important is a sensitivity to cultural differences that might affect the patient's expectations and reactions to care of the reproductive system. Providing privacy at all times is just as important as the physical care given to the patient. Because of the possibility of HIV/AIDS contamination, caregivers must wear protective gear where appropriate. Your immediate supervisor will assist you in identifying situations in which special protective gear must be worn.

NOTES

CHAPTER REVIEW

FILL IN THE BLANK Read each sentence and fill in the blank line with a word that completes the sentence.

1. The reproductive process begins with _____.

2. _____ is the group of characteristics that identify the differences between males and females.

3. Diseases that are acquired as a result of sexual intercourse are called _____ _____ _____.

4. HIV/AIDS is transmitted by _____ _____.

5. Cleaning of the perineum after delivery is called _____ care.

MULTIPLE CHOICE Choose the best answer for each question or statement.

1. Which of the following is not a part of the female reproductive system?
   a. Cervix
   b. Prepuce
   c. Hymen
   d. Ovary

2. Which of the following is not a part of the male reproductive system?
   a. Prostate
   b. Hymen
   c. Epididymis
   d. Scrotum

3. Which of the following is not a disorder of the female reproductive system?
   a. Dysmenorrhea
   b. Pelvic inflammatory disease
   c. Fibroids
   d. Hydrocele

4. Which of the following is not a disorder of the male reproductive system?
   a. Prostatitis
   b. Varicocele
   c. Cystocele
   d. Benign prostate hyperplasia

5. HIV/AIDS *cannot* be transmitted by
   a. blood transfusions.
   b. direct contact with body fluids.
   c. touching the skin of a patient who has the infection.
   d. being stuck by an IV needle used with an AIDS patient.

TIME-OUT

TIPS FOR TIME MANAGEMENT

At times you may be asked to work outside your "comfort zone." You may be sent to a unit different from your usual assignment. Be positive and cooperative, even if you would prefer not to go. Avoid time wasters such as arguing about going and complaining about being sent.

THE NURSING ASSISTANT IN ACTION

You are working in a community health center preparing Carrie Cooper, an 18-year-old woman, for a GYN exam. She is nervous about the pelvic exam and tells you her boyfriend is HIV positive, but refuses to use condoms when they have sex. Carrie says, "You know how men are, he will quit seeing me unless I do as he says. All my girlfriends keep telling me that he is so hot. I do not want to give him up!"

What Is Your Response/Action?

CRITICAL THINKING

CUSTOMER SERVICE Occasionally new infants have problems that require them to be in the nursery for observation. Anticipate that the walk to the nursery may be more exhausting if the mother has recently delivered. Offer to walk with her or take her in a wheelchair if it is some distance from her room. Be sure there is a chair in the nursery for the new mom to sit if she plans to stay there more than a few minutes.

CULTURAL CARE As a nursing assistant you will encounter many cultural differences related to the reproductive care of women. If you are not sure what the particular differences are, be sure to ask first if there are any particular things the patient can tell you that would help you to plan her care. If you are a male, it may be that a female should give personal care to your patient. Some patients will have very different views on the use of birth control or refuse to use condoms as some measure of protection from STDs because condoms are also a method of birth control.

COOPERATION WITHIN THE TEAM Some caregivers are more skilled or comfortable than others providing emotional support to patients. There may be times that assignments are uneven because the supervisor recognizes particular patients need extra attention. Caregivers often waste time comparing assignments and complaining about the fact they have one or two more patients than someone else. If you notice a colleague has been identified as particularly supportive, try to learn more from that person and ask advice about how he cares for patients you find difficult to manage.

EXPLORE MediaLink

Additional interactive resources for this chapter can be found on the Companion Website at www.prenhall.com/wolgin. Click on Chapter 25 and "Begin" to select activities for this chapter.

For chapter-related NCLEX-style questions and an audio glossary, access the accompanying CD-ROM in this book.

26 The Nervous System and Related Care

OBJECTIVES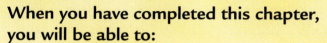

When you have completed this chapter, you will be able to:

- Describe the functions of the nervous system, the brain, and the spinal cord.
- List two divisions of the autonomic nervous system.
- List the five sense organs.
- Describe the care of a patient's artificial eye, eyeglasses, and hearing aid.
- Describe common age-related changes in the nervous system.
- List common diseases and disorders of the nervous system.
- Describe four types of seizures.
- Discuss five safety measures for the patient having a seizure.
- List four causes and results of a cerebrovascular accident (stroke).
- Describe the nursing assistant's role in care of a cerebrovascular accident patient.
- Describe the psychological aspects of caring for a patient who has had a cerebrovascular accident.
- Demonstrate how to communicate with an aphasic patient using correct technique.

MediaLink

www.prenhall.com/wolgin

Use the address above to access the free, interactive Companion Website created for this textbook. Get hints, instant feedback, and textbook references to chapter-related NCLEX-style questions. Link to other interesting sites.

AUDIO GLOSSARY:
Use the Companion Website, or the CD-ROM disk enclosed with your textbook, to hear the pronunciation of key terms in the chapter.

KEY TERMS

aphasia
autonomic nervous system
canthus
cerebral spinal fluid
cerebrovascular accident (CVA)
complex partial seizure
contracture
convulsive
deficit
embolus
environment
hemiplegia
hemisphere
hemorrhage
hypothalamus
impulse
intervertebral discs
involuntary
meninges
myelin sheath
nervous system
neuron
normal pressure hydrocephalus
osteoporosis
plaque
respond
rupture
seizure
simple partial seizure
spasm
stimuli
thrombus
vascular
vertebral bodies
voluntary

Caring for a patient with a neurologic condition is challenging and rewarding. Neurologic conditions can involve any part of the nervous system and are very frightening for most patients and their families. Patients and their families often need both emotional and physical support. In the course of helping with the care of these patients, the nursing assistant has a chance to provide much of this support.

Anatomy and Physiology of the Nervous System

nervous system The group of body organs consisting of the brain, spinal cord, and nerves that controls and regulates the activities of the body and the functions of the other body systems

voluntary Under control of the will; with conscious decision

involuntary Without conscious will, control, or decision

vascular Pertaining to blood vessels

neuron A type of nerve cell in the nervous system

The **nervous system** controls and organizes all body activity, both **voluntary** and **involuntary**. The nervous system is made up of the brain, the spinal cord, and the nerves. The nerves are spread throughout all areas of the body in an orderly way. The central nervous system is made up of the brain and spinal cord. The peripheral nervous system is made up of the nerves outside the brain and spinal cord.

The nervous system, and especially the brain, has a large **vascular** supply. That is, many blood vessels feed the brain so that it can carry out its many functions.

Nerve tissue is made up of cells called **neurons** and other supporting cells called neuroglia. A typical neuron consists of a cell body with one long column, called the axon, and many small outbranchings, called dendrites. Nerve impulses move from the dendrites through the cell body along the axon (Figure 26–1 ◆).

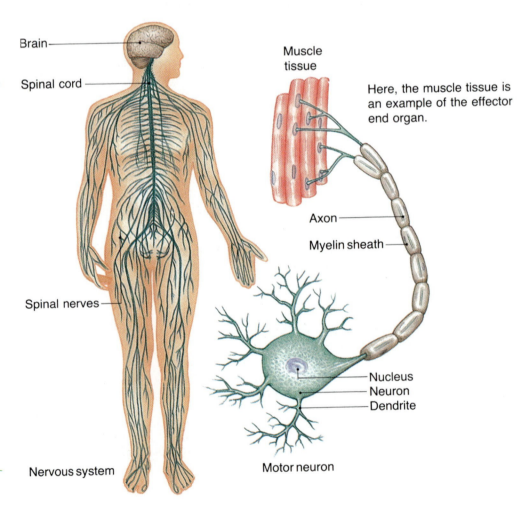

FIGURE 26–1 ◆
The nervous system and a motor neuron

Sensing and Responding to the Environment

Inside and outside our bodies, we have structures called receptor-end organs. Any change in our external or internal **environment** that is strong enough will set up a nervous **impulse** in these receptor-end organs. This impulse is carried by a sensory neuron to some part of the brain or spinal cord, where it connects with another neuron. The connection is called a synapse (Figure 26–2◆). Eventually the brain decides how to **respond** to the nerve impulse. This decision may come only after the interneuron has made hundreds of synapses (particularly in the cerebrum, the part of the brain in which we think). Once that happens, the proper impulses are sent down a motor neuron to the organ that will receive the impulse. When the organ (such as a muscle) receives the impulse, it responds. In the case of a muscle, it may contract or relax.

environment All the surrounding conditions and influences affecting the life and development of an organism

impulse An electrical or chemical charge transmitted through certain tissues, especially nerve fibers and muscles

respond React; begin, end, or change activity in reaction to stimulation

KEY IDEA

In the nervous system, when the body receives information, impulses travel from receptor-end organs through neurons to the brain. When the body responds to a stimulus, impulses travel from the brain through neurons to receiving organs, such as muscles.

Protection of the Nervous System

Most nerve cells outside the brain and spinal cord have a protective covering known as the **myelin sheath**. The task of the myelin sheath is to insulate the nerve cell. If you think of the nerve cell as an electrical wire, the myelin sheath is insulation that keeps the current in the correct pathway. This insulating sheath helps prevent damage to the cells and often helps the nerve return to healthy function, or regenerate, if it has been injured. Nerve cells with a myelin sheath also carry an impulse faster than those without myelin.

   The neurons in the brain and spinal cord do not have this kind of protection and are not able to regrow. When nerve cells are injured, as they are by a stroke, or **cerebrovascular accident (CVA)**, another part of the brain must take over the function of the part that has been damaged. The rehabilitation department in your health care institution helps patients learn to do things again after such damage has been done.

myelin sheath Protective covering around most nerves

cerebrovascular accident (CVA) Stroke; blockage or bleeding of blood vessels in the brain, interrupting the blood supply to that part of the brain and damaging the surrounding area of the brain

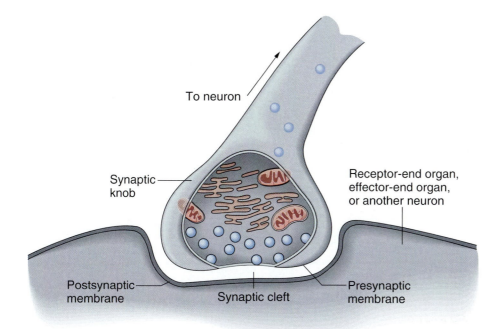

FIGURE 26–2 ◆

A synapse

To neuron

Synaptic knob

Receptor-end organ, effector-end organ, or another neuron

Postsynaptic membrane

Synaptic cleft

Presynaptic membrane

meninges The covering of the brain and spinal cord. There are three layers: the dura mater, the arachnoid, and the pia mater

cerebral spinal fluid The fluid that circulates around and within the brain and spinal cord

hemisphere Half of a sphere; in the nervous system, one-half of the brain

The brain is well protected by bones, membranes, the **meninges**, and a cushion of fluid called **cerebral spinal fluid**. This fluid circulates outside and within the brain, as well as around the spinal cord.

The Brain

The brain coordinates and controls all of the functions of the central nervous system such as memory, sight, and walking (Figure 26–3◆). The brain is a very complicated organ made up of five components: the cerebrum, the cerebellum, the midbrain, the pons, and the medulla.

The cerebrum is divided into two halves, called **hemispheres**. These hemispheres make up the top portion of the brain. The right hemisphere of the cerebrum controls most of the activity on the left side of the body. The left hemisphere controls activity on the right side of the body.

The cerebrum is where all learning, memory, and associations are stored so that thought is possible. Also, decisions are made for voluntary action. Certain areas of the cerebrum seem to perform special organizing activities. For example, the occipital lobe is the place that interprets what you see. The frontal lobe is the primary area of thought and reason. The cerebellum is the part of the brain that coordinates voluntary motion. It works with part of the inner ear, the semicircular canals, to enable you to walk and move smoothly through your world.

The midbrain, pons, and medulla are primarily pathways through which nervous impulses reach the brain from the spinal cord. Nerves throughout the body send messages through the spinal cord. The impulses then travel up the spinal cord to the higher centers of the brain. There are 12 pairs of cranial nerves and 32 pairs of spinal nerves through which these nerve impulses can travel. These nerves have branches that go to all parts of the body. The nerve impulses travel down from the brain through the spinal cord and out to the body.

There are many small structures in the brain. They screen all nerve impulses going to the brain, either getting them there faster or slowing them down. One of these tiny structures is the **hypothalamus**, which in times of stress, emergency, excitement, or danger

hypothalamus Area of the brain responsible for control of the pituitary gland

FIGURE 26–3 ◆

The brain

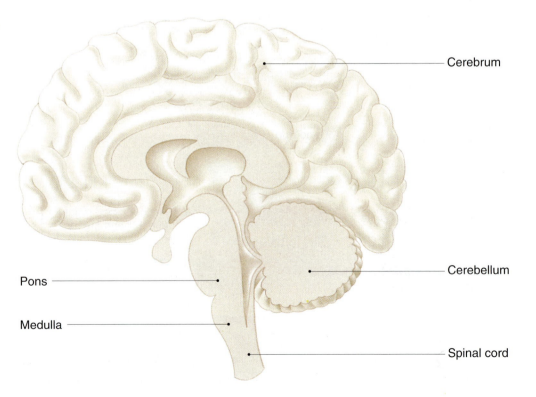

Cerebrum

Pons

Medulla

Cerebellum

Spinal cord

actually takes control of the body by controlling the pituitary gland, the body's master gland. We still know very little about the activity of the pituitary gland. We do know that it has tremendous control over most body activities. The hypothalamus seems to be the link between the mind and the body. It receives messages from the cerebrum, from the cerebellum, and from impulses coming up the spinal cord, and it has direct control over all the endocrine glands (glands that release hormones).

KEY IDEA

Among the activities of the cerebrum are learning, memory, and decision making. In general, the left hemisphere of the cerebrum controls the right side of the body, and the right hemisphere controls the left side. Thus, if the left side of the body were paralyzed, the right hemisphere is probably the affected side of the brain.

The Autonomic Nervous System

Much of the activity of the organs of the body is *involuntary*. In other words, we do not think about this activity, or we have little or no conscious control over it. The part of the nervous system that controls such involuntary activity as digestion and the functions of other visceral (abdominal) organs is the **autonomic nervous system**. This is really not separate from the brain and the spinal cord. The neurons that make up the autonomic nervous system use the same pathways as the neurons that control voluntary actions.

The autonomic nervous system has two divisions, which direct and control the activity of the internal organs. Each organ is supplied with neurons from each division of the autonomic nervous system.

One division is called the *sympathetic division*. The neurons that make up this division become active during stress, danger, excitement, or illness. These neurons cause the pupils of our eyes to become larger so that we can see more clearly and can see better at a distance. They also cause the heart to beat more strongly and to send more oxygen to the large muscles of the body in case it is necessary to fight or run. In today's fast-paced world, we are all subject to stress, and sometimes we cannot run away or fight. The action of the neurons from the sympathetic system responds by causing changes in the shape or activity of some of our organs. This action may also cause illness.

The *parasympathetic division* of the autonomic nervous system is in control when we are relaxed. It is known to conserve our energy.

Fortunately, a system of checks and balances operates between the two divisions. When one has been in action too long, the other automatically switches on. For example, during a stressful time when you may have been frightened, your heart rate increased. After you calmed down, your heart rate returned to normal. This is because stimulation of your sympathetic nervous system increases your heart rate and your parasympathetic nervous system causes your heart to return to normal functioning.

autonomic nervous system
The part of the nervous system that carries messages without conscious thought

KEY IDEA

The body's response to stress comes from the sympathetic nervous system. A response from this division of the autonomic nervous system prepares the body to fight or run. When the parasympathetic nervous system is stimulated, it helps the body return to normal functioning.

The Sense Organs

We are aware of our environment through our sense organs: eyes, ears, nose, tongue, and skin. The sense organs contain specialized endings of the sensory neurons, which are excited

FIGURE 26–4 ◆

Sensory and motor processes

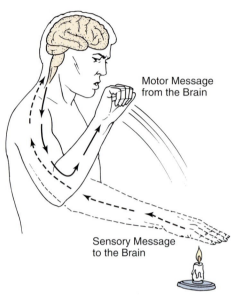

FIGURE 26–4 ◆

Sensory and motor processes

stimuli Changes in the external or internal environment strong enough to set up a nervous impulse or other responses in an organism

by changes in the outside environment. These changes are called **stimuli** (Figure 26–4◆). Each sense organ responds to a different category of stimuli:

- Eyes (Figure 26–5◆) respond to visual stimuli (what we see).
- Ears (Figure 26–6◆) respond mainly to sound stimuli (what we hear) and the body's position in space.
- Membranes of the nose respond to smell.
- Taste buds, located chiefly on the tongue, respond to taste sensations: sweet, sour, salty, and bitter.
- Skin responds to heat, cold, touch, pressure, and pain (Figure 26–7◆).

KEY IDEA

The sense organs are a person's sources of information about the environment. Thus, proper care of the sense organs is essential to good health and a feeling of well-being.

FIGURE 26–5 ◆

The eye

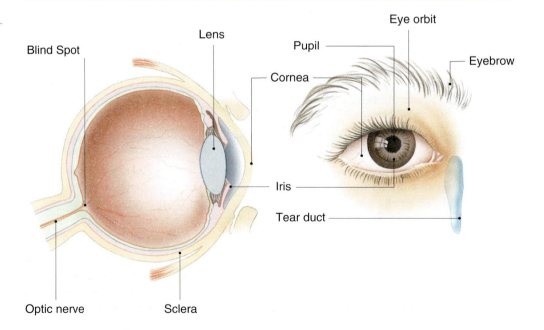

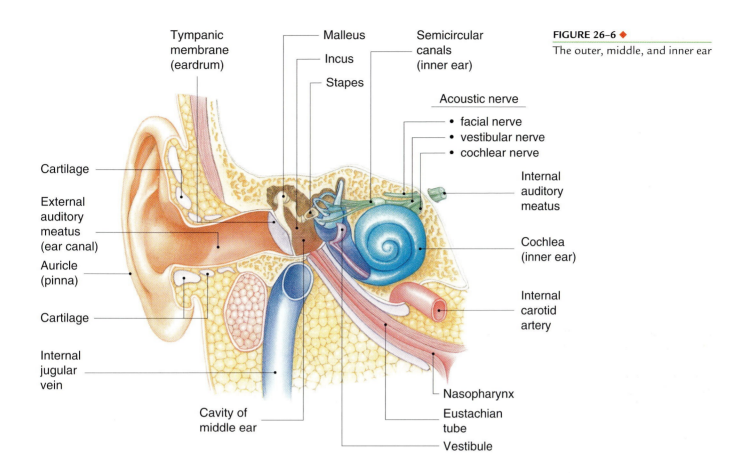

FIGURE 26–6 ◆
The outer, middle, and inner ear

Tympanic membrane (eardrum)

Malleus

Incus

Stapes

Semicircular canals (inner ear)

Acoustic nerve
- facial nerve
- vestibular nerve
- cochlear nerve

Cartilage

External auditory meatus (ear canal)

Auricle (pinna)

Cartilage

Internal jugular vein

Internal auditory meatus

Cochlea (inner ear)

Internal carotid artery

Cavity of middle ear

Nasopharynx

Eustachian tube

Vestibule

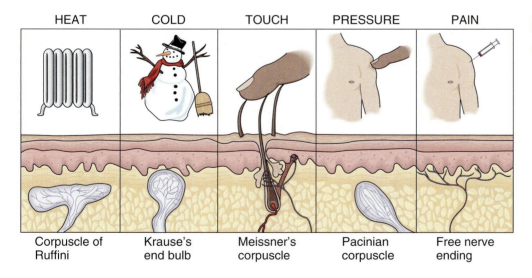

HEAT — Corpuscle of Ruffini

COLD — Krause's end bulb

TOUCH — Meissner's corpuscle

PRESSURE — Pacinian corpuscle

PAIN — Free nerve ending

FIGURE 26–7 ◆

The skin responds to heat, cold, touch, pressure, and pain

Care of the Artificial Eye

For a patient who has an artificial eye, cleaning the eye is part of daily personal hygiene. Proper care helps prevent infection and encrustation (formation of dried mucous material in the eye socket and around the artificial eye). Often a patient cannot care for his artificial eye himself. Encourage the patient to do as much as possible and assist as necessary.

CARING FOR THE ARTIFICIAL EYE

PROCEDURE

RATIONALE: Cleaning an artificial eye is part of the patient's daily care.

PREPARATION

1. Assemble your equipment on the bedside table:

   a. An eyecup half-filled with lukewarm water at 98° to 100°F (36.6° to 37.7°C) and labeled with the patient's name and room number (or, if no eyecup is available, use a clean denture cup)

   b. Gauze, 4" × 4" (3–4 pieces), for the bottom of the cup (or per your institution's policy)

   c. Small basin with lukewarm water

   d. Four cotton balls

   e. Special cleansing solution, if ordered by the doctor

2. Wash your hands.

3. Ask visitors to step out of the room, if this is your hospital's policy.

4. Identify the patient by checking the identification bracelet.

5. Tell the patient you are going to take care of his eye.

6. Pull the curtain around the bed for privacy.

STEPS

7. Help the patient lie down on the bed. This is to prevent accidental dropping of the artificial eye.

8. Put on gloves.

9. Have the patient close his eyes. Clean any external secretions from the patient's upper eyelid. Use cotton balls and warm water from the basin. Clean from the inner **canthus** to the outside of the eye area. This means you move from the nose to the outside of the eye. If you need to wipe more than once, use a clean (new) cotton ball each time. Use gentle strokes.

10. Remove the artificial eye. To do this, carefully depress the lower eyelid with your thumb. Lift the upper lid gently with your forefinger. The eye should slide out and down, into your hand. Have the patient do this, if he is able.

11. Place a 4" × 4" gauze in the cup and place the eye on the gauze. Let it soak in the water.

12. Wash off external matter and encrustations from the outside of the eye socket with cotton balls and warm water. Using gentle strokes, clean from the inner canthus to the outside of the eye.

13. Take the eyecup to the patient's bathroom. Close the drain in the sink. Fill the sink one-half full with water to prevent breakage if the eye is dropped.

14. Take the eye in your gloved hand and wash with running lukewarm water 98° to 100°F (36.6° to 37.7°C). Use plain water unless the doctor orders a special solution. Place the eye in the gauze from the eyecup and rub gently between your thumb and forefinger. *Do not use alcohol, ether, or acetone. These may dissolve the plastic of the artificial eye or dull the luster.*

15. Rinse the eye under running lukewarm water at 98° to 100°F (36.6° to 37.7°C), then dry it using the second 4" × 4" gauze. Discard the water from the eyecup. Place the slightly moistened eye on a dry gauze in the eyecup. A slightly moistened eye is easier to insert. Return to the patient's bedside.

16. If the patient cannot wear the eye immediately, store it by adding water to the eyecup and placing it in the bedside table drawer. Label the cup with the patient's name and room number.

17. Before inserting the artificial eye, remove your gloves and wash your hands thoroughly a second time. Put on clean gloves. If the patient is to insert the eye, have him wash his hands.

18. Insert the eye in the patient's eye socket. Have the notched edge toward the nose. Raise the upper lid with your forefinger. With your other hand, insert the eye. Place the eye under the upper lid. Then depress the lower lid. The eye should settle in place.

FOLLOW-UP

19. Make the patient comfortable.

20. Lower the bed to a position of safety for the patient.

21. Pull the curtains back to the open position.

22. Raise the side rails where ordered, indicated, and appropriate for patient safety.

23. Place the call light within easy reach of the patient.

24. Remove your gloves and wash your hands.

25. Report at once to your immediate supervisor:

   ■ That you have completed care of the artificial eye.

   ■ The time the procedure was done.

   ■ How the patient tolerated the procedure.

   ■ Your observations of anything unusual.

CHARTING EXAMPLE: 11/26/04 8am Artificial eye cleaned per procedure and inserted into Mr. Joseph's left eye socket. C. Best, CNA

canthus The inner aspect of the eye closest to the nose

Care of Eyeglasses

Proper care of a patient's eyeglasses is an essential task. Many patients find it difficult to function well without their eyeglasses because their vision is poor. Keeping the eyeglasses clean and scratch free is very important. Patients should always wear their glasses when they are walking or performing tasks if they cannot see well enough without them.

CARING FOR EYEGLASSES

PROCEDURE

RATIONALE: Dirty eyeglasses obstruct the patient's vision.

PREPARATION

1. Knock or ask permission to enter the patient's room.
2. Assemble your equipment on the bedside table or in the bathroom:
   a. A soft cloth
   b. Cleaning solution if needed
3. Wash your hands.
4. Identify yourself.
5. Identify the patient.

STEPS

6. Explain what you are going to do. Remove the patient's eyeglasses from the case or take them off the patient's face with the patient's permission and assistance. Handle the glasses by the frame only.
7. Inspect the eyeglasses. Do this by holding them up to the light and looking for scratches, smears, or soiling. Look for any loose screws in the hinges of the frame.
8. Clean the eyeglasses by polishing them with a soft cloth. If more cleaning solution is needed, run them under warm water or use the cleaning solution provided by your institution. Dry the eyeglasses with a soft cloth.
9. Return the eyeglasses to the case or to the patient. Assist the patient with putting them on as needed.
10. Remember to always keep eyeglasses in the case when the patient is not wearing them to avoid breaking or scratching them.

FOLLOW-UP

11. Wash your hands.
12. Report at once to your immediate supervisor:
    - That you have completed care of the eyeglasses.
    - The time the procedure was done.
    - How the patient tolerated the procedure.
    - Your observations of anything unusual such as scratches on the eyeglasses or loose hinge screws.

CHARTING EXAMPLE: 12/04/04
4pm Eyeglasses cleaned and placed in eyeglass case while Mr. Bright was asleep. Z. Zwicka, CNA

Hearing Aids

Even the best hearing aid cannot restore full, normal hearing ability. A patient who wears a hearing aid may still have trouble hearing. When talking to a patient who wears a hearing aid, face her and speak clearly. Speak in a normal tone of voice unless requested to speak louder by the patient.

Parts of the Hearing Aid

A hearing aid has several parts that a nursing assistant must recognize (Figure 26–8◆):

- **Microphone:** changes sound waves into electric signals and transmits sound
- **Amplifier:** uses battery energy to make the sound signals strong

FIGURE 26–8 ◆

A hearing aid

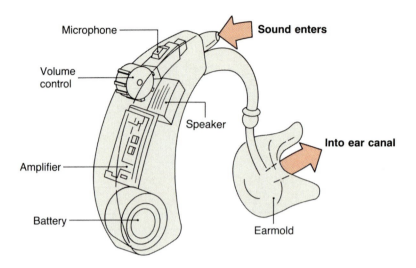

- **Earmold:** channels the sound through the external ear canal to the eardrum (tympanic membrane)
- **Cord:** connects the amplifier to the earmold
- **Volume control:** adjusts the volume level

Placement of the Hearing Aid

- Turn down the volume to the lowest or Off position.
- Place the hearing aid in the external ear canal; it should fit tightly but comfortably.
- After the hearing aid is in place, turn it on and adjust the volume so the patient can hear in a normal tone; the patient will tell you when she can hear comfortably.
- If the patient complains of an unpleasant whistle or squeal, check the placement in the ear and for a crack or break.

Checking the Batteries

- Before applying a hearing aid, check the batteries. There are many styles of hearing aids (Figure 26–9◆). Be sure the batteries are the right size for the hearing aid. The battery case must close easily; if not, something is wrong.

FIGURE 26–9 ◆

Types of hearing aids (Photo courtesy of SENSO by Widex)

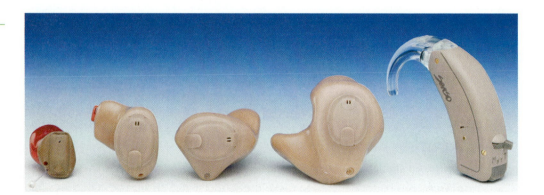

- To test the batteries, place the volume control switch to On and turn up the volume. Cup your hand over the hearing aid; you should hear a whistle. If you do not hear the whistle, change the batteries.

- If the patient complains that she cannot hear any sound, remove the hearing aid. Check the batteries and make sure the appliance is not broken.

- If the patient complains of hearing only intermittent (not always occurring) sound, remove and check the batteries.

CARING FOR AND STORING THE HEARING AID	GUIDELINES	OBRA
■ Caution: Never wash a hearing aid; you will ruin it. When the hearing aid needs cleaning, it must go back to the dealer to be cleaned properly. ■ Be sure to remove a hearing aid before the patient takes a shower or uses the bathtub or whirlpool.	■ Never drop the hearing aid. ■ Do not expose the hearing aid to heat. ■ Do not let moisture get into the hearing aid. Do not use any kind of hair spray or medical spray on a patient while her hearing aid is in place. The spray can clog the microphone opening.	■ Turn the hearing aid off when it is not in use. ■ Remove the battery from the battery case and leave the case open when the hearing aid is not in use. ■ Store the hearing aid in a container clearly marked with the patient's name and room number.

The Nervous System and the Normal Aging Process

As people age, the nervous system goes through changes. Age-related changes can be seen in the brain, the spinal cord, the peripheral nerves (the numerous nerves that send messages to the hands, feet, and throughout the body), and the senses. However, an inability to function is not considered a normal part of the aging process.

The weight and size of the brain decrease as a person ages. The ventricles, fluid-filled spaces in the brain, can enlarge and lead to a disorder called **normal pressure hydrocephalus**. People with this condition may have difficulty walking and become incontinent and confused.

Changes also occur in the chemicals of the brain that carry nerve impulses. If a patient is under stress, he may become confused because of these chemical changes. Nerve impulses are slower from the spinal cord to the brain and in the nerves outside the brain and spinal cord, which may lead to delayed responses.

Changes can occur in the **vertebral bodies**, the bones that surround the spinal cord, and the **intervertebral discs**, the material between the vertebral bodies that cushions the spinal column. There can be degeneration of the discs, and the bones can become thin and brittle (a condition known as **osteoporosis**). This may lead to fractures of these bones, causing pain.

Some of the sensory changes include decreased or blurred vision and diminished hearing. Decreased hearing can be from wax in the ear or changes in the structure of the ear.

normal pressure hydrocephalus A disorder caused by enlargement of the ventricles, fluid-filled spaces in the brain

vertebral bodies The bones around the spinal cord

intervertebral discs The material between the vertebral bodies that cushions the spinal column

osteoporosis Condition in which bones become brittle or thin and break easily

The number of taste receptors on the tongue decreases. Nerve endings in fingers and toes may be decreased, leading to changes in the sensation of touch.

AGE-SPECIFIC CONSIDERATIONS

Diseases and conditions of the nervous system require age-related care. Adolescents who have seizure disorders may be concerned with being different. Paraplegia and quadriplegia as a result of accidents, most common in adolescents and the adult ages, have a profound effect on the patients' sense of development, body image, sexuality, and sense of identity. For the elderly, strokes, dementias, and disabling diseases like multiple sclerosis are fraught with fears of helplessness and loss. As a caregiver, allow the patient to help in any way possible with her care. Patience and understanding are very important as the patient learns and/or relearns how to perform self care and adjust to the progressions of their disease.

KEY IDEA

Being aware of possible changes in the nervous system helps the nursing assistant recognize opportunities to assist patients with self-care activities. Recognizing which age-related changes are usual and which are not helps the nursing assistant reassure patients and families and makes it easier to detect problems early.

Common Diseases and Disorders of the Nervous System

- *Bell's palsy:* paralysis or weakness of one side of the face
- *Stroke or cerebrovascular accident (CVA):* reduction of blood supply to the brain due to cerebral thrombosis, cerebral embolism, or intracerebral hemorrhage (see the later section on cerebrovascular accidents)
- *Aphasia:* impairment of the ability to speak and sometimes listen, read, and comprehend
- *Brain tumor:* may be a benign or malignant growth of cells
- *Epilepsy:* a group of neurological disorders with recurrent episodes of convulsions or seizures; an electrical dysfunction of the nerve cells of the brain; may be related to cerebral trauma, infection, tumor, vascular (blood vessel) disturbances, chemical imbalance, or unknown causes
- *Parkinson's disease:* progressive disorder with loss of control of movement; a person walks with a shuffling gait
- *Dementia:* a disorder characterized by confusion, disorientation, a decline in the ability to function, and impaired memory
- *Multiple sclerosis:* chronic progressive disease of the nervous system that begins slowly and progresses throughout the life span but may have periods of remission; it causes fatigue (tiredness) and weakness in legs and arms, which leads to difficulty with daily functioning

- **Shingles (Herpes zoster):** disease characterized by blisters along the course (path) of certain nerves
- **Hemiplegia:** paralysis (loss of motion and sensation) on one side of the body
- **Paraplegia:** paralysis (loss of motion and sensation) on lower part of the body
- **Quadriplegia:** paralysis (loss of motion and sensation) of all four extremities
- **Detached retina:** separation of the sensory retina from the pigment epithelium (layers of cells)
- **Cataracts:** condition in which the crystalline lens of the eye becomes opaque
- **Glaucoma:** increase of pressure within the eye
- **Chronic otitis media:** infection caused by breaks in the eardrum
- **Meniere's disease:** disease that involves the inner ear and causes dizziness
- **Alzheimer's disease:** a disease that is a type of dementia; a person becomes confused and has impaired memory; treatment is to help maintain nutritional status and assist with daily functioning (i.e., toileting, bathing, dressing)

Care of the Seizure Patient

A **seizure** is caused by an abnormality within the central nervous system thought to be an electrical problem or disturbance in the nerve cells or activity of the brain. Seizures can begin at the time of birth or may be the result of cancer (tumor), cerebral trauma (head injury), infection, vascular disturbances, imbalance or abnormality in brain chemistry, cerebrovascular accident (stroke), or unknown causes.

There are three major categories of seizures: partial seizures, generalized seizures, and unclassified epileptic seizures. Under each category there are different types of seizures. Four of the most common types are simple partial seizures, complex partial seizures, absence seizures, and generalized tonic clonic seizures. The length of time each of these seizures lasts can vary greatly.

Simple partial and **complex partial seizures** fall into the broad category of partial seizures. These may also be known as focal or local seizures. During a *simple partial seizure* a patient's level of consciousness is unchanged. The patient may have uncontrolled movements of a body part, hear unusual noises, or see things such as flashing lights. When experiencing a *complex partial seizure*, a patient's level of consciousness changes. The patient will be unaware of anyone's presence. The patient may also have the same type of motor symptoms that are seen in simple partial seizures. A complex partial seizure may start out as a simple partial seizure and become complex.

A generalized seizure can be **convulsive** or nonconvulsive. An absence seizure is a nonconvulsive seizure where a patient's level of consciousness is decreased. There may also be some muscle twitching. A generalized tonic clonic (GTC) seizure is the other major type of seizure in this category. With this type of seizure, a patient will have a loss of consciousness followed by convulsions. She may be incontinent of urine or stool.

In caring for a patient having a seizure, the major role of the nursing assistant is to prevent the patient from being injured. Wherever you are, help the patient lie down. If she is not in bed, carefully help her to the floor. Loosen the clothing and move any equipment or furniture that the patient might bump. Place a pillow or something soft under the head. *Turn the head to the side to promote drainage of saliva or vomitus. Never place anything in the mouth of a patient having a seizure. Objects can break and obstruct the patient's airway. Never try to move or restrain the patient.*

Stay with the patient and pull the emergency signal cord for help. **Observe carefully what the seizure looked like.** Give this information to the nurse. After the seizure, assist the patient to a comfortable position, if possible. The patient may be very sleepy. If she has been incontinent, assist her to clean herself or do this for her if she is unable.

seizure An episode, either partial or generalized, that may include altered consciousness, motor activity, or sensory phenomena or convulsions

simple partial seizure A seizure when the patient is aware of his surroundings but experiences either motor (muscle twitching or movement) or sensory changes (see or hear things not present)

complex partial seizure Seizure with motor and possible sensory symptoms (such as muscle twitching and smelling a foul odor) and a change in the level of consciousness

convulsive Involving convulsions—rhythmic, involuntary contraction of muscles

KEY IDEA

When a patient has a seizure, the nursing assistant's chief role is to protect the patient from injury. In addition, the nursing assistant should observe the patient and give these observations to the nurse.

The Cerebrovascular Accident (Stroke) Patient

A **cerebrovascular accident (CVA)**, or stroke, is a disease or disorder of the circulatory system, but the results affect the nervous system. The term is defined as follows:

- **Cerebro:** dealing with the brain
- **Vascular:** dealing with the blood vessels
- **Accident:** an unpredictable and unexpected occurrence

A cerebrovascular accident occurs when a blocked blood vessel interrupts the blood supply to a part of the brain. When the tissue of the brain is not supplied with blood, which carries oxygen and nutrients, it dies.

The blood supply may be interrupted due to a blood clot or rupture of a blood vessel in the brain. The four main causes of CVA are:

1. **Plaque**, which accumulates in a blood vessel and eventually closes it so that no blood can pass through
2. **Rupture**, meaning a blood vessel breaks open and causes a **hemorrhage** into the brain tissue
3. **Embolus**, that is, a clot that forms elsewhere in the body, travels to the brain through the circulatory system, lodges in a small blood vessel, and causes an obstruction
4. **Thrombus**, meaning a blood clot that remains at the site of its formation

High blood pressure and atherosclerosis increase the risk of cerebrovascular accidents.

Common Results of Cerebrovascular Accidents

The results of a cerebrovascular accident depend on which blood vessel is blocked and where it is located in the brain. Sometimes blood vessels surrounding the damaged area of the brain take over to supply the injured tissues. This is called collateral circulation.

Frequently, following a large stroke, the patient remains paralyzed on one side of the body. This is called **hemiplegia**. The terms *left hemiplegia* or *right hemiplegia* describe the side of the body that is paralyzed. Loss of sensation may also result from the cerebrovascular accident. This includes loss of the ability to feel heat, cold, pressure, and pain in the affected areas.

When the face is involved, an eyelid may droop, or the patient may be unable to close the eyelid. The eye may become dry and irritated because of decreased or absent tearing. The patient may have difficulty chewing and swallowing. There is often an inability to feel the food on the paralyzed side, increasing the risk of burns, choking, and accumulating food inside the cheek. Weakening of the muscles on one side of the face may cause drooling.

plaque Fatty deposits within blood vessels attached to vessel walls

rupture Break open

hemorrhage Excessive bleeding

embolus Blood clot or mass of other undissolved matter that travels through the circulatory system from its place of formation to another site, lodges in a small blood vessel, and causes an obstruction

thrombus A blood clot that remains at its site of formation

hemiplegia Paralysis of one-half of the body

CARING FOR A CEREBROVASCULAR ACCIDENT PATIENT	GUIDELINES	OBRA

- Encourage the patient. Point out the positive aspects of his progress.
- Always show *patience* and *understanding*. A patient can become easily frustrated if he cannot perform a task.
- Use techniques that provide a safe and secure environment.
- To prevent disability:
  - Position the patient in proper alignment.
  - Provide good skin care and repositioning to prevent pressure

areas that contribute to the cause of pressure ulcers.
- Do complete, passive range-of-motion exercises to strengthen muscles and prevent contractures, or assist the patient as he is able with active range-of-motion exercises.
- Encourage a well-balanced diet.
- Prevent withdrawal by treating the patient as a unique person with potential to improve.
- When feeding, place food on the unaffected (not paralyzed) side of the mouth.
- Assist with ambulation if permitted to prevent falls.

- When assisting with dressing, always dress the affected (paralyzed) side first.
- To move the patient from the bed to the wheelchair when one side of the body has been affected by the stroke, position the wheelchair on the unaffected side of the patient's body. This permits the patient to see the wheelchair and lead with the stronger leg.
- Encourage involvement in self-care, allowing the patient to do as much of the care as possible.
- Provide a climate or environment where independence is praised and encouraged. This will give hope and motivation toward rehabilitation and self-care.

Spasm, an involuntary contraction of muscles, may occur in paralyzed limbs. The stimulation of exercise, bathing, or dressing may cause the muscles to spasm into a position of flexion or extension. Spasms are increased by nervous tension, cold temperature, and pain. This greatly increases the risk of **contractures**, if the limb remains fixed in one position.

Paralysis of the arm and leg interferes with the ability to perform all activities of daily living. The inability to move increases the risk of contractures, pressure sores, pneumonia, constipation, blood clots, and urinary retention.

A patient may also develop difficulty speaking or understanding what is being said to them (aphasia). This will be discussed in a later section.

spasm An involuntary sudden movement or convulsive muscular contraction

contracture Drawing together, bunching up, or shortening of muscle tissue because of spasm or paralysis, either permanently or temporarily

Psychological Aspects of Caring for a CVA Patient

When individuals experience a cerebrovascular accident, their lives change suddenly and drastically. The patient and family may grieve for the lost functions of paralyzed limbs, loss of ability to communicate, loss of independence, loss of control over his life, and lost hopes and dreams for the future.

The patient may experience multiple emotions, possibly including denial, anger, depression, acceptance, emotional instability, or overreaction to a stimulus. The patient may burst into tears or laughter for no apparent reason. This is frightening to both the patient and the family.

The loss of the ability to communicate also affects the patient in a variety of ways. Common responses include anger, fear, frustration, depression, and withdrawal.

KEY IDEA

Caring for someone who has experienced a stroke requires enormous patience. The patient and family may be grieving and experiencing difficult emotions. The nursing assistant should provide not only physical care but encouragement and praise, especially for efforts at self-care.

Patients with Aphasia

aphasia Loss of language or speech

Many patients who have a cerebrovascular accident experience **aphasia**—a loss of language. Aphasia occurs most commonly with the right hemiplegic, because, for most people, the language area of the brain is on the left (the hemisphere that controls the right side of the body). The patient may have difficulties in understanding what is heard, using numbers, reading, writing, or speaking. Types of aphasia are receptive (words are not understood), expressive (a patient can't form or express words), or global (difficulty in all areas of speech).

Usually, automatic speech is retained. The patient may sing, swear, or use common phrases like "yes" or "no," even though not used correctly. Words are said automatically.

The most important quality in caring for the aphasic patient is patience. Do not avoid the patient or attempt to anticipate all her needs. Speech may return completely or partially. Use the following techniques for talking with an aphasic patient:

- If the patient is able to read, communicate through writing.
- Allow enough time for a response.
- Trigger the word by saying the first sound. For example, say, "Do you want cr— in your coffee?" If the patient cannot find the word, tell her.

With patience and cooperation, communication may be established. Keys to communication with the aphasic patient should be written into the nursing plan of care or clinical pathway in order to maintain continuity of care on all shifts.

KEY IDEA

Aphasia involves a general loss of language. However, an aphasic patient may retain automatic speech, such as saying yes or no, singing, or cursing. These words and phrases are not used in a conscious way; that is why this speech is called "automatic."

Transient Ischemic Attacks

Transient ischemic attacks (TIAs) are sometimes called *mini strokes*. They occur when there is a partial blockage of a blood vessel that sends blood to part of the brain. Symptoms of a TIA can include a change in vision, weakness in an arm or leg, or aphasia. A TIA generally lasts only 10 to 15 minutes, sometimes longer, but never more than 24 hours. There are no permanent **deficits** following a TIA.

deficit A temporary or permanent negative change in a patient's usual neurologic function

A TIA can alert nurses and physicians to a potential problem with the patient. Therefore, report unusual weakness or changes in a patient's vision or speech.

SUMMARY

This chapter has covered the anatomy and physiology of the nervous system and the care of patients with nervous system disorders. Patients with neurologic conditions have many concerns and needs. The type and amount of assistance necessary to meet these needs will depend on the patient's limitations. The patient and the family should be included in planning and delivering the patient's care whenever possible. Working with neurologic patients will be challenging and will provide a great deal of satisfaction.

NOTES

CHAPTER REVIEW

FILL IN THE BLANK Read each sentence and fill in the blank line with a word that completes the sentence.

1. The nervous system controls and organizes all body movement, including _____ and _____

    types of movement.

2. The cerebrum is divided into two _____.

3. Changes in the external or internal environment strong enough to set up an impulse are called _____.

4. When a patient can only move one-half of his body, he has _____.

5. Loss of language or speech is called _____.

MULTIPLE CHOICE Choose the best answer for each question or statement.

1. The right hemisphere of the brain cerebrum controls
   a. the left side of the body.
   b. the right side of the body.
   c. a person's thought and reasoning ability.
   d. the hypothalamus.

2. The fight-or-flight response is activated
   a. in the parasympathic division of the nervous system.
   b. in the sympathic division of the nervous system.
   c. by the endocrine glands.
   d. None of the above.

3. When caring for a hearing aid,
   a. never wash it under water.
   b. check the batteries.
   c. do not expose it to heat.
   d. All of the above.

4. When caring for a patient who has had a seizure, do all of the following *except*
   a. note what kind of seizure the patient had.
   b. note what the seizure looked like.
   c. turn the patient's head to one side to prevent aspiration.
   d. protect the patient from injury.

5. You are working with a patient with aphasia. All of the following are helpful *except*
   a. communicating through writing.
   b. asking only yes/no questions.
   c. allowing enough time for a response.
   d. triggering the next sound for the patient.

TIME-OUT

TIPS FOR TIME MANAGEMENT

Allow others to give patient care differently than you do. It is easy to feel that your way is the best or right way. However, this is not true. Often, there is more than one right way to perform a task or give patient care. Do not waste your time criticizing others or forcing others to work the way you do.

THE NURSING ASSISTANT IN ACTION

Mr. Joseph is an elderly patient who requires hearing aids. He has just returned from a whirlpool treatment where another staff member was assigned to supervise him. He tells you that no one removed his hearing aid prior to the treatment. Somehow the hearing aid fell into the water while he was in the whirlpool and now it is not working properly.

What Is Your Response/Action?

CRITICAL THINKING

CUSTOMER SERVICE When working with patients who suffer from aphasia, anticipate that they will have difficulty communicating their needs to you. Allow the patient extra time to reply and give positive reinforcement to all efforts made by the patient.

CULTURAL CARE Patients may have variations in how frustrated they feel when trying to carrying out a task they were able to do prior to having a stroke or CVA. Some patients may just give up trying, while others will become angry or annoyed. Many patients are able to recover functioning with time and therapy. Do not expect each patient to handle feelings the same way.

COOPERATION WITHIN THE TEAM When caring for individuals with seizure disorders, it is important to take accurate notes as to how long a seizure lasts and any observations of the patient's movements. If you are the first person to respond in the emergency and are unsure about what to do, ask how you can best assist your coworker. Your coworker can direct you to go find the nurse, call for a doctor, take notes, or time the seizure while she is busy caring for the patient and protecting the patient from harm.

EXPLORE MediaLink

Additional interactive resources for this chapter can be found on the Companion Website at www.prenhall.com/wolgin. Click on Chapter 26 and "Begin" to select the activities for this chapter.

For chapter-related NCLEX-style questions and an audio glossary, access the accompanying CD-ROM in this book.

27 Warm and Cold Applications

KEY TERMS

compress
constrict
cyanosis
dilate
dry application
generalized
generalized application
hyperthermia
hypothermia
inflammation
intermittent
localized
localized application
moist application
sitz bath
soak

OBJECTIVES

When you have completed this chapter, you will be able to:

- Explain the principles of warm and cold applications.
- Explain the reasons warm and cold applications are used.
- Explain the difference between moist and dry applications.
- Explain the difference between generalized and localized applications.
- Demonstrate safe, correct, and comfortable applications.
- Demonstrate the application of the warm compress.
- Demonstrate the application of the warm soak.
- Demonstrate the application of the warm-water bottle.
- Demonstrate the application of the commercial unit heat pack.
- Demonstrate the application of the heat lamp.
- Demonstrate the application of the Aquamatic K-pad.
- Assist a patient with the disposable, portable, or built-in sitz bath.
- Demonstrate the application of the cold compress.
- Demonstrate the application of the cold soak.
- Demonstrate the application of the ice bag, ice cap, or ice collar.
- Demonstrate the application of the commercial unit cold pack.
- Perform the cooling bath.

MediaLink
www.prenhall.com/wolgin

Use the address above to access the free, interactive Companion Website created for this textbook. Get hints, instant feedback, and textbook references to chapter-related NCLEX-style questions. Link to other interesting sites.

AUDIO GLOSSARY:
Use the Companion Website, or the CD-ROM disk enclosed with your textbook, to hear the pronunciation of key terms in the chapter.

Warm and cold applications can decrease discomfort, reduce swelling, and promote the repair and healing of injured tissues or surgical areas. If the procedures are not done correctly, they can cause tissue damage. This chapter will provide you with the information you need to safely apply warm and cold applications.

Principles for Warm and Cold Applications

Blood vessels constrict in response to cold applications and dilate with heat applications (Figure 27–1◆). Heat may be applied to an area of the body to speed up the healing process. Heat **dilates** (expands) the blood vessels in the body and causes more blood to circulate to the injured tissues (Figure 27–2◆). Increased circulation can provide the body tissue with more food and oxygen which are needed for the repair (healing) of body tissue. Warm tub baths, sometimes with medication in the water, are often prescribed for this reason. A **sitz bath** is another example. In this procedure, warm water is applied to the patient's perineal or rectal area to speed healing after childbirth or surgery. Heat may also be applied to an area of the body to ease the pain caused by **inflammation** and congestion. When the blood vessels become dilated, the increased supply of blood may absorb and carry away the fluids that are causing the inflammation and pain. For example, people with certain bone and joint conditions often get relief from pain and can increase the movement of their body parts because of exercises in warm water.

Cold applications cause the blood vessels to **constrict** (Figure 27–3◆). This constriction may help to prevent or reduce swelling, as in the case of a sprained ankle or the beginning of a black eye. The constriction slows down the flow of blood, thereby reducing the amount of body fluids that are carried into the injured area. This may also reduce the pain that usually goes along with the swelling. Cold applications may be applied to control

ALERT

For all patient contact, adhere to Standard Precautions (🔗 Chapter 5, pages 83–85). Wear protective equipment as indicated.

dilate Get bigger; expand

sitz bath A bath in which the patient sits in a specially designed chairtub or a regular bathtub with the hips and buttocks in water

inflammation A reaction of the tissues to disease or injury; there is usually pain, heat, redness, and swelling of the body part

constrict Get narrower

FIGURE 27–1 ◆

Blood vessels constrict in response to cold applications and dilate with heat applications

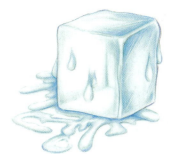

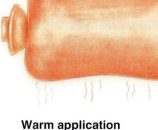

Cold application
Causes blood vessels to contract (get smaller)

Warm application
Causes blood vessels to dilate (get bigger)

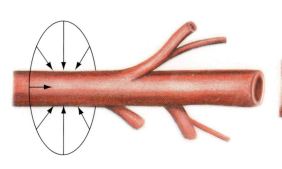

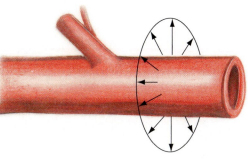

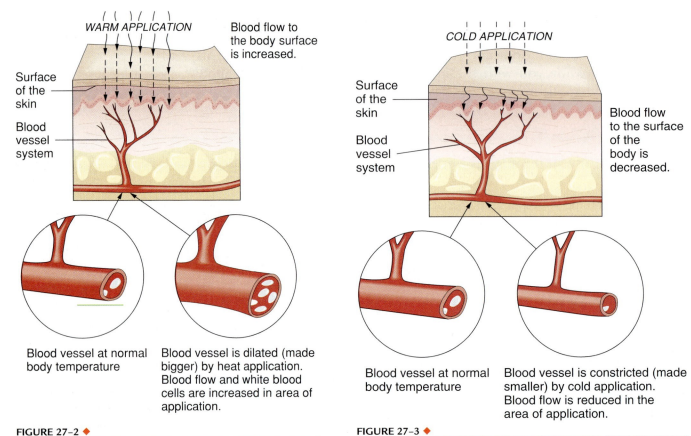

WARM APPLICATION

Blood flow to the body surface is increased.

Surface of the skin

Blood vessel system

Blood vessel at normal body temperature

Blood vessel is dilated (made bigger) by heat application. Blood flow and white blood cells are increased in area of application.

FIGURE 27–2 ◆

Principle of warm application

COLD APPLICATION

Surface of the skin

Blood vessel system

Blood flow to the surface of the body is decreased.

Blood vessel at normal body temperature

Blood vessel is constricted (made smaller) by cold application. Blood flow is reduced in the area of application.

FIGURE 27–3 ◆

Principle of cold application

hyperthermia A higher than normal body temperature

hypothermia A very low body temperature; cooling

bleeding. When cold is applied, the blood flow becomes slower and less blood is able to seep out through a cut or other wounds. For example, when a patient has had a tonsillectomy, an ice collar or ice pack may be applied to the neck region. Cold may be applied to a patient's entire body. This is usually done to lower a patient's body temperature when he or she has a fever or **hyperthermia**. Special equipment such as a **hypothermia** blanket is used to help lower the body temperature.

Moist and Dry Applications

moist application A warm or cold application in which water touches the body

dry application A warm or cold application in which no water touches the skin

All applications are either moist or dry. A **moist application** is one in which water touches the skin. A **dry application** is one in which no water touches the skin. Several types of both moist and dry applications are listed in Table 27–1 ◆.

TABLE 27–1

Types of Moist and Dry Applications

MOIST	DRY
Cool wet packs	Aquamatic K-pad
Compress: warm or cold	Commercial unit cold pack
Sitz bath	Commercial unit warm pack
Soak: warm or cold	Electric heat cradle
Tub bath	Heat lamp
	Hypothermia blankets
	Ice cap and ice collar
	Warm-water bottle

Compresses and soaks are both moist applications and can be either warm or cold. A **compress** is a localized application. A **soak** can be either localized or generalized. In applying a compress, a cloth is dipped into water, wrung out, and applied to the skin. To apply a soak, you immerse the body or body part completely in water. Warm-water bottles, ice caps, and Aquamatic K-pads are considered dry applications because they have a dry surface. Water is used only inside the equipment and never touches the skin. Warm dry applications are sometimes used to keep warm moist applications at the correct temperature (Table 27–2◆).

compress Folded piece of cloth used to apply pressure, moisture, heat, cold, or medication to a specific part of the body

soak Immerse the body or body part completely in water

KEY IDEA

The length of time an application is applied is a serious issue. Skin damage may result with misuse of application. Follow your immediate supervisor's instructions as to the exact time to begin the application and how long the application is to stay in place.

Keeping the Patient Safe and Comfortable

Be sure you know exactly where on the patient's body the warmth or cold is to be applied. A **generalized application** is one in which a warm or cold application is applied to a patient's whole body. A **localized application** is one that is applied to a specific part or area of a patient's body. Check the application often to keep it at the right temperature throughout the treatment. Suggested times for checking the temperatures of different kinds of applications are:

- Soaks and **intermittent** compresses: every 5 minutes
- Heat lamps: every 5 minutes

generalized Affecting, involving, or pertaining to the whole body

generalized application A warm or cold application applied to the entire body

localized Limited to one place or part; affecting, involving, or pertaining to a definite area

localized application A warm or cold application applied to a specific area or small part of the body

intermittent Alternating; stopping and beginning again

TABLE 27–2

Dry Heat Application

APPLICATION	USE	PRECAUTIONS
Infrared lamp	Provides heat to skin surface or mucous membrane	Be aware that heat penetrates only 3 mm of body tissue
Heat cradle	Supplies heat to abdomen, perineum, or chest	Use only 25-watt bulbs Ensure that temperature inside cradle does not exceed 125°F
Aquathermic pad	Supplies heat to small body part or to portions of back	Ensure that temperature does not exceed 105°F Do not secure with safety pins
Healing pad*	Supplies heat to any body surface	Do not secure with safety pins as could cause shock if wire were hit Set temperature control on medium

*Generally not used in hospitals due to safety problems (i.e., burns and electrical malfunctions).

SAFELY APPLYING COLD AND HEAT

GUIDELINES

- Avoid accidents.
- Be careful not to spill any water.
- Be sure electrical equipment does not come into contact with water.
- Be sure your hands are dry before touching electrical equipment.
- Be sure the bed is properly protected; put the side rails in the upright position if needed.

TABLE 27–3

Temperature Ranges

TEMPERATURE	CENTIGRADE (C)	FAHRENHEIT (F)
Cold	10–18°C degrees	50–65°F
Cool	19–27°C	65–80°F
Tepid	28–34°C	80–93°F
Warm	35–37°C	93–98°F
Hot	38–41°C	98–106°F
Very hot	42–46°C	107–115°F

- Ask your supervisor or an RN for direction if you are unsure how to operate any piece of equipment or commercial product. Review and follow your agency's policy for safe temperature ranges or settings (Table 27–3◆). Temperature ranges can vary slightly. Follow your agency's policy and carefully read the thermometer used.
- Be aware that older adults, infants, young children, persons with poor circulation, or those with diabetes are less able to tolerate cold or hot applications. The ordered application temperature will be less cold or warmer rather than hot for these individuals or others at risk.
- Cover cold or dry heat applications per policy with a cloth, flannel cover, towel, or pillowcase before applying it to the ordered site.
- Treatments should not be left on the patient longer than 20 minutes unless ordered differently. If this is the first ordered treatment, stay with or observe the patient's skin after 3–5 minutes to see how he is tolerating the treatment.
- Check the patient's skin under warm applications (Figure 27–4◆); watch for too much redness.
- Look for a dark discoloration, which might mean the patient is being burned.
- Listen when the patient complains.
- If you think that a patient is being burned, remove the heat application and report to your immediate supervisor at once.
- Check the patient's skin where cold is being applied. If the area appears to be blanched, very pale, white or bluish, tell you immediate supervisor at once.
- Watch for changes in color of parts of the patient's body. For example, if the patient's lips, fingernails, or eyelids look blue or turn a dark color, this is **cyanosis**, which is a sign of less oxygen getting to that part of the body. Stop the treatment immediately and report to your immediate supervisor.
- Always apply the ice cap and warm-water bottle with its metal or plastic stopper away from the patient's body. The stopper should never touch the patient's skin. It will be much warmer or colder than the application and could burn or freeze the patient's skin.
- You may be working with an unconscious patient. If so, you may be directed to protect him by putting a blanket between the skin and the warm-water bottle or ice cap.

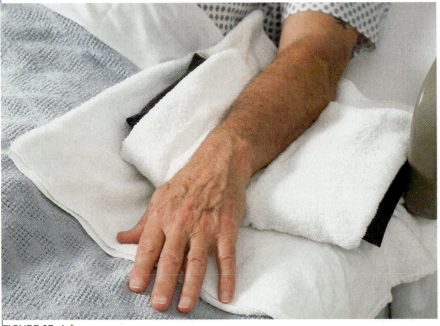

FIGURE 27–4 ◆
Check the patient's skin for redness or discoloration, signs the patient is being burned

KEY IDEA

Some patients may not complain when being burned or frozen, because they have no feeling in the body area where the application is applied. Such a situation may be due to a disease process.

Keeping the Patient Comfortable

Make sure the patient is in a position that is comfortable for him and convenient for your work. Keep the patient covered and warm during the treatment. Otherwise, the patient might become chilled and uncomfortable. If a patient shivers during the cold application, stop the treatment. Cover him with a blanket. Then report this at once to your immediate supervisor who will tell you what to do.

Be aware that the weight of the ice bag/warm-water bottle may increase the pain of the injured area. Never fill a warm-water bottle or ice bag more than half full. It gets too heavy.

Always dry the bottle or bag. Check it for leaks by turning it upside down. Place it in a flannel cover or a cloth case. Never let the patient lie on an uncovered warm-water bottle or ice bag.

cyanosis When the skin looks blue or gray, especially on the lips, nailbeds, and under the fingernails. In a black patient, it may appear as a darkening of color. This occurs when there is not enough oxygen in the blood

Heat Applications

In some institutions warm compresses are made by holding a cloth under running warm water or by microwaving a wet cloth. Sterile compresses are used in situations where there is an open wound or area of the body vulnerable to infection, for example, the eyes. If you are instructed to do this, be careful that you do not apply too much heat. Follow the instructions of your immediate supervisor.

APPLYING THE WARM COMPRESS (MOIST HEAT APPLICATIONS)

PROCEDURE

OBRA

RATIONALE: Heat applications are used to relieve pain, relax muscles, reduce tissue swelling, or decrease joint stiffness.

PREPARATION

1. Assemble your equipment:
   a. Disposable bed protector
   b. Basin
   c. Pitcher of water (98°F; 37°C)
   d. Washcloth, towel, or gauze pads (compress)
   e. Bath thermometer, if available
   f. Large sheet of plastic
   g. Bath towel
   h. Bath blanket
   i. Disposable gloves if any potential exists for exposure to body fluids

2. Identify the patient by checking the identification bracelet.

3. Wash your hands.

4. Tell the patient you are going to apply a warm compress.

5. Provide privacy for the patient.

6. Raise the bed to a comfortable working position.

STEPS

7. Help the patient into a comfortable, safe position. Have the body area exposed for application of a warm compress.

8. Place a disposable bed protector under the body area that is to be given the warm compress.

9. Fill the pitcher with warm water. Check the temperature of the water with a bath thermometer (98°F or 37°C). Then pour the water into the basin.

10. Dip the compress into the water and wring it out thoroughly. Apply gloves if soaks will be applied to any area where exposure to body fluid could occur.

11. Apply the compress gently to the proper area (Figure 27-5◆).

12. Wrap the entire area with a large towel or a blue pad, covering the

PROCEDURE *(continued)*

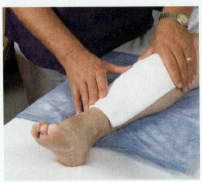

FIGURE 27–5 ◆
Apply the compress

wet compress. Cover the entire area, compress, and towel with a plastic sheet (Figure 27–6a–b◆). Be sure the plastic does not touch the patient's skin. This will keep the compress warm.

13. If the patient is cold or chilly, cover him with a blanket.

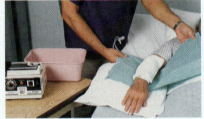

FIGURE 27–6a ◆
Wrap entire area with a towel or blue pad

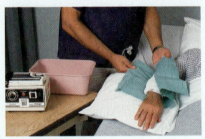

FIGURE 27–6b ◆
Cover with a plastic sheet or blue pad

14. Change the compress and re-moisten it, as necessary, to keep it warm. Sometimes a patient is able to apply the compress himself. If your immediate supervisor gives permission for this, position and assist the patient as necessary.

15. Check the skin under the application every 5 minutes. If the skin appears red, remove the compress. Cover the area with a towel or blanket. Report this to your immediate supervisor.

16. A warm compress is usually applied for 15 to 20 minutes. However, follow the instructions given to you by your immediate supervisor as to how long the warm compress is to be applied.

17. After the treatment is completed, remove the compress and gently pat the area dry with a towel.

FOLLOW-UP

18. Make the patient comfortable and replace the call light.

19. Lower the bed to a position of safety.

20. Raise the side rail when ordered or appropriate for patient safety.

21. Clean standard equipment and put it in its proper place. Discard disposable equipment and gloves if used.

22. Wash your hands.

23. Report to your immediate supervisor:

   ■ The time the warm compress was started.

   ■ How long the compress was in place.

   ■ The area of application.

   ■ How the patient tolerated the procedure.

   ■ Your observations of anything unusual.

CHARTING EXAMPLE: 12/09/04 11am Warm compress applied on Mr. Jasper's left forearm for 20 minutes. Mr. Jasper said the compress reduced his pain. C. Gentile, CNA

APPLYING THE WARM SOAK (MOIST WARM APPLICATION)

PROCEDURE   OBRA

RATIONALE: Moist heat applications provide penetrating heat to relieve pain, relax muscles, reduce tissue swelling, or decrease joint stiffness.

AGE-SPECIFIC CONSIDERATIONS

In adolescent patients, this is a time of concern over privacy. Be sure to take extra care to maintain an adolescent's privacy. This will increase their comfort and cooperation with the procedure. For geriatric patients, monitor the temperature of the soaks carefully. The aging process often results in a thinning of the skin, increasing the potential for burns. For patients of all ages, be very careful of treatments involving water. Leaking and melting bags or bottles lead to an increased potential for slipping and falling.

PROCEDURE *(continued)*

PREPARATION

1. Assemble your equipment:

   a. Basin, foot tub, or arm basin

   b. Bath thermometer

   c. Disposable bed protector

   d. Bath towel

   e. Bath blanket

   f. Disposable gloves, if any potential exists for exposure to body fluids

2. Identify the patient by checking the identification bracelet.

3. Wash your hands.

4. Tell the patient you are going to apply a warm soak.

5. Provide privacy for the patient.

6. Raise the bed to a comfortable working position.

STEPS

7. Help the patient into a safe, comfortable position. Expose the area to be treated.

8. Fill the basin one-half full with warm water (98°F; 37°C). Check the temperature with a bath thermometer. Apply gloves if soaks will be applied to any area where exposure to body fluids could occur.

9. Place a disposable bed protector under the body area that is to receive the soak.

10. Place the basin in a position so the patient's arm, leg, foot, or hand can be dipped into the basin easily.

11. Place the patient's arm or leg into the water gradually.

12. Check the temperature of the water every 5 minutes. When you need to change the water, take the patient's arm, foot, or leg out of the basin. Wrap it with a bath blanket or bath towel to keep it warm.

13. If the patient says he feels weak or cold, stop the treatment. Cover the patient with extra blankets and report this to your immediate supervisor.

14. Check the skin every 5 minutes. If the skin is red, stop the treatment. Report this to your immediate supervisor.

15. When the treatment is finished, dry the patient's arm or leg by patting gently with a towel.

FOLLOW-UP

16. Make the patient comfortable and replace the call light.

17. Lower the bed to a position of safety.

18. Raise the side rails when ordered or appropriate for patient safety.

19. Clean standard equipment and put it in its proper place. Discard disposable equipment and gloves, if used.

20. Wash your hands.

21. Report to your immediate supervisor:

   - The time the warm soak was started.

   - The length of treatment.

   - The area of application.

   - How the patient tolerated the procedure.

   - Your observations of anything unusual.

CHARTING EXAMPLE: 12/19/04 11am Soaked Mr. Jasper's left forearm in warm water for 20 minutes. Mr. Jasper said the soak felt good and reduced his pain. C. Gentile, CNA

APPLYING THE WARM-WATER BOTTLE (DRY HEAT APPLICATION)

PROCEDURE   OBRA

RATIONALE: Dry heat applications are used for longer periods of time to relieve pain, relax muscles, reduce tissue swelling, or decrease joint stiffness.

PREPARATION

1. Assemble your equipment:

   a. Warm-water bottle (may be disposable)

   b. Pitcher of warm water (98°F; 37°C). Note: Temperature for unresponsive adults and children is usually less (93°F to 97° F; 34°C to 36.8°C). If warm-water bottle is disposable, follow your institution's policies for the correct temperature of the water.

   c. Bath thermometer

   d. Flannel cover (or whatever type of cover is used in your institution)

2. Identify the patient by checking the identification bracelet.

3. Wash your hands.

4. Tell the patient you are going to apply a warm-water bottle.

5. Provide privacy for the patient.

6. Raise the bed to a comfortable working position.

STEPS

7. Fill the pitcher with water (98°F; 37°C). Check the temperature with a bath thermometer.

8. Fill the warm-water bottle half full of water (Figure 27–7◆).

PROCEDURE *(continued)*

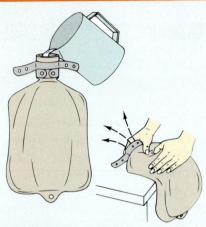

FIGURE 27–7 ◆

Fill bottle half full with warm water. Press excess air out of bag, then close the bag

9. Two methods of squeezing the air out of the bottle are:

- **Method A.** Place the bag on the edge of a counter. Have the part of the bag containing the water hanging down. Place the part of the bag without the water lying on the counter top. Put your hand on the top of the bag at the edge of the counter. Move your hand slowly toward the opening of the bag, pressing out the air. With the other hand, close the bag (see Figure 27–7).

- **Method B.** Place the warm-water bottle in a horizontal position on a flat surface. Hold the neck of the warm-water bottle upright until you can see water in the neck of the bottle. The water squeezes out the air.

10. Fasten the top tightly.

11. Dry the warm-water bottle. Check for leaks by turning it upside down.

12. Place the warm-water bottle in the type of cover used in your institution (Figure 27–8◆).

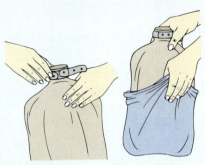

FIGURE 27–8 ◆

Place the warm water bottle in a cover

13. Help the patient into a safe, comfortable position. Expose the area to be treated. Apply the bottle gently to the proper body area (Figure 27–9◆). Use a pillow to support the bottle against the body area if necessary to keep it positioned.

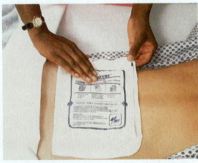

FIGURE 27–9 ◆

Apply the heat package or covered bottle to the proper area

14. Never place the warm-water bottle on top of a painful area. The weight will increase the pain. Place it on the side.

15. Check the warm-water bottle every hour to be sure the temperature is correct. Change the water in the bottle, when necessary, to continue the treatment at the same temperature.

16. Check the skin under the warm-water bottle after the first 5 minutes and then every hour. If the skin is red, remove the warm-water bottle and report to your immediate supervisor.

FOLLOW-UP

17. Clean standard equipment and put it in its proper place. Discard disposable equipment.

18. Make the patient comfortable and replace the call light.

19. Lower the bed to a position of safety.

20. Raise the side rails when ordered or appropriate for patient safety.

21. Wash your hands.

22. Report to your immediate supervisor:

- The time the warm-water bottle was applied.

- The length of treatment.

- The area of application.

- How the patient tolerated the procedure.

- Your observations of anything unusual.

CHARTING EXAMPLE: 12/19/04 11am Warm-water bottled applied on Mr. Jasper's left forearm for 20 minutes. Mr. Jasper said the heat reduced his pain. C. Gentile, CNA

APPLYING THE COMMERCIAL UNIT HEAT PACK (MOIST WARM APPLICATION)

RATIONALE: Heat applications are used to relieve pain, relax muscles, reduce tissue swelling, or decrease joint stiffness.

PREPARATION

1. Assemble your equipment:

   a. Commercial unit, single-use heat pack that has been warmed in the heating lamp unit; follow manufacturer's instructions

   b. Disposable bed protectors

   c. Bath blanket

   d. Gloves, if indicated

2. Identify the patient by checking the identification bracelet.

3. Wash your hands.

4. Tell the patient you are going to apply a warm pack.

5. Provide privacy for the patient.

PROCEDURE

6. Raise the bed to a comfortable working position. Apply gloves if indicated.

STEPS

7. Help the patient into a safe, comfortable position. Expose the area to be treated.

8. Place the bed protector under the body part that is to receive the warm pack.

9. Tear the foil covering from the warm pack.

10. Place the moist warm pack on the proper body area.

11. Cover the pack with the sheet of plastic or the disposable bed protector. This will keep the pack warm.

12. Check the skin under the application every 5 minutes. If the skin appears red, remove the pack and cover the area with a blanket. Report this to your immediate supervisor.

13. Follow the instructions of your immediate supervisor as to the length of application. Replace with a new warm pack as necessary.

FOLLOW-UP

14. When the treatment is finished, discard disposable equipment and gloves, if used.

15. Make the patient comfortable and replace the call light.

16. Lower the bed to a position of safety.

17. Raise the side rails when ordered or appropriate for patient safety.

18. Wash your hands.

19. Report to your immediate supervisor:

   - The time the warm pack was applied.
   - The length of treatment.
   - The area of application.
   - How the patient tolerated the procedure.
   - Your observations of anything unusual.

CHARTING EXAMPLE: 12/19/04 10am Heat pack applied on Mr. Jasper's left forearm for 20 minutes. Mr. Jasper said the heat reduced his pain. C. Gentile, CNA

APPLYING A HEAT LAMP (DRY WARM APPLICATION)

RATIONALE: Dry heat applications are used to relieve pain, promote healing, reduce tissue swelling, or decrease joint stiffness.

PREPARATION

1. Assemble your equipment:

   a. Heat lamp

PROCEDURE — OBRA

   b. Bath blanket

   c. Bath towel

   d. Tape measure

2. Identify the patient by checking the identification bracelet.

3. Wash your hands.

4. Tell the patient you are going to apply heat with a heat lamp.

5. Provide privacy for the patient.

6. Raise the bed to a comfortable working position.

7. Help the patient into a safe, comfortable position.

8. Expose only the body area that is to receive the heat. Drape the patient so that heat is directed to the proper area of the skin. Cover the rest of the patient's body with a bath blanket, sheet, or towel.

9. Check the electric cord to be sure it is in good condition and there are no frayed areas.

10. Plug in the lamp with the lamp turned off.

PROCEDURE *(continued)*

STEPS

11. Position the lamp so that heat will be directed to the proper skin area.

12. The part of the patient's body that is being treated should be at least 18 inches away from the heat lamp. Use a tape measure to check the distance.

13. Turn on the lamp. Be sure it is working properly.

14. Check the skin after 3 minutes. If the patient's skin becomes red, stop the treatment and report to your immediate supervisor.

15. There is a danger of fire when a heat lamp is being used. Therefore, keep all linen away from the lamp. Do not drape or cover the lamp. A cover on the lamp may catch fire. Tell patient to remain in position and not to touch the bulb of the heat lamp.

16. Leave the heat lamp on the patient from 5 to no more than 10 minutes, unless you have other instructions from your immediate supervisor.

FOLLOW-UP

17. After treatment is completed, unplug and remove the lamp.

18. Make the patient comfortable and replace the call light.

19. Lower the bed to a position of safety.

20. Raise the side rails when ordered or appropriate for patient safety.

21. Wipe the lamp with disinfectant solution and put it back in its proper place.

22. Wash your hands.

23. Report to your immediate supervisor:

- The time the heat was applied.
- The length of treatment.
- The area of application.
- How the patient tolerated the procedure.
- Your observations of anything unusual.

CHARTING EXAMPLE: 12/29/04 10am Heat lamp treatment given to Mrs. Drake for 10 minutes. She said the heat reduced her discomfort. C. Gentile, CNA

PROCEDURE

APPLYING THE AQUAMATIC HYDRO-THERMAL (K-PAD) (DRY HEAT APPLICATION)

OBRA

RATIONALE: Dry heat applications are used to relieve pain, promote healing, reduce tissue swelling, or decrease joint stiffness.

PREPARATION

1. Assemble your equipment (Figure 27–10a–b◆):

   a. Aquamatic Hydro-Thermal (K-pad) and control unit. (The temperature is preset by the central supply room. The container is filled with distilled water by central supply, or available in supply room.)

   b. Cover for pad (pillowcase, flannel cover, or cover from manufacturer)

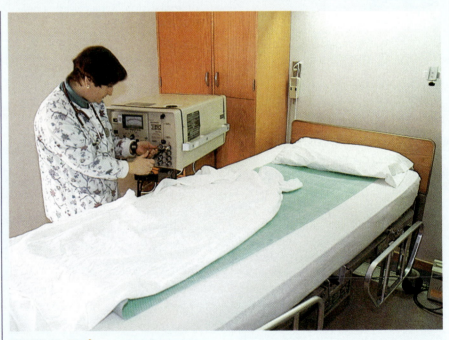

FIGURE 27–10a ◆
Aquamatic pads come in many different sizes and brand names. The pad should be covered before applying to the skin

PROCEDURE *(continued)*

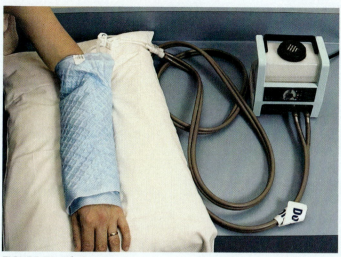

FIGURE 27–10b ◆
Aquamatic pad

2. Identify the patient by checking the identification bracelet.

3. Wash your hands.

4. Tell the patient you are going to apply the K-pad.

5. Provide privacy for the patient.

6. Raise the bed to a comfortable working position.

7. Help the patient into a safe, comfortable position. Expose the area to be treated.

8. Inspect the K-pad for leaks and make sure the cord and plug are in good condition.

9. Plug the cord into an electrical outlet.

10. Place the pad in the cover. *Do not use any pins!*

STEPS

11. Place the container on the bedside table. Arrange the tubing at the level of the pad. Do not allow the tubing to hang below the level of the bed.

12. Gently apply the pad in its cover to the proper dry body area.

13. Check the skin under the pad. Follow the instructions of your immediate supervisor as to how frequently to check the skin and the length of the application.

FOLLOW-UP

14. When the treatment is finished, return the equipment to its proper place.

15. Make the patient comfortable and replace the call light.

16. Lower the bed to a position of safety.

17. Raise the side rails when ordered or appropriate for patient safety.

18. Wash your hands.

19. Report to your immediate supervisor:

   - The time the K-pad was applied.
   - The length of treatment.
   - The area of application.
   - How the patient tolerated the procedure.
   - Your observations of anything unusual.

CHARTING EXAMPLE: 12/19/04 10am Aquathermia pad set at 98°F and applied on Mr. Jordan's back for 20 minutes. Mr. Jordan said the pad helped to reduce his pain. C. Gentile, CNA

USING THE DISPOSABLE SITZ BATH (MOIST WARM APPLICATION)

RATIONALE: Moist warm heat applications are used to relieve pain, promote healing, or reduce tissue swelling.

PROCEDURE   OBRA

PREPARATION

1. Assemble your equipment:

   a. Disposable sitz bath kit (Figure 27–11◆):
      - Plastic bowl with a large brim
      - Water bag
      - Tubing and stopcock (clamp)
   b. Plastic laundry bag

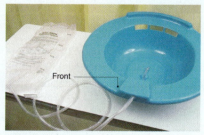

FIGURE 27–11 ◆
Disposable sitz bath kit

PROCEDURE *(continued)*

c. Bath thermometer

d. Bath towels

e. Pitcher of warm water (98°F; 37°C)

2. Identify the patient by checking the identification bracelet.

3. Wash your hands.

4. Tell the patient you are going to give him a sitz bath.

5. Provide privacy for the patient.

6. Help the patient to put on his slippers and robe.

STEPS

7. Help the patient into the bathroom.

8. Raise the toilet seat.

9. Check the temperature of the water with the bath thermometer. It should be 98°F (37°C).

10. Put the plastic bowl into the toilet bowl. Be sure that the opening for overflow is toward the front of the toilet.

11. Pour the water into the bowl, filling it half full.

12. Close the stopcock on the tubing. Fill the water bag with water (98°F; 37°C) from the pitcher. Close the bag.

13. Hang the container for water 12 inches higher than the bowl.

14. Help the patient remove his robe and pajamas and sit down into the sitz bath. Be sure the patient can reach the signal cord.

15. Place the tubing inside the bowl with the opening of the tube under the water level. The tube fits into a little groove in the front of the basin.

16. Open the stopcock and adjust the flow if necessary.

17. Have the patient sit in the sitz bath with water running in for from 10 to 20 minutes, as instructed by your immediate supervisor.

18. If the patient says he feels weak or faint, stop the treatment. Turn on the signal light if you need help getting the patient out of the bathroom.

19. When the treatment is finished, remove the tubing. Help the patient out of the sitz bath.

20. Pat the patient's body gently with a towel to dry.

21. Help the patient back into bed.

FOLLOW-UP

22. Make the patient comfortable and replace the call light.

23. Lower the bed to a position of safety.

24. Raise the side rails when ordered or appropriate for patient safety.

25. Clean your equipment and return it to its proper place. Discard disposable equipment.

26. Bag and dispose of the dirty towels in the laundry hamper.

27. Wash your hands.

28. Report to your immediate supervisor:

   ■ The time the sitz bath was started.

   ■ The length of time the patient was in the sitz bath.

   ■ How the patient tolerated the procedure.

   ■ Your observations of anything unusual.

CHARTING EXAMPLE: 12/19/04 10am Sitz bath treatment at 98°F given to Mrs. Black for 20 minutes. She said the treatment helped to reduce her episiotomy pain. C. Gentile, CNA

USING THE PORTABLE CHAIR-TYPE OR BUILT-IN SITZ BATH (MOIST WARM APPLICATION)

RATIONALE: Moist warm heat applications are used to relieve pain, promote healing, or reduce tissue swelling.

PROCEDURE

PREPARATION

1. Assemble your equipment:

   a. Portable chair or built-in sitz bath (Figure 27-12◆)

   b. Disinfectant cleaner

   c. Bath towels

   d. Bath blanket

   e. Bath thermometer

   f. Plastic laundry bag

   g. Disposable gloves

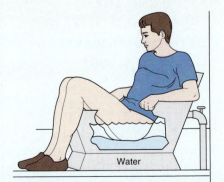

FIGURE 27-12◆
Patient using a built-in sitz bath

PROCEDURE (continued)

2. Clean the sitz bath with disinfectant cleanser and rinse it well.

3. Identify the patient by checking the identification bracelet.

4. Wash your hands.

5. Tell the patient you are going to give him a sitz bath.

6. Provide privacy for the patient.

STEPS

7. Bring the portable, chair-type sitz bath into the patient's room. Or help the patient (using a wheelchair if necessary) into the bathroom with the built-in chair-type sitz bath.

8. Fill it half full with water (98°F; 37°C).

9. Place a towel on the seat and on the front edge of the sitz bath. Apply gloves.

10. Help the patient undress, except for his gown and slippers.

11. Help the patient to sit down in the tub. Hold his gown up so it does not get wet.

12. Cover the patient's shoulders with a bath blanket if he complains of being cold.

13. Continue the treatment for 10 to 20 minutes, unless you have other instructions from your immediate supervisor.

14. Check the patient every 5 minutes.

15. If the patient feels weak or faint, stop the treatment. Turn on the signal light for help in getting the patient out of the tub. Let the water out of the tub.

16. When the treatment is finished, help the patient out of the tub.

17. Pat his body gently with a towel to dry.

18. Help the patient back into bed.

FOLLOW-UP

19. Make the patient comfortable and replace the call light.

20. Lower the bed to a position of safety.

21. Raise the side rails when ordered or appropriate for patient safety.

22. Clean the sitz tub with disinfectant cleanser.

23. Put the portable, chair-type tub back in its proper place.

24. Bag and dispose of the dirty towels in the laundry hamper.

25. Dispose of gloves. Wash your hands.

26. Report to your immediate supervisor:
    - The time the sitz bath was started.
    - The length of time the patient was in the sitz bath.
    - How the patient tolerated the procedure.
    - Your observations of anything unusual.

CHARTING EXAMPLE: 12/04/04 10am Portable sitz bath given for 20 minutes at 98°F to Mr. Bliss. His hemorrhoids are healing well. M. Pope, CNA

Cold Applications

| APPLYING THE COLD COMPRESS (MOIST COLD APPLICATION) | PROCEDURE | OBRA |

RATIONALE: Cold applications, which decrease circulation and bleeding, are used to treat sprains and fractures by reducing pain and tissue swelling.

PREPARATION

1. Assemble your equipment:
   a. Disposable bed protector
   b. Basin
   c. Washcloth, towel, or gauze pads (compress)
   d. Bath towel
   e. Bath blanket
   f. Pitcher of cold water (ice cubes, if ordered by your immediate supervisor)

2. Identify the patient by checking the identification bracelet.

3. Wash your hands.

4. Tell the patient you are going to apply a cold compress.

5. Provide privacy for the patient.

6. Raise the bed to a comfortable working position.

7. Help the patient into a comfortable, safe position. Expose the area to be treated.

STEPS

8. Place a disposable bed protector under the body area that is to be given the cold compress.

9. Put cold water in the basin (ice cubes only if ordered).

PROCEDURE (continued)

10. Dip the compress into the water and wring it out thoroughly.

11. Apply the compress gently to the proper area of the patient's body as quickly as possible. If you are slow, the compress will absorb heat from your hands and the air (Figure 27–13◆).

12. If the patient is cold or chilly, cover him with a blanket. Do not cover the compress or the area being treated.

13. Change the compress and re-moisten it, as necessary, to keep it cold. Sometimes a patient is able to apply the compress himself. If your immediate supervisor gives permission for this, position and assist the patient as necessary.

14. Check the skin under the application every 5 minutes. If the skin appears to be blanched or white, remove the compress. Cover the area with a towel or blanket. Report this to your head nurse or team leader.

15. A cold compress is usually applied for 15 to 20 minutes. However, follow the instructions of your immediate supervisor.

16. When the treatment is finished, remove the compress and gently pat the area dry with a towel.

FOLLOW-UP

17. Make the patient comfortable and replace the call light.

18. Lower the bed to a position of safety.

19. Raise the side rails when ordered or appropriate for patient safety.

20. Clean your equipment and put it in its proper place. Discard disposable equipment.

21. Wash your hands.

22. Report to your immediate supervisor:

   ■ The time the cold compress was started.

   ■ How long it remained in place.

   ■ The area of application.

   ■ How the patient tolerated the procedure.

   ■ Your observations of anything unusual.

CHARTING EXAMPLE: 12/19/04 10am Cold compress applied on Mr. Jenkins's right lower leg for 20 minutes. Mr. Jenkins's said the cold helped to decrease his pain. C. Gentile, CNA

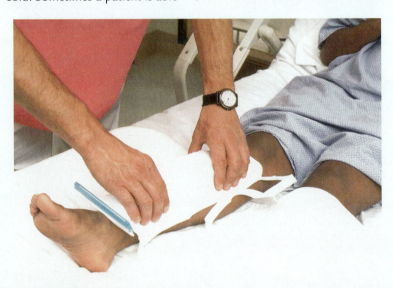

FIGURE 27–13 ◆
Apply compress to body area

APPLYING THE COLD SOAK (MOIST COLD APPLICATION)

PROCEDURE

OBRA

PREPARATION

1. Assemble your equipment:

   a. Basin, foot tub, or arm basin

   b. Disposable bed protector

   c. Washcloth, towel, or gauze pads (compress)

   d. Bath towel

   e. Bath blanket

   f. Gloves if indicated

2. Identify the patient by checking the identification bracelet.

3. Wash your hands and apply gloves if indicated.

4. Tell the patient you are going to apply a cold soak.

RATIONALE: Cold applications, which decrease circulation and bleeding, are used to treat sprains and fractures by reducing pain and tissue swelling.

PROCEDURE *(continued)*

5. Provide privacy for the patient.

6. Raise the bed to a comfortable working position.

7. Help the patient into a safe, comfortable position. Expose the area to be treated.

STEPS

8. Fill the basin half full with cold water (Figure 27–14◆).

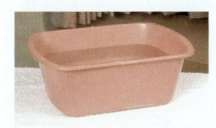

FIGURE 27–14 ◆
Fill the basin half full with water

9. Place a disposable bed protector under the body area that is to receive the cold soak.

10. Place the basin in a position so that the patient's arm, leg, foot, or hand can be dipped into the basin easily (Figure 27–15◆).

11. Gradually place the patient's arm or leg into the water.

12. When you have to change the water, take the patient's arm or leg out of the basin. Wrap it with a bath towel or bath blanket for comfort.

13. If the patient says he feels weak or cold, stop the treatment. Cover the patient with extra blankets and report this to your immediate supervisor.

14. Check the skin every 5 minutes. If the skin is blanched or white, stop the treatment. Report to your immediate supervisor.

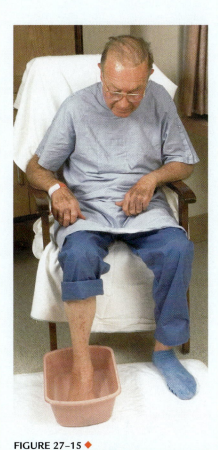

FIGURE 27–15 ◆
Place basin in position for patient to easily dip foot in it

15. When the treatment is finished, dry the patient's arm or leg by gently patting with a towel.

FOLLOW-UP

16. Make the patient comfortable and replace the call light.

17. Lower the bed to a position of safety.

18. Raise the side rails when ordered or appropriate for patient safety.

19. Clean standard equipment and put it in its proper place. Discard disposable equipment and gloves, if used.

20. Wash your hands.

21. Report to your immediate supervisor:

   - The time the cold soak was started.
   - The length of treatment.
   - The area of application.
   - How the patient tolerated the procedure.
   - Your observations of anything unusual.

CHARTING EXAMPLE: 12/19/04 10am Cold soak given to Mr. Perkins's right foot for 20 minutes. Mr. Perkins's said the cold helped to decrease his foot pain. The foot is still swollen and bruised. C. Gentile, CNA

APPLYING THE ICE BAG, ICE CAP, OR ICE COLLAR (DRY COLD APPLICATION)

PROCEDURE

OBRA

RATIONALE: Dry cold applications, which decrease circulation and bleeding, are used to treat sprains and fractures by reducing pain and tissue swelling.

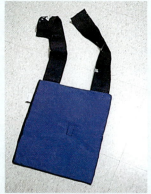

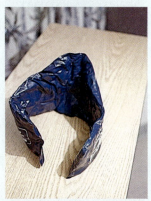

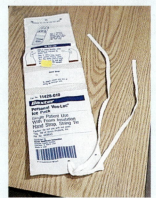

FIGURE 27–16 ◆

Examples of ice bag, ice collar and ice pack

PREPARATION

1. Assemble your equipment:

   a. Ice bag, ice cap, or ice collar (may be disposable) (Figure 27–16◆)

   b. Flannel cover (or whatever type of cover is used in your institution)

   c. Ice in a clean container

   d. Bath blanket

   e. Gloves, if indicated

2. Identify the patient by checking the identification bracelet.

3. Wash your hands. Apply gloves if indicated.

4. Tell the patient you are going to apply the ice bag, ice cap, or ice collar.

5. Provide privacy for the patient.

6. Raise the bed to a comfortable working position.

7. Help the patient into a safe, comfortable position. Expose the area to be treated.

8. Pour cold water over the ice to melt the sharp edges.

9. Fill the ice collar, ice bag, or ice cap one-half full of ice (Figure 27–17 ◆).

10. Squeeze the sides of the ice bag to force the air out of it.

11. Fasten the stopper tightly.

12. Dry the outside of the ice bag with a paper towel.

13. Invert the ice bag to test for leaking.

14. Place the ice bag into the type of cover used in your institution.

STEPS

15. Apply the ice bag to the proper area of the patient's body.

16. If the patient is cold or chilly, cover him with a blanket. Do not cover the ice bag or the area being treated.

17. Follow the instructions of your immediate supervisor as to the length of application. Replace the ice as necessary.

18. Check the skin under the application every 10 minutes. If the skin appears to be blanched or white,

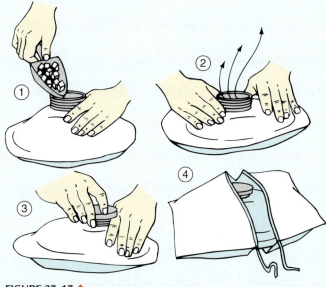

FIGURE 27–17 ◆

Preparing ice bag for use

PROCEDURE (continued)

remove the ice bag. Cover the area with a towel and report to your immediate supervisor or team leader.

FOLLOW-UP

19. Clean standard equipment and put it in its proper place. Discard disposable equipment and gloves, if used.

20. Make the patient comfortable and replace the call light.

21. Lower the bed to a position of safety for the patient.

22. Raise the side rails when ordered or appropriate for patient safety.

23. Wash your hands.

24. Report to your immediate supervisor:

   - The time the ice bag was applied.
   - The length of treatment.
   - The area of application.
   - How the patient tolerated the procedure.

   - Your observations of anything unusual.

CHARTING EXAMPLE: 12/18/04 10am Cold ice bag applied to Mr. Perkins's right foot for 20 minutes. Mr. Perkins's said the cold helped to decrease his foot pain. The foot remains swollen and bruised. C. Gentile, CNA

APPLYING THE COMMERCIAL UNIT COLD PACK (DRY COLD APPLICATION)

PROCEDURE

OBRA

RATIONALE: Dry cold applications, which decrease circulation and bleeding, are used to treat sprains and fractures by reducing pain and tissue swelling.

PREPARATION

1. Assemble your equipment:

   a. Commercial unit, single-use cold pack
   b. Cover used in your institution
   c. Bath blanket
   d. Gloves, if indicated

2. Identify the patient by checking the identification bracelet.

3. Wash your hands.

4. Tell the patient you are going to apply a cold pack.

5. Provide privacy for the patient.

6. Raise the bed to a comfortable working position.

7. Help the patient into a safe, comfortable position. Expose the area to be treated.

STEPS

8. Place the flannel cover on the cold pack (or whatever type of cover is used by your institution).

9. Hit or squeeze the cold pack to activate it according to the manufacturer's directions (Figure 27–18◆). Apply gloves, if indicated.

10. Apply the pack to the proper area of the patient's body.

11. Check the skin under the application every 10 minutes. If the skin appears blanched or white, remove the pack and cover the area with a blanket. Report this to your immediate supervisor.

12. Follow the instructions of your immediate supervisor as to the length of application. Replace with a new cold pack as necessary.

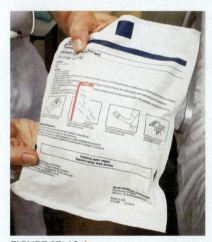

FIGURE 27–18 ◆
Disposable cold package

FOLLOW-UP

13. Discard disposable equipment and gloves, if used.

14. Make the patient comfortable and replace the call light.

15. Lower the bed to a position of safety for the patient.

16. Raise the side rails when ordered or appropriate for patient safety.

17. Wash your hands.

PROCEDURE *(continued)*

18. Report to your immediate supervisor:

    ■ The time the cold pack was applied.

    ■ The length of treatment.

    ■ The area of application.

■ How the patient tolerated the procedure.

■ Your observations of anything unusual.

CHARTING EXAMPLE: 12/19/04 10am Cold pack applied to Mr. Perkins's right foot for 20 minutes. Mr. Perkins's said the cold helped to decrease his foot pain. The foot remains swollen and bruised. C. Gentile, CNA

The Cooling (Tepid) Sponge Bath

You have had the experience of perspiring on a warm summer day. You often feel cooler as the moisture evaporates from your skin. As perspiration evaporates into the air, it carries some heat with it. This cools the body. A tepid (slightly warm) sponge bath cools a patient's body in the same way. Patients who run temperatures near 105°F (40.5°C) or higher are in danger of having convulsions in some cases. A tepid bath can lower the temperature to one more desirable. Generally, the bath is ended if the patient's temperature reaches 101°–102°F (38.3°–38.8°C). It is important to take the patient's temperature before the procedure is started, and then every 10 minutes during the procedure. Cold water, ice, or alcohol is not used since this can cause chilling or irritation of the skin. Cooling sponge baths are never used on infants, toddlers, or geriatric patients since such baths tend to cause chilling in these patients. Chilling can make them too cold too fast. Shivering can cause their temperatures to rise quickly.

KEY IDEA

All sponge baths require a doctor's order. The purpose of the tepid sponge bath is to lower the patient's body temperature.

GUIDELINES

GIVING THE COOLING (TEPID) SPONGE BATH

■ Place moist washcloths on the axillary area (armpits), the groin, the inner aspect of the elbows, and the back of the knees. These are places where many blood vessels are close to the surface of the body, and so evaporation can more quickly lower the body temperature at these places.

■ Place a covered hot-water bottle at the patient's feet to prevent chilling.

■ Use only tepid (slightly warm) water (80°–92°F; 27°–33°C).

■ If the patient becomes chilled or starts to shiver, stop the treatment, dry the patient, and cover him with a light blanket. Call your immediate supervisor at once.

■ Carefully monitor the patient's temperature before beginning the procedure, every 10 minutes during the 25–30 minute procedure, and 10 minutes after the procedure. Stop the procedure at once if the temperature reaches a low of 102°F (38.8°C). Once the bathing begins, do not take the temperature in the axillary area (armpit) because the moist cloths will alter the correct readings. Also, take the oral temperature with care because chilling or shivering can cause the patient to bite down on the thermometer and break it, or injure his teeth. A rectal temperature is advised to prevent injury.

■ To hasten the cooling, a moist bath towel can be placed on the trunk (chest and abdomen) of the patient's body. Also, the use of a fan to move the room air is helpful in evaporation. *Do not direct the air flow at the patient.*

GIVING THE COOLING (TEPID) SPONGE BATH

PROCEDURE

RATIONALE: Cooling sponge baths are given to reduce a person's body temperature.

PREPARATION

1. Assemble your equipment:

   a. Two hot-water bottles with covers

   b. Disposable gloves

   c. A waterproof sheet to protect the bed

   d. Two bath blankets

   e. One ice bag, covered

   f. Six washcloths

   g. One moist bath towel

   h. Two dry bath towels

   i. Oral or rectal thermometer (oral thermometer should not be glass)

   j. Basin with tepid water (80°–92°F; 27°–33°C)

   k. Bath thermometer

   l. Laundry bag

   m. Clock or wristwatch

2. Identify the patient by checking the identification bracelet.

3. Explain the procedure to the patient.

4. Provide privacy for the patient.

5. Wash your hands and put on gloves.

6. Raise the bed to a comfortable working position.

STEPS

7. Take the patient's temperature, pulse, and respirations. Record on a flow sheet.

8. Place protective waterproof sheet on the bed.

9. Cover patient with bath blanket. Slide top bed covers from under the bath blanket. Remove patient's gown and all other clothing without exposing the patient.

10. Place covered hot-water bottles at his feet to prevent chilling.

11. Place covered ice bag on his forehead.

12. Place moist washcloths on the axillary area (armpits), the groin, the inner aspect of the elbows, and the back of the knees.

13. A moist bath towel to hasten cooling can be placed on the trunk (chest and abdomen). This is optional.

14. Note the time on the clock or your wristwatch. Start by bathing (stroking the extremity with a washcloth moistened with tepid water from the basin) two extremities for 5 minutes each. *Take the temperature, pulse, and respirations. Record on flow sheet.*

15. Bathe two more extremities for 5 minutes each. *Take the temperature, pulse, and respirations. Record on flow sheet.*

16. Then bathe the chest and abdomen for 5 minutes if no moist towel has been used as stated in step 13.

17. Next bathe the back and buttocks for 5–10 minutes. *Take the temperature, pulse, and respirations. Record on flow sheet.*

18. Notify your immediate supervisor if the temperature doesn't *start* to drop within 30 minutes of beginning the bathing.

19. Repeat the procedure until the desired temperature is reached.

20. Dry the patient and cover him with a bedsheet. Remove the protective sheet. Remove bath blanket. Assist patient to put on gown and replace other covers.

FOLLOW-UP

21. Make the patient comfortable and replace the call light.

22. Lower the bed to a position of safety.

23. Raise the side rails when ordered or appropriate for patient safety.

24. Clean reusable equipment and return to its proper place. Discard disposable equipment according to your institution's policy.

25. Bag and dispose of dirty linen in the laundry hamper.

26. Dispose of gloves and wash your hands.

27. Copy onto a permanent record the vital signs you have taken, or include the flow sheet in the patient's record according to your institution's policy.

28. Report to your immediate supervisor:

    ■ The time the procedure started.

    ■ The length of the procedure.

    ■ Your observations of anything unusual.

CHARTING EXAMPLE: 12/19/04 10:30am Cooling sponge bath given to Mr. Hotman as ordered. His temperature was 105°F at 9:30am and 101°F at 10:30am. Vital signs documented on flow sheet. F. Peking, CNA

SUMMARY

This chapter has provided examples and procedures to safely apply warm and cold applications. You also learned that warm and cold applications may be either moist or dry and that they can be generalized or localized applications. The length of an application is always a serious issue since the misuse of an application may cause skin damage. You will follow the instructions of your supervisor as to the time to begin an application and how long the application should remain in place.

NOTES

_____

_____

_____

_____

_____

_____

_____

_____

_____

_____

_____

_____

_____

_____

_____

_____

_____

_____

_____

CHAPTER REVIEW

FILL IN THE BLANK Read each sentence and fill in the blank line with a word that completes the sentence.

1. When a blood vessel expands in size, it _____.

2. When a blood vessel gets smaller in size, it _____.

3. _____ occurs when the tissue reacts to disease or injury. There is usually pain, heat, redness, and swelling of the body part.

4. When something is _____, it means it is limited to one place or part, or affects a definite area of the body.

5. If a patients's lips, fingernails, eyelids, or skin look blue or a darker color, _____ is said to have occurred.

MULTIPLE CHOICE Choose the best answer for each question or statement.

1. Heat may be used as treatment to
   a. decrease blood pressure.
   b. speed the healing process.
   c. improve the appearance of the skin.
   d. decrease age of the skin.

2. Cold applications may be used to
   a. prevent or reduce swelling.
   b. decrease blood pressure.
   c. improve the appearance of the skin.
   d. dilate the blood vessels.

3. Which of the following is not a moist heat or cold application?
   a. Sitz bath
   b. Heat lamp
   c. Cool compress
   d. Tub bath

4. In order to keep the patient safe during hot applications, you should
   a. be careful not to spill any water.
   b. watch for too much redness or darkened area.
   c. go on break during the treatment.
   d. check the skin every 5 minutes.

5. When blood vessels become dilated,
   a. the increased blood supply carries away the fluids that cause inflammation.
   b. the increased blood supply increases inflammation.
   c. the decreased blood supply carries away the fluids that cause inflammation.
   d. the decreased blood supply increases inflammation.

TIME-OUT

TIPS FOR TIME MANAGEMENT

Arrive at work 10 minutes early to give yourself time to go to your locker, greet coworkers, and get something to drink before your shift begins. You will be organized and ready to work instead of straggling in at the last moment.

THE NURSING ASSISTANT IN ACTION

You are assigned to care for Curtis Brown, a 20-year-old man who has sprained his ankle. You are supposed to apply a cold pack to his ankle, but he does not want it on. He tells you, "Hey man, I am in serious pain and that is not helping. You can just get me some pain pills and take that thing out of here!"

What Is Your Response/Action?

CRITICAL THINKING

CUSTOMER SERVICE Some treatments can be uncomfortable or embarrassing. If you see that your patient is reluctant to accept your assistance with a sitz bath, allow her to have as much privacy as possible.

CULTURAL CARE If you are male and assigned to take care of a female patient who has a sitz bath ordered, you should check and see if the patient would prefer that a female staff member assist her with that procedure. Once a preference is determined, it should be noted in the patient's plan of care and efforts made to accommodate this cultural or personal preference.

COOPERATION WITHIN THE TEAM When you are performing heat or cold applications, it is important that the patient be checked frequently. If you find yourself taking longer than expected with another patient, call for assistance to have someone check in on your patient or relieve you for a few minutes to check on the patient. Offer to do the same for your coworkers.

EXPLORE MediaLink

Additional interactive resources for this chapter can be found on the Companion Website at www.prenhall.com/wolgin. Click on Chapter 27 and "Begin" to select the activities for this chapter.

For chapter-related NCLEX-style questions and an audio glossary, access the accompanying CD-ROM in this book.

28

Care of the Surgical Patient

MediaLink

www.prenhall.com/wolgin
Use the address above to access the free, interactive Companion Website created for this textbook. Get hints, instant feedback, and textbook references to chapter-related NCLEX-style questions. Link to other interesting sites.

AUDIO GLOSSARY:
Use the companion Website, or the CD-ROM disk enclosed with your textbook, to hear the pronunciation of key terms in the chapter.

INTRODUCTION

This chapter will prepare you to care for the surgical patient before surgery (preoperative) and after surgery (postoperative). Preparation of the patient for surgery includes patient education, psychological support, and completion of the procedures on the preoperative checklist. The patient's unit must be prepared to receive the patient after surgery. When the patient returns from surgery, he must be watched closely for any postoperative problems. Procedures that can help prevent respiratory problems following surgery are deep-breathing exercises and training.

Surgery

ALERT

For all patient contact, adhere to Standard Precautions (Chapter 5, pages 83–85). Wear protective equipment as indicated.

Surgery is a procedure that involves cutting the skin to remove a diseased organ, body part, tumor, or foreign object. It is used to repair injured tissue, diagnose a disease, improve appearance, or improve body functioning.

Reasons for surgery include the following:

- Remove or replace a diseased organ.
- Repair internal damage resulting from an accident or injury.
- Cosmetic or improve appearance (cornea lasix, botox injections, face-lifts, breast implants, nose reductions, liposuction, etc.)

Surgery Types

emergency surgery
Performed to save life or limb

Emergency surgery: performed to save life or limb (following gunshot wounds, explosions, car accidents, trauma, and knife wounds)

Urgent surgery: unexpected but not immediately life threatening, these surgical procedures must be done soon to restore health or prevent further damage

Scheduled surgery: routine procedures scheduled in a doctor's office, outpatient, or ambulatory surgical center, or hospital operating room (OR)

elective surgery Chosen and not vital for health

Elective surgery: refers to cosmetic or appearance-improving procedures that are usually not covered by health care plans; many of these are outpatient procedures. If performed in a hospital OR, these procedures will be delayed or rescheduled if the room is needed for emergency surgery.

Preoperative Care

preoperative Before surgery
postoperative After surgery

Two very important words are used often in this chapter. They are **preoperative** and **postoperative**.

- The word *operative* means an operation or surgery.
- *Pre* means before.
- *Post* means after.
- *Preoperative* means before surgery.
- *Postoperative* means after surgery.

Preoperative Patient Education

Preoperative patient education prepares the patient for surgery. Each step of the surgical experience is explained to eliminate fear of the unknown and to empower the patient to take an active part in his or her own care. A parent, family member, or friend is instructed when he will be responsible for supervising or providing care for children or elderly persons who are unable to care for themselves. Each member of the health care team is responsible for assisting with preoperative patient education. Your immediate supervisor will instruct you as to your role in this education. The patient will be instructed about the routine before surgery, the morning of surgery, what to expect upon arrival in the surgical suite, the recovery room, and postoperative care, including:

- Deep-breathing and coughing exercises
- Turning from side to side
- Patient participation in self-care
- Leg and foot exercises (see Chapter 33)
- Getting out of bed
- Pain or discomfort; how to ask for medication
- Safety: side rails in the up position
- Explanation of NPO (nothing by mouth)

Psychological Aspects of Preoperative Care

Almost every patient who enters a hospital or ambulatory surgical center for surgery will be a little nervous and upset. Part of your job as a nursing assistant is to help the preoperative patient feel as calm and relaxed as possible (Figure 28–1◆). For every successful surgical procedure shared or reported in the media, there are many more reporting any error or mistake that happens. Patients and families will tell all their friends and acquaintances when the wrong procedure was performed or the surgery was unsuccessful. Staff members will be quick to share stories of the case where things went wrong or a lawsuit followed. All these reports will increase a patient's anxiety when they are faced with surgery.

Some things that might worry the preoperative patient are:

- Concern for the family, pets, or significant friends
- The possibility of death or serious complications
- Not awakening from the anesthesia or dying on the table

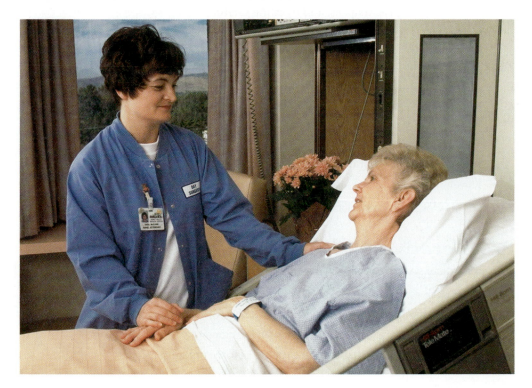

FIGURE 28–1 ◆

Part of preoperative care is helping the patient feel as calm and relaxed as possible

- Fear of the unknown or confirmation of cancer
- A possible disability because of the operation
- Concern the surgery will not correct the condition or problem
- Concerns about scars or the loss of a body part
- Pain or dependence on pain medications following surgery
- Fear of impotence following prostate surgery
- For women fear that they will no longer be attractive following breast surgery
- Being away from work; financial fears

AGE-SPECIFIC CONSIDERATIONS

Preparing to go to surgery is a nervous time for patients of all ages. Children wonder what might happen to them and may be frightened of the equipment and noises of the environment. Allow parents to stay with the child for as long as possible. Explain things to the child in simple language. Let the child touch as much equipment as possible. For the adolescent, avoid the use of medical jargon. Maintain privacy, but let them know their parent is available if they want them. For adults and the elderly, give them as much decision making as possible. Explain things in terms that they can understand and allow time for questions and concerns.

Good physical and emotional preoperative care can help reduce anxiety and fears. Give the patient all your attention. Make him feel that you care about him and how the operation comes out. Listen and show interest in what the patient says. Many frightened people relieve their tension by talking a lot and asking lots of questions. Others do not say anything. Alert your immediate supervisor if the patient appears abnormally upset or fearful.

KEY IDEA

You can give support to your patients by being there when they need assistance, by staying calm if they seem upset, and by being tactful.

Preventing Chest Complications

Preoperative patient education includes deep-breathing exercises. To prevent chest **complications** following surgery, watch for these symptoms of respiratory infection in preoperative patients:

complication An unexpected condition, such as the development of another illness in a patient who is already sick

- Sneezing, sniffling, or coughing
- Complaints or signs of chest pains
- Elevated temperature

Report any of these immediately to your immediate supervisor.

Preoperative Checklist

Your immediate supervisor will give you the preoperative checklist and instruct you as to:

- What each patient has been told about his operation
- What you are to tell the patient to prepare him for his surgery and postoperative care
- How to handle and answer the patient's questions
- What care to give the patient the evening before surgery

- What care to give the patient the morning of surgery
- What portion, if any, of the preoperative checklist you are to complete

Figure 28–2◆ is an example of a preoperative checklist. By filling out this checklist, the nursing staff can be sure the patient has been prepared properly for surgery. Report to

IMMEDIATE PREOPERATIVE CHECKLIST
Name   Date
_____

PATIENT IDENTIFICATION
   ID on and accurate (name and numbers)   ☐ Yes   ☐ No
   Comments _____

PLANNED PROCEDURE
   Patient's statement of: _____
   _____
Patient verifies side: ☐ Right   ☐ Left   ☐ N/A
ALLERGIES
   any known allergies: ☐ Yes   ☐ No
   Specify if yes _____
   _____

NPO STATUS
   NPO since midnight   ☐ Yes   ☐ No

PREGNANCY
   Patient   ☐ Denies   ☐ Confirms   ☐ Unsure   ☐ N/A
   Comments _____
PERSONAL POSSESSIONS
   Dental appliance   ☐ Yes   ☐ No   _____
   Prostheses/Implants   ☐ Yes   ☐ No   _____
                                            _____

   Valuables: Item   Disposition
   _____   _____
   _____   _____
   _____   _____

HEIGHT_____WEIGHT_____ lb/kg   ☐ Actual   ☐ Est.

VITAL SIGNS   B/P____   T____   P____   R ____   Time ____

PREOPERATIVE PREPARATION
   Physically prepared: ☐ Yes   ☐ No
      (personal clothes, glasses, contacts, nail polish, wigs,
      dentures, jewelry removed and hospital gown applied)
                          Yes   No   Comments
Med. sheets to OR   ☐   ☐   _____
Patient voided preop   ☐   ☐   _____
Preop meds given   ☐   ☐   _____
Meds/supplies to OR   ☐   ☐   _____
Side rails up   ☐   ☐   _____
Patient instructed   ☐   ☐   _____
to stay in bed
Preoperative treatments _____
PATIENT IDENTIFIED IN OR DEPT. BY DR. _____

COMMENTS: _____
_____

READY FOR OR   Date _____
   Preoperative unit RN/LPN (initials) _____
   Preoperative RN (initials)   _____

FIGURE 28–2 ◆

Sample preoperative checklist to be completed by the nursing assistant

your supervisor when you have completed the activities you are responsible for on the checklist. Medications are given upon completion of the checklist.

KEY IDEA

> The patient signs a surgical consent form prior to surgery. Obtaining the patient's written consent for surgery is the doctor's responsibility. However, the doctor often delegates this responsibility to the nurse. You are never responsible for securing the patient's signature on this form.

NPO (nothing by mouth)
Cannot eat or drink anything at all, usually past midnight the night before surgery or a procedure

You may be asked to take away the patient's water pitcher and glass at midnight and to post a sign saying **NPO** (Figure 28–3◆). NPO is taken from the Latin *nils per os*, which means "nothing by mouth." The sign is usually put at the head or foot of the bed; follow your immediate supervisor's instructions.

FIGURE 28–3 ◆

Nothing by mouth sign, usually posted at the head or foot of the patient's bed, if required

Skin Preparation

skin prep Shaving the area of the body where an operation is going to be performed in preparation for surgery

Close to the time of an operation, the patient's skin in the operative area must be free of hair that would interfere with the operative or surgical procedure. The skin must be as clean as possible. Hair on the body is a breeding place for microorganisms. Because hair cannot be sterilized, it must be removed by shaving. The **skin prep** covers the area on the body where the operation is going to be done. When you are shaving a patient before an operation, watch for scratches, pimples, cuts, sores, or rashes on the skin. If you see anything on the skin that looks unusual, be sure to report this to your immediate supervisor. *For many procedures, shaving is no longer performed.* The nicks caused by shaving may actually harbor more microorganisms than the skin and hair.

In some hospitals, the patient is sent to the operating room suite 1 hour before he is scheduled for surgery. At that time, the nurses in the operating room will prep the patient (shave the skin in preparation for surgery). This is done in those hospitals that have holding areas in the operating room suite. In the holding area, each patient has his own cubicle (sometimes an anteroom) where preparation for surgery, including administration of medications, starting of intravenous infusions, and skin preps, are done.

In other hospitals, the staff does the prep the evening before surgery. The operating room staff does another complete prep after the patient is on the operating room table.

The prep is done with a special prep kit, which is obtained from the central supply room for each patient. After it is used, it is discarded in the dirty utility room. Each kit contains a safety razor and a sponge filled with soap. Most health care facilities have a hazardous disposable sharps box or container to dispose of razors. If your health care facility does not supply a disposable prep kit, get the individual items from central supply. Be sure to follow Standard Precautions and use Blood-borne Pathogen Standards.

SHAVING A PATIENT IN PREPARATION FOR SURGERY

PROCEDURE

RATIONALE: Shaving the skin is done to remove hair that could interfere with the procedure.

PREPARATION

1. Assemble your equipment:

   a. Disposable prep kit (Figure 28–4a–b◆) containing:
   - Razor and razor blades
   - Sponge filled with soap
   - Tissues

   b. Basin of warm water (115°F; 46.1°C)

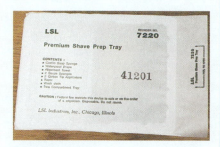

FIGURE 28–4a ◆
Shave prep tray

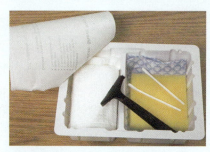

FIGURE 28–4b ◆
Open shave prep tray

   c. Bath blanket

   d. Towels

   e. Disposable gloves

Note: Some health care institutions do a "dry prep;" they shave the skin without soap. Follow the policies of your institution.

2. Identify the patient by checking his identification bracelet.

3. Tell the patient that you are going to shave him.

4. Provide privacy for the patient.

5. Wash your hands and put on gloves.

6. Raise the bed to a comfortable working position.

STEPS

7. Place the bath blanket over the bedspread and top sheet. Ask the patient to hold the blanket in place. Fan-fold the top sheets to the foot of the bed. Do this from underneath the blanket without exposing the patient.

8. Adjust the bedside lamp so that the area is well lighted. There should be no shadows where you will be working.

9. Open the disposable prep kit.

10. Wet the soap sponge in the basin of water. Next, soap the area to be shaved. Work up a good lather with the sponge.

11. Check to be sure the razor blade is in the correct position in the razor.

12. Hold the skin taut with a dry tissue. Shave in the direction the hair grows. Rinse the razor often. Keep the razor and the patient's skin wet

and soapy throughout the procedure.

13. Clean the patient's umbilicus (navel) if it is in the area to be shaved.

14. Rinse the soap off the patient's skin. Dry thoroughly with the towel.

15. Clean your equipment and put it in its proper place. Discard disposable equipment. Never throw razors in the garbage.

16. Cover the patient with the top sheet and bedspread. Ask him to hold them while you take the bath blanket from underneath without exposing the patient.

FOLLOW-UP

17. Make the patient comfortable and replace the call light.

18. Lower the bed to a position of safety.

19. Raise the side rails when ordered or appropriate for patient safety.

20. Dispose of gloves and wash your hands.

21. Report to your immediate supervisor:
   - The time at which you shaved the patient.
   - How the patient tolerated the procedure.
   - Your observations of anything unusual.

DOCUMENTATION: 12/23/04 5am Skin prepared and shaved as ordered. D. Hunter, CNA

Areas to Be Shaved in Preparation for Surgery

The areas to be shaved in preparation for various types of surgery are shown in Figures 28–5◆ through 28–11◆. The area not being operated on is called the *unaffected side*. The area where the operation will be done is called the *affected side*. Clipping, a common alternative to shaving, is gaining preference, as there is a reduced chance of introducing infection (Figure 28–12◆).

FIGURE 28–5 ◆

Prep for breast surgery. Shave from the nipple line of the unaffected side to the middle of the patient's back on the affected side. On the affected side, shave from the chin down to the umbilicus (navel), the axilla (armpit), and part of the upper arm.

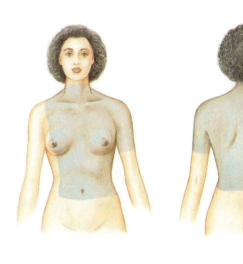

FIGURE 28–6 ◆

Chest prep for thoracic surgery. Shave the area extending from the nipple of the unaffected side, across the chest area of the affected side, and across the back, from the top of the shoulders down to the pubic hair.

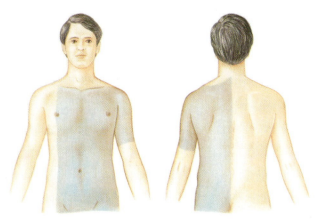

FIGURE 28–7 ◆

Abdominal prep. Shave from the nipple line on male patients and from below the breasts on female patients down to and including the pubic area. Shave the width of this area to each side of the body.

abdominal prep The procedure for making the patient's abdomen ready for surgery; includes thorough cleansing of the skin and careful shaving of body hair in the abdominal area

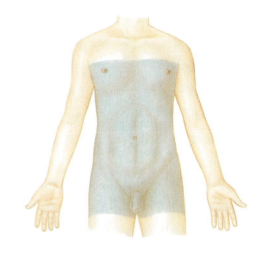

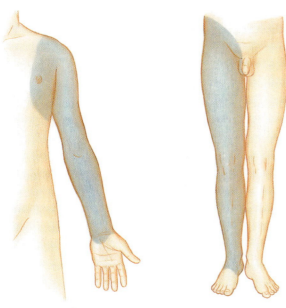

FIGURE 28–8 ◆

Prep for surgery of an extremity (arm or leg). If a joint such as an elbow or knee is going to be operated on, you will shave up to the next joint above and down to the next joint below. For example, if the patient's elbow is going to be operated on, you will shave the entire arm from the shoulder down to the wrist. If an area between joints is going to be operated on, you will shave the entire area, including the joints above and below. Shave all around an arm or a leg.

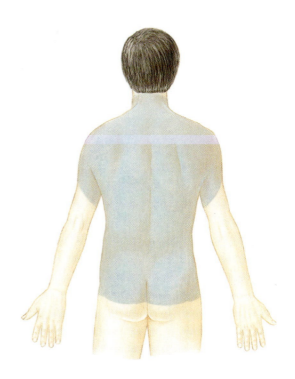

FIGURE 28–9 ◆

Back prep. Shave the patient's entire back, from the hairline on the neck down to the middle of the buttocks, including the axillary area.

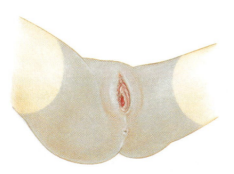

FIGURE 28–10 ◆

Vaginal prep, or the preparation of the genital area of female patients.

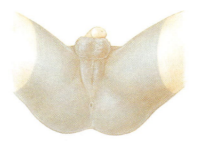

FIGURE 28–11 ◆

Scrotal prep, or the preparation of the genital area of male patients.

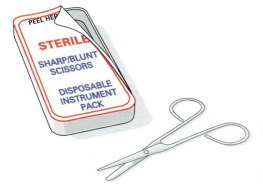

FIGURE 28–12 ◆

Clipping, a common alternative to shaving, is gaining preference as the chance of introducing infection is reduced.

vaginal prep The procedures for making the genital area of a female patient ready for surgery; the preparation includes thoroughly cleansing the skin and carefully shaving the pubic hair; it may also include a cleansing douche

scrotal prep The procedures for making the genital area of a male patient ready for surgery; the preparation includes thoroughly cleansing the skin and carefully shaving the hair in the area

The Morning of Surgery

After the patient has been given his preoperative medications by the medication nurse:

- Keep the side rails in the up position.
- Remind the patient that he or she is not to smoke, eat, or get out of bed.

The transportation attendant or the operating room assistant will come at the proper time to take the patient to the operating room suite. Move the furniture out of the way. Make the room ready for the stretcher to be brought into the room. Assist with moving the patient from the bed to the stretcher. Tell the patient that you or another nurse will see her in her room after the surgery.

The transportation assistant will then wheel the patient on the stretcher to the nurse's station (Figure 28–13◆). At this time, the nurse or unit clerk will give the attendant the patient's chart and check the name on the identification bracelet against the name on the chart. The attendant then takes the patient and chart to the operating room.

Readying the Postoperative Patient's Unit

Your next task is to strip the linen from the bed, make the OR or surgical bed, and prepare the unit to receive the patient postoperatively (Figure 28–14◆).

- Bring the IV pole to bedside (Note: Most portable IV pumps have an attached pole).
- Strip the linen from the bed; make the OR bed.
- Place tissues and an emesis basin on the bedside table, along with any other equipment requested by the nurse.
- Be sure to remove drinking water if so instructed.

FIGURE 28–13 ◆

When transporting the patient to the operating room, cover the patient with a blanket or sheet, be sure the straps are secure, stand at the patient's head, and push the stretcher slowly

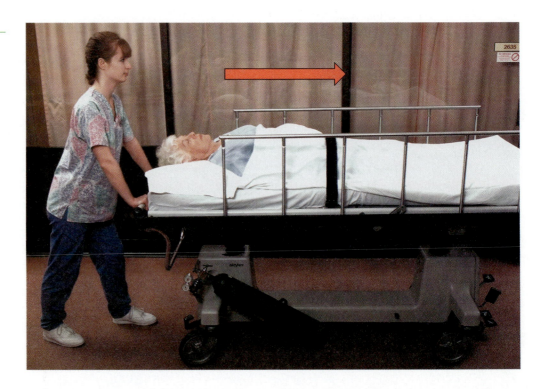

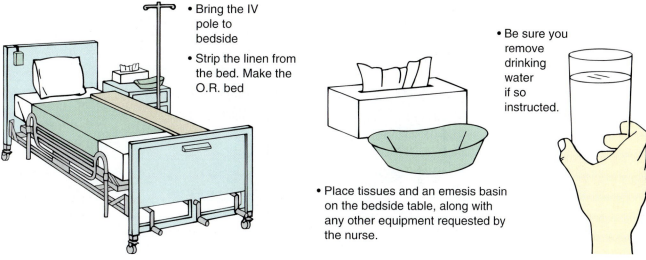

• Bring the IV pole to bedside

• Strip the linen from the bed. Make the O.R. bed

• Be sure you remove drinking water if so instructed.

• Place tissues and an emesis basin on the bedside table, along with any other equipment requested by the nurse.

FIGURE 28–14 ◆

Responsibility list for preparing for the return of the postoperative patient

 Postoperative Nursing Care

Postoperative care means taking care of a patient right after surgery. Most patients are taken to a surgical recovery room immediately following surgery. They remain in the recovery room until they begin to recover from the effects of anesthesia and vital signs have stabilized. When the patient returns to his room, you will begin assisting with postoperative nursing care. The patient must be watched closely for any complications such as fever, bleeding, extreme restlessness, choking, vomiting, or changes in vital signs. Report any such observations to your immediate supervisor immediately.

When the Patient Comes Back from Surgery

The patient will be coming back to his unit on a stretcher. Move the furniture out of the way and make sure the bedside area is clear. The stretcher can then be brought easily and quickly to its place next to the bed.

When the patient is brought back to the unit, you will do the following things:

- Help move the patient safely from the stretcher to the bed.
- Be sure the patient is covered with blankets to keep warm.
- Be sure the bedside rails are raised after the patient is in bed.
- Lower the bed to a position of safety.
- Measure the patient's vital signs (TPR and BP) as instructed by your immediate supervisor.
- Place the call light within the patient's reach (Figure 28–15◆).
- Be sure all drinking water has been removed.

Signal your immediate supervisor immediately if you observe any of the following signs or symptoms:

- Rise or fall of blood pressure
- Choking
- Pulse: fast (above 100), slow (below 60), or an irregular pulse beat
- Respirations: rapid (above 30), labored, very slow, or shallow

FIGURE 28–15 ◆

When the patient awakens from the anesthesia, call the patient by her preferred name; this reassures the patient that someone who knows her is present. Be sure the call light is within easy reach.

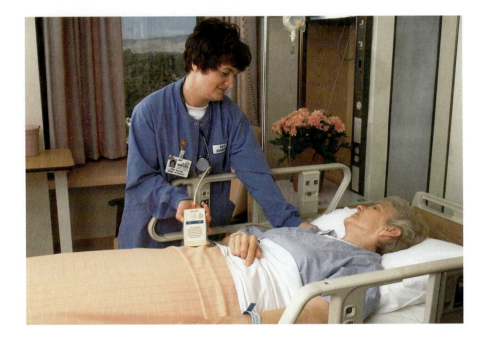

- Skin, lips, fingernails are very pale or turning blue (cyanosis)
- Thirst: patient asks for water often
- Unusual or extreme restlessness
- Moaning or complaining of pain
- Sudden, bright red bleeding on or near the dressing or surgical site
- Any other noticeable sudden changes
- Nausea or vomiting

The postoperative patient may appear to be unconscious, but not really be. He may be able to hear you. Say only those things you would want the patient to hear if he were fully conscious. Speak normally. Always tell the patient who you are and what you are doing. Figures 28–16◆ through 28–18◆ provide additional information on the techniques for postoperative care.

FIGURE 28–16 ◆

If the patient vomits, turn her head to one side to prevent vomitus from being drawn back into the lungs (aspiration); wipe the patient's mouth and chin. If the patient is conscious, rinse out her mouth with cold water. Caution: The patient is not to swallow the water.

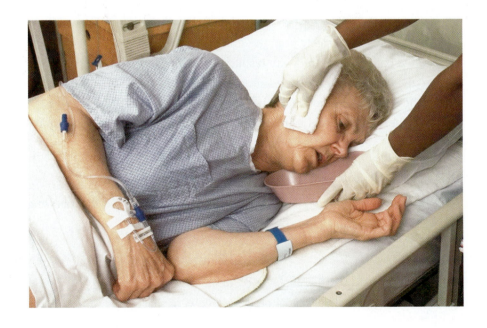

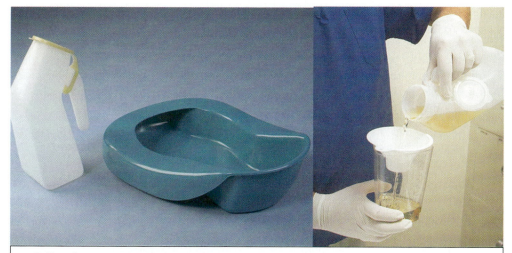

FIGURE 28–17 ◆
The first voiding after surgery

- Collect for a routine urine specimen
- Measure for amount
- Check for odor and color
- Record in a proper place on output side of I and O sheet
- Report if the patient has not yet **voided** on your shift
- Report if the patient voids only a few drops of urine
- If an indwelling urinary catheter is present:
  Be sure it is unclamped and draining
  Observe amount and color in the drainage bag

void To urinate, pass water

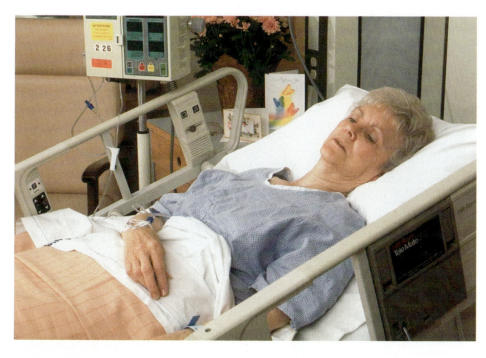

FIGURE 28–18 ◆
Keep side rails in the up
position for patients who are
coming out of an anesthetic

anesthetic A drug used to
produce loss of feeling; can
be given orally, rectally, by
injection, or by inhalation;
a person who has been given
an anesthetic is anesthetized

anesthesia Loss of feeling or
sensation in a part or all of the
body

general anesthetics General
anesthetics cause loss of
sensation in the entire body

Anesthesia

Before surgery, the patient is given special medications that cause a loss of feeling in all or part of the body, which means the patient feels no pain. When the patient is under the influence of these special medications, called **anesthetics**, he is in a state of **anesthesia**. Some anesthetics cause the loss of sensation in the whole body. These are called **general anesthetics**.

local anesthetics Local anesthetics cause numbness or a loss of sensation in only a part of the body

spinal anesthetics Anesthetics that cause a loss of feeling in a large area of the body, usually from the umbilicus down to and including the legs and feet

anesthesiologist The medical doctor who administers the anesthetic to the patient in the operating room

anesthetist The registered nurse who assists the anesthesiologist

unconscious Unaware of the environment; occurs during sleep and in temporary episodes ranging from fainting or stupor to coma

aspirate Material (vomitus, food, or liquids) inhaled into the lungs

Some anesthetics cause a numbness or loss of feeling in only a part of the body. These medications are called **local anesthetics**. A **spinal anesthetic** causes loss of feeling in a large area of the body, usually from the umbilicus down to and including the legs and feet.

The doctor who administers the anesthetic to the patient in the operating room is a medical doctor who is known as an **anesthesiologist**. The registered nurse who assists in administering the anesthetic to the patient in the operating room is known as an **anesthetist**.

Chest complications following anesthesia may happen for several reasons:

- The anesthetic may irritate the patient's respiratory passages (mouth, nose, trachea, lungs) and cause the secretions in these passages to increase. This might increase the chance of an infection in the lungs or other parts of the respiratory system.

- Smoking tends to irritate the whole respiratory system. Smoking may increase the secretion of mucus, which can also raise the chance of an infection.

- After surgery, many patients are so sore they cannot breathe deeply. They cannot cough up the increased amount of mucous material being secreted in the lungs. This can cause a respiratory infection, such as pneumonia. A patient might vomit while he is still **unconscious** after surgery. The vomitus (emesis, vomited material) might be **aspirated**, that is, drawn back into the lungs. This could very quickly cause an infection or even the patient's death. Saliva might also be drawn into the throat and block the air passages, which could cause an infection.

- Unconsciousness and inactivity during anesthesia allows mucus to accumulate in the patient's respiratory passages. If ordered by the physician, the head nurse or team leader will call the respiratory therapy department (pulmonary medicine). Staff persons from that department will treat the patient with chest complications.

Turning the Postoperative Patient

Unless you are instructed not to, you should move a postoperative patient into a new position every 2 hours (q2h). This protects his skin, promotes healing, prevents pneumonia, and increases blood circulation in the legs. Each time the patient is moved, he should be turned onto his opposite side so that he faces the other side of the bed (Figure 28–19◆). Move the patient's legs at the same time.

FIGURE 28–19 ◆

Turning the postoperative patient

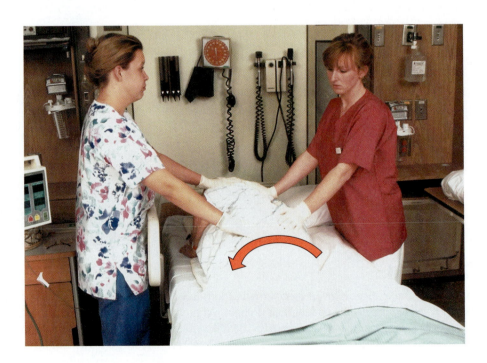

If the patient's gown becomes wet, change it immediately. Change the bed linens whenever they become damp or soiled. Take the blankets off the bed if the patient complains of being too warm. Keep the side rails up at all times.

Check dressings when you turn the patient. Report to your immediate supervisor if there is new drainage (clear or red), or if the dressing is soaked. Be sure to ask postsurgical patients about their level of pain. Report any changes to your immediate supervisor.

Coughing and Deep-Breathing Exercises

Deep-breathing exercises expand the lungs by increasing lung movement and assist in bringing up lung secretions. These exercises will help prevent postoperative pneumonia, or pneumonitis. In many institutions, the patient will use a handheld spirometer to breathe into for expanding the lungs. If no spirometer is ordered, the following procedure may be used.

AGE-SPECIFIC CONSIDERATION

Older persons have weak respiratory muscles and less elastic tissue. Coughing, deep breathing, and using an incentive spirometer after surgery are important to prevent complications.

ASSISTING THE PATIENT WITH COUGHING AND DEEP-BREATHING EXERCISES

PROCEDURE   **OBRA**

RATIONALE: These exercises are done to promote lung expansion, bring up secretions, and prevent pneumonia.

PREPARATION

1. Assemble your equipment:
   a. Pillow or folded bath blanket
   b. Specimen container, if a specimen is ordered
   c. Tissues
   d. Disposable gloves
2. Report to the medication nurse that you are ready to start deep-breathing exercises.
3. Identify the patient by checking her identification bracelet.
4. Tell the patient that you are going to help her with deep-breathing exercises.

5. Wash your hands and put on gloves.
6. Provide privacy for the patient.

STEPS

7. Raise the bed to a comfortable working position.
8. Offer the patient a bedpan or urinal.
9. Dangle the patient's legs over the side of the bed, if allowed. If not, place the patient in as much of a sitting position as possible (semi-Fowler's to full Fowler's).
10. If your patient had abdominal surgery, place the pillow or folded bath blanket on the patient's abdomen for support. Ask the patient to hold the pillow across the abdomen to splint the incision.
11. Ask her to breathe deeply 10 times. (*Explain:* Breathe slowly and evenly through your nose until your chest is fully expanded. Hold your breath 2–3 seconds and exhale through

your mouth. Continue exhaling until your chest is deflated. Repeat.) Use an incentive spirometer if ordered.
12. Count the respirations out loud to the patient as she inhales and exhales. If the patient cannot breathe deeply, ask her to cough. Coughing is just another way of breathing deeply.
13. Ask the patient to feel her abdomen as she breathes to encourage deeper breathing.
14. Tell the patient to cough up all loose secretions into the tissues, if a specimen is not necessary, or into a specimen container, if you have been instructed to collect a specimen.
15. Assist the patient to a position of comfort and safety in bed.
16. If a specimen has been collected, label it and send it to the laboratory with a requisition slip.

PROCEDURE (continued)

17. Discard disposable equipment.

18. Dispose of gloves and wash your hands.

FOLLOW-UP

19. Replace the pillow under the patient's head.

20. Lower the bed to a position of safety and replace the call light.

21. Raise the side rails when ordered or appropriate for patient safety.

22. Report to your immediate supervisor:

   ■ That you have helped the patient with coughing and deep-breathing exercises.

   ■ The number of breathing exercises.

   ■ The color, amount, and consistency of the secretions the patient was able to cough up.

   ■ That a specimen was collected and sent to the laboratory.

■ How the patient tolerated the procedure.

■ Your observations of anything unusual.

CHARTING EXAMPLE: 12/18/04 11pm Assisted Mrs. Smoke to cough and deep breathe. She was able to cough up some thick yellow secretions. She is resting comfortably now. H. Jinks, CNA

KEY IDEA

After surgical procedures requiring recovery in a hospital, some patients may have their pain medication administered by an infusion pump. The patient is able to push the attached button to have the pain medication automatically administered in small doses through the IV. This method of pain relief is effective, and the patient does not have to experience more intense pain while waiting for a nurse to bring ordered pain medication.

SUMMARY

Preoperative care includes educating the patient about the routine activities before and after surgery. Psychological support means listening to any concerns of your patient and getting any questions answered. Being sure the patient does not get any water or food if NPO is ordered; giving a bath, and properly caring for dentures, glasses, and jewelry are only part of the care which must be done and marked on the preoperative checklist. Postoperatively, vital signs and pain level must be checked frequently and the patient watched closely for any complications such as fever, bleeding, extreme restlessness, choking, vomiting, or changes in vital signs. Regularly asking about and reporting pain levels while taking vital signs can help provide the patient more timely pain relief. Any unusual observations must be reported at once. Turning the patient and assisting with deep breathing exercises as ordered can help prevent respiratory complications.

NOTES

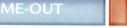

CHAPTER REVIEW

FILL IN THE BLANK Read each sentence and fill in each blank line with a word that completes the sentence.

1. A _____ is an unexpected condition, such as the development of an infection, in a patient who is already sick.

2. When a patient cannot eat or drink anything at all, it is called being _____.

3. Shaving the area of the body where surgery is to be performed is called a _____ _____.

4. Loss of feeling or sensation in a part or all of the body is called _____.

5. Exercises to expand the lungs after surgery are called _____ _____ exercises.

MULTIPLE CHOICE Choose the best answer for each question or statement.

1. Things that might worry the patient going to surgery are
   a. how his hair will look.
   b. a possible disability or death because of the operation.
   c. who his roommate might be.
   d. None of the above.

2. Which type of surgery is usually not covered by health insurance?
   a. Emergency
   b. Urgent
   c. Facial cosmetic surgical repair following a car accident
   d. Elective

3. Which of the following is not a type of surgical skin prep?
   a. Abdominal prep
   b. Vaginal prep
   c. Elbow prep
   d. Scrotal prep

4. All of the following is included in postoperative care *except*
   a. deep-breathing exercises.
   b. measurement of intake and output.
   c. skin prep.
   d. measurement of vital signs.

5. Notify your supervisor immediately for all of the following *except*
   a. rise or fall of blood pressure.
   b. patient questions.
   c. bleeding.
   d. cyanosis.

TIME-OUT

TIPS FOR TAKING CARE OF YOURSELF

You may not always be told that you are doing a good job. Patients who are ill or unhappy do not often say thank you. Your supervisor and fellow workers may seem to take your work for granted. Give yourself compliments when you know you have done a good job. You may want to ask for feedback occasionally from your supervisor as well. You will work hardest and manage your time best when you feel rewarded for your work.

THE NURSING ASSISTANT IN ACTION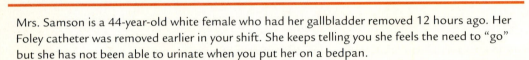

Mrs. Samson is a 44-year-old white female who had her gallbladder removed 12 hours ago. Her Foley catheter was removed earlier in your shift. She keeps telling you she feels the need to "go" but she has not been able to urinate when you put her on a bedpan.

What Is Your Response/Action?

CRITICAL THINKING

CUSTOMER SERVICE A child may want to see favorite toys or blankets when she returns from surgery. A religious person may be comforted by having his priest, minister, or rabbi bless him or pray with him prior to having a serious procedure performed. If the patient appears anxious, ask if there is something or someone who could provide him comfort and reassurance.

CULTURAL CARE Individuals approach surgery in different ways. Some cultures expect many family members to be nearby and visit, while others may prefer to be alone. Ask the patient if there are individuals who she would like you to contact if the patient is unable to do this on her own.

COOPERATION WITHIN THE TEAM Some caregivers are more skilled or comfortable than others when providing emotional support to patients who are afraid. If you notice a colleague has been identified as particularly supportive, try to learn more from him and ask advice about how he cares for patients and what things he says to provide reassurance.

EXPLORE MediaLink

Additional interactive resources for this chapter can be found on the Companion Website at www.prenhall.com/wolgin. Click on Chapter 28 and "Begin" to select activities for this chapter.

For chapter-related NCLEX-style questions and an audio glossary, access the accompanying CD-ROM in this book.

29 Special Procedures

OBJECTIVES

When you have completed this chapter, you will be able to:

- Label the parts of the intravenous infusion equipment on a diagram.
- Change the gown of the patient with an intravenous infusion.
- Check the intravenous bottle, drip chamber, tubing, and the patient's arm so that you can promptly report anything unusual to your immediate supervisor.
- List three reasons for the use of binders.
- Apply the three types of binders.
- Explain the purpose of antiembolism elastic stockings and elastic bandages.
- Apply elastic bandages and antiembolism elastic stockings.

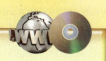

MediaLink
www.prenhall.com/wolgin

Use the address above to access the free, interactive Companion Website created for this textbook. Get hints, instant feedback, and textbook references to chapter-related NCLEX-style questions. Link to other interesting sites.

AUDIO GLOSSARY:
Use the Companion Website, or the CD-ROM disk enclosed with your textbook, to hear the pronunciation of key terms in the chapter.

KEY TERMS

antiembolism stockings
binder
infiltration
intravenous infusion
phlebitis
thrombophlebitis

While giving care to a patient receiving an intravenous infusion (IV), the nursing assistant must carefully observe the amount of liquid in the container, the tubing, and the needle site. Changing the gown of a patient receiving an IV requires special care so that you do not disturb the flow of the intravenous infusion solution. Binders are used to give support to a weakened body part, hold dressings in place, prevent or reduce swelling, or to put pressure on parts of the body. Elastic bandages and antiembolism elastic stockings are used to improve return circulation and are usually applied following surgery. The proper application of binders, elastic bandages, and antiembolism stockings promotes healing and adds to the comfort of the patient.

Intravenous Infusion (IV) Equipment

intravenous infusion The injection of fluids, nutrients, or medication into a vein

An **intravenous infusion** is often used in the hospital to put fluids into the patient's body. A tube is connected to a bottle or plastic container. The container holds a fluid that could be a solution of salt or sugar, a prescribed medication, or blood (Figure 29–1◆).

The other end of the tube is connected to a needle. The needle is inserted by the doctor or the nurse into the patient's vein to give fluids, nourishment, or medications to the patient. It may be used to change the balance of certain chemicals in the patient's body. The solution flows from the container into the patient's vein and is circulated through the body.

The amount of fluid that can flow into the patient's body is controlled by a clamp on the tube. This clamp allows only a certain number of drops per minute to flow from the

FIGURE 29–1 ◆

Intravenous (IV) infusion equipment

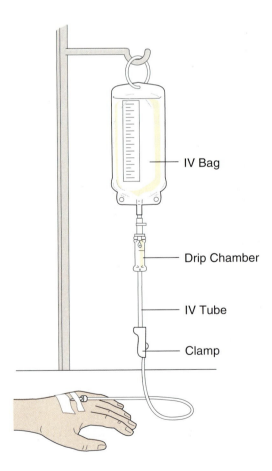

IV Bag

Drip Chamber

IV Tube

Clamp

container. The IV flow may also be regulated by an IV pump. You have to move the patient in bed or change his position without interrupting the flow of the solution. The pump may be moved to assist the patient out of bed or to walk.

Caring for the Patient with an Intravenous Infusion

Check the IV solution or blood transfusion to make sure it is flowing (Figure 29–2◆). Make sure the tubing is not kinked and that the patient is not lying on the tubing. Do not adjust the clamps or flow rate. Notify your supervisor immediately if the patient's skin around the needle is swollen or bleeding, if the fluid is not running properly, or if the patient complains of discomfort. It is possible that the solution is not running into the vein, but, instead, into the tissue nearby. This is called **infiltration** of an IV solution.

If available, choose a gown designed with snaps, Velcro®, or ties on the shoulders and sleeves. These types of gowns are designed for use with IV pumps to let you avoid lifting the patient's arm where the IV line is in place. When there are no gowns with shoulder ties or snaps available, a LPN or RN will change the gown of patients with IV pumps. Raising

infiltration Occurs when an IV solution runs into nearby tissue instead of into a vein

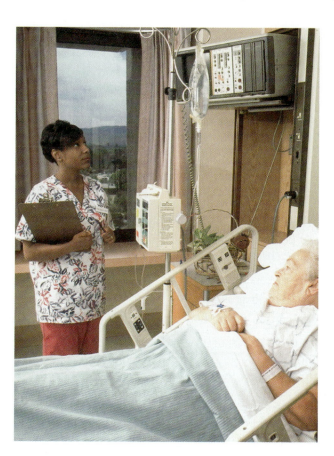

FIGURE 29–2 ◆

When a patient is receiving IV fluids, check the IV solution, drip chamber, and tubing

CHANGING A PATIENT'S GOWN

RATIONALE: The patient gown is changed when the patient is bathed or whenever the gown becomes soiled or wet.

PREPARATION

1. Place a clean gown and a laundry bag on the chair near the bed.
2. Untie the patient's gown.

STEPS

3. Remove the arm without the IV from the sleeve.
4. Remove the gown from the arm with the IV carefully, considering the tube and the container of fluid as part of the arm. Move the sleeve down the arm, over the tubing, and up to the bottle or container.
5. Remove the container or bottle from the hook, being careful not to lower the bottle below the area on the patient's arm where the needle is inserted.
6. Slip the gown over the bottle and return the bottle or container to its hook.
7. Place the soiled gown in the laundry bag on the chair.

    To put the clean gown on the patient, consider the bottle or container and tube as part of the patient's arm, and continue using these steps:

8. Lift the bottle from the hook carefully. Do not put the bottle or container below the area on the patient's arm where the needle has been inserted.
9. Slip the sleeve of the gown over the bottle or container quickly.
10. Replace the bottle on the hook.
11. Slip the gown down the tube and then over the patient's arm.
12. Slip the gown over the other arm without the IV.
13. Tie the back straps for the patient's comfort.
14. Make sure IV is running and the patient has no complaints.

FOLLOW-UP

15. Bag and dispose of soiled linen in the laundry hamper.

CHARTING EXAMPLE: 12/30/04 10am Bathed Mr. Amos and changed gown. IV is running in R arm. B. Cleary, CNA

the arm usually results in the patient's blood backing up into the IV tubing. If no IV gown is available and you need to change the patient's gown without disturbing the IV, use the procedure above. The nursing assistant should never remove the tubing from an IV pump. Consult with the nurse if you need assistance.

Binders

binder A type of bandage applied to a large body area (abdomen or chest) to secure a dressing in place or to put pressure on or support a body part

Binders are wide cloth bandages, usually made of cotton. They are applied mainly to the abdomen, chest, and perineal area of the patient for several reasons. Binders can be used postoperatively, or after childbirth, or whenever it is desirable to:

- Give support to a weakened body part
- Hold dressing and bandages in place
- Put pressure on parts of the body to make the patient more comfortable

Your immediate supervisor will tell you if a particular patient is to have a binder applied and what kind of binder is to be used. Remember, unless the binder is put on properly, it can be more uncomfortable for the patient than if it had not been used at all. Binders are obtained from central supply.

Straight abdominal binders are often ordered following lower back surgery. They provide needed support and can add to the patient's comfort. This binder is rectangular in shape, covers the area from the waist to the hips, and is fastened in the front.

<table>
<tr><td colspan="3">

BINDERS   **GUIDELINES**

</td></tr>
<tr>
<td>

- Keep the binder smooth and clean. Otherwise, it will be uncomfortable in the same way that crumbs or wrinkles in the patient's bed are uncomfortable. Bedsores (decubitus ulcers or pressure ulcers) can be caused by wrinkles or wetness of a binder.

</td>
<td>

- Watch for reddened areas on the patient's skin. Report these to your immediate supervisor.
- Use the correct type of binder. Be sure it is the correct size. Several different types of binders commonly used are:

</td>
<td>

- Straight abdominal binder
- T binder (Single T = female; Double T = male)
- Breast binders

</td>
</tr>
</table>

The *T binder* is used for males and females to keep dressings in place on the perineal (genital) area and rectal area. This binder is often used after a hemorrhoidectomy (an operation to remove hemorrhoids) or after the delivery of a baby. The binder is first wrapped around the patient's waist. Part of the binder then goes between the patient's legs and is brought back up to be fastened at the waist.

Breast binders are used for females following breast surgery.

Elastic Stockings and Elastic Bandages

Antiembolism elastic stockings and elastic bandages are applied to the body extremities (arms, hands, legs, feet). In postoperative care, they are most often used on the lower extremities or legs. They are used either as treatment for **thrombophlebitis** (blood clots in the veins) or for **phlebitis** (inflammation of the veins) or to prevent these conditions.

The purpose of antiembolism elastic stockings and elastic bandages is to compress the veins and, therefore, improve the return of venous blood to the heart, which improves circulation. In cases of sprain or strain at the joint, they are used to provide support and comfort.

thrombophlebitis Inflammation and blood clots in a vein

phlebitis Inflammation of a vein

<table>
<tr><td colspan="3">

APPLYING ANTIEMBOLISM/ ELASTIC SUPPORT HOSE   **GUIDELINES**

</td></tr>
<tr>
<td>

- Check that you have the correct size or type of support hose ordered for the patient. A nurse will measure the patient to determine the size.
- Apply the hose before the patient gets out of bed.
- Hold the heel of the stocking and

</td>
<td>

gather the leg portion of the stocking in your hand.
- Support the patient's foot at the heel as you slip the front of the stocking over his toes, foot, and heel.
- Pull the stocking firmly and evenly up over the leg.
- Check to be sure all wrinkles are smoothed out and that the hose is not twisted.

</td>
<td>

- Stockings are removed and reapplied when the patient is bathed and at least every 8 hours, or as ordered by the doctor.
- Check the patient for edema, complaints of pain, discolored or red areas. Document and report any changes to your immediate supervisor.

</td>
</tr>
</table>

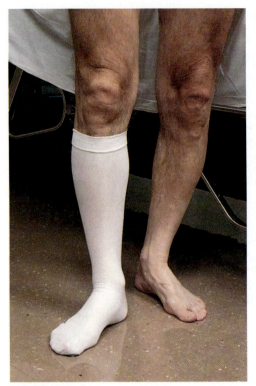

FIGURE 29-3a ◆

Knee-length antiembolism stocking

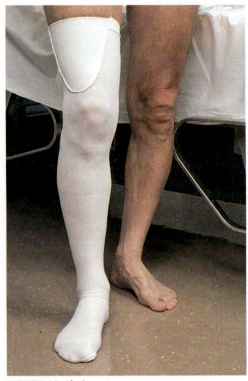

FIGURE 29-3b ◆

Full-length antiembolism stocking

Applying Antiembolism Elastic Stockings

antiembolism stockings
Designed to promote blood to flow and to prevent the formation of blood clots in the bloodstream

Antiembolism stockings are also called elastic support hose. These stockings can be either knee-length or full-length (Figure 29-3a◆ and 29-3b◆). ***Be careful to smooth out all the wrinkles. Be sure the stocking is pulled up firmly.*** Elastic stockings must be removed and reapplied at least once every 8 hours and more often if the doctor has so ordered. Always follow doctor's orders for application and removal. These stockings come in various sizes. When first ordered, the leg must be measured to be sure the stockings are the right size and fit the patient. They should be applied while the patient is lying down (not sitting in a chair) before getting out of bed. Elastic stockings should be applied only on the instructions of your immediate supervisor.

Applying Elastic Bandages

Elastic bandages (sometimes called ACE® bandages) are long strips of elasticized cotton (Figure 29-4◆). They are wound neatly into rolls, with a metal clip or Velcro® to keep the end in place. They provide support, hold dressings in place, apply pressure to a body part, and improve return circulation. Bandages may be ordered toes to knees, toes to mid-thighs, toes to groin, or heel-free (heel-free means heel uncovered). Follow the instructions given to you by your immediate supervisor. Use as many bandages as necessary to cover the area as ordered.

If the bandage has been wrapped too tightly, circulation may be impaired and the patient may develop symptoms such as paleness, coldness, blueness (cyanosis), pain, swelling, or numbness in the extremities. Be very careful to wrap these bandages firmly but not too tightly. Check the patient's condition frequently. Elastic bandages should be removed and reapplied once per shift, unless otherwise ordered. Observe the condition, color, and sensation of the skin every hour (qh). Also, check for movement of fingers or toes if applicable.

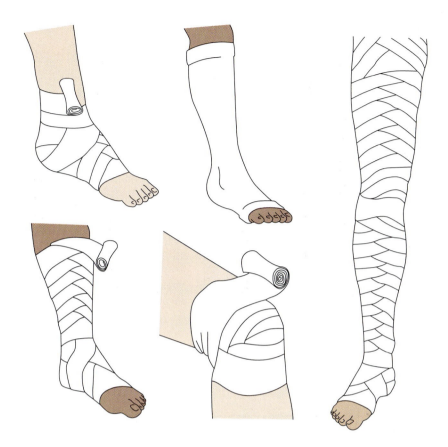

FIGURE 29–4 ◆
Elastic stockings and bandages

APPLYING ELASTIC BANDAGES

PROCEDURE   OBRA

RATIONALE: Elastic bandages are used to provide support or pressure to a body part, hold dressings in place, or improve return circulation in the legs.

PREPARATION

1. Assemble your equipment:

   a. Elastic bandages

   b. Clips or safety pins

   c. Disposable gloves

2. Identify the patient by checking the identification bracelet.

3. Explain to the patient that you are going to wrap his leg or arm (or whatever area is to be wrapped) with an elastic bandage.

4. Provide privacy for the patient.

STEPS

5. Wash your hands and put on gloves.

6. Raise the bed to a comfortable working position.

7. Place the patient in a comfortable position that is convenient for you to work. Expose the area to be wrapped.

8. Extend the part of the body to be bandaged. Support the patient's heel or wrist.

9. Stand directly in front of the patient or facing the part to be bandaged.

10. Hold the bandage with the loose end coming off the bottom of the roll.

11. Anchor the bandage by two circular turns around the body part at its smallest point. This usually is the ankle or the wrist.

12. Apply the bandage in the same direction as venous circulation, that is, toward the heart.

13. Roll the bandage smoothly and wrap it firmly but not too tightly.

14. Exert even pressure. Keep the bandage smooth. Be sure no skin areas show between the turns.

PROCEDURE *(continued)*

15. If possible, leave the toes or fingers exposed for observation of circulatory changes.

16. Continue wrapping upward with a spiral turn. Each turn should overlap the one before about one-half width of the bandage.

17. After applying the bandage, secure the terminal end by pinning it with a safety pin, applying bandage clips, or with Velcro®.

18. If more than one bandage is used, overlap them to prevent the bandages from slipping.

19. To remove the bandage, unwind it gently. Gather it into a loose mass, passing the mass from hand to hand as the bandage is unwound. Then roll the bandage smoothly so it is ready for the next application.

FOLLOW-UP

20. Make the patient comfortable and replace the call light.

21. Lower the bed to a position of safety for the patient.

22. Raise the side rails when ordered or appropriate for patient safety.

23. Dispose of gloves and wash your hands.

24. Report to your immediate supervisor:

    ■ That you have applied or removed the elastic bandages.

    ■ The area of application.

    ■ How the patient tolerated the procedure.

    ■ Your observations of anything unusual.

CHARTING EXAMPLE: 12/30/04 11am Elastic bandages applied to Mrs. Smith's legs. She has good circulation in her toes after bandages applied. B. Smart, CNA

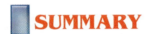

SUMMARY

In caring for a patient receiving an IV, the nursing assistant should check that the solution is dripping from the container, that the tubing is not kinked, and that there is no swelling or bleeding at the needle site. Straight, T, and breast binders are used to support or apply pressure to a body part or to hold a dressing in place. They must be applied without wrinkles. Antiembolism stockings and elastic bandages are two other types of binders that are frequently used to improve return circulation.

NOTES

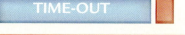

CHAPTER REVIEW

FILL IN THE BLANK Read each sentence and fill in the blank line with a word that completes the sentence.

1. The injection of fluids, nutrients, or medications into a vein is called an _____ _____.

2. Only a _____ or _____ may change or regulate the amount of flow from an IV solution.

3. An _____ occurs when an IV solution runs into nearby tissue instead of into a vein.

4. _____ is an inflammation of a vein.

5. Stockings that are designed to promote blood flow and prevent the formation of clots are called _____ stockings.

MULTIPLE CHOICE Choose the best answer for each question or statement.

1. All of the following are tasks a nursing assistant should do when caring for a patient with an intravenous therapy *except* for which one?
   a. Check to make sure the IV fluid or blood is flowing through the tubing.
   b. Make sure the tubing is not kinked.
   c. Adjust the rate if it is not flowing.
   d. Notify your supervisor if the skin around the IV is swollen.

2. When changing the gown of a patient who has an IV,
   a. remove the gown from the arm with the IV.
   b. move the gown down the tubing and up to the bag.
   c. unhook the IV bag from the pole and slide the gown off.
   d. All of the above.

3. Binders are wide cloth bandages applied mainly to the abdomen, chest, and perineum to
   a. secure a dressing.
   b. reduce pressure on a body part.

   c. stop circulation.
   d. increase pain and discomfort.

4. A medical condition in which there is inflammation of the vein is
   a. thrombophlebitis.
   b. diabetes.
   c. phlebitis.
   d. hepatitis.

5. When caring for a patient with antiembolism hose, make sure the stockings are
   a. pulled up firmly and twisted.
   b. changed and replaced every 8 hours or as ordered.
   c. in place during the bath.
   d. applied after the patient is out of bed.

TIME-OUT

TIPS FOR TIME MANAGEMENT

When superiors request something of you, give them your full attention. Repeat the request back, if needed, to clarify what you are being asked to do. If you are unsure of how to perform the task, say so. This will prevent misunderstandings and mistakes.

THE NURSING ASSISTANT IN ACTION

You are assigned to Mr. Smith who has antiembolism stockings ordered. His stockings are supposed to be on for 8 hours. You enter his room and see he has removed the stockings. He says, "I do not like wearing these things. I feel like a woman wearing these support hose and do not want them on when my friends and family are visiting me."

What Is Your Response/Action?

CRITICAL THINKING

CUSTOMER SERVICE If your patient has only one pair of support hose, inquire if another can be obtained for him. It is important that the hose be washed on a regular basis. Putting the patient's name on special-order hose would reduce the possibility of them being lost or misplaced.

CULTURAL CARE You may encounter patients who have different views based on their religious or cultural beliefs. They may decline treatment or special procedures if they decide to do so. It is important to respect their right to choose the treatments they desire and not try to force them to accept something, even if you think it better for them.

COOPERATION WITHIN THE TEAM Many special procedures require extra time to perform and should be completed once started. If you will be applying antiembolism stockings and anticipate that another patient will require your assistance during the time you need to apply the stockings, first attempt to take care of the need in advance. You can ask a coworker to watch for the light while you are busy, but respect that they have patients to care for as well.

EXPLORE MediaLink

Additional interactive resources for this chapter can be found on the Companion Website at www.prenhall.com/wolgin. Click on Chapter 29 and "Begin" to select activities for this chapter.

For chapter-related NCLEX-style questions and an audio glossary, access the accompanying CD-ROM in this book.

30 Other Patients with Special Needs

OBJECTIVES

When you have completed this chapter, you will be able to:

- Contrast benign and malignant tumors.
- Review risk factors and cancer prevention strategies.
- List the warning signs of cancer.
- Explain the psychosocial aspects of cancer.
- Give one example of a disease or treatment that results in immunosuppression.
- List three common misunderstandings about the transmission of AIDS.
- Name and describe a thought disorder and a mood disorder.
- Name the three spheres of orientation.
- List three signs or signals of substance abuse.

MediaLink

www.prenhall.com/wolgin

Use the address above to access the free, interactive Companion Website created for this textbook. Get hints, instant feedback, and textbook references to chapter-related NCLEX-style questions. Link to other interesting sites.

AUDIO GLOSSARY:

Use the Companion Website, or the CD-ROM disk enclosed with your textbook, to hear the pronunciation of key terms in the chapter.

KEY TERMS

acquired immune deficiency
    syndrome (AIDS)
benign tumor
cancer
chemotherapy
immunocompromised
lumpectomy
malignant (neoplasms)
mastectomy
mental health
mental illness
metastasis
neoplasm (tumor)
orientation
radiation therapy
substance abuse

In this chapter, you will learn about patients dealing with cancer, immunosuppression, AIDS, mental illness, and substance abuse. Each of these disorders will be defined, and special considerations for the nursing assistant in recognizing these conditions and in caring for patients will be described. It is important for you, as a nursing assistant, to understand that these conditions are diseases, to know how to recognize them, and to be aware of your own feelings and attitudes.

Cancer and Benign Tumors

neoplasm (tumor) New growth; the words *tumor* and *neoplasm* are interchangeable

benign tumor A tumor that stays at its site of origin and does not usually regrow once removed

cancer Refers to malignant neoplasms, or tumors

malignant (neoplasms) New growths that spread, invade, and destroy organs

Neoplasm means new growth. Normal cells reproduce because of need; however, when a neoplasm grows, the cells grow without any control, organization, or purpose. Neoplastic growth can be slow or rapid, benign or malignant. The words *tumor* and neoplasm are interchangeable.

A **benign tumor** stays at its site of origin and does not usually regrow once removed. It never invades surrounding tissue and grows slowly. It looks like the tissue it grew from.

Cancer refers to malignant neoplasms, or tumors. **Malignant neoplasms (tumors)** grow, spread, invade, and destroy organs. Cancer cells interfere with normal body function. If they are not controlled, they grow and spread between cells, invade surrounding tissues, and sometimes cause death. Malignant neoplasms can recur after surgical removal. **Metastasis** refers to the spreading of cancer cells through the systems of the body. Changing behavior to decrease risk factors (for example, stopping smoking) and early detection of cancer can reduce the risk of dying from cancer (see Table 30–1 ◆).

TABLE 30–1

Risk Factors and Cancer Prevention Strategies

RISK FACTOR	PREVENTION STRATEGY
Tobacco	Quit smoking/avoid secondhand smoke/reduce smoking or smoke the lower tar and nicotine cigarettes if you can't stop smoking.
Diet	Decrease high-fat diet, reduce consumption of nitrates/nitrites found in cured meats, bacon, and pickled foods. Increase fiber by eating more whole grains, cruciferous vegetables, i.e., broccoli, cauliflower. Reduce weight, if obese.
Sunlight	Use sunscreen of at least SPF 15, wear hat, protective clothing; avoid exposure 11AM–3PM, avoid tanning beds.
Alcohol	Avoid drinking and smoking in combination. Those who drink should limit alcoholic drinks (including beer) to 1–2/day. More excessive drinking increases the risk of mouth, throat, esophageal, larynx, liver, and breast cancer.
Radiation	Avoid unnecessary x-rays; use protective shields positioning patients.
Chemicals	In the workplace: Use protective masks, gloves; follow safety rules, avoid contact with dangerous chemicals: benzene, asbestos, nickel, vinyl chloride. Read/follow warning labels. Report exposures in workplace/follow OSHA guidelines/procedures.
Family Patterns	Be aware environmental exposure could affect everyone exposed; follow doctor's advice about prevention; seek routine tests and checkups, especially since some cancers seem to have higher incidence in blood relatives.
Sedentary Lifestyle	Increase exercise, walking.
Sexual/Lifestyle	Use condoms; practice safe sex.
Stress	Seek support, social services, pastoral, or mental health counseling.

EARLY WARNING SIGNS. Some cancers are not easily detected, or their symptoms are such that they are easily overlooked. Usually the sooner cancer is diagnosed and treatment begins, the better one's chances for recovery.

The signs listed in Table 30–2◆ may be associated with cancer and are signals to have a medical checkup. They can be remembered by the word CAUTION.

metastasis Refers to the spreading of cancer cells through the systems of the body

TABLE 30–2

Early Warning Signs of Cancer

1. Change in bowel or bladder habits:

   - Bleeding from the rectum; black stools
   - Elderly men: difficulty in urination, blood in urine
   - Diarrhea alone, with no sign of flu

2. A sore or skin ulcer that does not heal
3. Unusual bleeding or discharge: bleeding from the rectum; fluid discharge from a woman's nipples
4. Thickening or lump in any part of the body: breast, neck, head, vulva, testicles
5. Indigestion or difficulty swallowing
6. Obvious change in the size, color, or shape of a wart or mole
7. Nagging, persistent cough; cough producing blood in sputum; continuing hoarseness

Additional warning signs include pain that continues with no apparent cause and frequent infections.

Breast cancer is one of the leading causes of death among women. If detected early, breast cancer is treatable and curable. Early detection includes monthly self breast exams and mammograms every 1–2 years for women over 40 years of age. Treatment for breast cancer may include surgery, radiation therapy and chemotherapy, or a combination of the three. There are many surgical options for breast cancer treatment. Surgery that is limited to a small area of the breast is called a **lumpectomy**. Surgery that removes the total breast is called a **mastectomy**. It may be difficult for the woman to deal with this alteration to her body. Adjusting to body image changes takes time. You will need to be calm and accepting of the patient's responses.

lumpectomy Removal of a small part of the breast

mastectomy Removal of the entire breast

Prostate cancer is the most common cancer among men in the United States. The prostate gland is located between the bladder and the penis and surrounds the urethra. The prostate enlarges with age, and most men eventually experience symptoms of benign enlargements that usually cause difficulty in urination. Cancerous tumors require treatment with surgery, radiation, and hormone therapy. Frequent complications and side effects of treatment include impotence and incontinence. The survival rate is over 57 percent following treatment. Often, treatment is not recommended in men over 75 years of age, as the tumor is generally slow growing, and the side effects of treatment may cause greater problems than the disease.

Cancer is a leading cause of death in the United States. Many cancers are treatable if detected early. Surgery, chemotherapy, and radiation therapy are the main treatments for cancer. Often a combination of the three is used for the maximum cure or treatment benefit to the patient.

FIGURE 30–1 ◆

Often a word of encouragement will be enough to get the patient to take some nourishment

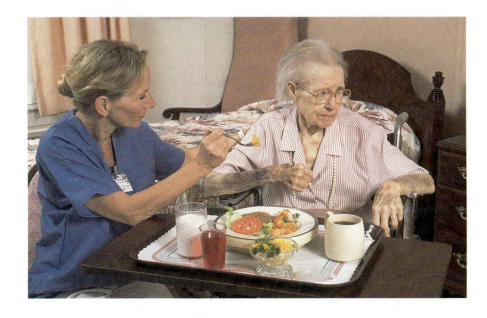

chemotherapy Refers to the use of drugs to treat cancer

radiation therapy The use of high doses of radiation, many times the dose used for x-ray exams, to treat the cancer

In surgery, the tumor is removed. Sometimes surrounding tissue is also removed to completely rid the area of any growing tumor. **Chemotherapy** is the use of drugs to treat the cancer. Chemotherapy may cure the cancer, stop it from spreading, or slow its growth. **Radiation therapy** refers to the use of high doses of radiation, many times the dose used for x-ray exams, to treat the cancer. Radiation kills the cells and stops them from growing. Because cancer cells divide so fast, radiation is effective in cancer treatment. Normal cells are also killed with radiation and therefore patients will have side effects from treatment.

Many people fear the side effects of cancer treatment. Radiation therapy and chemotherapy can cause unpleasant symptoms which the patient must cope with during treatment. Fatigue, diarrhea, nausea, and hair loss are common occurrences (Figure 30–1◆). Your role in assisting and supporting the patient and his family is crucial to the patient's health.

Psychosocial Aspects of Cancer

Every patient has a different personality and different coping patterns. The patient with cancer goes through the stages of denial, anger, depression, bargaining, and finally acceptance. When the cancer patient must undergo a surgical procedure that results in changes in bodily functions or form, acceptance is not easy to achieve. For example:

- Removal of the rectum due to cancer, including creation of an ostomy in the abdomen, necessitates wearing an appliance to collect waste from the bowel
- Total or partial removal of one or both breasts. Both men and women have difficulty in accepting this body change
- Amputation of an extremity
- Removal of the voice box (larynx); the patient loses the ability to speak

Immunosuppression

Immune disorders can be encountered in virtually every clinical situation from geriatrics, with the normal decline of immune defense mechanisms, to the high-tech situations of organ transplants. You must understand what it means to be immunocompromised and to be able to discuss special considerations when caring for patients without normal immunity.

The human body has many natural defense mechanisms to help fight off disease. Fever, for example, is a natural defense mechanism against infection. Fever is a sign that the body is responding to a virus or bacteria and defending against infection by raising the body's temperature. Other defense mechanisms are acquired after birth. Childhood immunizations and "flu shots" are examples of acquired defense mechanisms. These immunizations force the body to develop special cells called antibodies to fight off particular bacteria or viruses.

Several diseases and conditions can cause disorders of the immune system. In these cases, a patient is said to be **immunocompromised**, or immunosuppressed, which means that the immune system is not able to fight off bacteria and viruses. Cancer, AIDS, malnutrition, stress, infections, chronic illnesses such as diabetes, chemotherapy, and radiation are examples of immunocompromising conditions. Infections and poor wound healing are characteristic of these conditions.

Acquired immune deficiency syndrome (AIDS) is a condition caused by a virus that destroys a key part of the body's immune response system (Figure 30–2◆). This virus is called the human immunodeficiency virus or HIV. The AIDS virus can live in a number of human body fluids including blood, semen, and vaginal secretions. The AIDS virus can only be spread by direct blood-to-blood contact or close sexual contact with an infected person's body fluids. The two most common ways of getting AIDS are by having sex with an infected person and by sharing an intravenous needle with an HIV-infected person. Though much less common, AIDS can also be passed from an infected mother to an infant during pregnancy or childbirth. In the United States, it is highly unlikely to get AIDS from a blood transfusion, since all blood donors are questioned and all blood products are tested for the HIV virus.

Common Misunderstandings

It is important for the nursing assistant to be aware of some common misperceptions about AIDS. The AIDS virus is not passed on to others by coughing, sneezing, holding hands, hugging, touching, or being around someone with AIDS. It is not passed by silverware, drinking glasses, towels, bathtubs, showers, or toilet seats. The AIDS virus does not survive outside the human body fluids associated with sexual activity. AIDS is not a "gay disease." AIDS is primarily a heterosexual disease.

When the body is infected with the HIV virus, after an initial "flu"-like illness, there are no obvious signs of AIDS. After several years, the destruction of the immune system is so severe that the patient begins to develop complications, called opportunistic infections (OIS). Infecting organisms take advantage of the "opportunity," the damaged immune system.

immunocompromised
Means that the immune system is not functioning normally; immunocompromised and immunosuppressed mean the same and are used interchangeably

acquired immune deficiency syndrome (AIDS) Condition caused by a virus that destroys a key part of the body's immune response system

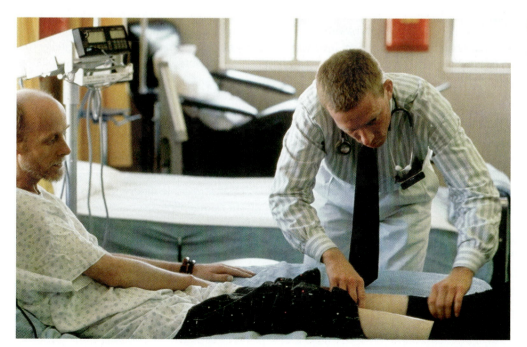

FIGURE 30–2 ◆

AIDS is caused by a virus that affects the body's immune system

These infections develop, or persist, because the body's immune or defense system is no longer working. Examples of these opportunistic infections are pneumonia, tuberculosis, cancer, thrush, meningitis, and encephalitis (brain infections). *Pneumoncystis carinii* pneumonia (PCP) is one of the most deadly of opportunistic infections, infecting 75 percent of AIDS patients at some point in the course of their disease. Side effects of medications commonly used to treat PCP include anemia and liver damage. While current drug combinations are offering hope, their long-term ability to treat AIDS is yet to be seen. Eventually, the immune system is so compromised (not working) that the person with the AIDS virus is not able to survive the infections. People with normal immune systems are either protected from getting these infections or would recover from them easily.

Research completed over the last 10 years has resulted in the development of drug treatments that allow a person with AIDS to live with the virus for a long time. Having AIDS can now be considered a chronic disease like diabetes or heart disease. It is important *to protect yourself from exposure to an infectious disease and also to protect the patient from exposure to bacteria,* or viruses, that are not harmful to you as a nursing assistant, but would be harmful to your patient. You must follow the Standard Precautions guidelines emphasized throughout this book in this regard. Nursing assistants need to be attentive to skin care, nutrition, mouth care, and emotional support when caring for patients with immunocompromised conditions.

KEY IDEA

You must also examine and discuss your own feelings about AIDS so that you can be accepting and nonjudgmental in your interactions with persons with AIDS. Should you be sick or recently exposed to an infectious disease, it is important to inform your employer when caring for AIDS patients as they are extremely susceptible to infection.

Mental Health and Mental Illness

Approximately 45 percent of the population will suffer from cancer over their life spans, while 15 percent will be affected by mental illness. This number increases in the aging population. Many older adults are depressed and others turn to alcohol to seek relief or to cope with chronic illness, social isolation, or boredom. Mental illnesses are medical disorders just like diabetes, high blood pressure, or heart disease. Mental illness is not the same as mental retardation, which involves impairments in learning ability and intellectual process. Your approach to patients and families of patients suffering from mental illness should be accepting and nonjudgmental.

mental health Describes the best adjustment an individual can make at a given time, based on internal and external resources

mental illness Describes a number of chemical imbalances in the brain or genetically based brain diseases that interfere significantly with people's abilities to live and work

Mental health is a term used to describe the best adjustment an individual can make at a given time, based on internal and external resources. **Mental illness** is a term used to describe a number of chemical imbalances in the brain or genetically based brain diseases that interfere significantly with one's ability to live and work. Mental illnesses that affect a person's mood and feelings are called *mood disorders*. Depression is an example of a mood disorder. Mental illnesses that affect thinking are called *thought disorders*. Schizophrenia is an example of a thought disorder. Mental illnesses are treatable illnesses. Stigma—negative attitudes, stereotypes, and misunderstandings about mental illness—create tremendous barriers for mentally ill people and their families. As a nursing assistant, you will need to be aware of your own thoughts, feelings, and beliefs about mental illness in your care of patients with mental illness.

Depression is a common illness that can affect anyone (Figure 30–3◆). About 19 million Americans get depressed every year. For older adults, depression is the most common psychiatric disorder, affecting 10 to 12 percent. Older adults with depression are more likely than younger persons to have repeated episodes or bouts of depression or to commit

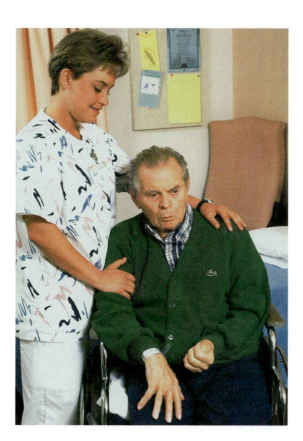

FIGURE 30–3 ◆
Depression can affect anyone

suicide. Another challenge is untreated anxiety disorders, which may prevent the individual from leaving home. Older adults are far more likely to report physical problems over psychiatric problems. Depression is not just having the "blues" or feeling "down" or sad. All people feel sad after a loss or "blue" or "down" at different times in their lives. A person with a depressive disorder has some of the following symptoms every day, all day, for at least 2 weeks:

- Persistent feelings of hopelessness
- Feelings of inappropriate guilt
- Noticeable increase or decrease in appetite
- Loss of interest in things they used to enjoy
- Tremendous feeling of sadness, worthlessness, or guilt
- Thoughts of death or suicide
- Problems concentrating or making decisions
- Trouble sleeping

Treatment for depression usually includes medications and talk therapy, known as psychotherapy or counseling. With psychotherapy and medication treatment, most people feel better in 3 to 4 weeks. There has been a dramatic increase in the number of adults and children who are taking prescribed antidepressants such as Prozac or herbal over-the-counter products like St. John's wort.

The ability to recognize possible signs of depression is important for a nursing assistant. You may see and talk with a patient every day and notice when he seems to be getting depressed. Inform your supervisor of conversations or observations you have with a patient that lead you to be concerned. Early recognition and treatment may prevent the depression from becoming more severe. Thoughts of suicide are common in depression, and suicidal thoughts will go away when the depression is treated.

PREVENTING DEPRESSION	GUIDELINES

- Keep, maintain, and develop new friendships over the years to prepare for major changes in life, such as job changes, loss of relationships or divorce, retirement, death of family or friends. Having friends or others you can confide in helps ease the loneliness of losing a spouse or others dear to you.
- Develop interests or hobbies.
- Keep your mind and body active, exercise regularly.
- Stay in touch with family members.
- Eat a variety of foods and a balanced diet to avoid illness.
- Avoid or limit use of medications that have depression as a side effect.
- Find ways to laugh (books, comics, funny movies, comedians, friends who share jokes).
- Volunteer or give of yourself to others.

Schizophrenia is a type of brain disease that affects the way a person thinks. A patient with schizophrenia often exhibits unexplained behaviors, such as talking aloud, being restless, or speaking in a confused manner that makes no sense. Schizophrenia occurs most frequently in young adults aged 16 to 25. Schizophrenia is not multiple, or "split," personality.

As a nursing assistant, it is important that you be aware of the patient's awareness or orientation. **Orientation** is an individual's ability to identify who she is, where she is, and some information about time (month, year, time of day). These three areas are known as "orientation to time, person, and place." The abbreviation "oriented X3" or "A (alert) + OX3" describes someone who is oriented. Report any changes in a patient's orientation to your immediate supervisor.

orientation An individual's ability to identify who she is, where she is, and some information about time (month, year, time of day)

Substance Abuse

Misuse and abuse of alcohol and other drugs, including prescription medications, can occur in people of all ages, walks of life, socioeconomic status, and ethnic backgrounds. The extent of substance abuse in the United States is staggering (Table 30–3◆).

Substance abuse is defined as the excessive use of mood-altering drugs that results in negative changes to an individual's life. Mood-altering drugs include a variety of legal and illegal substances, such as alcohol, prescription pain medications, cocaine, marijuana, and tobacco. People begin to use mood-altering drugs to feel good or to avoid, or ignore, uncomfortable feelings. People develop problems when they disregard low-risk drinking guidelines, ignore doctor's orders for prescriptions, and discount state and federal laws related to alcohol and other drug use. Like diabetes and heart disease, substance abuse is a lifestyle-related health problem that gets worse when personal health guidelines are ignored.

substance abuse The excessive use of mood-altering drugs such as alcohol, cocaine, tobacco, or caffeine that results in negative changes to a person's life

The person who develops a substance abuse problem begins to use mood-altering drugs in a higher quantity and to a greater frequency than the body can tolerate. For example, a normal drink is a single 12-oz. can of beer, a 4-oz. glass of wine or a 1-oz. shot of liquor. Social or low-risk drinking includes no more than one drink per hour, no more than two drinks per day, and a reduction of drinking based on current eating, health, and stress conditions. The person who has a substance abuse problem finds that the body gets used to the amount of alcohol or other drugs consumed, and then requires more of the substance to get the same feeling. (This is called *tolerance* and is a frequent reason why some patients need more pain medication than others in hospitals.)

As the person continues to use in high quantities, the substance begins to control the person, even though the person will often say that he can control the substance use. Family, friends, and coworkers of the person who is abusing a substance may know that the individual has problems, but they may not make the connection between the abuse of alcohol or other drugs and the difficulties the person is having. Helping the substance-abusing person

TABLE 30–3

Extent of Substance Abuse Problems

- Almost half of all people over age 12 are current alcohol users, 109 million people (U.S. Department of Health and Human Services, Substance Abuse and Mental Health Services Administration, 2001 National Household Survey on Drug Abuse [NHSDA]).

- In 2001, almost 17 million Americans aged 12 or older abused or were dependent on either alcohol or illicit drugs (*The NHSDA Report: Substance Abuse or Dependence,* October 11, 2002).

- Nearly one-fourth of all persons admitted to general hospitals have alcohol problems or are undiagnosed alcoholics being treated for the consequences of their drinking (National Institute on Alcohol Abuse and Alcoholism [NIAAA], 1998).

- A minimum of 3 out of 100 deaths in the United States can be attributed to causes linked directly to alcohol (NIAAA, 1996).

- Prior substance use increases the probability that an adolescent will initiate sexual activity, and sexually experienced adolescents are more likely to initiate substance use—including alcohol and cigarettes (National Center on Addiction and Substance Abuse at Columbia University, *Substance Use and Risky Sexual Behavior Fact Sheets,* 2002).

- Adolescents who drink are seven times more likely to have sex than those who do not, while those who use illicit substances are five times more likely—even after adjusting for age, race, gender, and parental educational level. (National Center on Addiction and Substance Abuse at Columbia University, *Substance Use and Risky Sexual Behavior Fact Sheets,* 2002).

- Fetal alcohol syndrome (FAS) is a pattern of birth defects that results from drinking alcohol during pregnancy. It occurs in 1 out of every 750 births (Michigan Substance Abuse and Traffic Safety Information Center).

- In 2001, an estimated 15.9 million Americans age 12 years or older used an illicit drug during the month immediately prior to the survey interview. These people are identified as current drug users. This estimate represents 7.1 percent of the population 12 years or older. By comparison, in 2000 the survey found that 6.3 percent of this population were current users of illicit drugs. The survey also found statistically significant increases between 2000 and 2001 in the use of particular drugs or groups of illicit drugs, such as marijuana (from 4.8 to 5.4 percent) and cocaine (0.5 to 0.7 percent), and the nonmedical use of pain relievers (1.2 to 1.6 percent) and tranquilizers (0.4 to 0.6 percent) (NHSDA, 2001).

    Of the 20 million Americans who have tried cocaine, by 1996 there were an estimated 6 million current or frequent users. Cocaine is a white powder produced from the leaves of the South American coca plant. Users refer to it as coke, C, toot, blow, nose candy, or The Lady. This stimulant drug produces a fleeting high after it is snorted in powder form through the nose or dissolved and injected into the muscle or vein. Crack is smoked and produces the most rapid high followed by a profound low. The brain experiences intense cravings for more of the drug, and this leads to dependency and addiction to achieve the rush, feeling of well being, and energy. Some users binge on the drug and require a couple of days to recover from the crash they experience when they quit taking the drug or collapse from physical exhaustion. Addiction leads to health problems, drains financial resources, and can drive away friends and family. Deaths can result when crack or cocaine triggers brain seizures or malfunctions in the electrical signals regulating the heart and muscles controlling breathing. It is important for the nursing assistant to be aware of signals of substance abuse in a patient or in a coworker.

and those around him make these connections is critical to the person being able to begin the process of breaking the cycle of abuse and addiction. Breaking this cycle frequently requires substance abuse treatment that may include detoxification, individual and group counseling, relapse prevention activities, and medication to counteract some of the effects of the drugs or provide assistance in early recovery.

An accepting, nonjudgmental, and understanding approach to patients, families, and coworkers is very important for the nursing assistant when dealing with substance abuse problems. You need to recognize your own life experiences with substance use and abuse and be aware of how these experiences may influence your thoughts and feelings about caring for patients with substance abuse problems.

As important as recognizing how your own life experiences may influence your patient care is, it is just as important for the nursing assistant to be aware of signs of substance misuse and abuse in a patient or in a coworker (Figure 30–4◆). Some examples of the behavior changes often associated with substance abuse are:

- Increased absences or tardiness
- Change in grades or quality of work
- Incomplete assignments

FIGURE 30–4 ◆

Signs of substance abuse

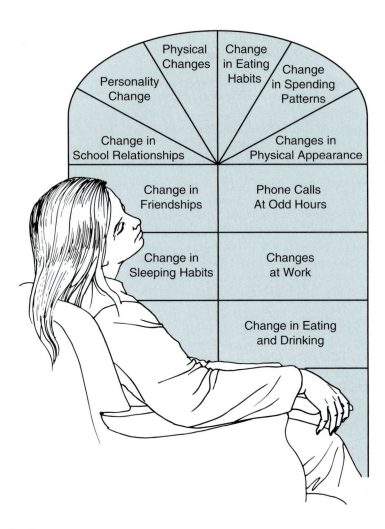

- Mood swings
- Change in eating habits
- Change in sleep habits
- Change in money spending habits
- Defensiveness or unprovoked angry outbursts

Such behavior changes can be observed at home, work, or school. Signs that someone is currently under the influence of a mood-altering substance include:

- Missing liquor or pills
- Odor of alcohol
- Unsteady gait or problems with coordination
- Tremors of the hands
- Forgetfulness or lack of concentration
- Distorted mental perceptions

When you observe such behavior changes or signs in your patient or a coworker, report this to your supervisor. Treatment is available for persons with a substance abuse problem. Pretending that the problem does not exist can lead to physical problems, as well as loss of family and work.

Problem or binge drinking is common with high-school and college students as well as adults of all age groups. Review the Guidelines on the next page to help identify the signs and symptoms of a drinking problem.

GUIDELINES

IDENTIFYING THE SIGNS AND SYMPTOMS OF A DRINKING PROBLEM

- Drinking to calm nerves, forget worries, or reduce depression
- Lack of interest in food or eating
- A tendency to gulp drinks
- Drinking alone, lying about or hiding drinks or alcohol

- Injuries from drinking or unexplained injuries
- Needing an increased amount of alcohol to get high
- Getting drunk more than 3–4 times per year
- Irritability, resentfulness, unreasonableness
- Medical, social, family, or financial problems caused by drinking

- Isolation or avoiding others who bring attention to the drinking

There are a variety of sources for help for both the drinker and those who live with or care for the problem drinker. Examples include counselors, clergy, Alcoholics Anonymous or other self-help groups, health care providers, and social service agencies.

SUMMARY

This chapter has given you information about natural defense mechanisms of the human body. You will need to keep this information in mind when caring for individuals who are immunosuppressed. These patients have lost some of those natural defenses either due to medications they are taking, such as chemotherapy, or a condition or disease they have, such as AIDS or diabetes. Care for patients with cancer, including special considerations for patients who are undergoing chemotherapy and/or radiation therapy, was also discussed in this chapter. Information about mental health and illnesses with behavioral changes, for example mental illness and substance abuse, was also covered in this chapter.

NOTES

CHAPTER REVIEW

FILL IN THE BLANK Read each sentence and fill in the blank line with a word that completes the sentence.

1. The word neoplasm means _____.

2. _____ is a leading cause of death in the United States.

3. When the immune system is not functioning normally and the body is unable to fight off infection, the patient is said to be _____.

4. Mental illnesses are _____ illnesses.

5. Abuse of alcohol, cocaine, and other drugs can occur in people of _____ ages.

MULTIPLE CHOICE Choose the best answer for each question or statement.

1. Treatment for cancer may include
   a. chemotherapy.
   b. radiation.
   c. surgery.
   d. All of the above.

2. Diseases that affect the immune system include
   a. cancer.
   b. HIV/AIDS.
   c. diabetes.
   d. All of the above.

3. HIV/AIDS is considered
   a. terminal.
   b. treatable with surgery.

   c. a chronic disease.
   d. an airborne infectious disease.

4. A person with depression has all of the following *except*
   a. persistent feelings of hopelessness.
   b. high blood pressure.
   c. tremendous feelings of sadness, worthlessness, or guilt.
   d. problems concentrating or making decisions.

5. Americans experience the highest rate of death and injury from
   a. anthrax.
   b. abuse of prescription drugs.
   c. abuse of illegal drugs.
   d. abuse of alcohol.

TIME-OUT

TIPS FOR TAKING CARE OF YOURSELF

Be sure that you are at a stopping point before you leave the unit for break or lunch. Do not leave until another staff member is able to take over a task you are performing. If no one is available, complete the task before you leave the unit. Likewise, when you return to the unit from a break or lunch, check to see if you need to relieve another staff member.

THE NURSING ASSISTANT IN ACTION
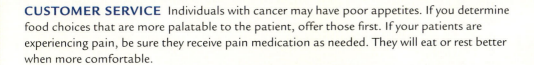

You are assigned to care for Mr. Underwood, a 70-year-old man who has cancer and is clinically depressed. He takes antidepressant medication and was admitted to begin a course of chemotherapy. You find a bottle of vodka in his drawer when you are gathering equipment for his bath. He says, "Please don't tell anyone about the bottle. It is hard to get someone to bring me a drink. I really need a couple of drinks to get through the day in this place. Give a dying man a break."

What Is Your Response/Action?

CRITICAL THINKING
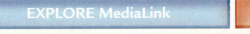

CUSTOMER SERVICE Individuals with cancer may have poor appetites. If you determine food choices that are more palatable to the patient, offer those first. If your patients are experiencing pain, be sure they receive pain medication as needed. They will eat or rest better when more comfortable.

CULTURAL CARE You may be assigned to care for patients who have sexual preferences different from your own. Some religions may teach that AIDS is God's punishment for homosexuals or persons who have sex outside marriage. Try to be nonjudgmental in your approach when you care for patients whose beliefs are different from yours.

COOPERATION WITHIN THE TEAM It is not uncommon to have a team member who has an alcohol or substance abuse problem. If you notice a coworker exhibiting signs of substance abuse, encourage him to get help. Covering up for a coworker is not cooperation. It enables him to continue drinking or abusing drugs without consequences. Working while impaired can endanger patients.

EXPLORE MediaLink

Additional interactive resources for this chapter can be found on the Companion Website at www.prenhall.com/wolgin. Click on Chapter 30 and "Begin" to select activities for this chapter.

For chapter-related NCLEX-style questions and an audio glossary, access the accompanying CD-ROM in this book.

31 Neonatal and Pediatric Care

KEY TERMS

circumcise
constipation
dehydrate
diaper
diarrhea
infant
pediatric patient
stool
umbilical cord

OBJECTIVES

When you have completed this chapter, you will be able to:

- Feed a baby using a bottle.
- Assist a mother to breast-feed.
- Feed and burp an infant.
- Describe a normal infant bowel movement.
- Diaper a baby.
- Demonstrate circumcision care.
- Demonstrate umbilical cord care.
- Demonstrate an infant bath.
- List five safety precautions when caring for infants.
- List eight safety precautions when caring for children.
- Measure vital signs in infants and children.
- List six things to remember when communicating with children.

MediaLink
www.prenhall.com/wolgin

Use the address above to access the free, interactive Companion Website created for this textbook. Get hints, instant feedback, and textbook references to chapter-related NCLEX-style questions. Link to other interesting sites.

AUDIO GLOSSARY:
Use the companion Website, or the CD-ROM disk enclosed with your textbook, to hear the pronunciation of key terms in the chapter.

In this chapter, you will learn about neonatal and pediatric care. Caring for infants and small children can be one of the most challenging opportunities you will encounter in your career as a nursing assistant. You will play a key role in modeling appropriate behaviors for the new mother. Key elements are to give safe care and to prevent accidents. Establishing a good relationship with the mother or caregiver and the small child will be of great importance. Understanding how to provide the basics of child care such as feeding, diapering, and bathing is essential to providing high-quality neonatal and pediatric care. The procedures you will use to measure vital signs of the pediatric patient are presented in this chapter.

INTRODUCTION

ALERT

For all patient contact, adhere to Standard Precautions (⊗ Chapter 5, pages 83–85). Wear protective equipment as indicated.

Neonatal Care

Neonatal care refers to the care given to newborn **infants**. This care includes feeding, burping, changing, and bathing. Care of the umbilical cord and observing bowel movements for possible problems are very important. Special attention is given to the safety of the newborn. Safety of the infant is a full-time job. Remember to wash your hands before and after each time you pick up, feed, bathe, or diaper an infant.

infant A baby aged 1 month to 1 year

Feeding the Infant

Infant feeding should be a relaxing experience. Most infants are fed at least six times a day, every 4 hours, but many infants need to be fed more often than that. If the mother is breast-feeding her baby, you may bring the baby to her when it is time for a feeding. If the baby is being bottle-fed, you may need to prepare the *formula*. Discuss the care of the newborn infant with the mother and your supervisor and follow their instructions. See Chapter 11 for preparing infant formula, including sterilizing bottles and tap water.

Feeding the Baby from a Bottle

The steps to follow when feeding a baby from a bottle are demonstrated in Figures 31–1◆, 31–2◆, and 31–3◆.

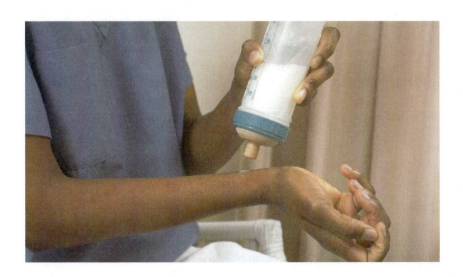

FIGURE 31–1 ◆

Check the temperature of the formula

Tilt the bottle so the nipple is always full of milk and the air in the bottle rises

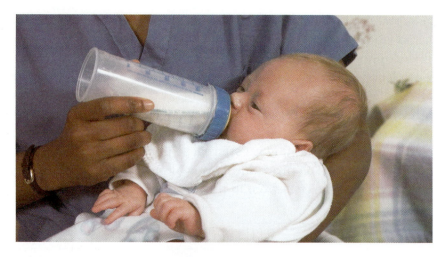

The infant should be held during feeding; do not prop the bottle and leave the baby

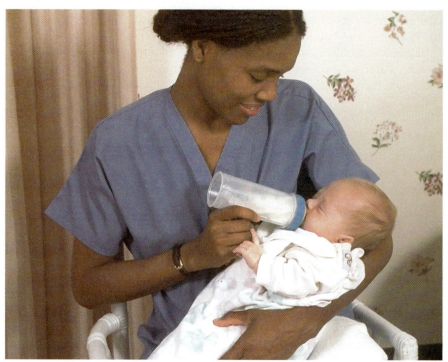

Helping a Mother Breast-feed

You can help a mother breast-feed by making sure the area she is in provides privacy and comfort. You can make the mother comfortable by helping to position her so that her back is supported, and the arm holding the baby is supported by a pillow or folded blanket. Make sure the mother has a call light if you leave the room, or stay close by in case she has difficulty. Never leave a sleepy mother alone while she is holding the baby. It is also important to raise the side rails for her protection.

Nurses will teach the mothers to breast-feed, and help them with any problems. If the mother states she is having difficulty, notify the nurse immediately.

Burping the Infant

Most infants, especially those who are bottle-fed, swallow some air while drinking. Air in the stomach can cause vomiting and abdominal pain. You can prevent a buildup of the air by feeding the infant slowly, stopping after every 1 to 2 ounces (30 to 60 cc) to burp the baby.

HELPING THE MOTHER WITH BREAST-FEEDING

GUIDELINES

- Give the mother a basin, washcloth, and soap to wash her hands.

- Position the mother in bed or in a chair.

- Have the mother hold the baby close to her breast, and with the nipple or her finger stroke the baby's cheek which is closest to her. This will stimulate the rooting reflex in the baby, which will cause it to turn toward the breast to nurse.

- Have the mother keep the breast tissue away from the baby's nose so the baby can breathe. (She can hold her finger or thumb above the baby's nose on the breast.)

- A diaper, small towel, or blanket can be draped over the exposed breast and the baby's head to promote privacy for the mother.

- Both breasts should be used at each feeding. Example: 10 minutes each breast; or 5 minutes right breast, then 15 minutes left breast. At the next feeding, the left breast will be used for 5 minutes and the right breast for 15 minutes. At the end of a feeding, some mothers put a safety pin on the bra strap to remind themselves which breast they want to use first (for 5 minutes) at the next feeding.

- When the mother wants to remove the breast from the baby's mouth, she must first push down on the breast tissue near the baby's

mouth with a finger to release the suction. She should never pull the breast out of the baby's mouth, as this can cause pain and irritate her skin.

- The baby should be burped between breast changes and after feeding. If the baby was crying before nursing, he may need to be burped to remove air he swallowed while crying. This will make the feeding more comfortable for the baby and prevent excessive spitting up of the milk after feeding.

- Change the baby and help the mother get comfortable after the feeding.

- Notify the nurse if the patient has breast-feeding questions.

There are two methods for burping the baby:

- **Method A:** Cover your shoulder with a clean cloth (a small towel or a cloth diaper). Hold the baby in an upright position, so the baby's head is resting on your shoulder (Figure 31–4◆). Gently rub and/or pat the infant's back until you hear the burp.

- **Method B:** Sit the infant on your lap so the baby's feet are dangling over the side of your legs. Put one of your hands on the infant's chest and lean the baby over so your hand is supporting him (Figure 31–5◆). Gently rub and pat the baby's back with your other hand until you hear the burp.

Observing the Infant's Stool

You will need to observe the infant's **stool** at each diaper change in order to detect a stool that is too hard, indicating possible **constipation**, or too liquid. When you observe a change from what has been normal for your patient, report your observations to the nurse.

The bottle-fed infant will have stools that are yellowish or mustard color. They will be lumpy but soft. One to three bowel movements each day is normal for an infant that is bottle-fed every 3 to 4 hours.

The breast-fed infant will have stools that are yellowish or mustard color, but the color may change slightly and may appear to have a greenish tint, depending on the mother's diet. The stools will be looser and smoother than the stools of a bottle-fed infant. It is not unusual for the stools to look like there are tiny seeds in them. A bowel movement after every feeding or only once or twice a day is normal for an infant that is breast-fed every 2 to 3 hours. Check with your supervisor if you suspect that the infant is not having bowel movements this often. Also, tell the supervisor if an infant's bowel movement is dry and formed. Often, all that is necessary to correct this situation is to offer the infant some plain sterile water between each formula feeding. Usually the infant will drink 1 ounce (30 cc) of water. If the condition doesn't change, report this to the nurse.

stool Solid waste material discharged from the body through the rectum and anus; other names include feces, excreta, excrement, bowel movement, and fecal matter

constipation Difficult, infrequent defecation with passage of unduly hard and dry fecal material

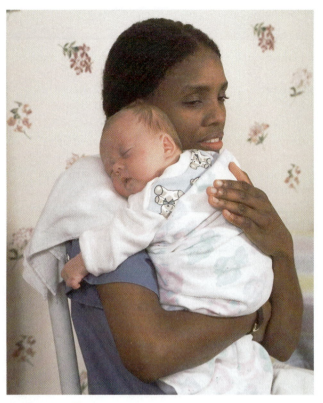

FIGURE 31–4 ◆
Gently rub and pat the infant's back until you hear the burp

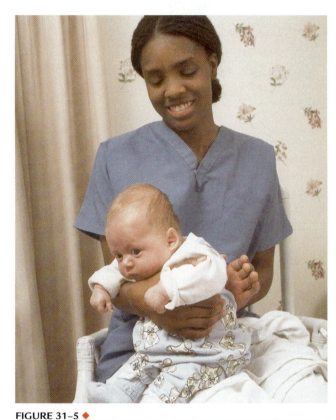

FIGURE 31–5 ◆
Support the baby with one hand while gently rubbing and patting the baby's back with the other

Diarrhea in Infants

dehydrate Loss of body fluids

diarrhea Abnormally frequent discharge of fluid fecal material from the bowel

Diarrhea in infants can be a very serious problem and requires immediate attention. Infants can lose a large amount of their body fluids and **dehydrate** very quickly. An infant with too many watery stools can become dehydrated within 2 days or less. You will be able to see a noticeable change in the infant's elimination pattern and in the actual color and consistency of the stools when an infant has **diarrhea**. The stools may appear green and watery, running right out of the diaper. There may be a distinct odor. The frequency of the stools may increase to two or three times within just a few hours. At the first sign of diarrhea, report to your immediate supervisor.

There are many causes for diarrhea in infants. It may be caused by equipment that was not sterilized (cleansed) properly, by carelessly prepared or spoiled formula, or by allergies. Much diarrhea is caused by passing bacteria to the infant from the caregiver's hands. This is the reason proper handwashing is so essential when caring for an infant. Encourage everyone who handles the infant to wash their hands frequently and certainly before handling the baby or equipment used in caring for the infant. Be sure to explain why you are asking them to do this, to avoid offending anyone. Frequent handwashing can prevent and limit unnecessary diarrhea.

Diapering

diaper Washable or disposable covering applied to the perineal area for the purpose of containing stool or urine

Traditionally, cloth **diapers** were used for babies. Today, although cloth diapers may be used in some cases, most diapers are of the disposable type. Use is so widespread that prices are quite competitive. Cloth diapers are held in place with safety pins, and need to be rinsed, stored, and washed. Additional waterproof pants go over the cloth diaper to prevent leakage. Disposable diapers are held in place with peel-and-stick tabs, are thrown away after use, and have the waterproof liners in place as part of the diaper. They are sold in sizes which match the infant's weight, such as "newborn to 10 pounds" or "16 to 24 pounds." Generally, using cloth diapers is less expensive than using disposable diapers.

Babies' diapers are changed whenever they become wet with urine or soiled with feces. Washing the genitals and perineum carefully and thoroughly from front to back is very important. If the baby is newborn, the cord and/or circumcision is to be cleansed at this time. Cream, lotion, or powder is applied after the area is cleaned. The clean diaper should fit well and not be too tight or too loose.

PROCEDURE

DIAPERING THE BABY

RATIONALE: Diapers are changed whenever they become soiled with urine of feces to reduce skin irritation.

PREPARATION

1. Assemble your equipment:
   a. Disposable gloves
   b. Clean prefolded cloth diaper or a disposable diaper
   c. Disposable baby wipes or cotton balls
   d. Baby soap
   e. Baby cream or powder
   f. Basin of warm water
   g. Waterproof changing pad
   h. Washcloth
2. Wash your hands.

STEPS

3. Place baby on pad.
4. Put on gloves.
5. Unfasten tabs or pins (keep pins out of reach of baby).
6. Remove as much feces as possible by wiping front to back.
7. Remove diaper, fold to enclose feces, and set aside.
8. Use disposable wipe or cotton balls with soap and water to clean from front to back. Use washcloth if there is a large amount of feces. Rinse well.

9. Clean the umbilical cord by wiping it with a disposable wipe or cotton ball moistened with soap and water. Ask the immediate supervisor if a cotton ball moistened with alcohol should be used.
10. Clean the circumcision gently with a disposable wipe or cotton ball moistened with soap and water.
11. Place diaper under the baby by raising the baby's legs and sliding the diaper under the buttocks.
12. Apply cream, lotion, or powder. (If using powder, never shake it onto the baby, because shaking makes it airborne and it can get into the baby's lungs. Instead, put powder in the palm of your hands and smooth onto baby's skin.)
13. Cloth diapers need to be folded before use. Fold so that there is more diaper thickness in the back for a female baby and more thickness in front for a male baby.
14. Bring the diaper up between the legs to cover the lower abdomen. If there is still an umbilical cord attached or the umbilicus has not healed, make sure the diaper lays across the abdomen but under the umbilicus.
15. Use the tabs to secure the edges of the diaper together at the hips (Figure 31-6◆). If pins are used, place the first and second fingers of your left hand between the skin and the diaper, holding the diaper edges in place with the thumb. Using the opposite hand, insert the

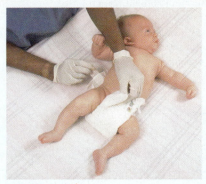

FIGURE 31-6 ◆
Diapering a baby

pin sideways (not up and down) and close it.
16. Apply waterproof pants over the cloth diaper.

FOLLOW-UP

17. Place the baby in a crib or other safe place.
18. Rinse feces from the cloth diaper in the toilet. Store in prepared diaper pail or plastic bag. Throw disposable diaper in covered trash can.
19. Dispose of gloves and wash your hands.
20. Document the urine, feces, appearance of the skin (rash, no rash, and so on), and whether cream or powder was applied.

CHARTING EXAMPLE: 12/09/04 11am Wet diaper changed, zinc oxide cream applied to buttocks and outer labia. H. Hand, CNA

Circumcision

circumcise Remove the foreskin of the penis by surgical procedure

In our society, it is customary to **circumcise** the foreskin from the end of the penis. It is thought that it promotes cleanliness, and some early studies supported the idea that this procedure prevents cancer of the penis. While this practice has not been shown necessary, many parents are still requesting it be done. In the Jewish culture circumcision is performed at a later age than at birth. For a few days the penis will look reddish and may be swollen. It will be sensitive to touch, so be gentle when changing diapers or cleaning the area. Some doctors prescribe an ointment to be applied with each diaper change. Check with your immediate supervisor for special directions. The area must be thoroughly cleaned with each diaper change.

Umbilical Cord

umbilical cord Rather long, flexible, rough organ that carries nourishment from the mother to the baby; it connects the umbilicus of the unborn baby in the mother's uterus to the placenta

Before birth, the **umbilical cord** serves as a lifeline, connecting the fetus with the mother's placenta. All nourishment is passed from mother to fetus through the umbilical cord. At the time of delivery, the cord is clamped and cut, and the healing process of the umbilicus begins. Within 5 to 10 days the cord will dry, turn black, and eventually fall off.

CARE OF THE UMBILICAL CORD	GUIDELINES	
■ Keep the diaper folded down away from the cord. A wet diaper on top of the cord could cause an infection. ■ At every diaper change, check the baby's cord. Wash the cord with	plain rubbing alcohol on a cotton ball or according to your institution's policy. The alcohol will help speed up the drying process and will keep the cord clean. Follow your supervisor's instructions regarding the use of alcohol.	■ Never pull on the cord. Let it fall off by itself. Laying the infant on the abdomen will not hurt the cord. Binders or belly bands are not advised.

Bathing the Infant

Bath time should be a pleasant and enjoyable time for mother and baby. Try to involve the mother as much as she is able and take the opportunity to teach her how to care for the baby. The infant's safety is your first responsibility. Keep your hands and eyes on the baby throughout the bath.

Sponge Bathing

While the umbilical cord is still attached, the baby can be washed using a sponge bath. A tub bath is not permitted until the cord has fallen off. The infant should receive a sponge bath at least once a day. Use soap, oils, or lotions sparingly. Soap tends to dry the skin; oils and lotions may clog pores or cause allergies. Do not use on the face. Follow your agency's policy on Standard Precautions and the use of protective equipment when bathing an infant. Some mothers and infants receiving home care services may be HIV positive. Information regarding the mother and infant's status may not be available when services are started; therefore, you must use precautions with all patients.

Sponge bathing an infant means gently washing each part of the baby's body with mild soap and warm water, but not submerging the infant in water. Maintaining the safety of the infant at all times is very important. A safe table or counter is a convenient place to give a sponge bath. Clear off the counter and wash it well. Spread a towel on the counter to make a soft and warm place on which to place the baby. Prepare warm water, mild soap, washcloth, blankets, and towels before bringing the baby to the counter. Only one part of the body is washed at a time. Wash, rinse, and dry each body part or area very well. Then cover the body part right away with the bath blanket. If you do not have a bath blanket, use a towel.

Report any signs of redness or drainage from the umbilicus, signs of severe diaper rash, and bruises or other signs of possible injury or abuse to your supervisor immediately.

GIVING THE INFANT A SPONGE BATH	PROCEDURE

RATIONALE: Bathing provides an opportunity to interact with the infant while cleaning the infant's body.

PREPARATION

1. Assemble your equipment on a chair or counter top:

   a. Bath basin or sink

   b. Two bath towels (soft)

   c. Cotton balls

   d. Washcloth

   e. Warm water (98°F; 37°C)

   f. Bath thermometer

   g. Baby soap

   h. Baby shampoo (optional)

   i. Baby powder, lotion, or cream

   j. Diaper

   k. Clean clothes

2. Wash your hands.

3. Identify the infant.

4. Place a towel on the counter next to the basin as you may want to lay the infant down to wash and dry him.

5. Fill the basin with 2 to 3 inches of warm water (100°F; 37.8°C). Use a tub thermometer or test on your wrist.

STEPS

6. Undress the infant. Wrap him in a towel or blanket: Fold the lower corner of the blanket over the feet and legs (Figure 31–7a◆), fold the

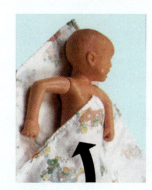

FIGURE 31–7a ◆

Place undressed infant on a towel

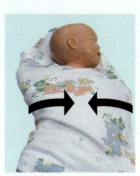

FIGURE 31–7b ◆

Wrap infant in the towel

two side corners under the arms and over the chest. Bring the infant to the table or sink (Figure 31–7b◆).

7. Using a cotton ball moistened with warm water and squeezed out, gently wipe the infant's eyes from the nose toward the ears. Use a clean cotton ball for each eye (Figure 31–8◆).

8. To wash the hair, hold the infant in the football hold with the baby's head over the sink or basin (Figure 31–9◆). This will free your other arm to wet the hair, apply a

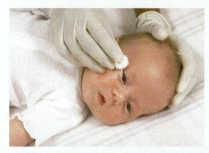

FIGURE 31–8 ◆

Use clean cotton ball for each eye

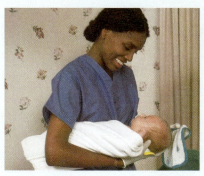

FIGURE 31–9 ◆

Use football hold while shampooing the baby's hair

small amount of shampoo, and rinse the hair.

9. Dry the infant's head with a towel.

10. Unwrap the infant and gently place him on the towel on a table. One of your hands should always be holding the baby. Never let go, not even for a second.

11. Wash the infant's body with the soap and your hands or the wash-cloth being careful to wash between the folds (creases) of the skin.

12. If the infant is female, always wash the perineal area from front to back.

PROCEDURE *(continued)*

STEPS

13. Rinse the infant thoroughly with warm water.

14. Dry the infant well, being careful to dry between the folds of skin.

15. Lightly apply powder, lotion, or cream to the infant, whichever the mother prefers or as instructed by the nurse.

16. Diaper and dress the infant (Figures 31–10◆ and 31–11◆).

17. Place the infant in his crib and raise the crib side rails or allow the mother to hold him. Show the mother how to hold the infant in either the upright position (Figure 31–12◆) or the cradle position (Figure 31–13◆).

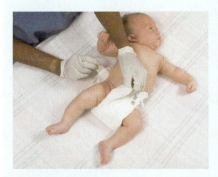

FIGURE 31–10 ◆
Diapering the infant

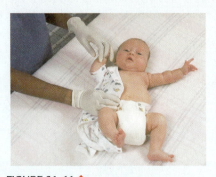

FIGURE 31–11 ◆
Dressing the infant

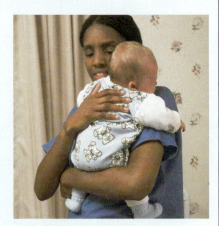

FIGURE 31–12 ◆
Holding the baby in the upright position

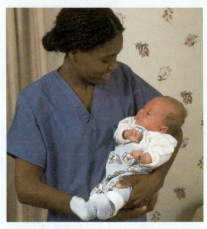

FIGURE 31–13 ◆
Holding the baby in the cradle position

FOLLOW-UP

18. Clean the counter, sink, equipment, and supplies and return them to their proper place.

19. Wash your hands.

CHARTING EXAMPLE: 12/04/04 10 am Sponge bath given. Baby returned to bed with side rails up. M. Poppin CNA

Tub Bathing

After the cord has fallen off, the infant can be given a tub bath in a large sink or baby bath tub. If you are using a sink, be sure to clean the sink and counter. Scrub the sink with a cleanser and rinse it thoroughly.

KEY IDEA

Assemble your equipment before you begin bathing the infant so you will not need to leave the baby to get anything. Do not leave the infant in the tub or on the counter at any time for any reason. Never fill the tub or sink with more than 1–2 inches of warm water.

Infant Safety

You must take special precautions to protect an infant from preventable accidents. Reinforce to the mother or family caregivers the precautions for safe handling of the newborn (keeping a firm grip on the wet infant and never leaving the infant unattended on a table

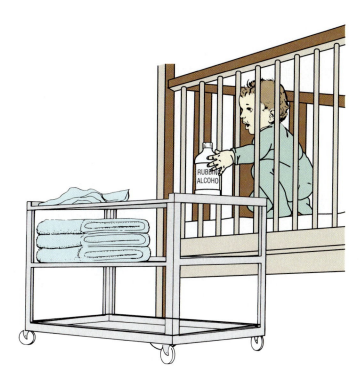

FIGURE 31–14 ◆

Keep hazards out of reach of all children

or couch). Even if an infant has not yet learned to roll over, she can wiggle and kick until she falls off beds, chairs, tables, or counters. Never leave an infant unattended on any of these surfaces. If you are far from the infant's crib and you must leave her unattended for a few seconds, put her on the floor. The safest place for an infant is in her crib, with the side rails up. Some people keep babies in a carriage because they do not have a crib. Other things you can do to prevent accidents when caring for an infant:

- Wash your hands before handling the infant or her supplies.
- Place the infant on her side or back after eating to prevent aspiration.
- Place the infant on her back or side to sleep, instead of her stomach.
- Keep the crib rails in the up position when the infant is sleeping or playing.
- Use only 1 or 2 inches of bath water and never leave the infant alone in the water.
- Never place the infant who is in an infant seat on tables, chairs, beds, or counters.
- Keep all medications and cleaning solutions out of the reach of all children (Figure 31–14◆).

 ## Pediatric Care

Pediatric patients are children (Figure 31–15◆). In most hospitals, anyone under age 16 is called a pediatric patient. These patients may be grouped in several ways. For example, pediatric patients are sometimes grouped according to age because children of different ages need different kinds and amounts of care. Children also may be grouped according to their medical or surgical condition.

These developmental age groupings are often used in referring to pediatric patients:

- Premature babies are born before the completion of 37 weeks of gestation (pregnancy) or 3 weeks less than full term (the normal gestation period is 40 weeks). Low birth weight babies are under 2,500 grams or 5.5 pounds in weight.
- Newborn babies (neonates) are full-term babies from birth until 1 month of age.
- Infants are babies from 1 month to 1 year old.

pediatric patient Any patient under the age of 16 years

FIGURE 31–15 ◆

Communicating with a
pediatric patient

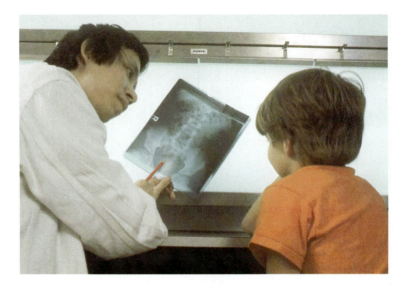

- Toddlers are children from 1 to 3 years of age.
- Preschoolers are children from 3 to 5 years old.
- School-age children are from 6 to 12 years old.
- Adolescents are children from 12 to 19 years old.

Pediatric patients are admitted to the health care facilities or require care at home for many reasons, for example, congenital defects, nutritional disorders, or accidents—falls, poisoning, fractures, or burns.

Nursing Care of Pediatric Patients

The nursing care of children is based on what is normal in terms of growth and development for a child of a certain age (see Chapter 15).

The three categories of nursing care for children are:

1. The things one normally does for a child at a certain age, such as feeding, bathing, keeping the child safe, communicating with both the child and the family, or providing opportunities for play
2. Nursing care related to the reason the child is in the health care institution, such as feeding a baby who has a cleft palate
3. Regular nursing care procedures that have to be adapted to children, such as collecting a urine specimen or measuring vital signs

Safety

There are several guidelines to follow to promote safety when caring for the child (see next page).

Measuring Vital Signs

Measuring vital signs (body temperature, pulse rate, respiratory rate, and blood pressure) may be a regular part of your duties as a nursing assistant, however, the pediatric patient requires special attention. Refer to Chapter 19 for more information about measuring vital signs. Be familiar with information that may be provided by your facility regarding the normal ranges for body temperature (see Table 31–1 ◆), pulse rate, respiratory rate, and blood pressure for the pediatric patient.

SAFETY WHEN CARING FOR THE CHILD	GUIDELINES

- Never use a heating pad on the baby or child.
- Never leave the child unattended in the bathtub.

- Use a bath thermometer when testing bath water.
- Keep small items out of reach to prevent choking.
- Keep dangerous or poisonous materials out of reach.

- Check the child often according to hospital policy, especially if the child is wearing a restraining device.
- Never prop a bottle and leave the child unattended.
- Keep the crib side rails up.

TABLE 31–1

Normal Temperature Readings

METHOD	CENTIGRADE	FAHRENHEIT
Oral	37.0	98.6
Axillary	36.4	97.6
Rectal	37.5	99.6

KEY IDEA

Always explain to the child and to the parent(s) or caregiver what you are going to do before providing care.

The *temperature* may be measured in the following ways:

- The *core (tympanic)* temperature is taken by placing an automatic device into the ear. Temperature is displayed within a few seconds. Read the result displayed on the device and record it. This has become a very popular method with the patient as well as the caregiver.

- The *rectal* temperature is taken by placing a lubricated thermometer into the rectum about 1/2 inch. The child may be on the back or stomach, but must be held securely to prevent movement. The thermometer should be shaken down before inserting, so that the reading is below 90 degrees. Leave in place for 4 to 5 minutes. Wipe off lubricant and read. Record the results. Remember to wear gloves and to wash your hands before and after the procedure.

- The *axillary* temperature is taken by shaking down the thermometer to below 90 degrees and placing it in the child's armpit. The arm is held close to the child's side or chest for about 10 minutes. Read the thermometer and record the results.

- The *oral* temperature is only taken if the child can understand and follow instructions to keep the thermometer under the tongue with the mouth closed for 4 to 7 minutes (above age 5) for glass thermometers. Remember to remain with the small child to prevent injury. The use of a digital thermometer requires the child to keep his mouth closed for 1 minute while the caregiver remains to hold the recording device.

In all of the above, handwashing and gloves are very important. Explain to the child and the child's parent(s) what you are going to do, and make sure to check the identification band before the procedure. After each use, clean and disinfect equipment (thermometer), and return it to the proper place. Discard disposable equipment in the place provided in your institution.

KEY IDEA

Remember to measure a child's pulse rate and respirations before you measure the temperature. Most children get upset when you measure the temperature, and this upset abnormally elevates the pulse and respirations.

Normal pulse rates (per minute) for different age groups:

- Before birth/birth: 120–160
- 4 weeks to 1 year: 80–160
- Childhood years: 80–115

Note: The radial pulse can be taken if the child is over 6 years old.

MEASURING THE CHILD'S PULSE RATE (HEARTBEAT)

PROCEDURE

RATIONALE: Apical heart rate measurements provide the most accuracy in infants and toddlers.

PREPARATION

1. Assemble your equipment:

   a. Stethoscope and antiseptic swabs

   b. Watch with a second hand

   c. Pad and pencil

2. Wash your hands.
3. Identify the child by checking the identification bracelet.

STEPS

4. Explain to the child what you are going to do.
5. Place the diaphragm of the stethoscope over the heart.
6. Count the beats for 1 minute.
7. Immediately record the full-minute count.

FOLLOW-UP

8. Clean the earplugs of the stethoscope. Return equipment to its proper place.
9. Wash your hands.

CHARTING EXAMPLE: 12/04/04
12 noon Heart rate: 153 regular beat. M. Poppins, CNA (Or the number may be recorded in a box on a vital signs sheet)

MEASURING THE CHILD'S RESPIRATORY RATE

PROCEDURE

RATIONALE: Respirations are counted to monitor the infant or child's breathing patterns.

PREPARATION

1. Assemble your equipment:

   a. Watch with a second hand

   b. Pad and pencil

2. Wash your hands.
3. Identify the child by checking the identification bracelet.

STEPS

4. Do not tell child that you are going to count respirations. If the child is sleeping, count his respirations before he wakes up.
5. For infants and toddlers *watch the stomach and chest.*
6. For children over 4 years *watch the chest.*
7. Count the number of times the stomach and/or chest rises during one minute.
8. Immediately record the full-minute count.

FOLLOW-UP

9. Wash your hands.

CHARTING EXAMPLE: 12/04/04
12 noon Respiration rate: 28. M. Poppins, CNA (Or the number may be recorded in a box on a vital signs sheet)

MEASURING THE CHILD'S BLOOD PRESSURE

RATIONALE: The blood pressure indicates a measure of heart function.

PREPARATION

1. Assemble your equipment:
   a. Blood pressure cuff (correct cuff size for size of child)
   b. Watch with a second hand
   c. Pad and pencil
2. Wash your hands.
3. Identify the child by checking the identification bracelet.

STEPS

4. Tell the child what you are going to do, explaining that he might feel a squeeze on his arm.

5. Wrap the cuff securely on the arm above the elbow area.
6. Feel for the brachial pulse on the inner aspect of the elbow below the cuff.
7. Place the stethoscope in your ears and the diaphragm over the area where you felt the pulse (Figure 31–16◆).

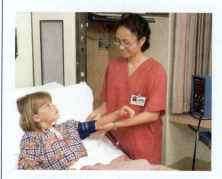

FIGURE 31–16 ◆
CNA taking child's blood pressure

8. Pump up the cuff until the pulse is no longer felt. If it is a manual blood pressure cuff, release the valve until you can hear the systolic and diastolic sounds. Count the beats for one minute. Many devices are automatic and will pump up the cuff, release the valve at the right time, and count and display the results.
9. Immediately record the results.

FOLLOW-UP

10. Clean the earplugs of the stethoscope. Return equipment to its proper place.
11. Wash your hands.

CHARTING EXAMPLE: 12/04/04 12:05pm BP = 64/48. M. Poppins, CNA (Or the number may be recorded in a box on a vital signs sheet)

Communicating with Pediatric Patients

The child's parents are the primary care givers and as such play a key role in communicating with the child. The younger the child, the more important the family is in easing the child's fears. Many hospitals and pediatric patient care units have a policy of allowing a family member to stay with the child. *Most* facilities encourage this. When it is not possible, it is important to make the child feel as safe and protected as possible (Figure 31–17◆).

Engage the child's parents and family members in supporting and calming the pediatric patient when possible and appropriate. It will be beneficial to the child, the parents, and you (Figure 31–18◆).

KEY IDEA

Family members are normally concerned and often are worried and frightened. Family members need to be with their children, and children need their families.

Things you can do to help are:

- Do the best possible job of caring for the child. This is usually reassuring to the family members.
- Show interest and concern about the family members' welfare. Ask, "Is there something we can do?"

FIGURE 31–17 ◆

CNA communicating with a
child

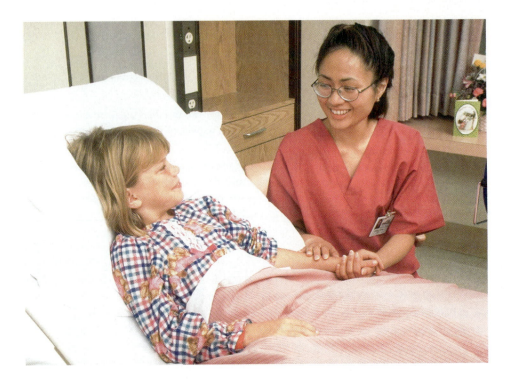

- Do not make judgments about the family members' attitudes or behavior, even if they seem strange to you.
- Encourage and allow the family members to help take part in the child's care when possible and if permitted.
- Sometimes family members seem to be worried about something concerning their child in the hospital and are afraid to talk about it. If you suspect this, tell your immediate supervisor.

FIGURE 31–18 ◆

Encourage family members to
take part in the child's care and
provide comfort to the child

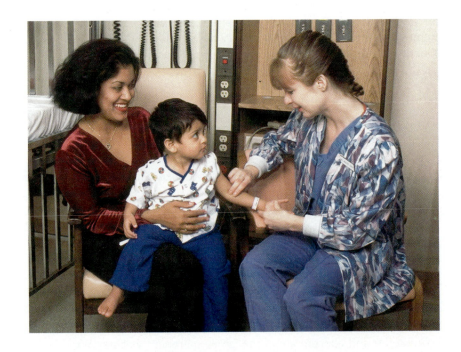

KEY IDEA

This may be the first time the child has been away from home. The child may be frightened or may view hospitalization as punishment. Such a patient needs to be held, touched, and talked to in order to be comforted and reassured.

There are several helpful guidelines to help you in your communications with young children. Refer to Chapter 3 for additional information on communicating with pediatric patients.

COMMUNICATING WITH PEDIATRIC PATIENTS	GUIDELINES	
■ Introduce yourself to the child. ■ Use the name or nickname the child prefers when addressing him. ■ If a child is toilet trained, find out what words he uses for urinating and bowel movements.	■ Expect that the child may not do as well with toilet training as he did at home. Praise him if he is successful, and do not scold him if he makes a mistake. ■ Allow the child to do as much as he can to maintain his independence, such as eating and dressing.	■ Avoid frustrating situations by allowing some choices and enough time to complete tasks. ■ Give explanations that are honest and simple. ■ Talk to the child during playtime, not just when you are providing care.

SUMMARY

Care of the infant and pediatric patient requires an understanding of the developmental age of the patient. It also requires sensitivity to how vulnerable, sick, or injured the child may be. Communication is vital to providing care. Always remember that the parents and family of the child are usually more than willing to be of help in providing support to the child. Whether caring for a newborn, infant, or child, *safety* is the most important part of your job. It is part of any procedure you perform. Because children can be unpredictable, safeguards must be taken to prevent injury. The different age groups require their own unique care, but safety will always be the key to good care.

NOTES

CHAPTER REVIEW

FILL IN THE BLANK Read each sentence and fill in the blank line with a word that completes the sentence.

1. Neonatal care refers to care given to newborn _____.

2. Diarrhea in the infant can result in _____.

3. Never _____ on the umbilical cord. Let it fall off naturally.

4. Never _____ a bottle and leave a baby unattended.

5. When taking a rectal temperature on a child, insert the thermometer _____ inches.

MULTIPLE CHOICE Choose the best answer for each question or statement.

1. You can prevent a buildup of air in the baby's stomach by doing all of the following *except*
   a. feeding the infant slowly.
   b. feeding the infant with its head elevated.
   c. burping the baby every 1–2 ounces.
   d. burping the baby only before feedings.

2. The normal color of a breast-fed baby's stool is
   a. dark black.
   b. brown.
   c. mustard yellow.
   d. green.

3. The umbilical cord will generally dry and fall off in how many days?
   a. 1–2 days
   b. 3–5 days
   c. 5–10 days
   d. 14–20 days

4. When giving an infant a bath, you should do all of the following *except*
   a. assemble all of the equipment that you will need.
   b. line the sink or tub with a towel.
   c. fill the sink or tub with 4–5 inches of water.
   d. dry the infant well, including between skin folds.

5. When taking a rectal temperature in a baby, insert a well-lubricated thermometer
   a. 1/2 inch.
   b. 1 inch.
   c. 1-1/2 inches.
   d. None of the above.

TIME-OUT

TIPS FOR TIME MANAGEMENT

When you need a piece of equipment that is being used by another staff member, continue to work while you wait. For example, if another nursing assistant is using the electronic thermometer, ask her to bring it to your patient's room when she is finished. Then proceed to the patient's room and take the rest of his or her vital signs while you wait.

THE NURSING ASSISTANT IN ACTION

You are assigned to care for Marta James, a new 20-year-old mother and her infant. Marta is to be discharged home tomorrow and she has not yet changed a diaper or fed her baby. Each time you try to encourage her to participate in the care of her newborn daughter, she says: "Leave me alone. I am too tired, and besides it is your job to care for my baby."

What Is Your Response/Action?

CRITICAL THINKING

CUSTOMER SERVICE When working with a child you may usually address him by his first name. You may find that he wishes you to call him a preferred nickname. If you need to ask any questions of parents that could be frightening to the child, it is better to do that in an area away from the child.

CULTURAL CARE Children may not be as aware as their parents of various cultural or religious food restrictions. Encourage the parents to assist with any meal menu choices if you are unsure of their preferences. Do not offer a child food items or snacks that you know are not part of his designated diet.

COOPERATION WITHIN THE TEAM There may be times when a child or parent confides in you that they do not understand why some test or procedure is needed. You can help reinforce why certain treatments are needed, if you know the reason. When unsure, offer to inform other care providers that the child or parent needs additional information or would like some aspect of the care explained again.

EXPLORE MediaLink

Additional interactive resources for this chapter can be found on the Companion Website at www.prenhall.com/wolgin. Click on Chapter 31 and "Begin" to select the activities for this chapter.

For chapter-related NCLEX-style questions and an audio glossary, access the accompanying CD-ROM in this book.

32

The Older Adult Patient and Long-Term Care

KEY TERMS

dangling position
dementia
deteriorate
disoriented
dysphagia
flammable
geriatric
pathologic
pouching
restorative care
sundowning syndrome
validation therapy
vertigo

OBJECTIVES

When you have completed this chapter, you will be able to:

- Describe the older adult patient in terms of physical and emotional changes.
- Define common chronic conditions of the older adult patient.
- Describe validation therapy.
- Provide opportunities to foster health and well being in the older adult patient.
- Provide functional or restorative care.
- Assist with reality orientation.
- Create a safe environment for the older adult patient.
- Assist with ambulation.
- Understand nutrition for the older adult patient.
- Provide skin care appropriate for hygiene as well as prevention of pressure ulcers.
- Describe patient rights.

MediaLink
www.prenhall.com/wolgin

Use the address above to access the free, interactive Companion Website created for this textbook. Get hints, instant feedback, and textbook references to chapter-related NCLEX-style questions. Link to other interesting sites.

AUDIO GLOSSARY:
Use the Companion Website, or the CD-ROM disk enclosed with your textbook, to hear the pronunciation of key terms in the chapter.

Geriatric care refers to health care provided for adults, usually age 65 and older. This population requires care to meet changing physiological and psychological needs that are related to age. There are further divisions within this age group; specifically high-functioning older adults and the frail elderly. The frail elderly are older and struggle to maintain their health. Health care workers who care for older adults practice the specialty of geriatric care. They must be sensitive to the needs of this population and alert to subtle changes in condition. Many older adults are cared for in long-term care facilities. In this case, the adult or patient is referred to as a resident. Many employing agencies refer to the patients cared for in the home as clients. Regardless of where you work or whether the older adults are referred to as patients, residents, or clients, you must have genuine respect for these older adults, valuing each person and providing each with quality care.

INTRODUCTION

Physical Changes of the Geriatric Person

As we grow older, many physical changes take place that make functioning independently more and more difficult. The body's central nervous system slows down. This can create problems in detecting heat, pain, and cold, and cause slower reflexes. Thought processes may be slow and memory may become poor. All the senses (hearing, sight, taste, touch, and smell) may not be as sharp as they once were. Muscle tone may be poor due to lack of exercise and muscle atrophy. A disturbed sense of balance might make older adults unsteady on their feet or cause a change in walking patterns. The bones tend to become brittle and break easily. Quick changes in position can cause the blood pressure to drop and, as a result, the patient will feel dizzy or faint. Posture may become more stooped. Circulation becomes less efficient and bodily processes slow down. The skin loses elasticity and some fat. Because of decreased circulation, along with these skin changes, older patients will get cold quicker.

Table 32–1 ◆ lists common physical changes experienced by and often observed in the older adult (**geriatric**) person. These changes may or may not occur in all persons.

ALERT

For all patient contact, adhere to Standard Precautions (∞ Chapter 5, pages 83–85). Wear protective equipment as indicated.

geriatric An aged person; elderly; over 65 years of age

TABLE 32–1

Common Physical Changes in the Older Adult Person

SYSTEM	PHYSICAL CHANGES
Skeletal	■ Softening of the bones (osteoporosis), bones become more brittle and can break easily ■ Decreased flexibility of joints (arthritis) ■ Changes in vertebrae and feet (difficult ambulation) ■ Decreasing strength
Muscular	■ Decrease in muscle mass and muscle tone ■ Decreased elasticity of tendons and ligaments
Cardiovascular	■ Decreased cardiac output ■ Decreased elasticity of blood vessels (poor circulation; edema)
Respiratory	■ Reduced tone of respiratory muscles and diaphragm ■ Decreased lung capacity ■ Increased risk of upper respiratory disease
Endocrine	■ Increased incidence of metabolic disease (diabetes) ■ Decreased hormonal functioning (post menopause) ■ Decreased ability to heal

(continued)

TABLE 32–1 (continued)

Common Physical Changes in the Older Adult Person

Nervous	■ Decreased touch sensation (hot, cold, pain) ■ Decreased equilibrium or motor coordination (can cause dizziness) ■ Decreased reaction and response time ■ Decreased taste perception ■ Decreased sense of smell ■ Decreased visual perception (night vision, depth and color perceptions, drying of cornea) ■ Decreased elasticity of eardrum (alteration in hearing; delayed auditory impulse) ■ Shorter memory, forgetfulness
Integumentary	■ Hair becomes more gray or white and thinner ■ Decreased fat cells ■ Decreased elasticity of skin ■ Decreased sweat and sebaceous gland secretions (loss of ability to regulate body temperature, therefore more tendency to be cold) ■ Increased pigmentation (aging spots) ■ Thinning of skin layers, dry skin develops ■ Nails become thick and tough
Urinary	■ Decreased kidney function (urinary output) ■ Decreased bladder tone (incontinence) ■ Urine can become more concentrated
Gastrointestinal	■ Alteration in metabolic rate ■ Alteration in bowel habits, decreased peristalsis ■ Decreased saliva production ■ Difficulty swallowing ■ Decreased appetite ■ Loss of teeth
Mental Health	■ Increased incidence of depression (loneliness, decrease in socialization, loss of friends or spouse) ■ Changes in sleeping patterns ■ Decrease in coping mechanism (stress response)

Psychosocial and Psychological Aspects of Aging

- **Psycho:** mental, spiritual, or emotional processes
- **Social:** interactions and relations among people

Social changes may be caused by physical problems, life crises, or the pressure of society. These may include:

- Retirement
- Change in income
- Fear of illness

Psychosocial changes include:

- Disruption of independence
- Increasing dependency
- Isolation from friends and family
- Death of a spouse, significant other, or close friends and family (Figure 32–1◆)
- Change in housing
- Increased dependence on others

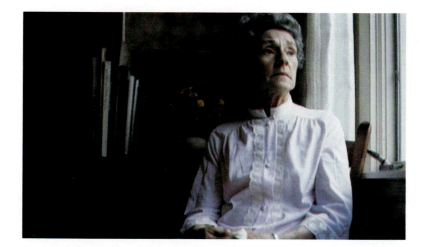

FIGURE 32–1 ◆
Losing one's spouse and
friends occurs as one ages

Common Disease Conditions

Along with the normal body changes that occur as a person grows older, there are many disease conditions that may result in **pathologic** behavior. The aging process is inevitable but it occurs at different rates in each person, as well as in each body system.

The terms **dementia** and delirium refer to a large group of acute and chronic mental disorders caused by or associated with brain damage or impaired cerebral function. Alzheimer's disease is the most common cause of dementia in the older adult patient. The cause of Alzheimer's disease is not known. With today's increasing life span, there is an increased incidence of this disease. Nursing care of patients with this disease is based on the signs and symptoms displayed.

Contribute to the well-being of these patients by creating a safe environment, including careful observation to prevent the patients from harming themselves and protecting patients from falls. Follow the principles of **validation therapy** or reality orientation, and encourage these patients to do as much for themselves as possible and praise their efforts. In addition, treat every patient with care, concern, and respect. The nursing assistant must approach every patient with respect, whether demented or not.

Table 32–2◆lists some common diseases and conditions associated with the older adult patient and the symptoms or changes that occur as a result of the diseases and conditions.

pathologic Involved with or caused by a disease

dementia An irreversible mental condition in which intellectual abilities are continuously reduced

validation therapy A way of communicating with confused people

deteriorate To make or grow worse; degenerate

AGE-SPECIFIC CONSIDERATIONS

AMD (Age-related macular degeneration) threatens the eyesight of millions of older Americans. The macula is the tiny, central portion of the light-sensing retina in the back of the eye. AMD involves the breakdown of cells in the macula. The macula provides the sharp, straight ahead vision needed for reading, doing detail work, and driving a car. Most people with AMD have a "dry" form of the disease which progresses slowly. Many retain good eyesight, and others can be helped by vision aids. In a minority of cases, though, this gives way to the "wet," rapidly worsening form of the disease. Abnormal blood vessels grow beneath the macula. These may leak, damaging nearby light-sensitive cells. Serious vision loss can occur.

TABLE 32–2

Common Disease Conditions of the Older Adult Patient

DISEASE CONDITION	WHAT OCCURS AS A RESULT OF THESE DISEASE CONDITIONS
Alzheimer's disease	Alzheimer's disease is a degenerative disorder that produces progressive dementia. This **deterioration** in mental function causes an inability to perform the activities of daily living; a lack of orientation to time, place, and person and of memory, judgment, and understanding; mood changes; a general inability to care; and death. Alzheimer's disease is divided into two classifications: 1. presenile dementia (before age 65) 2. senile dementia (after age 65)
Dementia and delirium	*Dementia* is an irreversible deteriorative mental state. The causes of dementia include multiple strokes, hardening of the arteries, and Alzheimer's disease. The patient suffering from *delirium* is often confused as a result of a temporary medical condition such as a fever, dehydration, or infection. *Delirium* is a sudden change in mental status and is often misdiagnosed as dementia. In many cases delirium is reversible. Signs and symptoms are: ■ Loss or decrease in orientation ■ Decrease in ability to do simple calculations ■ Loss of memory ■ Decrease in general information When the acute condition is treated, the symptoms disappear or are reversible. In the chronic stages there is a loss of cells in the cortex of the brain. Alzheimer's disease is one of the most common causes of irreversible mental impairment.
Arteriosclerosis	A pathologic condition in which there is a thickening, hardening, and loss of elasticity of the walls of the arteries. This results in altered function of the artery, that is, decreased flow of blood to parts of the body supplied by that artery.
Arthritis	Inflammation of the body joints causing pain, swelling, loss of movement, and changes in structure.
Atherosclerosis	A form of arteriosclerosis in which the arteries become clogged or blocked with various substances, such as plaque, calcium, or fat, which can result in sluggish circulation.
Cataracts	Clouding of the lens of the eye, causing decreased vision.
Cerebral vascular accident (CVA)	Blood supply to the brain is reduced. This may be due to cerebral thrombosis, cerebral embolism, or intracerebral hemorrhage. It is called a stroke.
Congestive heart failure	The inability of the heart to pump out all the blood returned to it from the veins. The vital organs of the body do not receive an adequate supply of blood. As a result, fluid backs up into the lungs and body. Signs and symptoms of congestive heart failure are: ■ Congestion in the lungs ■ Weakness, fatigue ■ Difficulty breathing ■ Dizziness ■ Restlessness, anxiety ■ Chest pain ■ Edema of the legs, feet, hands, face, buttocks ■ Confusion ■ Weight gain (from build up of fluid)
Diabetes mellitus	A disturbance of the carbohydrate metabolism because of an imbalance of the hormone insulin. The body is unable to process sugar appropriately.
Emphysema	The tiny bronchioles of the lungs become plugged with mucus. The lungs becomes less elastic and air inhaled is trapped in the lungs, making breathing difficult, especially during exhalation. Signs and symptoms of emphysema are: ■ Persistent cough (moist cough and wheezing) ■ Anxiety due to difficult breathing ■ Fatigue ■ Coughing up thick secretions ■ Loss of appetite ■ Breathing with pursed lips ■ Weight loss
Fractures	Breaks in bone due to loss of mineralization or injury.
Gallstones	Crystals that settle out of the bile stored in the gallbladder. Stones often block the secretion of bile. This causes pain, nausea, and vomiting. Surgical or nonsurgical removal may be necessary.

TABLE 32–2 (continued)

DISEASE CONDITION	WHAT OCCURS AS A RESULT OF THESE DISEASE CONDITIONS
Gastritis	Inflammation of the stomach caused by bacteria, viruses, vitamin deficiency, excessive eating, or overindulgence in alcoholic beverages.
Glaucoma	A genetic condition wherein there is elevated pressure in the eyes. Fluid builds up in the eye and is unable to drain. A variety of eyedrops can be used to reduce the pressure.
Hemorrhoids	Engorged, blood-filled vessels around the anus or inside the rectum. Hemorrhoids are painful and may bleed, causing the stool to become blood tinged.
Hypertension	High blood pressure. Signs and symptoms are: ■ Headache ■ Vision changes ■ Problems with urinary output ■ Slurred speech Treatment may include medication, diet, and exercise. In many cases, hypertension has no symptoms. The patients who have no symptoms will be tempted to stop taking medication. These patients should be encouraged to continue their medication, as hypertension is still present.
Macular degeneration	Loss of central vision.
Multiple sclerosis	Chronic condition that begins in middle age. Muscles lose tone due to damage to the nerves that control them.
Myocardial infarction (heart attack)	Arteries that supply the heart muscle become blocked; the heart muscle does not receive an adequate blood supply and parts of the heart muscle die or infarct.
Parkinson's disease	A chronic disease of the central nervous system, causing tremors in the body. Characterized by a peculiar gait or shuffling of the feet when walking and an expressionless face.
Pneumonia	Acute inflammation or infection in the lungs. Deep breathing and coughing are necessary to prevent the pooling of secretions (hypostatic pneumonia), which is a common condition occurring in older adult patients who remain in the same position for long periods.
Stomach (gastric) ulcer	An open sore or lesion that develops on the mucous membrane of the stomach. Ulcers are very painful and require special medications, diets, and occasionally surgical removal.
Urinary incontinence	Inability to control urination. This may be due to physical or mental conditions, such as stroke or Alzheimer's disease. It may also be caused by the inability to get to the toilet or decreased muscle tone (stress, urge, or overflow incontinence).
Varicose veins	Type of vascular disease. The veins are distended or swollen, especially in the legs.

Meeting the Older Adult Person's Psychosocial Needs

To foster health and well-being you should provide opportunities for the patient to participate in a variety of activities that will be mentally stimulating and meaningful. Purposeful activity should be designed to involve the patient with other people (Figure 32–2◆). This will encourage older adult patients to live their lives to the fullest. The feeling of being needed will stimulate feelings of self-accomplishment and satisfaction for the patient. By persuading the patient to participate and interact with others the nursing assistant can possibly decrease loneliness in the older adult patient. Such rehabilitative measures help to eliminate the physical dependency and mental depression commonly seen in the older adult patient. Use the guidelines that follow for meeting the older adult person's psychosocial needs to foster health and well-being in the patient.

In long-term care settings, an Activities or Recreation Therapy Department will offer structured activities to help keep older adult patients active, involved, and oriented. The nursing assistant should supplement this department by providing one-to-one stimulation for patients. Keep your conversations with other staff to a minimum; spend your time engaging your patients in conversations about their families, current events, upcoming holidays, items in the news, and so on. You can play a key role in getting patients to participate in meaningful activity, thus increasing their feelings of self-worth and self-esteem.

FIGURE 32–2 ◆
Involve the patient with others in stimulating activity

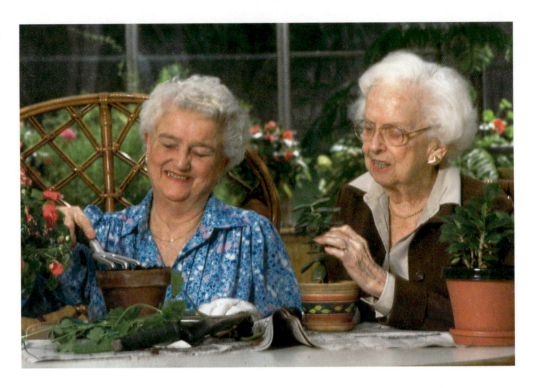

Spiritual needs can be met through visits from priests, ministers, or rabbis. Helping older adults attend services available within the care setting is another way to meet their needs.

Restorative Care

restorative care Care given to help patients attain or maintain their highest level of function and independence

Restorative care is described as care given to help a patient attain or maintain their highest level of function and independence. To provide restorative care, the health care team must consider every aspect of the patient's life. Nursing assistants have an important role in helping with restorative care, especially in long-term care facilities or in home care. Nursing assistants

MEETING THE OLDER ADULT PERSON'S PSYCHOSOCIAL NEEDS	GUIDELINES	
■ Maintain a safe environment. ■ Help the patient to feel confident in the health care team. ■ Pay attention to the patient and make him feel important. ■ Encourage the patient to do as much as he is able to do. ■ Show respect for the individual patient. ■ Provide care with a gentle touch and in a kind and considerate manner.	■ Be a good listener (pay attention to what the patient is saying). ■ Provide for the patient's privacy. ■ Accept the person as he is now, without passing judgment. ■ Call the patient by the patient's preferred name at each contact. ■ Touch the patient when you speak to him, if acceptable to the patient. ■ Talk directly to the patient in a respectful manner. ■ Keep the room well lighted. ■ Have the patient's personal belongings where the patient wants them.	■ Encourage the patient to interact with family, visitors, and other patients. ■ Assist the patient to see himself as a valuable, needed, and successful person. ■ Provide opportunities for the patient to make decisions and to be independent. ■ You may be one of the few persons your patient sees and talks to. Provide socialization by being friendly, understanding, and patient while completing your work with the patient. ■ Encourage writing, journal keeping, using audiotapes, and other artistic self-expression.

provide care and communicate in ways designed to maintain, or improve as much as possible, the functional ability in elderly patients encountered in all settings (see Chapter 33).

Reality Orientation for the Confused Patient

Sometimes the older adult patient is confused for short or long periods. A patient may not know where he is. He may speak to people who are not in the room. Report any new episodes of or changes in confusion to your supervisor. They may be caused by any number of things, many of which are reversible. Make an effort to orient this kind of patient. Tell the patient the time of day and where he is. Tell him who you are and why you are there (Figure 32–3◆). Always make sure the patient is wearing his ID band. There are some confused patients who will not benefit from reality orientation.

KEY IDEA

Never pressure the disoriented person to respond correctly. This may increase the anxiety disorientation, provoke anger, or lower self-esteem.

Patients who are **disoriented** may have difficulty remembering, recognizing, or describing people, places, or times. They may be unable to tell others who they are, where they are or the day, date, or time. These patients benefit from a consistent calm environment and routine. Display a clock and a calendar in a prominent place. Repetition is

disoriented Unaware of or unable to remember, recognize, or describe people, places, or times; confused perception of reality

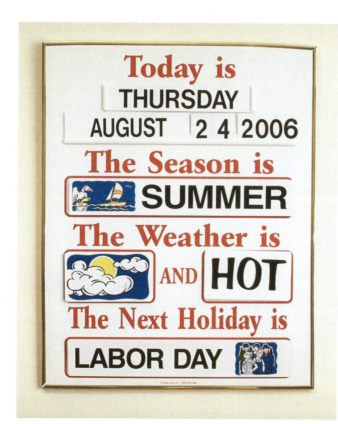

FIGURE 32–3 ◆
Reality boards are helpful in reality orientation

important. Remind the patient frequently of who he is, where he is, and the date and time. For example:

- Include the time when talking to the patient. "Good morning, it's 8 o'clock and breakfast is ready."
- Introduce yourself repeatedly.
- Avoid rushing or urging the patient to repeat what you said.

When a disoriented patient asks for or speaks to persons who are no longer living, gently remind him that this person has passed away. Going along with the patient may only increase his disorientation. However, do not pressure a disoriented person to respond correctly. This also may increase anxiety disorientation, provoke anger, or lower self-esteem. If a calendar is displayed, the patient may find it helpful to mark off each day, to assist in remembering days. In your conversation with the patient, it may be of benefit to make reference to current events in order to continually orient the patient.

sundowning syndrome A term used to describe a state of increased confusion and disorientation that usually occurs in persons with cognitive dysfunction as evening approaches

Sundowning syndrome is a term used to describe a state of increased confusion and disorientation that usually occurs in persons with cognitive dysfunction as evening approaches. It is characterized by *wandering, talking, or inappropriate behaviors at the usual evening bedtime*. Sundowning is a common problem encountered by many older adults. Sundowning is seen in older adults who become confused in the late afternoons or early evenings. Caregivers and family will notice that this is the only time when the older adult is likely to appear confused. The confused behavior is not seen in the mornings or during the night. The nursing assistant can play a key role in providing or recording observations about the behavior that occurs and how the older resident or patient responds. Risk factors that have been shown in the development of sundown syndrome include:

1. Recent changes in location or room within the facility
2. Visual impairment
3. Low environmental light
4. Older age (>74 years)
5. Disturbed sleep cycles
6. Dementia

The nursing assistant will need to be alert to these risk factors and observe if sundowning behavior occurs. If noted, record it if it continues on a daily basis or waxes and wanes intermittently. Some measures that can be used to help prevent the syndrome are:

- Avoiding relocation or changing rooms whenever possible
- Using soft music, singing, or other social sensory stimulation in the late afternoons
- Offering fluids frequently
- Turning on lights before it is dark
- Providing environmental clues such as a large clock, a bright distinctive way to identify their door, or a large print calendar in the person's room

Validation Therapy

Validation therapy is a therapeutic approach based on the theory that confused residents have their own reality. It also teaches that as the thinking processes of confused residents become weaker, the strength of their feelings becomes stronger. The goal of validation therapy is to attempt to discover these feelings so meaningful contact can be made with the confused resident. In this way, we recognize and confirm—or validate—their feelings. Validation therapy does not restore mental functioning. However, people who have used this type of therapy with confused residents often find that these residents have less anxiety, are less hostile and exhibit fewer abusive behaviors. Validation therapy can also reduce the caregiver's stress. When we no longer try to convince confused residents of our reality but accept and validate their reality, a more trusting relationship develops, making care giving more rewarding. Validation therapy reinforces the idea that it is never okay to argue with a resident or to lie to a resident.

Validation therapy is a way of communicating with confused people. It is based on the theory that the behavior of confused people is the result of an inner reality that makes sense to them—care providers do not know what that reality is. Validation therapy was pioneered by Naomi Fell, a social worker with extensive experience in working with the elderly. It is a program designed to be used to communicate with confused residents. Validation therapy does not restore mental functioning but it often reduces residents' anxiety and lessens disruptive behavior.

Stages of Confusion—Helping Measures

Validation therapy describes four stages of confusion. There is no clear-cut division between the stages. Residents may show signs of more than one stage as their confusion progresses.

Stage One—Malorientation Description

In Stage One, called *malorientation,* the person knows the time, date, place, and who they are. However, they may have some degree of recent memory loss. Often they give a detailed description of an event that may or may not have happened in an attempt to cover the fact that they have forgotten what did happen. People in the malorientation stage often appear tense. They try to establish schedules and rules to follow in an attempt to maintain control because they are aware of their occasional confusion. They can do their own personal care although they may need some reminders. They can read and write and sing familiar songs. They walk with purpose. They are continent and make good eye contact. The people in this stage generally do not like to be around people who are less oriented than they are. They may also accuse others of taking their things when they cannot find them. ***Helping Measures:*** The best way to help people in this stage of confusion is to avoid confronting them. Use words that help them clarify what is happening. For instance, ask Who? What? Where? When? and How? Instead of saying "No, it didn't happen that way," ask "Why did it happen that way?" or "Who else was there when it happened?" This is less threatening to them. Listen to them vent their feelings, but do not try to explore the feelings.

Stage Two—Time Confusion Description

In Stage Two, time-confused residents give up trying to hang on to reality and no longer attempt to follow outside rules and schedules. They retreat inward. Their bodies become more relaxed, they walk more slowly, their eyes become unfocused, and their voices soften. They may be incontinent, but are aware when they are. Their speech may be garbled, although frequently they can still sing familiar songs. Often, early memories become their reality. Their speech and behavior reflect their inner reality. They are feeling sad because their mother just scolded them. They are trying to leave the facility because they have to get home to feed their baby. ***Helping Measures:*** The goal when working with someone in Stage Two is to build a trusting relationship rather than insisting that they recognize your version of reality. We should try to provide stimulation by touching them gently and responding to their emotional needs. It is best to approach these residents from the front to avoid startling them. Get close enough to make eye contact and let them hear you clearly. Bend down if necessary. Attract their attention by a gentle touch and a clear, nonharsh voice. Recognize their world and help them clarify it. Respond to the feelings they express and forget the facts as you see them. When the person states "I am gone, gone, gone," you might respond "Where have you gone?" If the person sounds frightened, the response might be "Is it frightening to be gone?" This type of response will help people in Stage Two more than "Mrs. Jones, you have not gone anywhere. You are sitting right here in this chair."

Stage Three—Repetitive Motion Description

In Stage Three, repetitive motion, residents usually pace restlessly or slump forward in their chair with their eyes closed. They do not listen or talk with others. They are unaware of being incontinent. In essence, they are unaware of their bodies. They may perform the same motions over and over, which has meaning to them although we do not know what it is. It is likely that these motions have a goal. ***Helping Measures:*** When working with residents in Stage Three, attempt to relate to them at some level. A gentle touch may result in a moment of recognition that another person is present. A reassuring voice may help reduce feelings of anxiety. Use a calm voice when you ask questions about what the person is doing, such as "Are you making a pie crust?" You may occasionally happen on the right action or feeling. If you do, the person may respond. If you do not, they will ignore you. When words do not work, try copying their motion. If they are rubbing their fingers, rub your fingers in the same way. This can let them know that you accept them and what they are doing. In this way, you validate their feelings. The resident may also respond well to having something like a ball, a towel, a pocketbook or a doll to hold.

Stage Four—Vegetation Description

In Stage Four, vegetation, there is little movement. The eyes are usually closed, there is no facial expression and little body movement. There is little to indicate whether or not there is any thought process occurring. ***Helping Measures:*** Comforting touches, a reassuring tone of voice, and good physical care are the most we can do at this stage.

The essence of validation therapy is that for each confused person's behavior, there is a reason, although we may not know the reason. Confused residents, whether or not they understand what you say to them, will understand a caring touch and tone of voice.

KEY IDEA

Validation therapy is generally used with residents who are confused with no hope of recovery from their confusion, as in dementia, organic brain syndrome, Alzheimer's disease, etc. In contrast, reality orientation is used with residents where some recovery may be realized, for example: head trauma, stroke, and postoperative situations.

Safety for the Older Adult Patient

In creating a safe environment for the older adult patient, be diligent in your efforts to protect your patient from accidents, especially falls. Every patient is an individual and has different needs. Some patients may need your assistance to get in and out of bed or to walk from room to room. If you notice that your patient is unsteady, report this to your supervisor. The unsteady patient may benefit from the use of a cane or a walker or regular exercise. A sturdy, hard chair placed beside the bed will give the patient something to hold on to when getting out of bed. Be sure the patient's clothing is not so long that it might cause the patient to trip and fall. If the height of the bed is adjustable, make sure it is in the lowest position at all times and the wheels are locked.

To keep the older adult patient safe, the nursing assistant must continually observe the patient and the environment. For example:

- Bed-bound older adult patients should be protected by side rails, when ordered, that are kept in the up position on both sides of the bed at all times. If the bed is adjustable, keep it at its lowest level in a position of safety for the patient at all times. With an agitated patient, side rails may make their state of mind worse. Check with your supervisor to see how this patient should be handled. Elevated side rails are considered restraints and require orders and documentation (see Chapter 6).

- Before the patient moves out of bed, she should come to a full sitting (**dangling position**) before standing. Patients who are weak or mentally confused may have **vertigo** dizziness or an inability to maintain normal balance when sitting or standing. Carefully lower the patient to a sitting or safe position if they become dizzy or appear unable to maintain their balance.

  dangling position Sitting up on the edge of the bed with the feet hanging down loosely

  vertigo Dizziness

- When the patient gets out of bed, the nursing assistant must check to see that both of the patient's feet are firmly on the floor before the patient begins to stand. Assist the patient in securing shoes before walking whenever possible.

- The older adult patient who is permitted to smoke alone should be checked frequently. Provide a large ashtray to prevent ashes from falling on the bed or on any **flammable** article. Most facilities have limited smoking areas and do not allow patients or residents to smoke in their rooms.

  flammable Something that can be easily set on fire and burns quickly

- Remove harmful substances from the confused patient's reach, such as sharp equipment, Clinitest or Acetest supplies, matches, cigarette lighters, knives, and unauthorized medications.

- Monitor at all times any patient who may wander away. Some health care facilities use an alarm or security system with ankle bracelets to help monitor the whereabouts of patients who wander.

- Use a room closest to the nursing station and away from exits for the confused patient, so he can be monitored more frequently.

- Protect the patient from overexposure to sunlight.

- Keep frequently used articles within reach of the patient.

- Be alert at all times for any condition that might cause an accident or injury to the patient.

- Keep the patient's environment free from clutter. Keep the path from the bed and chair to the toilet clear.

Refer to Chapter 6 for more details on creating and maintaining a safe environment.

Ambulation Safety With and Without the Walker

- An unsteady patient using a walker should be accompanied by the nursing assistant.

- A walker provides support for the unsteady patient (Figure 32–4◆). Make sure there are rubber tips on the legs of the walker so that it cannot slide. The patient is supported on both sides as she holds on to the walker with both hands and lifts it slightly ahead.

- When assisting the patient, use an ambulation or gait belt on the patient and hold it lightly from behind (Figure 32–5◆).

- Some walkers have wheels and are used with patients who cannot lift the walker.

- If the walker is being moved, the patient's feet should be stationary. If the walker is stationary, the patient may move his feet forward.

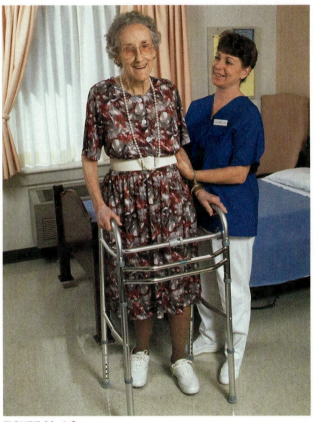

FIGURE 32–4 ◆

Using a walker for support

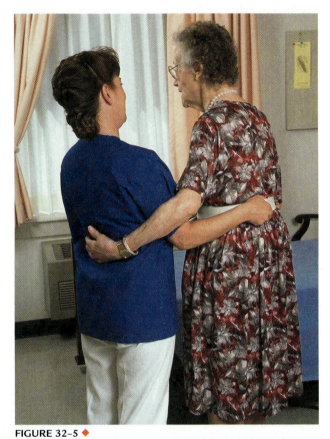

FIGURE 32–5 ◆

Steady the patient by holding the belt at the patient's back

Assisting the Older Adult Resident with Nutrition

Older adults, because of the physical changes they have experienced, may need the nursing assistant's help in meeting their nutritional needs. Make mealtime a positive experience and encourage the patient to eat (see Figure 32–6◆). Proper nutrition aids the healing process and maintenance of health. The box, *Tips for Improving the Older Adult Patient's Nutrition,* on the next page, provides some simple but effective tips for assisting the patient in getting proper nutrition.

FIGURE 32–6 ◆

A positive or encouraging word may coax a reluctant patient to eat

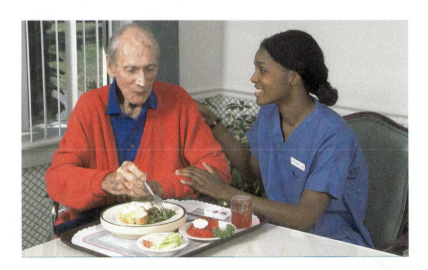

TIPS FOR IMPROVING THE OLDER ADULT PATIENT'S NUTRITION

- To reduce the risk or possibility of food aspiration, be sure the patient is sitting in an upright position. Offer fluids and solid food separately. (Refer to *Guidelines: Feeding a Patient with Dysphagia* in Chapter 21.)

- Observe for difficulty in swallowing or for signs of possible food aspiration, watch for **pouching** of food, gurgly voice quality and cough. Discontinue feeding if any of these swallowing problems occur. Pouching, or pocketing of food, is the retaining of food between the cheek and teeth or holding in the mouth.

- Patients should always be fed with the nursing assistant seated at eye level to the patient.

- Set up the tray, remove wrappers and lids, cut up meat and large items.

- Identify the foods and tell patients with visual impairments where in relation to a clock face to find them on the tray.

- Make sure dentures or dental work are in place.

- Verify that the diet served is appropriate to the patient's ability (soft foods, full thickened liquid, etc.)

- Be sure items are positioned within the patient's reach.

- Assist the patient, as needed. If the patient is to be totally fed, work at the patient's pace and do not rush. Offer liquids periodically between bites of solid food. Remind the patient to chew and swallow food.

- Report to your supervisor any change in appetite, food intake, nausea, or vomiting.

- If patient's appetite is poor, check with your supervisor to see if between-meal nourishment, such as milkshakes or snacks, should be provided. It may be appropriate to offer small, more frequent meals instead of three large meals per day.

- Encourage socialization during mealtime to stimulate the patient's appetite. Eating in a dining room with other patient's or having the television news on are two ways to offer stimulation for mealtime.

- Acquaint yourself with special diets so you know what patients can and cannot have.

- Be aware of which patients are diabetic. Notify the supervisor of what amounts of food were eaten.

- Find out the patient's food preferences and favorites and have those available for meals.

- Check to see if foods can be seasoned to enhance flavor for patients whose smell or taste are diminished.

- Encourage fluids throughout the day, not just with meals.

dysphagia Difficulty in swallowing usually requiring evaluation by speech therapist to prescribe a certain diet and method of feeding

pouching Also known as pocketing of food; the retaining or holding of food in the mouth between the cheek and teeth

Nursing Care for the Older Adult Patient

Restoring or Fostering Independence

Nursing assistants can use the following guidelines to assist in restoring or fostering independence in the older adult.

1. Encourage the older adult or resident to do as much as possible for themselves.

2. Allow the patient to set the pace and avoid rushing him through his activities of daily living (ADLs).

3. When assisting with care for older adults, allow them some choices in the care they receive, clothes they wear, or their food or beverages.

4. Be alert to changes in function as the patient or resident performs his ADLs.

Skin Care

Use the following guidelines in providing skin care for the older adult:

- The older patient's skin may be extremely dry, flaky, and wrinkled. This is due to the decreased amounts of oils being produced by the oil glands and poor circulation.

- Dry skin is less elastic and more sensitive than normal skin.

- Circulation tends to slow down in the older patient. Lack of frequent movement and exercise can contribute to problems.

- Aging skin and circulation problems make the older adult patient especially susceptible to pressure ulcers.

- Give thorough skin care frequently and urge the patient to move about as often as he is able.

- Different patients will need varying amounts of assistance from you when changing position. You will need to turn the nonambulatory patient many times each day. Practice good body mechanics and use a pull (turn) sheet to avoid friction.

- Sharpen your nursing skills concerning skin care by reviewing pressure ulcer care in Chapter 17.

- Use powder or lotion to protect the skin, depending on the patient's preference and skin condition. Note that powder has the tendency to cake on the skin, especially when used in combination with lotion. Lotion alone can effectively be used to protect the skin. Studies have shown that powder increases upper respiratory infections and increases the incidence of asthma as the dust is inhaled. When used in excess and inhaled, powder may cause calcification of the lungs.

- Report any skin tears, or reddened areas, bruises, rashes, and so on to your supervisor immediately.

The Bed-Bound Older Adult Patient

The bed-bound patient has the same needs as the ambulatory patient, but will require more help in meeting those needs (Figure 32–7◆). Emotional support and encouragement can be very helpful. If family members are visiting the facility often, involve them in the care of the patient by permitting them to suggest the patient's favorite foods, feed the patient, shave the patient, comb the patient's hair, or do simple tasks.

Proper positioning in bed increases the patient's comfort. Be sure the back and joints are supported to prevent unnecessary strain. Changing the patient's position at least every 2 hours will promote circulation and help in preventing pressure ulcers. Support the patient's arms and legs. Pillows can be used for support, but never put the support behind the knees unless you have specific instructions to do so. At all times bed coverings should be smooth, clean, dry, and free from wrinkles.

Assist the bed-bound patient with the activities of daily living. Many facilities have schedules for moving bed-bound patients to the bath or shower. Use available lifting equipment and practice good body mechanics when doing so. A daily bed bath will not only keep the patient clean, but also will help him to feel relaxed and refreshed. Oral hygiene, back rubs, and care of the hair and nails all help the patient look and feel better. The bed-bound patient may need less food than before illness due to a lack of physical activity. Meals should be well balanced and served attractively. Constipation may be aggravated by the lack of exercise.

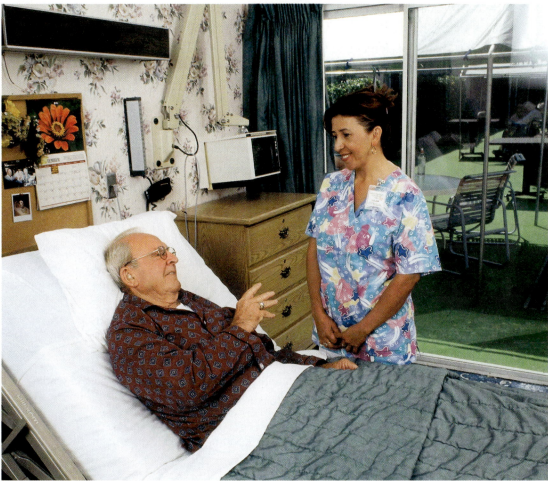

FIGURE 32–7 ◆
Bed-bound patients have the same needs as the ambulatory patient, but will require additional help

 # Maintaining Dignity and Quality of Life

As you provide care to older adults, you will want to ensure privacy, dignity, and the same quality of care you would want for yourself. Geriatrics is a specialty within health care, with a specialized body of knowledge and patients who have very important needs. Over the years, there have been health care providers who have taken advantage of the elderly. If you witness this, or know of anyone who might be a party to unethical or inappropriate care of the older adult patient, report it immediately to the supervisor.

Long-term care (nursing care) facilities are required by federal and state law to inform residents and their families of these rights orally and in writing at the time of admission. These rights are described in the 1987 Omnibus Budget Reconciliation Act (OBRA) which requires long-term care facilities to provide care and services that maintain, and in some cases improve, the quality of life, health, and safety of the residents in their facilities. Many health care institutions have a document known as a patient's bill of rights, which serves to protect all patients (see Chapter 2). Become familiar with this document, as well as its intent. Here are some of the residents' rights that long-term care facilities must protect and promote.

Residents have the right to:

1. A safe and clean living environment
2. Courteous and respectful treatment at all times

3. Adequate and appropriate medical treatment and nursing care

4. Prompt responses to all reasonable requests and inquiries

5. A change of clothes and bed sheets as needed

6. Communicate with the physician or other persons responsible for their care

7. A choice of doctors

8. Access to information in their medical records

9. Confidential treatment of personal and medical records

10. Withhold payment for physician visits if there were none

11. Privacy during medical examinations or treatment and in personal care

12. Refuse to participate (as a subject) in medical research

13. Be free from physical or chemical restraints or prolonged isolation unless medically indicated

14. Select a pharmacist of their choice

15. Vote and exercise all civil rights

16. Consume a reasonable amount of alcoholic beverages at their own expense unless medically contraindicated

17. Use tobacco at their own expense unless medically contraindicated

18. Retire and rise in accordance with reasonable requests

19. Observe religious obligations and participate in religious activities

20. Privacy in communications with family and other persons, in receiving and sending mail

21. Have access to private use of the telephone

22. Private visits at any reasonable hour

23. Privacy for visits by spouse or to share a room, if possible, if both are residents in the health care center

24. Have room doors closed

25. Retain and use personal clothing and possessions

26. Be fully informed of the facility's basic rates upon admission

27. Receipt of an itemized bill at least monthly by the person paying the bill

28. Manage personal financial affairs or to have an accounting if the facility manages the patients' finances

29. Be allowed unrestricted access at reasonable hours to property on deposit

30. Not be transferred or discharged from the home without cause

31. Voice grievances and recommend changes in policies and services

32. Be told of any significant change in health status or have reports sent to family or sponsor

AGE-SPECIFIC CONSIDERATION

Encourage older adults to do as much as they possibly can do for themselves. Independence is a basic desire in most adults and when independence is threatened, many residents feel saddened and depressed and feel at a loss as to what is happening to them. As a result, recovery is compromised. Encouraging older adults to participate in activities such as eating, drinking, toileting, and other personal care gives them a feeling that they have some control of their environment and they can see progress toward a goal of returning to their former activities and recovery and eventually going home.

One of the biggest challenges when caring for elderly patients is they can unexpectedly become angry, verbally abusive, or combative. Usually these things occur when they are afraid, think you plan to harm them, or think that the caregiver is someone else with whom they are angry. Patients with hearing loss or poor vision are more easily confused and often misunderstand what is said to them. Frustration over the loss of control over your life, being removed from loved ones, feeling rushed or forced to comply with the facility's or caregiver's schedule can all lead to anger in any patient. Pay attention when you sense or see that a patient is becoming tense, clenching the teeth, pacing, kicking or speaking in a loud or rapid voice. These signs of anger can quickly lead to aggressive or combative behavior including injury to yourself or others.

SUMMARY

This chapter focused on the care of older adults, known as the geriatric population. Changes in physiological and psychosocial needs were identified, along with conditions and diseases that can result from these changes. The nursing assistant should be aware of how the older person differs from younger adults and adapt care accordingly. Care of older adults may take more time and patience, but good care will be every bit as appreciated. This group of patients, who may be less able to care for themselves, will need considerable help from nursing assistants.

NOTES

CHAPTER REVIEW

FILL IN THE BLANK Read each sentence and fill in each blank line with a word that completes the sentence.

1. As patients age, there are many _____ changes that occur in the body.

2. _____ is an irreversible mental condition in which intellectual abilities are continuously reduced.

3. _____ is when a person is unable to remember, recognize, or describe people, places, or times.

4. The specialty within health care that cares for the older adult is known as _____.

5. A patient _____ of _____ is a document that outlines ways the institution will protect the dignity and privacy of the older adult.

MULTIPLE CHOICE Choose the best answer for each question or statement.

1. Which of the following is not generally a major life change for a geriatric patient?
   a. Isolation from friends and family
   b. Change in income
   c. Fear of illness
   d. Child care pressures

2. Which of the following is not a common disease of the elderly?
   a. Dementia
   b. Head injuries
   c. Emphysema
   d. Cataracts

3. Alzheimer's disease is a degenerative disorder that produces
   a. dementia.
   b. diabetes mellitus.
   c. delirium.
   d. double vision.

4. To meet the needs of the older adult, you should
   a. provide a variety of activities that are mentally stimulating.
   b. provide purposeful activities.
   c. encourage the patient to participate and interact with others.
   d. All of the above.

5. Reorienting the disoriented person includes all of the following except:
   a. telling the patient what day it is.
   b. telling the patient who you are.
   c. requiring the patient to verify the correct day, time, etc.
   d. making sure they have an accurate name band on.

TIME-OUT

TIPS FOR TAKING CARE OF YOURSELF

Confused patients with dementia may have no recollection of the event or the combative behavior once it has passed. Remind yourself that they are confused and really did not mean the things that were said.

THE NURSING ASSISTANT IN ACTION

An 85-year-old, Hispanic woman, Maria De Rosa, is admitted to your Long-Term Care unit. While in the hospital, she had been in bed for several days and became quite weak. Her English is very poor. Her family expresses concern that she has not been eating or drinking very much and, since her admission, appears confused at times.

What Is Your Response/Action?

CRITICAL THINKING

CUSTOMER SERVICE If you are having difficulty communicating with a patient, a language board can be created using pictures and words in both English and the patient's language. There may be another staff member who speaks the language who can assist with this project. If not, arrangements can be made to call a family member or interpreter when it is necessary to communicate important information or ease anxiety. Include a caregiver name space on the board so the patient can recall the caregiver's name.

CULTURAL CARE As a nursing assistant you will encounter many cultural differences among patients. If you are not sure what the particular differences are, be sure to ask first if there are any particular things the patient or family can tell you that would help you to plan the patient's care. Sometimes family members can bring in ethnic seasonings or foods the patient prefers.

COOPERATION WITHIN THE TEAM Many older patients benefit from having consistent caregivers who they come to know and trust. If the patient complains to you when another caregiver is assigned to care for him instead of you, reassure the patient that your coworker will provide the care needed. Your coworker will not appreciate hearing that you agreed that she is not as skilled. You can offer to check in with the patient when you are covering your coworker during her lunch or breaks.

EXPLORE MediaLink

Additional interactive resources for this chapter can be found on the Companion Website at www.prenhall.com/wolgin. Click on Chapter 32 and "Begin" to select activities for this chapter.

For chapter-related NCLEX-style questions and an audio glossary, access the accompanying CD-ROM in this book.

33 Rehabilitation and Return to Self-Care

KEY TERMS

active motion
apathy
depression
fatigue
holistic
incontinence
mobility
mobilization
motivation
occupational therapist
orthotics
passive motion
physical therapist
prosthetics
psychological
psychosocial
range-of-motion (ROM)
    exercises
rehabilitation
rehabilitation nurse
restorative care
subacute care
suppository
unilateral neglect
ventilator

OBJECTIVES

When you have completed this chapter, you will be able to:

- Explain the goals of a holistic rehabilitation program.
- List key members of the rehabilitation team.
- Describe the roles of the rehabilitation nurse, physical therapist, and occupational therapist, as well as your role in helping them.
- Define your role in the rehabilitation and restorative care process.
- Describe psychological aspects of rehabilitative care.
- Discuss how you can help address psychosocial concerns related to rehabilitation.
- Help the patient with a disability bathe, dress, and groom.
- Assist the patient with a disability to eat and drink.
- Assist with bowel and bladder rehabilitation and retraining for the incontinent patient.
- Insert nonmedicated rectal suppositories.
- Explain the principles and rules of range-of-motion exercises.
- Perform active or passive range-of-motion exercises with a patient.
- Explain the difference between subacute and acute care settings and the reasons for growth in subacute care.
- Follow guidelines when caring for a patient on a ventilator.

MediaLink
www.prenhall.com/wolgin

Use the address above to access the free, interactive Companion Website created for this textbook. Get hints, instant feedback, and textbook references to chapter-related NCLEX-style questions. Link to other interesting sites.

AUDIO GLOSSARY:
Use the Companion Website, or the CD-ROM disk enclosed with your textbook, to hear pronunciation of key terms in the chapter.

In this chapter you will learn about the vital role of the nursing assistant as part of the rehabilitation team. As a nursing assistant, you help patients regain self-care abilities they may have lost through illness or injury. This chapter introduces the functions of the members of the rehabilitation team, emphasizing the functions of the nursing assistant. It details how you can help patients care for themselves, rebuild muscle strength, and stay motivated to participate in the rehabilitation process.

INTRODUCTION

The Holistic Approach to Rehabilitation

An accident, injury, illness, disability, or chronic condition brings the patient into the health care institution. Family relationships, patients' feelings about themselves, and their physical, emotional and medical needs are all affected. **Rehabilitation** means helping the patient regain a state of health. Its goal is to return the patient to the highest level of function while maintaining the abilities that have not been lost. The rehabilitation team helps the patient and family set and reach realistic goals and enjoy any progress made toward regaining self-care skills.

Restorative care refers to the care given to help patients keep their current level of independence or regain the highest level of function and independence. It requires planning, an understanding the rehabilitation process, and ongoing staff commitment.

When planning rehabilitation or restorative care, the health care team must consider every aspect of the patient's life.

In the **holistic** approach, the health care team is concerned with every aspect of the patient, not just the injury or disease for which the patient was admitted to the health care institution. Thus, the holistic approach to rehabilitation requires meeting the total needs of the patient, including the following:

- Physical needs
- Emotional needs
- Social and economic needs
- Spiritual needs

This comprehensive effort seeks to restore patients to a medical, physical, psychological, psychosocial, and spiritual state of wellness. The goal is to help patients do as much as they can, as well as they can, for as long as they can.

ALERT

For all patient contact, adhere to Standard Precautions (Chapter 5, pages 83–85). Wear protective equipment as indicated.

rehabilitation The process by which people who have been disabled by injury or sickness are helped to recover as much as possible of their original abilities for the activities of daily living

restorative care Care given to help a patient attain and maintain the highest level of function and independence

holistic Intended to meet the needs of the whole patient; based on the belief that human beings function as complete units and cannot be effectively treated part by part

KEY POINTS OF RESTORATIVE CARE

GUIDELINES

- Use holistic care—treat the whole person.
- Start rehabilitation as soon as possible.
- Focus on ability over disability.
- Perform tasks consistently to reinforce the steps.

- Promote activity.
- Encourage patient decision making.
- Maintain your belief that restorative care will help the patient.
- Practice patience because the

process will take time and encouragement.
- Encourage and teach family members how they can help promote independence.
- Be watchful for patient fatigue, frustration, or exhaustion.

Cultural Care

There are wide variations in cultural and religious beliefs. If you are unfamiliar with the culture, rituals, or religious beliefs of a patient, check with the patient, his family, or your supervisor to determine if there are particular things you need to know to provide restorative care and support during this difficult time. There may be religious items that a patient would like to hold, wear, have near him, or placed on the bedside stand. A patient who believes that God punishes for misdeeds may believe that his disability, injury, or illness is God's will. If you notice a patient has no desire to participate in the rehabilitation, try asking if something is bothering him, or if he would like to talk to you or someone else.

Often patients are depressed, have accepted their fate, or are in pain. If a patient fears he could become addicted to pain medicine, he may not tell you how much pain he is experiencing. Some Native American Indian patients may have a totem or carving of an animal that brings strength or good luck. Chinese patients may desire specific hot or cold foods that will assist their recovery. Other patients may believe crystals have healing powers. Do not ignore the influence a particular item or belief may have. Most alternative medicines and practices can be used in conjunction with the rehabilitation program. It is important to be aware of any specific herbs or drugs the patient takes because some can interfere with prescribed medications.

KEY IDEA

Rehabilitation takes time and patience, and it often does not bring about a complete return to normal. A patient may have to accept a little progress at a time. The patient, as well as family members, must be aware that only minor gains may be possible. Rehabilitation therefore includes the patient's acceptance—and even enjoyment—of learning to accomplish small goals.

The Rehabilitation Program

Helping the patient return to the optimum level of wellness may require a rehabilitation program. This program is designed to lessen the effects of physical illness or trauma. It addresses the consequences of negative factors such as the following:

- Illness or trauma that has kept the patient inactive for a period of time and has resulted in weakness and lost function
- Surgery (for example, hip or knee replacement)
- Poor positioning for long periods of time
- Lack of weight bearing and disuse of muscle groups
- Catastrophic illness such as stroke
- Excessive stress
- Inability to perform activities of daily living

Rehabilitation begins when the acute phase of an illness or condition has passed. It follows the stage of illness when short- and long-term realistic goals are set for the patient. The patient acquires or relearns skills and gains strength through repetition and practice. As the patient reaches goals and becomes more independent, the patient will feel more confident and will try to reach additional goals.

You, as a nursing assistant, help the patient gain skill in dressing, personal hygiene tasks, and feeding by making sure the patient has access to all needed supplies and by allowing enough time for the patient to accomplish tasks. You should encourage the patient, praise any accomplishments, remind the patient of what has been taught and accomplished, and report reactions to your immediate supervisor.

It is important that you praise all accomplishments, no matter how small, and handle failures by providing encouragement to try again or overlooking the failures. This helps to prevent **apathy**—a lack of feeling or interest in things.

apathy A lack of feeling or interest in things

Obra Requirements

Nursing facilities are required by OBRA to provide professional rehabilitative services. These services may be provided by facility staff members or an external provider may be contracted to provide these rehabilitative services. For example, the facility may collaborate or develop a shared services agreement with a partner or nearby hospital to obtain services from a physical therapist. The key requirement to be in compliance with OBRA rules is that those rehabilitative services identified and required in the resident's rehabilitation plan must be provided for the resident. This requirement holds true for physical therapy, speech therapy, recreational or activity services, and occupational therapy. A doctor's order is needed to provide rehabilitation services. Each facility is also required to maintain a rehabilitation/restorative nursing program to prevent deterioration and maintain optimal levels of functioning and independence.

KEY IDEA

To meet OBRA requirements, residents must receive the therapy outlined in their care plan.

The Professional Rehabilitation Team

In the holistic approach to rehabilitation, the professional rehabilitation team can have many members. Key team members are the following:

- Rehabilitation nurse
- Physical therapist
- Occupational therapist
- Nursing assistant
- Physician
- Speech therapist
- Social worker

Other rehabilitation team members may include:

- Rehabilitation psychologist
- Cardiac rehabilitation nurse
- Staff nurse
- Recreational therapist
- Case manager
- Activities director or assistant
- Vocational counselor
- Rehabilitation therapist
- Specialist(s)—orthopedist, neurologist, internist, and/or family practitioner
- Patient educator

- Physiatrist, or doctor of physical medicine and rehabilitation
- Spiritual counselor (priest, minister, or rabbi)
- Other professional personnel, where indicated

In keeping with the aim of holistic care (caring for all aspects of a person's needs), members of the rehabilitation team will provide a variety of services. As needed, their services may include medical care, surgical care, occupational therapy, rehabilitation nursing services, recreational activities, social services, remedial and continuing education, speech therapy, **prosthetics** (artificial limbs) and **orthotics** (making and fitting prosthetic devices), psychological care, volunteer services, outpatient diagnostic and therapeutic services, inpatient diagnostic and therapeutic services, medical and paramedical services for acute and chronic rehabilitative care, vocational counseling, podiatry care, dental care, nutritional services, pastoral care, and beautician services.

prosthetics Artificial limbs or substitutes for missing body parts

orthotics The science concerned with making and fitting prosthetic devices

The Role of the Rehabilitation Nurse

The **rehabilitation nurse** plays an important role in planning the care patients require. This member of the rehabilitation team establishes a routine for the patient, taking into consideration the following categories of patient needs:

rehabilitation nurse A nurse with special training in the causes and treatment of disabilities; may be certified in this specialty with the title certified rehabilitation registered nurse (CRRN)

- Physical
- Psychological
- Socioeconomic
- Spiritual
- Environmental

The rehabilitation nurse then writes a plan of care. This plan includes all the members of the rehabilitation team, the patient, and the patient's family or significant other. It can establish a length of time for each step of the rehabilitation process. In writing the plan, the nurse considers a patient's abilities, attitudes, and resources, such as the following:

active motion Producing, involving, or participating in activity or movement

passive motion Not active, but acted upon; enduring with effort or resistance

- The degree of **active motion** (motion generated by the patient) or **passive motion** (motion applied to a patient's body part) the patient has
- The patient's sensory deficits in vision, hearing, speech, touch, and balance
- The patient's perception of the disability
- The patient's attitude, which includes:
  - Depression
  - Euphoria
  - Anger
  - Cooperation
  - Resentment
  - Frustration
  - Motivation
  - Acceptance of what has happened to him
- Other factors:
  - Activities the patient can do and will attempt to do for himself
  - Level of functioning before becoming disabled
  - Priorities
  - Barriers or obstacles to rehabilitation
  - Available support system

The rehabilitation nurse evaluates a multitude of factors about the patient and the patient's condition to develop a rehabilitation plan. Each plan is tailored to a particular patient's needs and abilities.

The Role of the Physical Therapist

The **physical therapist** is trained to assist patients with activities related to motion. The physical therapist and physical therapy assistants use special training and equipment to help the patient strengthen muscles and regain physical independence. Responsibilities of the physical therapist include the following:

- Evaluate muscle strength and **mobility** (ability to move).
- Help the patient regain muscle strength and mobility.
- Measure, fit, and help the patient to use a prosthesis (an artificial body part).
- Teach the use of canes, crutches, and walkers.

physical therapist Person trained to assist the patient with activities related to motion

mobility Ability to move

The Role of the Occupational Therapist

The **occupational therapist** focuses on increasing the functional ability of the patient within the environment. In other words, the occupational therapist helps the patient learn to carry out activities of daily living. The therapist will teach the patient to work with and learn to adapt to new skills. The occupational therapist generally works in several areas:

- **Mobilization:** teaching the patient techniques to use to change position or to reach, grasp, or turn while sitting, or to maintain balance during an activity
- **Activities of Daily Living Tasks:** teaching the patient tasks to be performed each day, such as toileting, bathing, dressing, feeding, grooming, homemaking, and leisure activities
- **Coordination, Strength, and Activity Tolerance:** teaching the patient techniques to conserve energy, to perform the task to the patient's own satisfaction, and to use all physical resources to the fullest without tiring quickly

occupational therapist Person trained to assist the patient with performing activities of daily living

mobilization Making movable; putting into action

ASSISTING THE OCCUPATIONAL THERAPIST	GUIDELINES	

- Completely understand what the patient is allowed to do.
- Help the patient perform activities of daily living as taught by the occupational therapist.
- Assist the patient to function independently following the occupational therapist's instructions.
	- Keep the environment safe.
	- Discuss the outside world with the patient with regard to:
	  - Change of seasons
	  - Events in the community
	  - Sports or other activity in which the patient is interested
	  - Other areas in which the patient can be involved with the whole world.
		- Help the patient with daily needs by providing access to equipment and needed supplies.
		- Report observations of the patient to the occupational therapist:
		  - Signs of pain
		  - Signs of being tired
		  - Signs of achievement of each task
		  - Tolerance of each procedure
		  - Any attempt at a newly taught procedure.

KEY IDEA

The occupational therapist helps the patient learn to perform activities of daily living. The nursing assistant supports this effort by encouraging the patient to be actively engaged in the world.

The Nursing Assistant's Role in Rehabilitation

In addition to the previous examples of supporting the occupational therapist, the nursing assistant supports various members of the rehabilitation team. When other team members work with the patient, the nursing assistant's role is to help in the following ways:

- Repeat exercises with the patient to achieve the best result possible.
- Maintain a safe environment.
- Offer **psychological** support.
- Contribute information about the patient's condition and progress.
- Observe the patient.
- Listen to the patient.
- Establish a relationship with the patient.
- Maintain a positive attitude.
- Allow the patient to regain some degree of independent activity within the limitations of the disease or injury.
- Motivate the patient to achieve the highest possible level of wellness.

psychological Involving aspects of the mind, such as feelings and thoughts

KEY IDEA

Because nursing assistants interact closely with patients, they are in a good position to support the rehabilitation program through careful observation and the establishment of a therapeutic relationship.

Psychological Aspects of Rehabilitative Care

Rehabilitation is influenced by psychological factors, particularly depression and motivation. **Depression** is a persistent sad mood or feeling of low spirits. It can be a significant factor in the rehabilitation process (see Chapter 30).

All members of the team must be alert to signs of depression in the patient. The following signs may indicate that a patient is depressed:

- Pessimism (a tendency to see or anticipate the worst)
- Unhappiness
- Persistent feelings of hopelessness
- Low self-esteem
- Withdrawal or isolation
- Loss of interest (apathy)
- Loss of appetite or excessive appetite with weight gain or significant weight loss

depression Low spirits that may or may not cause a change in activity

- Constant **fatigue** (a feeling of excessive tiredness or weariness)
- Slow movement or constant movement
- Excessive irritability
- Recurring thoughts of suicide or death

Another psychological factor influencing the outcome of a rehabilitation program is **motivation**—the reason, desire, or purpose that causes a person to do something. To be motivated, a person must understand what the goal is and have a sincere desire to reach it. In rehabilitation, the nursing assistant is in a unique position to support motivation by providing a safe, positive atmosphere in which the patient can gain confidence in developing self-care abilities.

fatigue A feeling of tiredness or weariness

motivation Reason, desire, need, or purpose that causes a person to do something

The Role of the Nursing Assistant

There are a number of specific ways in which you can support motivation:

- Involve the patient in recreational activities to provide a creative change of pace (Figure 33–1◆).
- Offer choices whenever possible and encourage the patient to make decisions.
- Involve the patient in programs that involve decision making.
- Constantly display a positive attitude toward rehabilitation and the patient's success.
- Establish a trusting relationship with the patient by providing consistent care, listening to the patient, and respecting the patient's rights to privacy and dignity.
- Carefully observe and report any change in physical or mental condition to your immediate supervisor

The Role of the Activity Director or Recreational Therapy Department

Most long-term care facilities have an activity director or Recreational Therapy Department to provide residents with programs that help promote socialization, encourage mobility, or improve self-esteem. Often a calendar or flyer is posted to remind residents and staff of when day trips, special holiday, birthday, or theme parties, exercises or dance, and crafts or games are scheduled. The activities director will coordinate outside groups coming in to sing, visit, or entertain any residents or family members who wish to attend.

Meeting Recreational Needs	
TYPE OF ACTIVITY	**EXAMPLES**
Passive recreation	Movies, television, radio, audio recordings
Arts and crafts	Handicrafts, gifts, decorations
Physical activities	Games such as shuffleboard or croquet, nature walks, exercise or dance classes
Mental activities	Board games, word puzzles, lectures, art and music programs, discussion groups, reading, pet therapy
Hobbies	Gardening, writing, collecting, art, music, theater
Community service	Work with youth groups, present programs for youth or disabled groups, "adopt" foster grandchildren

FIGURE 33–1 ◆

Meeting the patient's recreational needs is one way of supporting motivation

KEY IDEA

Maintaining a positive attitude and establishing a trusting relationship are two ways in which you can combat the development of depression in a patient and enhance motivation. You, as a nursing assistant, can also enhance motivation by getting the patient involved in doing activities and making decisions.

Psychosocial Aspects of Rehabilitative Care

psychosocial Involving aspects of living together in a group of people

The **psychosocial** aspects of rehabilitative care are all the aspects that relate to living together in a group with other people. The rehabilitation plan for the patient will include care of psychosocial concerns and will outline the nursing assistant's role.

One important aspect of the nursing assistant's role is to develop a therapeutic, or helping, relationship with the patient. There are several ways you can accomplish this:

- Encourage the patient to actively participate in his plan of care.
- Help and encourage the patient to participate in a variety of activities that provide sensory stimulation such as interacting with others, reading the daily newspaper, watching television, and listening to the radio.
- Facilitate interaction between the patient and family and friends.
- Help the patient develop a sense of belonging, self-fulfillment, and responsibility for actions and feelings by protecting the patient's right to respect and dignity at all times.
- Identify and encourage the coping mechanisms that help the patient tolerate stress and develop a stronger belief in the patient's own ability to regain functional independence.

Also, the nursing assistant should watch for signs and symptoms of psychosocial problems. If you observe any of the following signs, you must report them to your supervisor as soon as possible:

- Depression or discouragement
- Hopelessness or isolation
- Fear or distrust
- Extreme hostility, anger, or demanding behavior
- Total dependency without any effort toward self-care
- Apathy
- Hyperactivity

Social workers provide counseling to both patients and families as they struggle with feelings related to changes in independence, health, disability, or the need to change living arrangements. Social workers can also refer the family to community support groups and resources or provide information on available financial assistance programs.

Personal Care of the Patient Who Has a Disability

Personal care includes bathing, grooming, eating, and using the toilet. Depending on the disability, a patient may be able to handle some or all of these tasks. The nursing assistant should encourage the patient to handle the personal care tasks the patient is capable of performing. Often, however, the nursing assistant must help with or perform at least some of them. The goal is to assist the patient to achieve optimum independence related to the condition.

Assisting the Patient with Bathing and Grooming

Good grooming and hygiene are important to persons who are ill or have a disability because they contribute to a positive self-image. The nursing assistant should be sure the patient has all necessary items in easy reach for each task. Patients should be encouraged to dress in street clothes. Being up and dressed enhances not only the patient's feelings of self-esteem but also the family's perceptions about the patient's health.

Some disabling conditions such as stroke may cause the patient to forget that the weakened side of the body exists, so the patient will not dress, bathe, or otherwise care for that side. This condition is called **unilateral neglect**. Simply reminding the patient will not take care of the problem. Instead, you must provide practical help with those tasks.

unilateral neglect Failure of a patient disabled on one side of the body to dress, bathe, or otherwise care for that side because the patient forgets that side exists

GUIDELINES

BATHING THE PATIENT WHO HAS A DISABILITY

- Do not attempt any technique that has not been taught or outlined to you or to the patient by the occupational therapist, physical therapist, nurse, or team leader.
- Provide a safe environment.
- Assemble all equipment, placing it where the patient can reach it.

- Thin washcloths and small face towels may be easiest for the patient to use.
- Place soap on a dampened sponge or face cloth, where it will be less likely to slide.
- Assist the patient or permit the patient to undress following the instructions of the occupational therapist or your immediate supervisor.
- Always wash the involved arm first, reminding the patient to rinse off the

soap and dry each part of the body, if the patient is washing in bed or at a sink.
- If the patient is learning to turn on the water faucets, be sure the patient turns on the cold water first to avoid burns. Also be sure the patient turns off the hot water first.
- Wash any areas the patient cannot reach.

GUIDELINES

DRESSING AND GROOMING

- Let the patient select clothing and do as much of the dressing as possible, no matter how long it takes.
- Dress the weakest or most involved extremity first, and undress this extremity last.
- Position the patient in front of a mirror. If the patient is a woman, encourage her to put on makeup.
- The occupational therapist may suggest certain tools to assist the patient to care for herself (Figure 33–2◆).

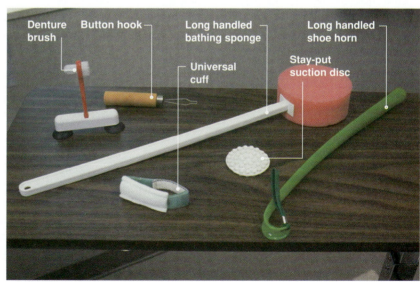

FIGURE 33–2 ◆

Some grooming and dressing devices

Feeding the Patient Who Has a Disability

When feeding any patient, it is important to provide privacy for one who has unpleasant eating habits or is unable to control drooling. A pleasant, odor-free environment with adequate lighting is needed to provide a satisfying mealtime experience.

The nursing assistant is responsible for observing and documenting the patient's food and fluid intake. Foods and fluids are an important part of rehabilitation because they help patients gain the nutrients they need to gain strength. Because patients will eat more and feel better emotionally and physically when feeding themselves, the occupational therapist will assist each patient to gain many of the motor skills needed to perform this activity of daily living. Learning these skills will motivate the patient to perform other activities of daily living.

Patients who have sensory deficits that affect eating may lack sensation if the facial muscles are weak on one side. This will affect the way they eat. Speciality products may be ordered to thicken fluids and reduce swallowing difficulties for some patients. If they cannot swallow easily, they may tend to pocket food between their cheeks and teeth on the involved side of their face. This can cause them to gag and choke as the food builds up. Place a mirror in front of the patient so the patient can see and be aware of what occurs during eating. The patient may begin to automatically use a napkin or to search with the tongue to dislodge stored food that remains on the lips. Fluids are more easily handled, but choking again may be a concern. Be sure to assist the patient when necessary.

ASSISTING WITH FEEDING

GUIDELINES

- Set up the tray or table so that it is convenient and attractive to the patient.

- The occupational therapist may suggest devices to make eating easier. Enlarging the gripping surface of the utensils may enable the patient to hold and lift them. Another suggestion may be a plate guard, a plastic ring that slips over the edge of a plate and creates a bumper for the patient to push food against. This will make it easier for her to pick up her food (Figure 33-3◆).

- Use cups with handles to help the patient hold the cup or take a drink by herself.

- Food should be easy to chew and easy to swallow.

- Encourage family or friends to join the patient during a meal. This will help make the patient more independent when eating.

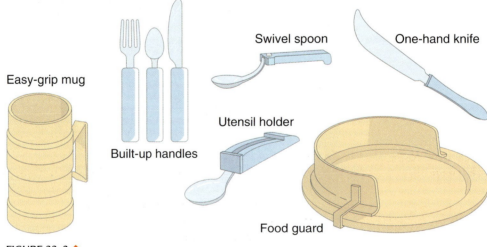

Easy-grip mug

Built-up handles

Swivel spoon

One-hand knife

Utensil holder

Food guard

FIGURE 33-3 ◆
Devices to make eating easier

KEY IDEA

Many of the guidelines for assisting with eating are designed to make mealtimes more pleasant. Relearning feeding skills and using them in a pleasant environment with loved ones can enhance the patient's physical health and mood at the same time.

PROCEDURE   OBRA

ASSISTING WITH FEEDING

RATIONALE: Assisting with feeding provides an opportunity to use restorative care as your focus. Allow the patient to do as much as he can.

PREPARATION

1. Provide an opportunity for the patient to go to the bathroom and take care of all personal needs.
2. Help the patient with hand washing.

STEPS

3. If the patient is eating in bed, position the patient in the supine position with the head of the bed elevated as high as is comfortable. If the patient is to eat at a table, make sure the patient is properly positioned and aligned in the chair with feet supported.

4. If the patient is on a feeding/dining program, obtain specific instructions from the rehabilitation nurse or therapist before you start feeding. The nurse or therapist will also have information about how much help each patient will need with feeding.
5. Wash your own hands.
6. Check the diet card and the patient's wrist band to make sure you are with the right patient.
7. If the patient can handle finger foods but cannot grip a spoon or hold a glass or cup, arrange the plate so the finger foods are in reach.
8. Sit down, at eye level, to assist with meals.
9. Offer choices about seasonings and beverages.
10. When offering food on a spoon, touch the tip of the spoon on the patient's tongue and gently press down. If the patient has weakness on one side, place the food on the opposite side.
11. Allow the patient time to taste, chew, and swallow. If a patient doesn't drink a sufficient amount of fluids during the meal, tell the nurse so that additional fluids can be offered between meals.
12. Focus your attention on the patient you are feeding. Be alert for signs of choking.

FOLLOW-UP

13. Document or report patient's progress and any unusual observations.

CHARTING EXAMPLE: 8/23/04 9am Assisted Mr. Kent with breakfast. He was able to use left hand to feed himself about 10 minutes. He could not hold cup but was able to drink from a straw when milk and coffee were offered to him. L. Lane, CNA

Bowel and Bladder Rehabilitation for the Incontinent Patient

Incontinent patients are those who have lost all or part of their control over their bowel and bladder functions. In some cases of **incontinence**, bladder or bowel training may be used to help the patient regain some or all of this control. Offering the patient the bedpan or urinal at regularly scheduled intervals may help the patient avoid incontinence.

A patient who is incontinent may suffer embarrassment and decreased self-image. It is vital for the rehabilitation team to work toward assisting the patient to regain control as much as possible. The process of retraining requires that everyone work toward that goal. The retraining program usually includes increased activity, adequate fluid intake, and a high-fiber diet.

incontinence Inability to control the bowels or bladder; inability to control urination or defecation

Enlist the cooperation of the patient by explaining what can be accomplished with patience and commitment. Begin by keeping a log for 3 or 4 days, indicating what time the patient voided or has a bowel movement, whether it was during toileting or in between, in order to establish a voiding or evacuation pattern. If the patient is able to hold urine or stool for periods of time and to indicate the need to void or defecate, the patient may be a candidate for a retraining program.

The patient with an indwelling catheter (Foley) may also be on a restorative bladder program. In this case, the goal is to remove the catheter and prevent incontinence. The catheter may be clamped for a period of time, so that urine will not drain. The clamp is opened at specific times to allow the bladder to empty. The nursing assistant may be asked to clamp or unclamp the catheter. Report any complaints of pain or discomfort to the nurse. Remember, while the catheter is clamped, urine cannot drain from the bladder. Clamping and unclamping the catheter as scheduled will prevent injury to the bladder, which could occur from overfilling. Wear gloves and follow Standard Precautions when performing this procedure.

Some patients benefit from bowel movement programs, using rectal suppositories to cause the patient to evacuate bowel contents at predictable times, thereby helping to prevent accidents.

KEY IDEA

Helping a patient learn to regain control over bladder and bowel functions not only allows the patient to perform a routine task but can boost self-esteem. The nursing assistant plays an important role in this aspect of rehabilitation by keeping records to establish a voiding or bowel pattern; helping the patient use the bedpan, bedside commode, or toilet; and inserting suppositories, if prescribed by the patient's physician.

BOWEL AND BLADDER REHABILITATION AND TRAINING

PROCEDURE

RATIONALE: This training is designed to help the patient regain control of bowel and bladder function.

PREPARATION

1. Assemble your equipment:

   a. Urinal, if appropriate

   b. Bedpan or bedside commode

   c. Container of warm water at 98°F (37°C)

   d. Towel

   e. Suppositories, as ordered by the physician

2. Wash your hands.

3. Knock on the door and identify yourself to the patient. Explain your purpose.

4. Identify the patient by checking the identification bracelet.

5. Ask visitors to step out of the room, if this is your hospital's policy.

6. Tell the patient that you are going to assist with use of a bedpan, bedside commode, or toilet.

7. Pull the curtain for privacy.

8. Raise the bed to a comfortable working position.

STEPS

9. Place the patient on a bedpan or on the bedside commode, or walk the patient to the bathroom every 2 hours to stimulate evacuation of the bowel and bladder.

10. If the patient has difficulty in voiding, pour warm water at 98°F (37°C) over the genital area into the bedpan to stimulate elimination.

11. Dry the patient with toilet tissue when finished.

12. Remove the bedpan.

13. Help the patient back into bed from the bedside commode or toilet.

14. Wash the patient's hands.

FOLLOW-UP

15. Make the patient comfortable.

16. Lower the bed to a position of safety for the patient.

PROCEDURE (continued)

17. Pull the curtains back to the open position.

18. Raise the side rails where ordered, indicated, and appropriate for patient safety.

19. Place the call light within easy reach of the patient.

20. Wash your hands.

21. Report to your immediate supervisor:

- That the patient was placed on the bedpan, commode, or toilet on a regular basis.

- The time this was done.

- Whether the patient urinated or had a bowel movement into the bedpan, commode, or toilet.

- How the patient tolerated the procedure.

- Your observations of anything unusual.

CHARTING EXAMPLE: 7/03/04 3:30pm Assisted Mr. Evans to bedside commode at 9am, 11am, 1pm, and 3pm. He was able to urinate at 1pm, but had no bowel movement this shift. R. Rogers, CNA

Rectal Suppositories

If prescribed by the physician, a rectal **suppository** ordered on a regular schedule can help train the patient to empty the rectum while on the bedpan. A single- or double-cone shape is used for adults; a long thin one is used for children. Simple, nonmedicinal suppositories are made of soap, glycerine, or cocoa butter. Medicinal suppositories that contain drugs are not administered by nursing assistants.

    Rectal suppositories are inserted into the rectum to aid in elimination, to assist in healing, to relieve pain, or to re-toilet train an incontinent patient (Figure 33–4◆). Typically, suppositories are considered a medication and are usually given by a nurse, except in home care situations. The nursing assistant should follow the instructions of the immediate supervisor for the time and type of suppository to be used.

suppository A semisolid preparation, sometimes medicated, that is inserted into the vagina or rectum

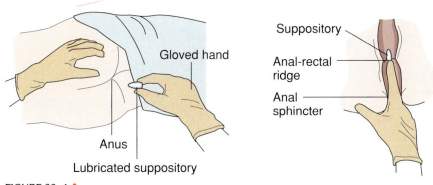

Gloved hand

Anus

Lubricated suppository

Suppository

Anal-rectal ridge

Anal sphincter

FIGURE 33–4 ◆

Inserting a rectal suppository

INSERTING A RECTAL SUPPOSITORY

RATIONALE: Rectal suppositories are inserted into the rectum to aid in elimination, assist in healing, relieve pain, or re-toilet train a patient.

PROCEDURE

PREPARATION

1. Assemble your equipment:

   a. A pair of disposable gloves

   b. Water-soluble lubricant such as K-Y jelly

   c. Bedpan and cover

   d. Protective covering for the bed

   e. Suppository

2. Check the physician's order to be certain you are giving the suppository that was ordered.

3. Wash your hands.

4. Identify the patient by checking the identification bracelet.

5. Ask visitors to step out of the room, if this is your hospital's policy.

PROCEDURE *(continued)*

STEPS		FOLLOW-UP

STEPS

6. Tell the patient that you are going to insert a rectal suppository.

7. Pull the curtain for privacy.

8. Raise the bed to a comfortable working position.

9. Help the patient to roll to the left side and, if possible, raise the right knee toward the patient's chest. This is called the *left Sims's position*.

10. Put on the gloves and apply a small amount of lubricant to the tip of the suppository.

11. With one hand, hold the right buttock up to expose the anus. Insert the suppository with your free hand, gently pushing it up into the rectum about 2 inches, as far as your index finger will reach.

12. Keep the patient in the side-lying position for 5–10 minutes to allow the warmth of the body to melt the suppository. If you leave the room, place the call light within easy reach of the patient. It is best to leave side rails up for safety during this procedure.

13. Assist the patient onto the bedpan or to the toilet.

14. Remove the bedpan, cover it, and take it to the bathroom.

15. Assist the patient with hygiene if needed.

16. Remove your gloves and wash your hands.

17. If the patient was in the bathroom, assist the patient back to the bed or chair and make the patient comfortable.

FOLLOW-UP

18. Wash your hands again.

19. Report to your immediate supervisor:

- The time the suppository was inserted.

- The type of suppository used.

- The patient's reaction, including any cramping or discomfort.

- The results of the procedure— amount and color of stool.

- Any unusual observations.

CHARTING EXAMPLE: 7/03/04 5:30pm Inserted a glycerine rectal suppository into Mr. Evans' rectum. He was able to have a bowel movement when assisted to the commode and says he is feeling more comfortable now. W. Kane, CNA

Range of Motion

Exercise is an important part of restorative care. The benefits of exercise include stress reduction, increased mental alertness, improved appetite, and sound sleep. Exercise reduces joint stiffness and maintains muscle strength. A patient who is confined to bed or is unable to move about freely will not be getting enough exercise. Therefore, the nursing assistant may have to help the patient exercise muscles and joints. This is accomplished through **range-of-motion (ROM) exercises**. These exercises move each muscle and joint through its full range of motion using the basic movements of adduction, abduction, extension, hyperextension, pronation, supination, flexion, dorsal flexion, and rotation (see also Chapter 16).

range-of-motion (ROM) exercises Exercises that move each muscle and joint through its full range of motion and help a confined patient exercise the muscles and joints

The nursing assistant's part in range-of-motion exercises will depend on the patient's level of ability and the physician's orders. According to these criteria, range-of-motion exercises will be one of the following types:

- *Active range of motion (AROM):* The patient is able to move limbs through their range of motion unassisted

- *Passive range of motion (PROM):* The nursing assistant moves the patient's limbs through the range of motion because the patient is unable, for whatever reason, to do it

- *Active assist range of motion (AAROM):* The patient participates to the extent that the patient is able

RANGE-OF-MOTION EXERCISES

GUIDELINES

- Do each exercise three times. (Follow the supervisor's instructions.)
- Follow a logical sequence so that each joint and muscle is exercised. For instance, start at the head and work your way down to the feet.
- If the patient is able to move some body parts, encourage the patient to do as much as possible.
- Be gentle. Never bend or extend a body part farther than it can go. Never exercise to the point of pain.
- If a patient complains of unusual pain or discomfort in a particular body part, be sure to report this to your immediate supervisor.
- Never exercise a reddened, swollen, or painful joint.
- Support all joints when exercising.

RANGE-OF-MOTION EXERCISES

PROCEDURE   OBRA

RATIONALE: Range-of-motion exercises are done to exercise the patient's muscles and joints.

PREPARATION

1. Assemble your equipment:
   a. Blanket
   b. Extra lighting, if necessary
2. Wash your hands.
3. Knock on the door and identify yourself and your purpose.
4. Identify the patient by checking the identification bracelet.
5. Ask visitors to step out of the room, if this is your hospital's policy.
6. Explain to the patient that you are going to help her exercise her muscles and joints while he is in bed.
7. Pull the curtain around the bed for privacy.
8. Raise the bed to a comfortable working position.

STEPS

9. Place the patient in a supine position (on his back) with her knees extended and his arms at her side.

10. Loosen the top sheets, but don't expose the patient.
11. Raise the side rail on the far side of the bed.
12. Exercise the neck (Figure 33–5a and b◆, Figure 33–6a and b◆, and Figure 33–7a and b◆).

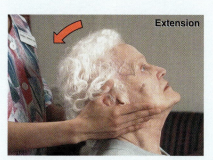

FIGURE 33–5a ◆
Extension

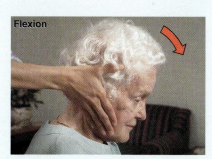

FIGURE 33–5b ◆
Flexion

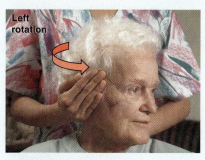

FIGURE 33–6a ◆
Left rotation

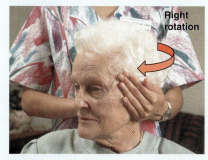

FIGURE 33–6b ◆
Right rotation

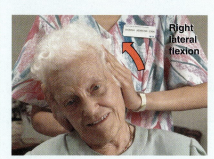

FIGURE 33–7a ◆
Right lateral flexion

PROCEDURE *(continued)*

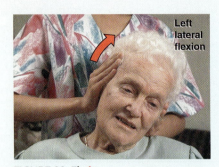

FIGURE 33–7b ◆
Left lateral flexion

13. Hold the extremity to be exercised at the joint (for example, the knee, wrist, elbow).

14. Exercise each shoulder (Figures 33–8◆ and 33–9a and b◆).

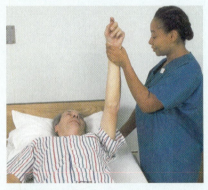

FIGURE 33–8 ◆
Hold arm at the wrist

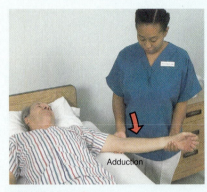

FIGURE 33–9a ◆
Adduction

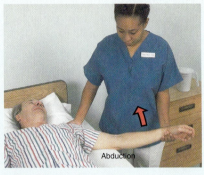

FIGURE 33–9b ◆
Abduction

15. Exercise each elbow (Figure 33–10◆).

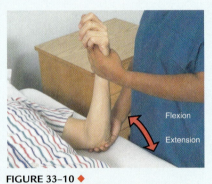

FIGURE 33–10 ◆
Flexion and extension of the elbow

16. Exercise each wrist (Figures 33–11a and b◆ and 33–12a and b◆).

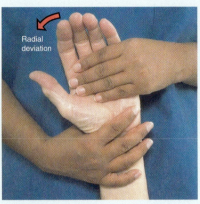

FIGURE 33–11a ◆
Radial deviation

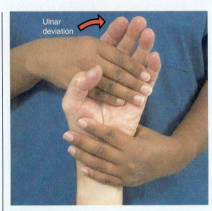

FIGURE 33–11b ◆
Ulnar deviation

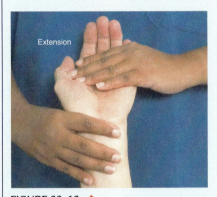

FIGURE 33–12a ◆
Extension of the fingers

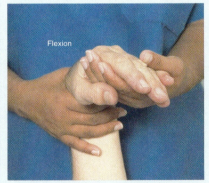

FIGURE 33–12b ◆
Flexion of the fingers

17. Exercise each finger (Figures 33–13◆ and 33–14a and b◆).

PROCEDURE *(continued)*

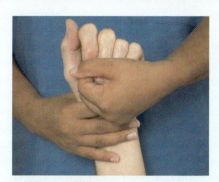

FIGURE 33–13 ◆
Support the wrist

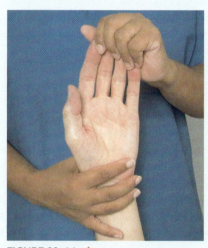

FIGURE 33–14a ◆
Extending and exercising fingers

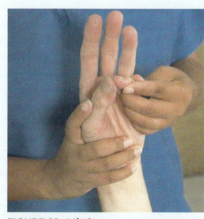

FIGURE 33–14b ◆
Exercising the thumb and small finger

18. Exercise each hip (Figures 33–15◆ through 33–18◆).

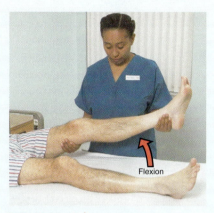

FIGURE 33–15 ◆
Exercise each hip and leg

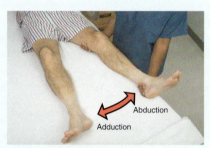

FIGURE 33–16 ◆
Abduction

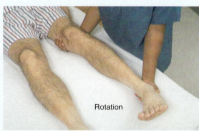

FIGURE 33–17 ◆
Rotation

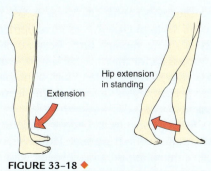

FIGURE 33–18 ◆
Extension and hip extension

19. Exercise each knee (Figure 33–19◆).

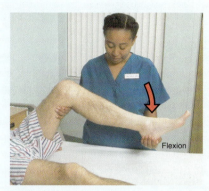

FIGURE 33–19 ◆
Knee flexion

20. Exercise each ankle (Figures 33–20◆ and 33–21◆).

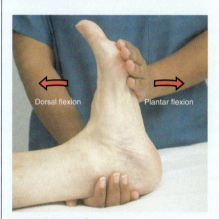

FIGURE 33–20 ◆
Dorsal flexion

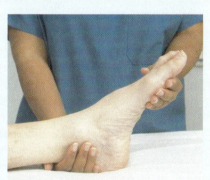

FIGURE 33–21 ◆
Planter flexion

PROCEDURE *(continued)*

21. Exercise each toe (Figures 33–22a and b◆).

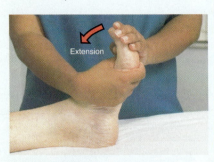

FIGURE 33–22a ◆
Toe extension

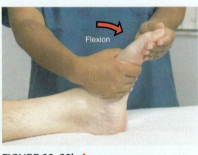

FIGURE 33–22b ◆
Toe flexion

FOLLOW-UP

22. Make the patient comfortable.

23. Replace the sheets if a blanket was used. Fold and return the blanket to its proper place.

24. Lower the bed to a position of safety for the patient.

25. Pull the curtains back to the open position.

26. Raise the side rails where ordered, indicated, and appropriate for patient safety.

27. Place the call light within easy reach of the patient.

28. Replace any extra lighting in its proper place after washing with an antiseptic or disinfectant solution.

29. Wash your hands.

30. Report to your immediate supervisor:

    ■ That you have completed range-of-motion exercises with the patient.

■ The time the exercises were done.

■ How the patient tolerated the exercises.

■ Your observations of anything unusual.

CHARTING EXAMPLE: 7/04/04
10am Passive range-of-motion exercises performed for 20 minutes on Mrs. Oakley. She tolerated the exercises and is resting comfortably.
G. Gunn, CNA

Pediatric Rehabilitation

Usually the process of rehabilitation is easier in children than in adults because of the child's age and stage in growth and development. In many cases, a child is learning activities of daily living for the first time. Because children are adaptable, they can easily learn ways to compensate for their disabilities. For example, a child who was born with a certain spinal defect may never be able to kick a football but may learn to be an expert swimmer. A child who is born with a deformed limb learns to regard it as a natural part of developing self-image.

A child's natural curiosity can be very helpful in the rehabilitation process because it can get the child interested in treatment. However, this curiosity may also have led to an injury, for example, getting burned while playing with matches.

Your positive attitude will encourage positive attitudes in the child and the child's family. Remember to praise the child for anything done well, and help when the child needs assistance. The key is to focus on the child's possibilities, not disabilities.

A child's natural curiosity and eagerness to learn can make rehabilitation of children easier than rehabilitation of adults. The nursing assistant can build on these advantages by adopting a positive attitude and providing appropriate levels of praise and assistance.

 # Subacute Care

When patients' immediate health needs have been met after an injury or illness, they often need continuing care. **Subacute care** refers to caring for a patient who requires less care than regular acute care. In other words, subacute care serves as a transition from regular hospital care to the time when patients can manage on their own or be helped by long-term care. For example, the patient whose surgery is over but requires several days or weeks of daily dressing changes, IV therapy, and medications needs continued care. This patient is discharged from an acute care bed and either transferred to a subacute bed within the same hospital or to a separate free-standing skilled nursing facility (SNF). The patient is cared for outside the acute care area of the hospital because it is not cost effective to care for the patient there. Keeping costs down and still providing high-quality health care is called *managed care*. Managed care is responsible for much growth in the subacute care services in this country.

As hospitals continue to discharge patients who require increasingly complex follow-up care, the demand for subacute care will increase. Likewise, as more insurance companies agree to pay for this care, the subacute segment of health care will grow.

Also important to growth in subacute care is the aging of the population. The elderly are an increasing part of subacute care services. Many of the services they require can be provided through subacute care facilities. However, one of the big problems is how to pay for this kind of care. Although subacute care is less costly than hospital care, it still is very expensive. Medicare and Medicaid, at this time, will not pay for subacute care unless special arrangements are made ahead of time with state or federal government agencies. Many subacute care facilities are linked with a hospital or a health system to help them pay for some of the costly care required by patients.

Similar to acute care, subacute care has its routine components, but medical and nursing care are still primary concerns. Medications, rehabilitation care, physical therapy services, nursing assessment and care, dietary guidance, ventilator support, IV therapy, and other services are included. Subacute care patients tend to be unstable and need to be closely watched. Nursing assistants need to be skilled in their ability to provide assistive subacute care.

Documentation of subacute care is very important and detailed so that patients and facilities can be reimbursed by insurance payers. The nursing assistant must be thorough in documenting care given.

Both hospitals and skilled nursing facilities offer subacute care services. Although the subacute services may be offered in different settings and by different providers, it is important to define subacute care clearly but still be comprehensive (include all types). Figure 33–23◆ lists standards of care for subacute care categories. It defines the type of subacute care, the criteria for putting a patient in this category, the number of care hours required per day, and an estimate of how long the patient might remain in each category. Some patients may start out in one category and move to another. (See also Chapter 28, "Care of the Surgical Patient," and Chapter 29, "Special Procedures.")

As a nursing assistant, you play an important role in caring for patients in subacute care. Opportunities for employment in subacute care will grow as managed care increases and the population continues to age.

subacute care Ongoing medical, nursing, rehabilitative, or dietary care provided to patients who need a lower level of care than an acute care (i.e., hospital) setting provides; categories of subacute care are based on the patient's health status and the type of care and length of care needed

STANDARDS OF CARE FOR SUBACUTE PATIENTS		Nursing Hours PPD	Average Length of Stay
Type of Subacute Patient	Clinical Criteria for Admission		
I. Transitional Subacute:		5-8 hours	5-40 days
A. Definition: Serves as substitute for continued hospital stay rather than alternate hospital discharge placement. B. Facility Requirements: 1. Physician program director or consultant 2. Dedicated RN staff of acute or CCRN with ACLS certification 3. 24-hour respiratory therapy 4. 7 days/week rehabilitation therapies 5. Nutritional therapist C. Goals: 1. Manage patient's care and therapy in a less expensive setting for cost-effectiveness 2. Discharge patient to home or in other alternative less expensive setting such as assisted living or long-term care	1. Wound management for burns 2. Stroke patients by 5th day of hospitalization 3. Coronary bypass patients, not off ventilator within 4-5 days for weaning 4. Pulmonary management of tracheostomies 5. Multiple stage III and IV decubiti 6. Cardiac patients recovering from heart attack or cardiac surgery 7. Oncology surgery, including chemotherapy 8. Rehabilitation for CVAs or for complications following orthopedic surgery 9. Medically complex patients with diabetes, digestive disorders or renal disorders/failure 10. Following vascular or other surgeries.		
II. General Medical-Surgical Subacute		3-5 hours	7-21 days
A. Definition: Provides care for patients who require medical care and monitoring at least weekly, certain rehab therapies, and moderate nursing care services. B. Facility Requirements: 1. Physician consultant 2. RN staff with acute or CCRN background 3. 6 days/week rehabilitation therapies 4. Respiratory therapy consultant 5. Nutritional therapist/dietitian 6. Medicare certified beds C. Goals: 1. Manage patient's care in a cost-effective manner 2. Discharge patient to home or assisted living facility	1. Patients requiring I.V. therapy for septic conditions without other significant medical complications 2. Patients with tracheostomy who require monitoring and tending or trach care 3. Stabilized medical patients with cardiac problems, diabetes, digestive disorders or renal disorders 4. Stroke, CVAs requiring continued rehab therapies, e.g., PT, OT, ST, (1-3 hrs. PPD) 5. Orthopedic patients requiring physical rehab therapies of 1-3 hrs. PPD 6. HIV patients		
III. Chronic Subacute		3-5 hours	60-90 days
A. Definition: Provides care for patients with little hope of ultimate recovery and functional independence. B. Facility Requirements: 1. Physician consultant 2. RN and LPN with medication certification 3. Restorative Nursing 4. PT, OT, ST consultants	1. Ventilator-dependent patients 2. Long-term comatose patients 3. Patients with progressive neurological disease 4. Patients in need of restorative care provided by RN/LPN with assistance from PT, OT, ST.		
IV. Long-Term Transitional Subacute		6.5-9 hours	25 days or more
A. Definition: Provides care for medically complex patients or acute ventilator-dependent patients, e.g., Vencor Hospital. B. Facility Requirements: 1. Physician director 2. Pulmonologist, physiatrist, cardiologist, endocrinologist, cardiovascular surgeon, gastroenterologist consultant 3. Nutritional therapist/dietitian 4. Respiratory therapist 5. RN with acute care experience, CCRN certification preferred	1. Acute ventilator-dependent patients requiring intensive daily care and management 2. Medically complex patients with at least two medical or surgical concurrent diagnoses requiring medical specialists and primarily RN interventions.		

FIGURE 33–23 ◆

Standards of care for subacute care categories. (Reprinted with permission of Springhouse Corporation from the Oct. 1994 edition of *Nursing Management.* Copyright 1994.)

Ventilator Care

ventilator Machine that mechanically breathes for and provides oxygen to sustain a patient unable to inhale and exhale on his own

Ventilator-dependent patients require subacute care. They are attached to a machine that breathes for them, providing artificial respirations. The ventilator will not provide a cure for the coma, respiratory disease, injury, or condition, that is causing patients to be unable to breathe on their own. There are a variety of ventilators, but they all have tubes connecting the patient to the machine. Many of the patients who require ventilators are unconscious. When patients are conscious it is likely they will be anxious or frightened. They are unable to speak and know that, should the machine not function properly or the tube become

GUIDELINES

CARING FOR A PATIENT ON A MECHANICAL VENTILATOR

- Remember, the unconscious patient is still a person, not the "ventilator in room 208A."
- Get help whenever you move the patient. Avoid twisting, turning, disconnecting, or bending the tubing.
- Check the controls and tubes after you complete any task where the patient is moved or turned.
- Turn or reposition the patient at least every 2 hours.

- Notify the nurse immediately when the alarm sounds, the pressure gauge drops, or you observe a change in the patient's condition.
- Provide frequent oral care.
- Keep the call light in reach of conscious patients and respond immediately to their lights.
- Offer support and reassurance to the patient.
- Talk to the patient while you are providing care. Remember that unconscious persons can sometimes hear what you are saying, even

though they cannot respond to you.
- Never remove a resident from the ventilator.
- Accurately record all vital signs.
- Assist conscious patients with communication.
- Notify the nurse or your supervisor immediately if you observe cyanosis, confusion, or increased restlessness in a patient who is being weaned (taken off the ventilator for prescribed periods of time).

disconnected, they will stop breathing and can die. Even the very basic tasks such as changing their beds, providing baths, or personal care is complicated by their situation. As a nursing assistant you will be working closely with a nurse when caring for a patient on a ventilator. The guidelines above can assist you in planning the patient's care.

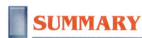

SUMMARY

Rehabilitation affects every aspect of a patient's life and requires considerable planning and coordination. This chapter introduced the key members of the rehabilitation team and the jobs they do to assist patients who have disabilities with learning self-care skills. New skills and procedures such as range-of-motion exercises and personal care for persons with disabilities were covered. All these tasks must be carried out within the context of building a trusting, therapeutic relationship.

NOTES

_____

_____

_____

_____

_____

_____

_____

_____

CHAPTER REVIEW

FILL IN THE BLANK Read each sentence and fill in the blank line with a word that completes the sentence.

1. The process of helping a person regain a state of health is called _____.

2. The _____ _____ is trained to assist patients with activities related to motion.

3. The _____ _____ is trained to increase the functional ability of patients to do their activities of daily living.

4. Low spirits that may or may not cause a change in activity are called _____.

5. _____ is a feeling of tiredness or weariness.

MULTIPLE CHOICE Choose the best answer for each question or statement.

1. Rehabilitation
   a. usually is a waste of time.
   b. is a process done to the patient.
   c. can help the patient recover as much as possible.
   d. is not influenced by cultural and religious beliefs.

2. Activities of daily living include all of the following *except*
   a. toileting.
   b. bathing.
   c. computer skills.
   d. homemaking.

3. In a rehabilitation program, the nursing assistant should
   a. do as much as possible for the patient.
   b. instruct the patient in exactly what to do.
   c. watch for signs that the patient is tired.
   d. All of the above.

4. A condition that occurs when the patient who is disabled on one side of the body forgets that side of the body exists is called
   a. exercise neglect.
   b. exhaustion.
   c. exercise fatigue.
   d. unilateral neglect.

5. Subacute care is appropriate in all the following cases *except*
   a. long-term transitional care (ventilator-dependent patients).
   b. Critical Care unit (newly admitted trauma victims).
   c. chronic subacute (long-term comatose patients).
   d. transitional subacute (stroke patients with >6 days hospitalization).

TIME-OUT

TIPS FOR TIME MANAGEMENT

Help other staff members when you observe the opportunity. For example, if you ask another nursing assistant to help you transfer a patient, help him or her finish making the bed first. If you have finished your tasks, look for ways to help other staff members finish their work. The spirit of cooperation will come back to you.

THE NURSING ASSISTANT IN ACTION
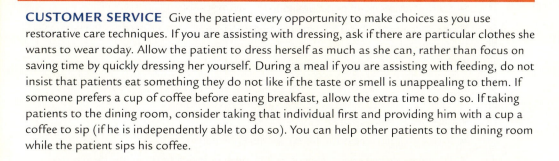

Mrs. Williams is an 88-year-old woman who has been in good health. She was living independently and able to drive her car prior to a fall this week. She had surgery to repair her broken hip. Part of her rehabilitation includes getting her up walking. Mrs. Williams has been in pain and is afraid to allow you to get her up.

What Is Your Response /Action?

CRITICAL THINKING

CUSTOMER SERVICE Give the patient every opportunity to make choices as you use restorative care techniques. If you are assisting with dressing, ask if there are particular clothes she wants to wear today. Allow the patient to dress herself as much as she can, rather than focus on saving time by quickly dressing her yourself. During a meal if you are assisting with feeding, do not insist that patients eat something they do not like if the taste or smell is unappealing to them. If someone prefers a cup of coffee before eating breakfast, allow the extra time to do so. If taking patients to the dining room, consider taking that individual first and providing him with a cup a coffee to sip (if he is independently able to do so). You can help other patients to the dining room while the patient sips his coffee.

CULTURAL CARE There are wide variations in cultural and religious beliefs. If you are unfamiliar with the culture, rituals, or religious beliefs of a patient, check with the patient, the family, or your supervisor to determine if there are particular things you need to know to provide restorative care and support during this difficult time. There may be religious items that a patient would like to hold, wear, have near, or placed on the bedside stand. If you notice a patient has no desire to participate in the rehabilitation, try asking if something is bothering him, or if he would like to talk to you or someone else.

If a patient fears he could become addicted to pain medicine, he may not tell you how much pain he is experiencing. Some Native American Indian patients may have a totem or carving of an animal that brings strength or good luck. Chinese patients may desire specific hot or cold foods that will assist their recovery. Other patients may believe crystals have healing powers. Do not ignore the influence a particular item or belief may have. Most alternative medicines and practices can be used in conjunction with the rehabilitation program. However it is important to be aware of any specific herbs or drugs the patient takes because some can interfere with prescribed medications.

COOPERATION WITHIN THE TEAM Rehabilitation and restorative care require teamwork. When caring for adult patients who need to be lifted, be sure to have help from a coworker or use back-saving devices when available in the facility.

EXPLORE MediaLink

Additional interactive resources for this chapter can be found on the Companion Website at www.prenhall.com/wolgin. Click on Chapter 33 and "Begin" to select the activities for this chapter.

For chapter-related NCLEX-style questions and an audio glossary, access the accompanying CD-ROM in this book.

34 The Terminally Ill Patient and Postmortem Care

acceptance
advance directive
anger
bargaining
denial
depression
expired
hospice
morgue
palliative care
postmortem
rigor mortis
terminally ill

OBJECTIVES

When you have completed this chapter, you will be able to:

- Cite an advantage of organ donation.
- Assist in meeting the psychological, spiritual, or psychosocial needs of the terminally ill patient.
- List common feelings of a patient who is dying.
- Assist in meeting the special care needs of the elderly patient's family or significant other.
- Describe hospice care.
- Identify comfort measures for the terminally ill patient.
- Describe *palliative care,* care designed to comfort, instead of cure, the patient.
- Identify the signs of approaching death.
- Explain *DNR* (do not resuscitate) status.
- Give postmortem care gently and respectfully.
- Explain how to protect the patient's valuables.

MediaLink
www.prenhall.com/wolgin

Use the address above to access the free, interactive Companion Website created for this textbook. Get hints, instant feedback, and textbook references to chapter-related NCLEX-style questions. Link to other interesting sites.

AUDIO GLOSSARY:
Use the Companion Website, or the CD-ROM disk enclosed with your textbook, to hear the pronunciation of key terms in the chapter.

Patients who are terminally ill will behave in ways that help them to accept the fact that they are dying. The nursing assistant must recognize this and provide emotional support. There are emotional experiences that are common to terminally ill patients. They are described by the stages of denial, anger, bargaining, depression, and acceptance. The patient's family or significant other must receive emotional support while you are caring for the emotional and physical needs of the patient. Hospice care is an option for dying patients who wish to remain at home. Signs of approaching death are observations that you will be making.

   The doctor may order not to resuscitate a dying patient. If there is no order, every effort is made to keep the patient alive. After a patient has been pronounced dead by a physician, postmortem care is given by the nursing assistant.

INTRODUCTION

ALERT

For all patient contact, adhere to Standard Precautions (⚭ Chapter 5, pages 83–85). Wear protective equipment as indicated.

 ## Care of Dying Patients

Patients have the right to determine how they will be cared for as they near death. In many cases they have an **advance directive** or living will, their prewritten instructions regarding withholding resuscitation and life-prolonging measures and equipment (Figure 34–1◆).

advance directive Prewritten instructions on withholding resuscitation and life-prolonging measures and equipment

---

CITY MEMORIAL HOSPITAL

Advance Directive for Health Care (Living Will)

I, _____, understand that I have the right to make voluntary, informed choices to accept, reject, or choose among alternative courses of treatment. I make this Advance Directive for Health Care to declare my wishes for use in the event that I am no longer able to participate actively in making my own health care decisions as determined by the physician who has primary responsibility for my care. I direct that this document become part of my permanent medical records.

Life Sustaining Treatment means the use of any medical device or procedure, artificially provided fluids and nutrition, drugs, surgery, or therapy that uses mechanical or other artificial means to sustain, restore, or supplant a vital bodily function, and thereby increase the expected life span of a patient.

Fluids and Nutrition. I request that artificially provided fluids and nutrition, such as by feeding tube or intravenous infusion: (Initial one.)

— shall be withheld or withdrawn as "Life Sustaining Treatment."

— shall be provided to the extent medically appropriate even if other "Life Sustaining Treatment" is withheld or withdrawn.

Directive as to Medical Treatment. I request that "Life Sustaining Treatment" be withheld or withdrawn from me in each of the following circumstances: (Initial all that apply.)

— If the "Life Sustaining Treatment" is experimental and not a proven therapy, or is likely to be ineffective or futile in prolonging my life, or is likely to merely prolong an imminent dying process;

— If I am permanently unconscious (total and irreversible loss of consciousness and capacity for interaction with the environment);

— If I am in a terminal condition (terminal stage of an irreversibly fatal illness, disease, or condition); or

— If I have a serious irreversible illness or condition, and the likely risks and burdens associated with the medical intervention to be withheld or withdrawn outweigh the likely benefits to me from such interventions.

— None of the above I direct that all medically appropriate measures be provided to sustain my life, regardless of my physical or mental condition.

— **Cardiac Arrest.** In the circumstances checked above my attending physician may issue an order not to attempt cardiopulmonary resuscitation (Do Not Resuscitate or "DNR") in the event I suffer a cardiac or respiratory arrest.

— **Pregnancy.** If I have been diagnosed as pregnant, I direct that all "Life Sustaining Treatment" be continued during the course of my pregnancy.

Lack of Health Care Representative. This Advanced Directive shall be legally operative even if I have not designated a Health Care Representative or if neither my representative or any alternative designee is able or available to serve. This Directive shall be honored in accordance with its terms by all who act on my behalf. If this directive is not specific to my medical condition and treatment alternatives, then my physician, in consultation with my Health Care Representative, or if none, then my family, shall exercise reasonable judgment to effect-ate my wishes, giving full weight to the terms, intent, and spirit of this Directive. I release all physicians and other health personnel of all institutions and their employees and members of my family from egal culpability and responsibility.

By signing below, I indicate that I understand the contents of this Advance Directive for Health Care.

Dated: _____ Signature: _____

Witness Statement. We attest to the fact that the person who signed this directive is of sound mind and free of duress and undue influence. We also state that we have not been designated herein as Health Care Representative.

Name: _____ (print) _____ (sign)

Name: _____ (print) _____ (sign)

FIGURE 34–1 ◆

A living will

Advance directives can be individualized. They usually include a list of preferred alternative courses related to life-sustaining and medical treatments and fluids and nutrition. A health care representative may be designated who serves in place of the patient when the person is unable to make informed decisions.

Organ and Tissue Donation

There is a shortage of available organs and tissue that can be used to enhance or improve the lives of others. You may be asked when you renew or acquire your driver's license if you would like to be an organ donor. State and national organizations work with hospitals to meet the federal requirements to give patients and families the opportunity to donate organs or tissue following their deaths. It is better to have the decisions about organ donation made at the same time you are preparing your advance directive. Most facilities have a policy that includes asking patients or families if they are interested in donation when death is inevitable. Organ donation requires some planning. Each have criteria that must be met for the individual to qualify as an organ donor. Harvesting of organs needs to occur after the brain is no longer functioning, while the heart and other systems are kept functioning with ventilator support. It is not uncommon in the cases of teenagers who have suffered brain death in a car or motorcycle accident to be able to provide numerous organs (heart, liver, kidneys) and tissue (cornea, lens, skin) to individuals on waiting lists hoping to receive the organ transplants that can save or prolong their lives. Organs are extracted in an operating room and sent to be transplanted in individuals for whom there is a match.

The decision to participate in organ or tissue donation is often influenced by personal, religious, and cultural beliefs. Some family members may fear that organ donation will make having an open-casket funeral a problem. This fear is unfounded. Some families receive solace or comfort knowing their loved one has helped others through his or her organ or tissue donation.

Psychological/Psychosocial Aspects of Caring for a Terminally Ill Patient

terminally ill Having an illness that can be expected to cause death, usually within a predictable time

Some patients who enter a health care institution are **terminally ill**, that is, dying. Sometimes death is sudden or unexpected. More often it is not. Your first responsibility to the terminally ill patient is to help make the patient as physically comfortable as possible. Your second responsibility is to assist in meeting the emotional needs of the patient and the patient's family or significant other.

The most important single fact to remember when you are caring for dying patients is that they are just as important as the patients who are going to recover. You will not have the satisfaction of contributing to recovery, but you will know that you have helped your patients face the end of their lives in peace, comfort, and dignity. Everyone must die. Surely we would all prefer to die in reassuring and comfortable surroundings.

Try to be very understanding. The patient may want to believe he will get well. He may want people around him to reassure him that he won't die. When a dying patient talks to you, listen. But don't give him false hopes. Don't tell him that he is getting better. Your supervisor can help you know what to say.

KEY IDEA

People have different ideas about death and the hereafter. These ideas depend on their beliefs and background. You must show respect for patients' beliefs. Be careful not to impose your own beliefs on them, their families, or significant others.

When a patient suspects he is going to die, he may react in various ways. The patient may:

- Ask everyone about his chances for recovery
- Be afraid to be alone and want a lot of attention from you
- Ask a lot of questions
- Seem to complain constantly
- Signal members of the staff often
- Make many apparently unreasonable requests
- Rest and prefer to be left alone

When a patient is told that he has a terminal disease or condition, the patient enters a very difficult time of life. Death may be frightening and the patient's reactions reflect the quality of emotional support provided by everyone interacting with him, as well as his culturally determined attitudes. Feelings of isolation, hopelessness, despair, sorrow, and uselessness affect the coping mechanisms displayed by the patient and family members.

Stages of Dying

Elizabeth Kübler-Ross describes five "stages" of dying in her book, *Death and Dying* (Figure 34–2◆). These are not intended to be stages that the patient must go through. Rather, they are emotional experiences that are common to terminally ill patients. This is especially true for the newly diagnosed patient and much less so for the patient who has known he is dying for a while.

These "stages," or feelings common to terminally ill patients, are:

- **Denial:** This is a reaction to the shocking news. The patient may say, "No, this is not happening to me, this is something that happens to other people." This is sometimes the first reaction on the part of the patient.

  denial Refusal to admit the truth or face reality

- **Anger:** The patient resents what has happened—all the unfinished plans and the realization that he will be unable to finish or enjoy life's activities. It is at this point that the patient will begin to react to everything, making demands and asking for

  anger A strong emotional response of displeasure, irritation, and resentment

FIGURE 34–2 ◆

The five stages of dying

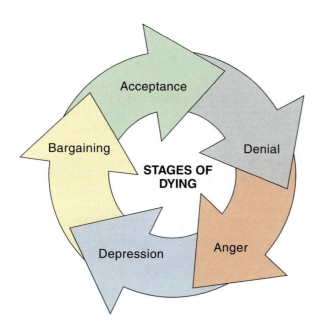

additional attention. The patient now is beginning to feel that soon he will be forgotten and that all is over.

bargaining Trying to make a deal to change the situation

- **Bargaining:** This is an attempt to make a bargain with God to postpone the inevitable. This bargaining may be connected with guilt for not having done what religious teachings tell us to do. It is here that the patient may request that a priest, minister, or rabbi be called.

depression A state of sadness, grief, or low spirits that may or may not cause change of activity

- **Depression:** The patient reaches some acceptance of death. He may begin to grieve, to talk about his innermost feelings, and may want you to listen. By being a good listener at this point, you can help the patient.

acceptance Admitting, understanding, or facing the truth or reality of the situation, for example, one's death

- **Acceptance:** Communication often becomes difficult. Some patients become quiet and withdrawn, while others may become more talkative after accepting the inevitable. The patient may communicate his needs to you through body language or gestures. Your job as a nursing assistant is to make the patient as comfortable as possible.

The Patient's Family or Significant Other

When it is known that death is approaching, the dying patient's family may want to spend a lot of time with the patient. This should be encouraged and permitted as much as possible.

Everyone on the staff should respect the family's need for privacy during their visits. If a private room is not available, the patient's area should be screened so that they will have the privacy they need. When the patient is visited by his pastor, priest, rabbi, or minister, assure them that they will not be disturbed.

Don't stop doing your work just because the patient's family is present. Carry out your job quickly, quietly, and efficiently. Don't wait until the family has gone before taking care of the patient. They might think that, because the patient is dying, he is being neglected by the hospital staff.

The patient's family may ask you many questions. Respond to their questions. Answer any you can. Also, do whatever is asked of you, if it is allowed.

There will be some questions that you can't answer. For example, you may be asked, "What did the doctor say today about the patient's condition?" Refer the family to your immediate supervisor.

Even if the patient becomes unconscious, the family may want to stay with him. Family members may continue to hope for his recovery. They will watch you perform your patient care procedures. They will want you to make the patient comfortable, even if you cannot help him recover.

Unconscious patients require as thorough care as those who are conscious. Their needs must still be met. Sometimes you must ask the family to leave the bedside while you are giving care to the patient. Explain this to the family. Tell them that you will let them know when you have finished.

Some visitors stay with the patient for many hours at a time. Be as helpful to them as you can. You might suggest that they have some nourishment. Tell them where the cafeteria, vending machines, or coffee shop is located. Also, learn the policy in your institution on serving meals to visitors. You may be able to arrange for trays to be delivered to the patient's family at mealtimes. If this is not allowed, tell the visitors where they can find the cafeteria or a nearby restaurant. Make sure the visitors know the location of the washroom, lounge, and telephones.

Remember at all times to be quietly courteous, understanding, sympathetic, and willing to help (Figure 34–3◆). These are the marks of a competent nursing assistant.

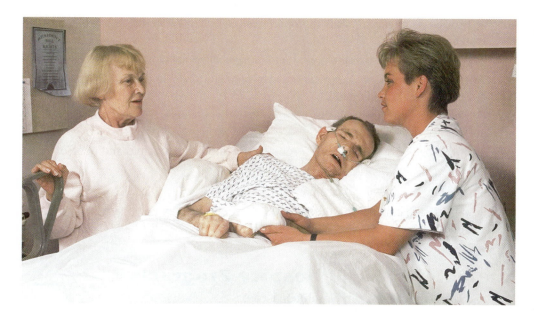

FIGURE 34–3 ◆
Supporting the family of the terminally ill patient is very important

KEY IDEA

Don't feel helpless or guilty because you can't improve the patient's condition. You can help the patient and family most by maintaining a concerned and efficient approach to your work.

 # Hospice Care

Hospice care is a method of health care delivery used to ensure individualized and humane care for the terminally ill. Hospice care is an option for patients expected to die within 6 months. Hospice facilities or rooms in long-term care facilities are designed to provide a comfortable, less frightening homelike setting. Families are encouraged to spend as much time as they wish with their loved one and are included in all aspects of the patient's care. Hospice staff and volunteers provide nursing care, financial counseling, and emotional, psychological, and spiritual support to the family and patient. Some patients or families arrange to have hospice care provide in their own homes.

hospice Program that allows a dying patient to remain at home or in a nonhospital environment and die there while receiving professionally supervised care

The philosophy of hospice stresses:

- Assisting with psychological, physiological, and spiritual problems
- Using a family-oriented approach
- Alleviating pain and other symptoms in the advanced stage of disease
- Offering professional and voluntary services to meet individual needs
- Making the patient as comfortable as possible

Principles of Hospice Care

- To provide physical comfort
- To provide psychological counseling
- To assist the patient to maintain ability to participate in life

- To provide an environment that emphasizes the quality of life on a daily basis, rather than longevity
- To provide assurance that the patient and family will not be alone in a moment of crisis
- To provide the patient with evidence that family, friends, and staff care about what the patient thinks and feels
- To provide an environment that permits the patient to return to his own schedule of activities of daily living
- To encourage the patient to be surrounded by familiar belongings and people
- To provide assessment of changing needs
- To facilitate the grieving of the patient and family
- To provide the patient with the opportunity to die with dignity in familiar and caring surroundings

Characteristics of Hospice Programs

- Coordination of home and institutional care
- Patient and family regarded as one unit
- Physician and other health care provider availability
- Care provided by an interdisciplinary team
- Control of symptoms and pain
- Availability of care 24 hours a day
- Volunteer involvement
- Follow-up care for bereaved families
- System of open communication between staff, volunteers, patient, and family

Making the Patient Comfortable

palliative care Care designed to comfort, instead of cure, the patient

Remember that caring for the terminally ill patient is just as important as caring for a patient who is going to recover. Table 34–1 ◆ identifies the care needs of a terminally ill patient and gives a description of the care to be given. This care is often referred to as **palliative care**.

Signs of Approaching Death

Death comes in different ways. It may come quite suddenly. Or it may come after a long period during which there has been a steady decline of body functions. Death also may result from complications during convalescence. Here are some signs showing that death may be near:

- Blood circulation slows down. The patient's hands and feet are cold to the touch. If the patient is conscious, he may complain that he is cold. Keep the patient well covered. If possible adjust the room temperature as needed.
- The patient's face may become pale because of decreased circulation.
- The patient's eyes may be staring blankly into space. There may be no eye movement when you move your hand across her line of vision.
- The patient may perspire heavily, even though his body is cold.
- The patient loses muscle tone and her body becomes limp. The jaw may drop and the mouth may stay partly open. Eyes may not close in sleep.

TABLE 34–1

Meeting the Terminally Ill Patient's Needs—Palliative Care

PATIENT NEED	DESCRIPTION
Personal	A patient approaching death continues to be given routine personal care, such as baths and mouth care. That is, the patient receives the same care that would be given if she were expected to recover. Members of the nursing staff should stay calm and sympathetic. This may help to relieve some of the patient's fears and make this time easier. As the patient becomes weaker, her condition may require more of your time. You may need to do many things that the patient is no longer able to do for herself.
Positioning	The patient will tell you what position is most comfortable. It is important that the patient remain active as long as possible, and his position in bed be changed regularly to protect the skin (Figure 34-4◆).
Communication	Speak to the patient in your normal voice, even if she appears to be unconscious. You should still tell the patient who you are and what you are doing. The dying patient's hearing is usually one of the last senses to fail. We do not know how much an unconscious person hears or understands. It could be a great deal. Encourage the family to continue to talk to the patient unless she is sleeping.
Visual	Adjust the light in the room to suit the patient. For some, bright lights are irritating; for others, a dark room is frightening.
Elimination	As death comes closer, the sphincters relax and the patient may lose control of the bowels and bladder. Your job is to keep the patient's body clean at all times. Change the bedding whenever necessary. This will keep the patient's skin from becoming irritated and will help to keep the patient comfortable. You may also be giving more back rubs than usual. The urine may become concentrated and strong smelling, and it is especially necessary to keep the skin clean. Foley catheters are rarely necessary with the use of incontinent pads and bed pads.
Nutrition	Usually the patient is allowed whatever foods he desires. However there is often a decreased appetite. Semisoft foods or semi-frozen liquid may be easier to handle than liquids.
Oral Hygiene	The patient approaching death needs special mouth care. The mouth may be dry because the patient is breathing through it. You might use an applicator with glycerine (or other lubricant) to swab the patient's mouth and lips. If the patient's mouth has a large amount of secretions in it, tell the nurse. The nurse may use suction to remove the secreted material. If the patient has dentures, ask your immediate supervisor if you should leave them in the patient's mouth or take them out. If you remove the dentures, place them in a denture cup half filled with water, with the patient's name on the cover. If the patient has cancer or AIDS, watch for and report sores in the mouth. Often persons near death have gums or lips that bleed. Using a dark-colored towel or washcloth may make this less frightening. A moist mouth will make it easier for the patient to eat.
Treatment: Oxygen Therapy	A patient may be receiving oxygen through a nasal catheter or mask. If so, check the nostrils from time to time. Tell your immediate supervisor if the nostrils are dry and encrusted. Check the tops of the ears or any other place the tubing contacts as it can cause skin irritation. A patient's nostrils also may become dry and encrusted because he has difficulty breathing. If you notice dryness, with your immediate supervisor's permission, clean the nostrils with cotton swabs moistened slightly with glycerine (or other lubricant).
Spiritual	Respect the patient's and family's need for spiritual support (Figure 34-5◆). Learn the policy in your institution concerning religious observances and requirements at the time of death. If the patient has particular beliefs or practices relative to death, such as the care of the body, it is important to know these before death occurs.

- Respirations may become slower and more difficult or faster, or there may be brief periods of no breathing. Mucus collecting in the patient's throat and bronchial tubes may cause a sound that is sometimes called the "death rattle."

- The pulse may be rapid or may become weak and irregular.

- Just before death, respirations stop and the pulse gets very faint. You may not be able to feel the patient's pulse at all.

- Contrary to popular belief, a dying person is rarely in great pain. As the patient's condition gets worse, less blood may be flowing to the brain. Therefore, the patient may feel little or no pain.

FIGURE 34–4 ◆

Changing the patient's position every 2 hours protects the patient's skin

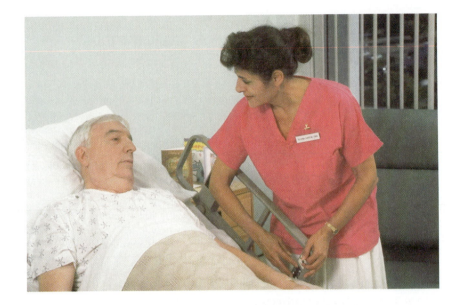

FIGURE 34–5 ◆

The dying patient may find spiritual comfort in a visit from the chaplain

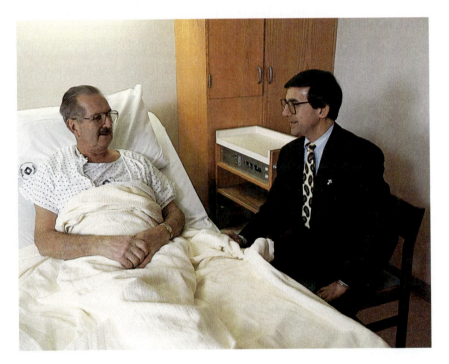

■ The patient may talk to persons who have died.

■ The patient's urine output may decrease.

■ The patient's swallowing ability may decrease.

■ The patient may have periods of confusion and/or agitation.

If you notice any of these signs or any changes in the patient's condition, report them to your supervisor immediately. Sometimes the patient requests, and the physician orders, that no resuscitative measures be taken when the patient's lungs and heart cease to function. This is referred to as *DNR (Do Not Resuscitate) status*. Your immediate supervisor will be aware of this and will not initiate resuscitative procedures. Follow your supervisor's instructions.

Refer to Chapter 2 for information regarding living wills and other advance directives, for example the decision to refuse to be fed by artificial means such as a nasogastric or gastric feeding tube.

Postmortem Care (PMC)

If you observe any signs of approaching death, tell the nurse immediately. The nurse will examine the patient and confirm what you have found. In some health care institutions, a nurse, after confirming that a patient has no pulse or has stopped breathing, calls a "code." This code (Code Blue or some other term) is an emergency announcement to the entire staff. A preassigned team will come to help the patient and use every means available to keep the patient alive. Only when all efforts fail to keep the patient alive is the patient declared to be dead by a physician. In some cases, if it is known in advance that the patient may die, the physician may write a DNR (Do Not Resuscitate) order. In such cases the patient's death is not an emergency, and no code is called.

When the patient has **expired**, **postmortem** care is given. The patient's body still must be treated with respect and must be given gentle care. The patient's family will be allowed to view the body again if they wish after you have completed postmortem care. Ask them if they would like to be alone with their loved one or if they would like you or another member of the health care team to stay with them.

Sometimes the family is not present when the patient dies. In this case, either the doctor or the nurse then notifies the family and finds out whether any family members wish to view the patient's body before it is sent to the **morgue**. If so, the body usually stays in the room until the family arrives.

expired Deceased, dead

postmortem After death

morgue A place for temporarily keeping dead bodies for identification, autopsy, retrieval by funeral home staff, and burial

PROCEDURE — POSTMORTEM CARE — OBRA

RATIONALE: Postmortem care is done to prepare the body for viewing by the family and for transfer to the morgue.

PREPARATION

1. Assemble your equipment:
   a. Soap
   b. Washcloth
   c. Towels
   d. Wash basin with warm water
   e. Bed protectors
   f. Clean gown
2. Wash your hands and put on gloves.

STEPS

3. Turn off oxygen, suction, or IVs at the nurse's or doctor's instructions.
4. Raise the bed to a comfortable working position.
5. Lower the head of the bed so the patient is lying flat with the pillow under the head. This will keep the blood from pooling in the face and neck.
6. Replace dentures if they are not in the patient's mouth.
7. Gently close the eyelids if they are open. If they do not remain closed, notify your supervisor before the family comes to be with the body.
8. If the body is soiled with urine or feces, clean gently to remove odor. Place clean bed protectors under the body.
9. Straighten the body in a dignified position.
10. Cover the body with clean bed linen, but do not cover the head.
11. Straighten the room and remove any emergency equipment.
12. Turn off the bright light over the bed.

FOLLOW-UP

13. Remove gloves and wash your hands.
14. Provide privacy and support for the family's visit.

CHARTING EXAMPLE: 10/31/04 10:30pm Mr. Jasper's belongings given to wife. Dentures left in place and wedding ring taped in place on left hand. Postmortem care completed. C. Harris, CNA

When the family is present, they are given the patient's personal belongings. These items are checked against the admission valuables list to be sure that everything is accounted for. Jewelry remains on the patient unless the family requests its removal. Jewelry left on the body is taped in place and documented on the patient's record. Be specific describing the jewelry. You will learn the procedure in your health care institution for taking care of the deceased patient's clothes and belongings.

rigor mortis The natural stiffening of a body and limbs shortly after death

Postmortem care should be done before **rigor mortis** sets in. Each institution will have its own specific policies and procedures you must follow. Some general principles will apply in most institutions. For example, you may not remove some types of tubes, bandages, and so on from the body. Check with your immediate supervisor.

SUMMARY

Terminally ill patients need psychological and psychosocial support as well as physical care. Being a good listener is the best way to provide psychological support. Recognizing the five stages of dying will help you be even more supportive of your patients, their families, and significant others. The patients may choose hospice care so they can remain at home. The signs of approaching death include changes in circulation, breathing, vital signs, and consciousness. Know which patients have a "do not resuscitate" order. Postmortem care should be given in a caring, respectful manner according to the policy and procedures of your institution.

NOTES

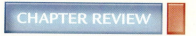

CHAPTER REVIEW

FILL IN THE BLANK Read each sentence and fill in the blank line with a word that completes the sentence.

1. When a patient is _____ ill, they have an illness that is expected to cause death, usually within a predicted time.

2. When a patient is dying, respect the patient's and family's need for _____ as much as possible.

3. A program that allows a dying patient to remain at home or in a nonhospital facility is called _____.

4. Care designed to comfort rather than cure is called _____ care.

5. Rigor mortis is the natural _____ of the body after death.

MULTIPLE CHOICE Choose the best answer for each question or statement.

1. People have different ideas about death and dying. As a nursing assistant, it is important that you
   a. impose your ideas and religious beliefs on patients.
   b. respect the cultures and religious beliefs of others.
   c. say "no" or "you must follow policy" when patient or family requests pose a problem or inconvenience for you.
   d. All of the above

2. The most common stages of dying are
   a. denial, anger, depression, bargaining, and acceptance.
   b. denial, depression, anger, bargaining, and acceptance.
   c. anger, denial, depression, repression and acceptance.
   d. anger, repression, denial, bargaining and acceptance.

3. All of the following are signs of approaching death *except*
   a. the hands and feet become cold to the touch.
   b. the patient's face may become pale.
   c. the arms and legs become stiff.
   d. the patient may perspire heavily even though his body is cold.

4. A physician's order that states that emergency care must be given to a patient is
   a. DNR.
   b. advanced directive.
   c. slow code.
   d. None of the above.

5. Postmortem care should be completed
   a. after rigor mortis has set in.
   b. only in the morgue.
   c. by a funeral attendant.
   d. before rigor mortis has set in.

TIME-OUT

TIPS FOR TIME MANAGEMENT

Keep personal phone calls and messages to a minimum while you are at work. Some facilities have policies prohibiting personal calls. Your family should contact you only if an urgent or emergency situation arises. Keep your work time focused on patients and their care.

THE NURSING ASSISTANT IN ACTION

Mr. Justice is a patient on your unit who is terminally ill with an advance directive in place. His son who lives in another town has arrived to visit and just learned his father is dying. The advance directive states you are not to give fluids or nutrition to Mr. Justice. His son is upset and tells you he will have you fired from your job if you do not start giving his father some water immediately.

What Is Your Response/Action?

CRITICAL THINKING

CUSTOMER SERVICE There are wide variations in cultural and religious beliefs. If you are unfamiliar with the culture, rituals, or religion of a dying patient, check with the patient, the family, or your supervisor to determine if there are particular things you need to know to provide the most compassionate and considerate care during this difficult time. There may be religious items that a patient would like to hold, wear, have near them, or placed on the bedside stand. Some patients may have no particular religion but would prefer to watch videos, hear music they like, or have their bed positioned so they can see out the window. Any reasonable request should be accommodated or granted.

CULTURAL CARE As a nursing assistant you will encounter many variations and cultural differences related to death and dying. Some families will grieve loudly and others will be very quiet. A patient may wish to have many visitors and family nearby or prefer to be alone. Recognize that it is their choice. Be respectful when touching or moving any religious item.

COOPERATION WITHIN THE TEAM If you have not had the experience of having patients die while you are assigned to care for them, it can be unnerving. Some people are afraid when they are alone in a room with a dead person or uncomfortable touching the body. The experience of giving postmortem care happens rarely while you are a student. Talk to your supervisor or preceptor and request that when you need to perform postmortem care, you would appreciate it if an experienced coworker could assist you the first time to be certain you correctly learn the procedure. Should you notice that a coworker is uncomfortable, extend an offer to assist her. She will probably accept your offer and later be more eager to help you when you need her assistance.

EXPLORE MediaLink

Additional interactive resources for this chapter can be found on the Companion Website at www.prenhall.com/wolgin. Click on Chapter 34 and "Begin" to select the activities for this chapter.

For chapter-related NCLEX-style questions and an audio glossary, access the accompanying CD-ROM in this book.

35 Beginning Your Career as a Nursing Assistant

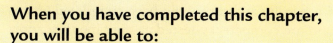

OBJECTIVES

When you have completed this chapter, you will be able to:

- List the steps to be taken in completing competency evaluation and testing.
- Describe the function of the state Nurse Aide Registry.
- Select a method of preparing for competency testing.
- Successfully complete a model test.
- Identify job opportunities and be prepared for an interview.
- Write one or two possible career plans using the career options chart provided.
- Describe how your competencies can be assessed in an employment setting.

KEY TERMS

competency
continuing education
evaluation
staff development

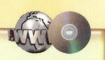

MediaLink
www.prenhall.com/wolgin

Use the address above to access the free, interactive Companion Website created for this textbook. Get hints, instant feedback, and textbook references to chapter-related NCLEX-style questions. Link to other interesting sites.

AUDIO GLOSSARY:
Use the Companion Website, or the CD-ROM disk enclosed with your textbook, to hear the pronunciation of key terms in the chapter.

In this chapter you will learn about the process of competency evaluation for nursing assistant candidates mandated by OBRA, the Omnibus Budget Reconciliation Act of 1987. This act requires nursing assistants employed in long-term care to demonstrate that they are capable of carrying out specific care-related tasks at the minimal level prior to having their name placed on the state's Nurse Aide Registry.

It is anticipated that all areas of health care will require a competency test for all nursing assistants in the future. Many institutions, including acute care hospitals, prefer to hire nursing assistants who have completed an approved training program and are competency-tested at the time they apply for employment.

This chapter will also help you identify where to look for employment opportunities and describe the ways you can continue to develop and grow in your career.

Preparing for the Competency Evaluation Exam

> **ALERT**
>
> For all patient contact, adhere to Standard Precautions (🔗 Chapter 5, pages 83–85). Wear protective equipment as indicated.

competency A demonstrable skill or ability

evaluation Assessment of one's ability or skill to perform a given task

The Ominbus Budget Reconciliation Act of 1987 made many changes in the care and treatment of people who are cared for in long-term care and nursing facilities. OBRA regulations also require health care facilities to hire nursing assistants who hold certificates or licenses from state-approved training programs and have completed the Nursing Assistant Competency Evaluation as described in this chapter.

The Nursing Assistant **Competency Evaluation** is administered in two parts: a clinical/practical test and a written test. The candidate usually must successfully complete part one before progressing to the second test.

Candidates for the competency examination must have completed a state-approved training course consisting of a minimum of 75 hours of theory, lab practice, and supervised patient care. Based on written test scores, demonstration of skills learned, and observation of care given to assigned patients/residents during the required 75 hours, the student will be given a certificate or verification, indicating the satisfactory completion of the training course (Figure 35–1◆). Usually candidates may then begin the testing process.

There is variation by state as to how the competency evaluation tests are administered. Your instructor will be aware of the current process. Some states require that the clinical skills section of the test be successfully completed before the second test is administered. Other states allow you to take both parts of the test and will only require retests of the failed section of the test. You may find that the written test is administered prior to the clinical skills test. The amount of information the candidate is given following each skill will also vary. The process will be explained prior to the test. The candidates are told when they can expect to find out if they have successfully completed or failed any of the skills.

Clinical Skills Examination

Usually, the first portion of the testing process is the skills demonstration, *Clinical Skills Examination* (CSE), *Nurse Aide State Examination,* or some similar examination. The CSE is administered in a skills lab or other area where needed supplies are at hand. The test-taker (you), a trained observer, and an actor (if one is used) are the only people present during testing. Any tasks that require the actor to be exposed in any way are performed on a mannequin. The care tasks the test-taker is required to perform are designed to demonstrate competencies you have acquired during training.

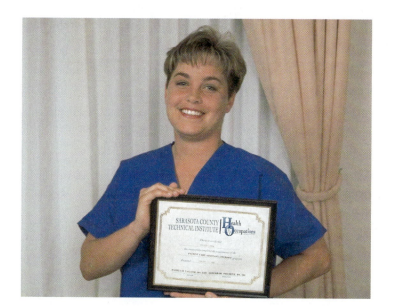

FIGURE 35–1 ◆
Certificate received upon completion of Patient Care Assistant program

Remember this is not the time to ask questions! The observer will observe and document the steps you take in demonstrating your skills. No advice or prompting may be given during testing. Usually, the observer will not be able to tell you whether or not you have "passed." The test-scoring of the *Clinical Skills Examination* is done by an independent agency. Some national testing services, for example, in Vermont, offer same-day scoring and reporting.

There are variations in how actors are used in the examination process. If child actors are used, their parents must have provided consent for them to participate. Actors may be other students or, if permitted, the actor may be a patient/resident or an employee of the facility where the test is being administered or someone else known to the test-taker. The actor may NOT be anyone unable to give informed consent or another nursing assistant student who has not yet taken the test. Do not bring an actor to the test site unless your instructor tells you to do so. The actor must remain impartial, giving no assistance or clues to the test-taker.

Some of the tasks you may be asked to demonstrate are:

- Making an occupied or unoccupied bed
- Measuring and recording temperature, pulse, and respiration
- Toileting
- Transfer and positioning
- Applying a safety device
- Personal care and grooming tasks
  - Hair and nail care
  - Denture care and oral care
- Feeding or assisting with a meal
- Dressing
- Measuring and recording height and weight
- Giving a bed bath

Your training course provided you with demonstrations of these care skills and an opportunity to practice and demonstrate the skills yourself. It will help you to review the steps of each procedure in your textbook prior to taking the *Clinical Skills Examination/ Skills Demonstration Examination*. In some states, the skills and written exams may be given at the same time, for example, the ASI test for long-term care facility competency evaluation program.

Written/Oral Examination

As previously mentioned, this part of the testing process may take place after you have successfully taken the *Clinical Skills Examination*. The written examination is also given in oral form in certain circumstances. Your instructor will provide you with information about the oral form of the test if necessary. The written test is administered by a national testing service, for example, the American Red Cross in some areas and by the State Board of Nursing in others. Your instructor will have specific information on how to register for the examination.

The test consists of 50 or more multiple choice questions. A sample test is provided in this chapter following the section on the Nurse Aide Registry. These questions test your knowledge of care tasks and procedures you have learned as well as concepts like infection control, safety, ethics, and communicating with others. You may find it helpful to study with classmates in small groups, or have someone quiz you on topics in your textbook. Regardless of how you prepare for the written examination remember to review the medical terms and abbreviations included in the training course—many of them are included in the multiple choice test questions.

Some important terms to know:

- abuse
- ADL
- ambulate
- body mechanics
- dignity
- edema
- elimination
- ethics
- infection
- isolation
- privacy
- pulse
- Standard Precautions
- therapeutic
- transfer
- void

Test Fees and Time Requirements

Fees for the *Clinical Skills/Skills Demonstration Examination* and the *Written/Oral Examination* vary from state to state. Your instructor can advise you of the fee requirements in your area. Payment must be made by money order or cashier's check; no cash or personal checks are accepted. Test fees must be paid upon registration or at the time you take each test.

Both the *Clinical Skills Examination* and the *Written/Oral Examination* are given by appointment. It is important that you keep your appointments and arrive on time, and be prepared to take the examination. Upon completing your training course, you have a specified amount of time called a "window of opportunity" within which you must complete the testing process and register with the Nurse Aide Registry. Candidates who go past this "window" may be required to retake the training course before being tested. Your instructor will provide you with information in your area.

Some states do not certify nurse assistants. For example, in Pennsylvania nurse assistants are placed on a registry as nurse assistants and use NA as their title. In states where there is a certification process, once you have passed both portions, of the competency examination your title will be certified nursing assistant (CNA) or CENA. CENA stands for competency evaluated nursing assistant. You will be able to care for patients/residents at the basic level, providing personal care within your training (Figure 35–2◆). Some home health agencies will require you to "recertify" within their organization by building on the skills you have learned to be able to provide care, usually without direct supervision in the home. The home health agency may require you to take a separate skills examination prior to working with patients in the home.

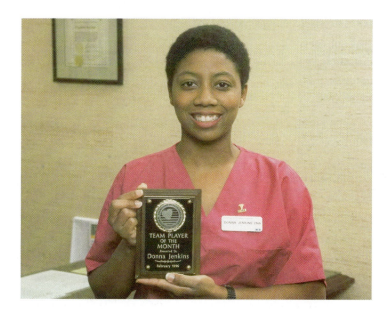

FIGURE 35–2 ◆

CNA receiving team player of the month award

Nurse Aide Registry

All states are required to maintain a Nurse Aide Registry. After successfully completing the Nursing Assistant Competency Evaluation, your name may be placed on the Nurse Aide Registry. Employers can contact the agency to verify if you or anyone else they are considering for employment is properly certified/listed.

If a nursing assistant is involved in a situation involving the theft of a patient's property or suspected patient abuse, the employer reports this to the registry. The registry document of a nursing assistant who is convicted of misconduct is "flagged," and the individual is not permitted to work as a nursing assistant. Certain information is considered confidential and therefore is not given to prospective employers. However, the "flag" indicates that there is proof that a serious incident has occurred.

Some states have recently begun to require that registry documents be renewed every 1 to 2 years. A renewal form is mailed to your home and you will be instructed to complete a section indicating any changes such as your name, address, or telephone number. Your current or most recent health care employer may need to complete a section indicating that you meet the requirements for renewal.

Sample Test

This sample test contains questions similar to those that appear on the Nursing Assistant Competency Evaluation test. Read carefully each question and all the possible answers before choosing the *one* correct answer.

1. Cyanosis means

   a. a bluish color to the skin.

   b. difficulty breathing.

   c. a colorless, odorless gas.

   d. abnormally high blood pressure.

2. Body temperature can be increased by

   a. dehydration.

   b. cold environment.

   c. medications.

   d. shock.

3. The first step in any procedure is to

   a. gather your supplies.

   b. wash your hands.

   c. explain what you will do.

   d. lower the side rail.

4. When moving and lifting a patient, the nurse assistant should

   a. plan all moves.

   b. be alert to safety.

   c. let the patient help if possible.

   d. All of the above.

5. The best definition of the word "emergency" is

   a. an unusual event or occurrence.

   b. a source of potential danger.

   c. an event that calls for immediate action.

   d. None of the above.

6. Pathogens can be destroyed by

   a. sterilization.

   b. handwashing.

   c. disinfection.

   d. careful handling.

7. You can maintain your own good health by

   a. getting enough rest and sleep.

   b. eating properly.

   c. washing your hands frequently.

   d. All of the above.

8. Select the example of a barrier to conversation.

   a. Speaking slowly and clearly.

   b. Avoiding eye contact.

   c. Identifying yourself.

   d. Calling the patient by name.

9. Elderly persons do not need a complete bath or shower every day because

   a. they might become chilled.

   b. their skin has less oil and is drier.

   c. they are too tired.

   d. None of the above.

10. You find a small blister on the buttock of your patient; your first action should be to

   a. apply a hot compress.

   b. report it to the nurse.

   c. massage the area.

   d. apply a bandage.

11. The brachial pulse is found

   a. inside the elbow.

   b. on the top of the foot.

   c. inside the wrist.

   d. behind the knee.

12. In caring for a hearing aid you should
   a. rinse with water daily.
   b. never remove it from the ear.
   c. avoid dropping it.
   d. keep the volume on high.

13. Your first action in case of a fire is to
   a. learn to use the fire extinguisher.
   b. rescue the patient.
   c. call for help.
   d. pull the fire alarm.

14. Which statement is true about physical restraints?
   a. They do not require a doctor's order.
   b. They must be removed every half hour.
   c. They can cause injury to a patient.
   d. They can be left on for up to four hours at a time.

15. The longest and strongest muscles in your body are
   a. in your buttocks.
   b. in your back.
   c. in your abdomen.
   d. in your thighs.

16. The proper positioning of a patient's body is called
   a. body mechanics.   c. body alignment.
   b. range of motion.   d. positioning.

17. Pressure ulcers are
   a. also called bedsores.
   b. always infected.
   c. prevented by frequent baths.
   d. only found in elderly people.

18. The term "ad lib" means
   a. immediately.   c. only once.
   b. as desired.   d. as necessary.

19. Miss Taylor's orders state "May have juice ac and hs"; you would give the juice
   a. morning and evening.   c. whenever she asked for it.
   b. before meals and at bedtime. d. twice a day.

20. You find a resident who has fallen on the floor; your first action is to
   a. assist the resident to a chair.   c. find someone to help lift her.
   b. call for help.   d. call the doctor.

21. Another word for high blood pressure is
   a. hypotension.   c. hypertension.
   b. hypothyroid.   d. systolic pressure.

22. Elderly people may eat less because
   a. they have poorly fitting dentures.
   b. their sense of smell is decreased.
   c. they may be depressed.
   d. All of the above.

23. An example of an objective statement would be

a. "Mr. Smith has a fever."

b. "Miss Godfrey is in a bad mood."

c. "Mr. Smith's temperature is 101."

d. "Mrs. Davis is tired."

24. An example of meeting patients' spiritual needs is

a. taking them to church with you.

b. providing privacy when their clergyman visits.

c. talking to them about your religion.

d. telling them their beliefs are old fashioned.

25. What equipment would you expect to find in a nursing home resident's unit?

a. A bed, overbed table, and nightstand.

b. A blood pressure cuff, oxygen tank, and sink.

c. A clock, calendar, and bulletin board.

d. A stretcher, bed, and mechanical lift.

Answer Key

1. a	6. a	11. a	16. c	21. c
2. a	7. d	12. c	17. a	22. d
3. b	8. b	13. b	18. b	23. c
4. d	9. b	14. c	19. b	24. b
5. c	10. b	15. d	20. b	25. a

Pursuing Employment Opportunities

Almost everyone has had the experience of pursuing employment opportunities once and perhaps several times during her lifetime. Some things are the same whether the person, a nursing assistant for example, is looking for that first job after course completion/certification, returning to work after several years' absence from the workplace, or looking for a position in another facility. Let's consider the situation of the nursing assistant looking for that first job after course completion/certification.

Where to Look for Jobs

Successful completion of your patient care attendant (PCA)/nursing assistant (NA) training may be part of your orientation and career development. If not, you will need to find employment. There are several places to look, and it is best to try as many as possible. Here are some places to start your search for employment.

- Personal contacts:
  - Educational and professional contacts
  - Family and friends
- Want ads/classifieds
- Employment agencies
- Local hospitals, nursing homes, other health care facilities; many post vacant positions on their websites

Personal Contacts

Your instructor is an excellent place to start. Sometimes employers who have openings will contact training programs to alert the faculty and students that they are seeking applicants or have current open positions. Your instructor can tell you if there is a place where these requests are posted. You can also talk to your instructor about her willingness to provide a reference for you.

Family and friends are probably your best advocates since they know you personally and are aware that you have been preparing for a career in health care. Broadcast the fact that you will soon be available to work as a patient care attendant/nursing assistant. Let everyone you know, even casual acquaintances from your church, community group, or a day care center, that you are looking for employment. Leads may come from any of these sources. Be sure to thank anyone who helps you and let him know if you are interviewed or offered a position.

Want Ads/Classifieds

The Sunday papers are a good resource to check regularly. Many of the positions will be listed under health care or nursing. Some states have monthly publications with many health care positions or the names, addresses, and phone numbers of recruiters.

Employment Agencies

Most cities or towns have employment agencies or specialty placement agencies that routinely look for health care workers. These agencies may also hire and staff temporary placements or agency employees in positions. Most agencies prefer to hire people with experience. If there is a high demand for nursing assistants, you may be considered with little experience.

Local Hospitals/Nursing Homes/Facilities

Call the recruiters or personnel/human resources offices at local facilities and ask if they have or are expecting any openings for nursing assistants. Request an application be sent to you or ask when you may go to the office to complete an application. Be sure to ask directions if you are going to an unfamiliar place.

Application Process

If you have not seen a health care facility application, refer to Figure 35–3◆. It is representative of many institutions' applications for employment. Once you have the application in hand, read it carefully and fill in the requested information. Most applications ask fairly common questions and request similar information. It is best to type or print the information on the application. Follow the instructions and complete the application as fully and accurately as you can. Return it in person or by mail as directed.

Preparing a Résumé

Prepare a simple one-page résumé giving your name, address, and phone number; your objective, education, and previous jobs, especially those where you used people skills and had to work with others. It is best to type the résumé or have someone type it for you. The information should be presented as follows:

Name:

Address:

Phone:

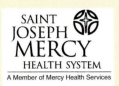

APPLICATION FOR EMPLOYMENT

SAINT JOSEPH MERCY HEALTH SYSTEM
A Member of Mercy Health Services

Please indicate Unit desired:

- ❑ St. Joseph Mercy Hospital, Ann Arbor
- ❑ McPherson Hospital, Howell
- ❑ Saline Community Hospital, Saline
- ❑ Other_____
  please specify

We are an equal opportunity employer. Qualified applicants are considered for employment without regard to race, color, religion, sex, height, weight, national origin, age, marital or veteran status, or the presence of a non-job-related medical condition or disability. It is the applicant's responsibility to notify Saint Joseph Mercy Health System of any reasonable accommodation necessary to perform the essential duties of the position for which the applicant has applied.

Important - Please Type or Print Clearly in Ink

PERSONAL DATA

Date

Social Security Number

Last Name   First   Middle

Address   City   State   Zip Code

Home Telephone (   )   Work or Alternate Telephone (   )

Are you age 18 or older? ❑ Yes ❑ No   Are you currently authorized to work in the U.S.?   ❑ Yes   ❑ No

Have you ever been convicted of a crime other than a minor traffic violation?   ❑ Yes   ❑ No

If yes, give circumstances, place, and date:

Have you ever been employed at a Saint Joseph Mercy Health System Unit?   ❑ Yes   ❑ No

If yes, give date(s) and location(s):

Do you have any relative(s) working at Saint Joseph Mercy Health System?   ❑ Yes   ❑ No

List Name(s)/Relationship/Unit/Department

Have you ever been employed by Mercy Health Services?   ❑ Yes   ❑ No

If yes, give date(s) and location(s):

Have you ever worked or attended school under another name?   ❑ Yes   ❑ No

If yes, what name(s):

JOB INTEREST

Position Desired:

Department or Clinical Area Preferred (if applicable)

Indicate your availability to work (check all that apply) ❑ Full-time ❑ Part-time ❑ Contingent ❑ Temporary

❑ Days ❑ Afternoons ❑ Midnights ❑ Weekends ❑ Holidays ❑ Shift Rotations

If Part-time, specify days and hours available:

Earliest Date Available_____   Minimum Pay Required $ _____ Per Hour

How did you hear of this position?   ❑ Newspaper/Journal*   ❑ School*   ❑ Recruitment visit/job fair*

❑ Employee   ❑ Relative   ❑ Friend   ❑ Other*

*Please Specify_____

Are you currently employed?   ❑ Yes   ❑ No

May we contact your present employer?   ❑ Yes   ❑ No   *Contact must be made before an employment offer is finalized

01030R 8/97 (PC)D

FIGURE 35–3 ◆

Application for Employment (Courtesy of Saint Joseph Mercy Health System, Ann Arbor, MI)

EDUCATION AND TRAINING

	Date Started	Date Finished	School Name and Location	Major	Graduated	Degree/ Diploma	GPA
High School	███████████				❏ Yes ❏ No Yrs. Completed____		
College/ University					❏ Yes ❏ No Yrs. Completed____		
College/ University					❏ Yes ❏ No Yrs. Completed____		
Technical/ Vocational					❏ Yes ❏ No Yrs. Completed____		
Other					❏ Yes ❏ No Yrs. Completed____		

	Date Started	Date Finished	Name of Facility	Type of Clinical			
Student Clinical Rotations, Internship Programs							

Describe work related skills, qualifications, achievements and contributions that you would bring to Saint Joseph Mercy Health

System: _____

_____

_____

PROFESSIONAL CERTIFICATION REGISTRATION DATA

What profession(s) are you licensed, certified or registered to practice? _____

_____

By examination in: State _____   Number _____   Expiration date _____

By endorsement in (reciprocity): State _____   Number _____   Expiration date _____

Are there restrictions on your license?   ❏ Yes   ❏ No   If yes, please explain: _____

Are you eligible for licensure, certification or registry?   ❏ Yes   ❏ No

Profession _____   Anticipated Date of Exam _____

List any current memberships in professional or technical associations. (Those which indicate race, color, religion, sex, or national origin may be excluded.)

_____

_____

_____

_____

_____

FIGURE 35–3 ◆ (continued)

Application for Employment

EMPLOYMENT HISTORY

Beginning with your CURRENT or most RECENT employer, list the last four positions held including Military Service in date order. (Should you choose to list volunteer activities, those which indicate race, color, religion, sex, national origin may be excluded.)

Name of Employer	Position Held	From (Month/Year) To (Month/Year)
Address	Name and Title of Supervisor	Hours Per Week
City State Zip	Telephone # ( )	Base Hourly Rate/Salary
Type of Business	Reason for Leaving	
Duties		

Name of Employer	Position Held	From (Month/Year) To (Month/Year)
Address	Name and Title of Supervisor	Hours Per Week
City State Zip	Telephone # ( )	Base Hourly Rate/Salary
Type of Business	Reason for Leaving	
Duties		

Name of Employer	Position Held	From (Month/Year) To (Month/Year)
Address	Name and Title of Supervisor	Hours Per Week
City State Zip	Telephone # ( )	Base Hourly Rate/Salary
Type of Business	Reason for Leaving	
Duties		

Name of Employer	Position Held	From (Month/Year) To (Month/Year)
Address	Name and Title of Supervisor	Hours Per Week
City State Zip	Telephone # ( )	Base Hourly Rate/Salary
Type of Business	Reason for Leaving	
Duties		

Please Read The Following Carefully And Sign Where Indicated Below:

I have read all the questions and answers, and certify that the information given by me in this application is correct to the best of my knowledge. I understand that any false statements or answers or omissions may be grounds for dismissal. I further understand that my employment is contingent upon the satisfactory completion of a physical examination, including a drug screen, to be conducted by Saint Joseph Mercy Health System. I specifically authorize Saint Joseph Mercy Health System and Mercy Health Services to release all records or other information pertaining to any disciplinary action taken against me during my employment. I hereby release Saint Joseph Mercy Health System and Mercy Health Services, and their agents and employees from any liability whatsoever resulting from the release of such records or information. I hereby waive my right to written notice from my present and/or former employers whenever a disciplinary report, letter or reprimand, or other disciplinary action regarding me is divulged by my present or former employers, including but not limited to reports of disciplinary action which by law must be disclosed pursuant to M.C.L. 333.20175(5).

Signature of Applicant_____ Date_____

FIGURE 35–3 ◆ (continued)

Application for Employment

TO BE COMPLETED BY HIRING DEPARTMENT

Position Title	Base Hourly Rate of Pay
Department Name	Position Code Pay Grade
Department/Cost Center Number	Hours/pay period

Employment Status

❏ New Hire   ❏ Rehire

Starting Date and Time _____

❏ Full-time   ❏ Non-Exempt   ❏ Hourly

❏ Part-time   ❏ Exempt   ❏ Salaried I

❏ Contingent   ❏ Salaried II

❏ Term   Expires ___/___/___

❏ Temporary   Expires ___/___/___

Shift Hours

_____ AM / PM   to   _____ AM / PM Days

_____ AM / PM   to   _____ AM / PM Afternoons

_____ AM / PM   to   _____ AM / PM Midnights

(Work hours and/or work days may change according to department needs.)

Special Conditions of Employment, If Any

(Weekends, holidays, shift rotation, etc.)

_____

_____

_____

❏ Offer reviewed by Human Resources _____ (Specialist initials)

Authorized Management Signature _____ Date _____

I accept the above offer and in consideration of my employment I agree to conform to the rules, regulations and policies of Saint Joseph Mercy Health System. I understand the first 180 days of employment are designated as an orientation period.

New Employee Signature _____ Date _____

FIGURE 35–3 ◆ *(continued)*

Application for Employment

Objective: To obtain a nursing assistant or patient care assistant position in a health care setting.

Education:

High School:

Training Program:

Work Experience:

References: Available upon request/or list one or two people who have supervised you, for example, your instructor. Be sure to ask permission to use a person as a reference in advance of offering the person's name.

The Job Interview

If possible request a copy of the job description and review it before your interview. When you have an interview scheduled, check to be sure you know where to go and plan to arrive early. Write down the name and phone number of the person who will interview you, in case you get lost or need assistance finding the office when you arrive at the facility.

There is only one chance to make a good first impression. Dress conservatively in a suit or dress, if possible. Look as businesslike as you can. It is best to not wear jeans and casual clothes. Ask to see a job description if one has not already been provided. Discuss the duties listed, asking for clarification when necessary. Make notes on the job description, if appropriate.

If you have had very little experience, it is important to be as flexible as possible regarding what hours and days you are available to work. Health care systems need employees who are available to work on weekends, holidays, and over a 24-hour period. Usually, the open positions will be on the less desirable or rotating shifts. Experienced workers transfer to openings or positions that are more desirable or choose schedules with hours that are better suited to their life styles and personal needs.

After your interview, smile and shake the hand of the interviewer (Figure 35–4◆). Thank the person for the opportunity to interview for the position and in particular for the time the interviewer took to answer your questions and provide details and explanations you requested. If the person interviewing you would not be your supervisor, ask to meet that individual. Such meetings or interviews with possible supervisors are often part of the

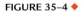

FIGURE 35–4 ◆

The job interview

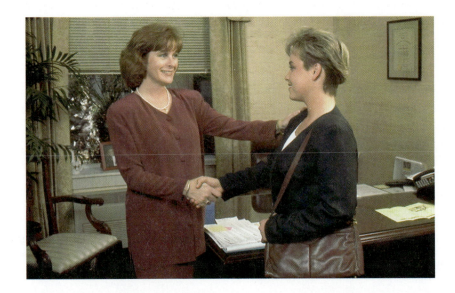

interview process in some institutions; other organizations plan such a meeting at the time of the second interview.

You may be told to call if you have questions, or in rare cases you may be offered a position at the time of the interview. On-the-spot hiring is infrequent since there are usually several applicants for each position and employers require time to check references. You will probably be told that someone, possibly the interviewer, will get back to you. Ask for a time frame, for example, 5 to10 days or 2 to 3 weeks, within which you can expect to hear whether you will be offered the job.

Job Offer

The job offer may come in the form of a phone call or letter. It is best to get an offer in writing to be sure there are no misunderstandings about salary, hours or shifts you are to work, and the date you start. If the job offer is verbal or if the letter does not include these details, request that a letter covering these items be sent to you. Preferably, you should accept the offer in writing. In some situations, a verbal acceptance is acceptable. The advantage of a written acceptance is that it provides you the opportunity of expressing your pleasure at receiving the job offer and restating the circumstances—salary, hours or shift you will work, and the date you are to start—of your acceptance as you understand it. This clarifies the issue for both you and the facility (personnel representative) hiring you. Some organizations do not require a written acceptance prior to hire.

Orientation

When you begin work in a facility, move to a new position within your department, or take a position in another department, there is some form of orientation. *Orientation* refers to the period of time in which your employer orients or familiarizes you with your work environment, your benefits, organizational or facility policies, work rules, and your role and responsibilities in your new job. Usually, your immediate supervisor will discuss specific job expectations with you. Classroom or one-to-one sessions or a combination of both may be given by a staff development educator or trainer.

Most employers have a probationary period during which specific skills and competencies required for patient care in your setting are validated. Classroom and/or on-the-job performance during this probationary period are evaluated. Once you have successfully demonstrated your skills and competence to perform your job duties, you will have completed your orientation. During this period of orientation, ask questions and learn as much as you can about your role and responsibilities. Often someone is assigned to help you as you learn about and put into actual practice the policies and procedures in your new employment setting.

Continuing to Learn

Continue your education! To keep up with new developments, all health care workers are expected to take refresher courses. As you continue to learn, your job will become more rewarding personally and professionally. Many agencies have a staff development or training person, group, or department. Services or training include orientation, inservice education, and ongoing **staff development**. Examples of inservice education include:

- Learning a new procedure or technique
- Learning to use new equipment
- Learning about a change in a particular procedure that requires staff to do a task differently
- Training in doing a new procedure

staff development On-the-job training or classes provided to enhance or expand an employee's skills or abilities

Every year there are required mandatory training classes in fire, safety, CPR, infection control, patients' rights, and confidentiality. There are some state to state variations in mandatory requirements.

Other examples of ongoing staff development training include:

- Communication
- Computer training
- Cultural diversity awareness
- Domestic violence
- Sensitivity training

continuing education
Formal classes, courses, or training programs to develop new knowledge or qualify one for career advancement

The staff development specialist or human resources representative can tell you about other educational benefits or refer you to available training programs or other **continuing education** options. It is important that you share your career goals with those people in your facility who can help you identify resources, support, and programs. Your supervisor may also offer you advice.

You can continue to learn while you are on the job. You can expand your knowledge of nursing care procedures, find better ways to do your work, and learn more about other aspects of health care. All this can make you a more effective nursing assistant, and you will become more secure in your job.

Planning Your Career Path

Figure 35–5◆ presents numerous career opportunities for the nursing assistant to consider in planning a career path. Some people know at an early age exactly what position or level they want to attain in the health care field. For others the path is not so clear. Take every opportunity to speak to friends, family, and coworkers in the health care field. Discuss the options and possibilities with education and career counselors at school or in the institution where you work. The opportunities are numerous.

If you enjoy your work as a nursing assistant, you may be interested in advancement where you are employed. Maybe you would like to be a multiskilled worker, advanced nursing assistant, or licensed practical (vocational) or registered nurse (Figure 35–6◆). The

FIGURE 35–5 ◆

Health care options to consider as you chart your career path

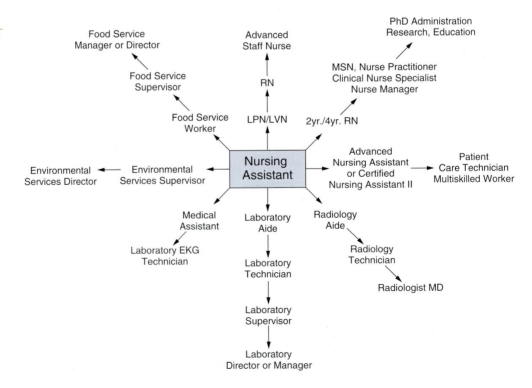

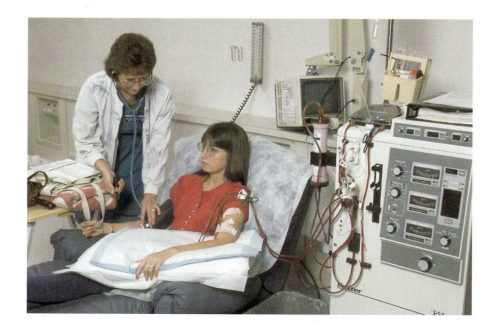

FIGURE 35–6 ◆

Work with a patient receiving kidney dialysis

career path shown in Figure 35–5 can guide you in planning your advancement. You can modify your career path to meet your long-term and short-term *goals* or to address changing needs and new opportunities. Skills, time, hard work, and planning are needed to advance to the work and educational level you set for yourself. When you reach your work and educational goals, you may choose to set new goals requiring more education or training to further develop your skills and improve your nursing techniques, or you may choose to remain indefinitely at the level you have just reached.

If you do not have a high school diploma, attaining one should be your first goal. Adult education programs at local high schools offer basic education programs that lead to a high school equivalency diploma. Community colleges offer prerequisite courses necessary to enroll in licensed practical nurse or registered nurse programs. Education or career counselors are available at community colleges to advise you along the way. Take advantage of such resources.

The director of nursing education in your health care institution is the person to ask about planning your career path. You can find career satisfaction in your role as a nursing assistant or choose to continue your education and prepare yourself for an ever increasing number of health care career possibilities.

 # Positioning Yourself for Promotion

Changing Jobs

Gaining experience working as a nursing assistant will open many opportunities to you. Once you have demonstrated good work habits and have received positive evaluations from your employer, you will find there are many employers in a variety of work settings seeking to hire individuals into open positions. In many cases, better pay, improved benefits, closer proximity to your home, or more desirable hours motivate job searches.

There may be career opportunities within your place of initial employment. Some larger facilities have internal training and development staff who provide training to become advanced nursing assistants or patient care technicians. Entry into these programs requires a willingness to learn, the same good work habits and satisfactory attendance, and no disciplinary actions in your record or file.

Many local community colleges offer courses or training programs that can lead to career advancement. Some employers have arrangements to pay or reimburse your tuition

KEEPING A JOB   GUIDELINES

- Maintain at least a satisfactory or good work record.
- When you can, volunteer to work overtime or fill staffing needs.
- Problem solve using your best communication skills and the formal process within your work place.
- Be sure to call your employer when you are sick or unable to get to work for any reason.
- Excessive tardiness or being late to work is one of the biggest causes of job termination.
- Recognize that most employers do not view accumulated "sick time"

as an earned right for employees to use whenever needed for personal convenience. It is better to request time off in advance or trade with coworkers than to call in whenever your scheduled time to work conflicts with your personal life.

- Do not drink alcohol before work or come to work high. It is usually grounds for discipline or can be automatic dismissal. If you have a problem with substance abuse, seek help.
- Seek opportunities to learn new skills and keep up with the constant changes in health care.

- Ask for feedback from coworkers and your supervisor as to your performance and listen to suggestions or recommendations for improvement.
- Request and keep a copy of work rules. Ask questions about any rules or policies you do not understand. Many employers view stealing, lying on an application, and violating confidentiality of or abusing patients as automatic grounds for dismissal. Policies are usually reviewed in orientation but many employees forget them until there is a big problem.

costs for attending programs. Your manager, staff development or human resource personnel usually know if such programs with tuition assistance are available. Colleges may be able to identify opportunities or programs where full or partial scholarships are available. If your supervisor is aware that you are interested in continuing your education, he or she is more likely to inform you of advanced training programs or other opportunities.

Resignation Letters

Once you have a new job offer in writing or need to leave your job for any reason, it is best to give your current employer at least 2 weeks notice. Leaving a position with little or no notice is reflected in your employment records and can make getting a positive reference a problem. It is best to be as positive as possible in your resignation letter and briefly state the reason you are leaving, for another job, relocation or personal or family reasons.

SUMMARY

This chapter has presented information to help prepare you to take your competency evaluation and test to become a nursing assistant. It described how you can find and apply for job opportunities. The importance of continuing education was also discussed, along with career path or lattice possibilities. As you become involved in your career there will be increasing opportunities to learn and grow.

NOTES

CHAPTER REVIEW

FILL IN THE BLANK Read each sentence and fill in each blank line with a word that completes the sentence.

1. A demonstratable skill or ability is called a _____.

2. The _____ _____ _____ is a list kept by each state to show who is certified in that state.

3. A _____ is a one-page description of who you are and what kind of skills you have.

4. The period of time that the institution teaches you about your new job is called _____.

5. On-the-job training of classes to enhance or expand an employee's skills or abilities is called _____.

MULTIPLE CHOICE Choose the best answer for each question or statement.

1. When taking the clinical examination portion of the Nurse Aide State Examination
   a. you may ask questions of the observer.
   b. you may not ask questions of the observer.
   c. say you "must always follow policy" anytime you do not know the correct steps.
   d. request prompting only on those skills confusing to you.

2. All of the following except one are good places to look for employment.
   a. Want ads
   b. Personal contacts
   c. Local hospitals, nursing homes, facilities
   d. Book store

3. Include all of the following on your resume except
   a. your name.
   b. your address.
   c. your health history.
   d. your work history.

4. After a job interview you should
   a. tell the interviewers you will not believe anything they tell you if it is not in writing.
   b. demand to be told immediately if the job will be offered to you.
   c. wait to hear from the interviewer before you contact the agency.
   d. smile and thank the interviewers for their time.

5. Which of the following is not considered in a promotion?
   a. Your attendance including tardiness
   b. Your willingness and ability to learn new skills
   c. The reason you were off sick for 2 days last year
   d. Your most recent performance evaluation or references

TIME-OUT

TIPS FOR TIME MANAGEMENT

When you go to a job interview, bring the names, addresses, and phone numbers of your references with you. This will prevent the delay of looking them up during or after the interview. Also, the interviewer will notice that you have planned ahead.

THE NURSING ASSISTANT IN ACTION

You are scheduled to work the night shift and are attending a birthday party prior to going to work. Your host is passing out shots of tequila to toast the guest of honor. Everyone else at the party accepts a glass for the toast. You decline telling your host you are going to work shortly and should not be drinking now. Your friend says, "Don't be such a jerk. Call in sick or chew some breath mints. No one at your job will know the difference."

What Is Your Response/Action?

CRITICAL THINKING

CUSTOMER SERVICE Prospective employers are very concerned about your interpersonal skills and your ability to provide customer or patient-focused care. Be sure to identify on your résumé if you have had customer-service training in another job such as the retail, restaurant, or fast-food businesses. These skills will be seen as assets. Write down two or three examples of situations where you had success resolving a problem or dealt with difficult patients or customers. When asked in an interview about how you would handle situations that may present themselves, you will have good examples to offer. Your critical thinking skills will be more evident to the interviewer.

CULTURAL CARE Being bilingual can be an advantage if you are applying for a position in a facility where the patients speak different languages. Learn some of the most important aspects of their cultures and words to better communicate with the patients. This skill can become the reason you are offered a position or promotion over an equally qualified and experienced candidate.

COOPERATION WITHIN THE TEAM There will be times in your career when you and another coworker apply for the same job or promotion. If you are not the candidate chosen, talk to the hiring person and find out what you need to do to better prepare for the next time you apply for a similar job. Do what you can to be supportive of the coworker who received the promotion. How you handle yourself in disappointing situations can influence future decisions.

EXPLORE MediaLink

Additional interactive resources for this chapter can be found on the Companion Website at www.prenhall.com/wolgin. Click on Chapter 35 and "Begin" to select activities for this chapter.

For chapter-related NCLEX-style questions and an audio glossary, access the accompanying CD-ROM in this book.

Medical Terms, Abbreviations, and Specialties

This appendix provides abbreviations and medical terms commonly used in the health care field. They are used regularly in charting, doctor's orders, nursing instructions, taking notes, and so on. You will find you are already familiar with many of the abbreviations and medical terms; others you will have to learn. A list of specialties, for example dermatology and pathology, gives the corresponding physicians' titles and brief descriptions of each specialty. In addition, word elements—roots, prefixes, and suffixes—are reviewed. Understanding these elements will assist you with the medical terms presented here and with new or unfamiliar terms you encounter in your work in the health care field. Your supervisor will advise you of reference manuals, *common* approved abbreviations, and terminology dictionaries that are used in your facility or unit.

Abbreviations and Their Meanings

Abbreviations are the shorthand of the health professions. They are clear and efficient tools for the nurse to tell you quickly what to do. As a nursing assistant, you will use these abbreviations in your daily work. They will help you to understand instructions from your immediate supervisor. Abbreviations help you when you are receiving reports about your patients and in keeping your notes on your daily assignments.

Abbreviations Used in Charting, Reporting, and Keeping Notes

ABBREVIATION	MEANING
aa	Of each, equal parts
abd.	Abdomen
ac	Before meals
AD	Admitting diagnosis
A&D	Admission and discharge
ad lib	As desired, if the patient so desires
ADL	Activities of daily living
AIDS	Acquired immune deficiency syndrome
AKA	Above knee amputation/also known as
A.M. or a.m., AM or am	Morning
amb.	Ambulation, walking, ambulatory, able to walk
amt.	Amount
AP or A.P.	Appendectomy
aqua	Water or H_2O
Approx.	Approximately
ASAP	As soon as possible
@	At
ATC	Around the clock
bid or B.I.D. or b.i.d.	Twice a day
b.m. or B.M.	Bowel movement, feces
B.P. or BP	Blood pressure
BRP or B.R.P. or brp	Bathroom privileges
BR or br or B.R. or b.r.	Bedrest
BSC or bsc	Bedside commode
°C	Celsius degree (or centigrade)
c̄	With
Ca or CA	Cancer
Cal	Calorie
Cath.	Catheter
CBC or C.B.C.	Complete blood count
CBR or C.B.R. or cbr	Complete bed rest
cc or c.c.	Cubic centimeter
CCU or C.C.U.	Cardiac care unit/coronary care unit
Chol	Cholesterol
Cl liq	Clear liquids
CM or cm	Centimeter
C/O or c/o	Complaint of
CO_2	Carbon dioxide
CPR or C.P.R.	Cardiopulmonary resuscitation
CSR or csr and C.S.R.	Central supply room
CVA or C.V.A.	Cerebrovascular accident or stroke
DBP	Diastolic blood pressure
dc or d/c or D/C	Discontinue
D&I	Dry and intact
Disch. or dish or D/C	Discharge
D. & C. or D&C	Dilatation and curettage
DM	Diabetes mellitus
DOA or D.O.A.	Dead on arrival
Dr. or Dr	Doctor
DRG	Diagnostic-related group
drsg.	Dressing
DX	Diagnosis
E. or E	Enema
EBL	Estimated blood loss

Abbreviations Used in Charting, Reporting, and Keeping Notes *(contd.)*

ABBREVIATION	MEANING
ECG or EKG	Electrocardiogram
ED or E.D.	Emergency department
EEG or E.E.G.	Electroencephalogram
EENT or E.E.N.T.	Eye, ears, nose, and throat
ER or E.R.	Emergency room
ETOH	Alcohol
°F	Fahrenheit degree
F. or Fe. or F or Fe	Female
FBS or F.B.S.	Fasting blood sugar
FF or F.F.	Forced feeding or forced fluids
ft	Foot
Fx	Fracture
Fx urine	Fractional urine
gal	Gallon
GI or G.I.	Gastrointestinal
gt	One drop
gtt	Two or more drops
Gtt or G.T.T.	Glucose tolerance test
GU or G.U.	Genitourinary
Gyn or G.Y.N.	Gynecology
H/A	Headache
H_2O	Water or aqua
HIPAA	Health Insurance Portability and Accountability Act
HMO	Health maintenance organization
HOB	Head of bed
HOH	Hard of hearing
H & P	History and physical
hr	Hour
HS or hs	Bedtime or hour of sleep
ht	Height
HTN	Hypertension
hyper	Above or high
hypo	Below or low
ICU or I.C.U.	Intensive care unit
I&O or I.&O.	Intake and output
Irr	Irregular
Isol. or isol	Isolation
IV or I.V.	Intravenous
L	Liter
Ⓛ	Left
Lab. or lab	Laboratory
lb	Pound
Liq or liq.	Liquid
LPN or L.P.N.	Licensed practical nurse
LVN or L.V.N.	Licensed vocational nurse
M	Male
Mat	Maternity
MD or M.D.	Medical doctor
Meas	Measure
med	Medicine
MI	Myocardial Infarction
min	Minute
ml	Milliliter
Mn or mn or M/n	Midnight

Abbreviations Used in Charting, Reporting, and Keeping Notes *(contd.)*

ABBREVIATION	MEANING
N.A. or N/A	Nursing aide or nursing assistant
NAS	No added salt
n/g tube or ng. tube or N.G.T.	Nasogastric tube
NKA	No known allergies
noct	At night
NP	Neuropsychiatric; or nursing procedure
NPO or N.P.O.	Nothing by mouth
nsy	Nursery
N & V	Nausea and Vomiting
O_2	Oxygen
OB or O.B.	Obstetrics
Obt or obt.	Obtained
OJ or O.J.	Orange juice
Ord.	Orderly
OOB or O.O.B.	Out of bed
OPD or O.P.D.	Outpatient department
OR or O.R.	Operating room
Ortho	Orthopedics
OT or O.T.	Occupational therapy; or oral temperature
oz or O.Z.	Ounce
pc	After meals
Ped or Peds	Pediatrics
per	By, through
p.m. or P.M., pm or PM	Afternoon
PMC or P.M.C.	Postmortem care
PN or P.N.	Pneumonia
po	By mouth
post or $\bar{p}$	After
postop or post op	Postoperative
PP	Postpartum (after delivery)
PPBS	Postprandial blood sugar
pre	Before
preop or pre op	Before surgery
prep	Prepare the patient for surgery by shaving the skin
prn or p.r.n.	Whenever necessary, when required
Pt or pt	Patient; pint
PT or P.T.	Physical therapy
q	Every
qam or q am or q.a.m.	Every morning
qd	Every day
qh	Every hour
q2h	Every 2 hours
q3h	Every 3 hours
q4h	Every 4 hours
QHS or qhs	Every night at bedtime/hour of sleep
QI	Quality improvement
qid or Q.I.D.	Four times a day
qod or Q.O.D.	Every other day
qs	Quantity sufficient; as much as required
qt	Quart
r or R	rectal
®	Right
Reg	Regular
Rm or rm	Room
RN or R.N.	Registered nurse

Abbreviations Used in Charting, Reporting, and Keeping Notes *(contd.)*

ABBREVIATION	MEANING
R/O	Rule out
rom or R.O.M.	Range of motion
RR or R.Rm.	Recovery room
Rx	Prescription or treatment ordered by a physician
s or s̄	Without
SCD	Sequential compression device
S&A or S.&A. Test	Sugar and acetone test
S&K or S.&K. Test	Sugar and ketone test
SO	Significant other
SOB	Shortness of breath
sos	Whenever emergency arises; only if necessary
Spec or spec.	Specimen
ss or s̄s̄	One-half
SSE or S.S.E.	Soapsuds enema
stat	At once, immediately
STD	Sexually transmitted disease
Surg	Surgery
TB	Tuberculosis
TBI	Traumatic brain injury
tid or T.I.D.	Three times a day
TLC or tlc	Tender loving care
TPR	Temperature, pulse, respiration
TWE	Tap water enema
tx	Treatment
U/a or U/A or u/a	Urinalysis
VDRL	Test for syphilis
V.S. or VS	Vital signs
WBC or W.B.C.	White blood count
w/c	Wheelchair
wc or W.C.	Ward clerk
wt	Weight

Roman numerals are the letters used to represent numbers in the ancient Roman system. The dots or "eyes" are used to eliminate a margin of error:

$$1 = \text{I or } \dot{\text{I}} \quad 2 = \text{II or } \ddot{\text{II}} \quad 3 = \text{III or } \dddot{\text{III}}$$
$$4 = \text{IV or } \overline{\text{IV}} \quad 5 = \text{V or } \overline{\text{V}}$$
$$10 = \text{X or } \overline{\text{X}} \quad 50 = \text{L or } \overline{\text{L}} \quad 100 = \text{C or } \overline{\text{C}}$$

Word Elements: Roots, Prefixes, and Suffixes

Many medical terms are composed of several smaller, simpler words or word elements. This discussion describes and shows how to use three primary word elements that are combined frequently to form medical terms. These three word elements are the prefix, the root, and the suffix.

- The **root** is the body or main part of the word. It denotes the primary meaning of the word as a whole.

- The **prefix** is a word element combined with the root. It changes or adds to the meaning of the words. A prefix is always added to the beginning of a root.
- The **suffix** is a word element used to change or add to the meaning of a root. It is always added to the end of the root.

Examples of Similarity Between Terms

WORD ELEMENT	EXAMPLE	MEANING
ante	antefebrile	**before** onset of fever
a	afebrile	**without** fever
cysto	cystogram	x-ray record of the **bladder**
cyto	cytogenesis	production (origin) **of the cell**
hyper	hypertension	**high** blood pressure
hypo	hypotension	**low** blood pressure
inter	interstitial	lying **between** spaces in tissue
intra	intracranial	**within** the skull
macro	macroscopy	seen **large,** as with the naked eye
micro	microscopy	seen **small,** as by microscope
pre	preclinical	**before** the onset of disease

The study of **medical terminology** can aid you in understanding the name of the specific disease for which the patient has been hospitalized. The suffix **itis** means "inflammation." Almost every organ in the body is subject to infection by disease organisms that will cause an inflammatory reaction. The word to describe a diagnosis of this nature is formulated simply by adding the suffix *itis* to the word for the body organ affected.

Medical Terms With the Suffix –itis

MEDICAL TERM	DESCRIPTION
appendicitis	inflammation of the appendix
dermatitis	inflammation of the skin
hepatitis	inflammation of liver tissue
rhinitis	inflammation of nasal mucosa
stomatitis	inflammation of the mouth

The suffix **ectomy** means "surgical removal." When used in combination with any word element denoting an organ or other body part, the term formed means that the organ or body part has been removed.

Medical Terms With the Suffix –ectomy

MEDICAL TERM	DESCRIPTION
gastrectomy	surgical removal of the stomach
thyroidectomy	surgical removal of the thyroid gland
colectomy	surgical removal of the large intestine

In many cases, an organ may be removed only partially. To indicate this procedure, other words are used to modify the medical term, for example:

- subtotal thyroidectomy
- partial cystectomy

Other modifying words may precede the medical term. This identifies the surgery performed even more accurately.

Detailed Medical Terms

MEDICAL TERM	DESCRIPTION
left salpingo-oophorectomy	removal of the left ovary and Fallopian tube
vaginal hysterectomy	removal of the uterus through the vagina
transurethral prostatectomy	removal of the prostate through the urethra
total abdominal hysterectomy	removal of the entire uterus through abdomen

Medical Specialties

Medical Specialty, Physician's Title, and Description of the Specialty

SPECIALTY	PHYSICIAN'S TITLE	DESCRIPTION
Allergy	Allergist	A subspecialty of internal medicine dealing with diagnosis and treatment of body reactions resulting from unusual sensitivity to foods, pollens, dust, medicines, or other substances.
Anesthesiology	Anesthesiologist	Administration of various forms of anesthesia in operations or procedures to cause loss of feeling or sensation.
Cardiology; cardiovascular diseases	Cardiologist	A subspecialty of internal medicine involving the diagnosis and treatment of diseases of the heart and blood vessels.
Dermatology	Dermatologist	The diagnosis and treatment of disorders of the skin.
Gastroenterology	Gastroenterologist	A subspecialty of internal medicine concerned with diagnosis and treatment of disorders of the digestive tract.
General practice: family medicine	General practitioner	The diagnosis and treatment of disease by medical and surgical methods without limitations to organ systems or body regions and without restriction as to age of patients.
General surgery	Surgeon	The diagnosis and treatment of disease by surgical means without limitation to special organ or body regions.
Gynecology	Gynecologist	Diagnosis and treatment of diseases of the female reproductive system.
Internal medicine	Internist	The diagnosis and nonsurgical treatment of illness of adults.
Neurology	Neurosurgeon	Diagnosis and surgical treatment of brain, spinal cord, and nerve disorders.
	Neurologist	Diagnosis and treatment of disease of brain, spinal cord, and nerve disorders.

Medical Specialty, Physician's Title, and Description of the Specialty *(contd.)*

SPECIALTY	PHYSICIAN'S TITLE	DESCRIPTION
Obstetrics	Obstetrician	The care of women during pregnancy, childbirth, and immediately following.
Oncology	Oncologist	Diagnosis, study, and treatment of cancer, benign or cancer-related tumors.
Ophthalmology	Ophthalmologist	Diagnosis and treatment of diseases of the eye, including prescribing corrective lenses.
Orthopedics	Orthopedist	Diagnosis and treatment of disorders and diseases of muscular and skeletal systems.
Otolaryngology	Otolaryngologist	Diagnosis and treatment of diseases of the ear, nose, and throat.
Pathology	Pathologist	Study and interpretation of changes in organs, tissues, and cells and alterations in body chemistry to aid in diagnosing disease and determining treatment.
Pediatrics	Pediatrician	Prevention, diagnosis, and treatment of children's diseases.
Physical medicine and rehabilitation	Physiatrist	Diagnosis of disease or injury in the various systems and areas of the body and treatment by means of physical procedures, as well as treatment and restoration of the convalescent and physically handicapped patient.
Plastic surgery	Plastic surgeon	Cosmetic, corrective, or reparative surgery to restore deformed parts of the body.
Psychiatry	Psychiatrist	Medical branch concerned with diagnosis and treatment of mental disorders.
Radiology	Radiologist	Use of radiant energy, including x-rays, radioactive substances, and magnetic imagery in the diagnosis and treatment of diseases.
Thoracic surgery	Thoracic surgeon	Operative treatment of the lungs, heart, or the large blood vessels within the chest cavity.
Urology	Urologist	Diagnosis and treatment of diseases or disorders of the kidneys, bladder, ureters, urethra, and the male reproductive organs.

This appendix has introduced you to many of the abbreviations, medical terms, and specialists you will need to know to function successfully in the health care field. It is just the start. Be open to learning and seek out other medical reference materials in your health care facility. Your supervisor will assist you with explanations of specific terminology used in your work.

Appendix B

What's New in Patient Restraints

Appendix B, "What's New in Patient Restraints," is an example of St. Joseph Mercy Health System patient restraint procedures. Each facility will have a written policy or procedure for employees to follow.

 ## Two Sets of Restraint Standards

Once the alternatives to restraints have failed and the nurse has decided that restraints need to be used, a determination must be made of whether to apply the medical-surgical (Med-Surg) standards or the Behavioral Management standards. The location of the patient in the hospital is no longer the prime determining factor. Instead use the following criteria to determine which set of standards to apply in each patient situation:

- When use of a restraint is an emergency measure, an unplanned, unanticipated situation with a patient exhibiting severely aggressive, violent, assaultive or destructive behavior that places the patient, staff, or others in imminent danger, use the behavioral management standards.
- Use of leather restraints indicates the need for behavioral management standards.
- For all other restraint situations, use the Med-Surg standards.

New Definitions

- **Physical restraint:** Involuntary use of any manual method or physical or mechanical device that restricts freedom of movement or normal access to one's body, material, or equipment, attached or adjacent to the patient's body that he or she cannot easily remove.
- **Chemical restraint:** A drug used as a restraint is a mediation used to restrict the patient's freedom or movement in a medical/postsurgical situation (Med-Surg standard) or for the emergency control of behavior (behavioral management) and is not a standard treatment for the patient's medical or psychiatric condition.
- **Restraints for acute medical surgical care:** Physical or chemical restraints used to limit mobility, temporarily immobilize a patient related to a medical/postsurgical procedure. The primary reason for use directly supports medical healing. It is used for nonviolent or nonaggressive patients.
- **Restraints for behavioral management:** Applies to emergency situations where the patient's behavior is violent, aggressive, or assaultive, and the least restrictive measure that will assure the patient or others safety is a restraint or seclusion. This is behavior that presents an *immediate and serious danger* to the safety of the patient, other patients, or staff. Restraints can be chemical or physical. Drugs used as restraints for behavior management are medications used in addition to or in

replacement of the patient's regular drug regimen to control extreme behavior during an emergency.

■ **Seclusion:** The involuntary confinement of a person in a room or an area where the person is physically prevented from leaving. This is not done outside of the behavioral health setting (six thousand) and is not addressed in the St. Joseph Mercy Health System policy.

New Rules for Use of Side Rails

Use of all four side rails or two full side rails, except in the instances below, limits freedom of movement and constitutes restraint.

Bed rails are **not** a restraint in these situations:

1. When voluntarily permission is granted by the patient and to comply with patient requests.
2. When patients are sedated, including preoperatively and postoperatively.
3. Whenever the bed is in the high position such as for a procedure. After the procedure, the bed should be returned to the appropriate position and the appropriate number of side rails should be determined.
4. When seizure precautions are used; additionally the side rails should be padded.
5. When used for any semi-comatose or comatose patient.
6. Full side rail stretchers are used in transport (not when stationary).
7. In peds, at night, and whenever the patient conditions warrants. When awake, children in junior or adult beds may have one or both side rails lowered at the nurse's discretion with the bed in the lowest position.
8. In peds, with the use of a crib for infants less turn or equal to 6 months old, the canopy must be down, in place. Infants up to 25 lbs may be in pediatric bassinets.

Protocol Orders

Protocol orders are no longer allowed for use. They are no longer legal authority for orders.

New Thoughts About Restraint Devices

"Posey" style vests are no longer going to be purchased (except for zipper vests in Rehab) due to high incidence of strangulation in other hospitals. Use waist belts instead.

Procedure Highlights for Medical-Surgical and Behavioral Management Standards

Alternatives to restraints will be used and documented *before* the least restrictive method of restraint is utilized.

Use of alternatives to restraint are based on respecting the patient's dignity, understanding behavior as a symptom of an unmet need, freedom of choice, and optimum patient outcomes. Alternatives include:

■ Collaborate, if possible, with patient and family to try to make sense of agitation or worrisome behavior.

- Careful assessment to attempt to make sense of the patient's behavior.
- Individualized care planning that attempts to correlate behavior with the unmet need.

1. ***A RN will participate in the assessment of the need for restraints***. If restraints are needed, the RN will determine if Med-Surg or Behavioral Management standards apply.

2. Use of physical restraint may be initiated before obtaining a physician's order only when the assessment by a RN determines the need for immediate intervention to prevent the patient from harming self or others (Behavioral Management). The RN or designated member of the health care team will apply the necessary physical restraint. In case of emergency, security personnel may be requested to assist the team.

3. The individual RN caring for the patient is responsible for the correct, safe application of restraints and safety devices, no matter who applies them. The least restrictive type of restraint that may meet the patients needs will be tried first. Special consideration and risks must be planned with the use of restraints for vulnerable patient populations including:

   - History of abuse, because such a history places that patient at greater psychological risk.
   - Physical conditions, because this may exacerbate symptomatology (i.e., arthritis)
   - Age-related considerations
   - Cognitively limited patients

   Restrained patients are identified in a central location on each nursing unit. This alerts staff in case of an emergency. In the event of fire/disaster, the staff member monitoring observation and physiological needs of the patient is responsible for removing the restraints and moving the patient to a safe location.

4. Secure restraint to the moveable frame (**not a side rail**) when an adjustable bed is used.

5. ***Leather restraints are secured with a lock and key and only used for behavioral management***.

6. The following must be documented by the individual initiating the application:

   - Events leading up to the intervention
   - The prior use of alternative measures
   - The patient's response to those measures
   - The time restraint was initiated
   - The time restraint was terminated

7. A physician's order for restraint must be obtained.

MEDICAL-SURGICAL STANDARDS	BEHAVIORAL MANAGEMENT STANDARD
An order must be obtained within 12 hours for all restraints/seclusion.	An order must be obtained within 1 hour for all restraints/seclusion. This requires a face-to-face assessment by a licensed independent practitioner (LIP).
The order must include the specific type of restraint, specific duration of restraint, and the reason for the restraint. Verbal orders must be signed within 24 hours. A licensed independent practitioner must give all orders, and the order must be time-limited, dated, and signed. If a physician other than the attending writes the restraint order, the attending physician must be consulted as soon as possible. The patient's plan of care will be modified to include use of restraints.	The order must include the specific type of restraint, specific duration of restraint, and the reason for the restraint. A licensed independent practitioner must give all orders, and the order must be time-limited, dated, and signed. If a physician other than the attending writes the restraint order, the attending physician must be consulted as soon as possible. The patient's plan of care will be modified to include use of restraints.

MEDICAL-SURGICAL STANDARDS	BEHAVIORAL MANAGEMENT STANDARD
The physician must perform a face-to-face assessment of the patient and write and order for restraints within 24 hours from the original initiation of restraints. If there is a continued need for restraints based on the assessment of the patient, a physician's written order is required daily.	The order may not exceed **4** hours for age 18 or over, **2** hours for children and adolescents age 9–17, and **1** hour for children under 9. In-person reevaluation must occur including efficacy of the treatment plan and work with the individual to identify ways to regain control. When the original order expires, a RN can telephone the physician, report the results of his/her most recent patient assessment, and request the original order be renewed.
	The **physician must conduct an in-person evaluation at least every 8 hours for individuals 18 or older and every 4 hours for age 17 or younger or** on six thousand unit and document a new order if needed. If the order is from a physician other than the attending, the attending must be notified. **If the individual is no longer in restraint or seclusion when an original verbal order expires** the licensed independent practitioner conducts an in-person evaluation of the individual within **24 hours** of the initiation of restraint or seclusion.
Restraint orders must not be written as a PRN order.	Restraint orders must not be written as a PRN order.
A new order **is not required** for restraints if the restraint is removed before the expiration of the original order, but later needs to be reapplied for the same reason and is within the time frame of the original order	A new order **is required** for restraints if the restraints are removed before the expiration of the original order, but later needs to be reapplied, or if the patient's behavior requires a more restrictive type of restraint.
A face-to-face assessment by a licensed independent practitioner must be done daily, with a progress note/order that states the reason for the restraint.	

8. The RN shall complete the initial assessment upon initiation of restraints and reassessment every 2 hours. This should include:

- Appropriate application
- Physical and emotional well-being, signs of injury from restraint
- Patient rights, dignity, and safety are maintained
- Least restrictive method employed
- Continued need for restraint.
- RN assesses effects of medication including side effects and half-life of medications, if used as a restraint.

9. In addition, the RN is responsible for updating the plan of care to incorporate the use of restraints and revise the plan of care when the restraints are discontinued.

10. The RN has accountability for informing the patient (or, in case of a patient with impaired decision making, the next of kin or designee) of a change in the patient condition or behavior warranting restraint. This should be done as soon as possible. If using Behavioral Management standards, attempt to notify the family if the patient has consented to have the family kept informed and the family has agreed to be notified.

11. The RN, LPN, PCT/Tech, or PCA II can monitor and provide patient care for a restrained patient.

MEDICAL-SURGICAL STANDARDS	BEHAVIORAL MANAGEMENT
■ Observation q 1 hour	**CONTINUOUS IN-PERSON OBSERVATION**
■ Circulation and skin check q 2 hours	
■ **VS q 4 hours**	■ Circulation and skin check **q 15 minutes**
■ Offer ROM with release of restraint and repositioning q 2 hours	■ **VS q 2 hours**
	■ Offer ROM with release of restraint and repositioning q 2 hours
■ Offer fluids and toileting q 2 hours	
■ Provision for meals	■ Offer fluids and toileting q 2 hours
■ Provision for regular hygiene, skin care.	■ Provision for meals
	■ Provision for regular hygiene, skin care.

EXPECTED OUTCOMES

■ Skin color, temperature, and integrity are according to patient's baseline
■ Absence of numbness, tingling, and vascular compromise
■ Patient is free from physical injury
■ Environmental safety is maintained
■ Restraints are discontinued at the earliest possible time

12. Monitoring/reassessment may permit the reduction to a less restrictive device or early termination of restraint. Inform the patient and family of the criteria for early release. Staff may release/reduce restraint before the time limit based on reassessment. Document discontinuation of restraints and rationale. For behavioral management, the patient will be made aware of behavioral criteria he or she must meet to have restraints discontinued and staff will work with patient throughout the restraint period to achieve criteria.

13. Watch for distress from patients in restraints: Changes in vital signs/circulation/breathing/ range of motion as well as any signs of dehydration indicate a need to further assess the patient by an RN and/or notification of the physician.

Glossary

Following the definition of each term, the number(s) of the chapter(s) in which the term is defined appears in parentheses.

abbreviation   A shortened form of a word or phrase used to represent the complete form (Appendix A)

abdominal prep   The procedure for making the patient's abdomen ready for surgery; includes thorough cleansing of the skin and careful shaving of body hair in the abdominal area (28)

abdominal respiration   Breathing in which the patient is using mostly the abdominal muscles (19)

abduction   Movement of an arm or leg away from the center of the body (16)

absorb   To take or soak in, up, or through (22)

absorption   Part of the digestive process in which digestive juices and enzymes break down food into usable parts (20)

acceptance   Admitting, understanding, or facing the truth or reality of the situation, for example, one's death (34)

accountable   To be answerable for one's behavior; legally or ethically responsible for the care of another (2)

accuracy   The quality of being exact or correct; exact conformity to truth and rules; free from errors or defects (2)

acquired immune deficiency syndrome (AIDS)   A condition caused by a virus that destroys a key part of the body's immune response system; viral infection characterized by decreased immunity to opportunistic infections (25, 30)

active motion   Producing, involving, or participating in activity or movement (33)

activities of daily living (ADL)   The activities or tasks usually performed every day, such as toileting, washing, eating, or dressing (12)

adduction   Movement of an arm or leg toward the center of the body (16)

admission   The administrative process that covers the period from the time the patient enters the institution door to the time the patient is settled (8)

Advance Directive   Prewritten instructions on withholding resuscitation and life-prolonging measures and equipment (34)

AIDS   Acquired immune deficiency syndrome. A condition caused by a virus that destroys a key part of the body's immune response system; viral infection characterized by decreased immunity to opportunistic infections (25, 30)

alternating-pressure mattress   A pad similar to an air mattress that can be placed beneath the patient to reduce pressure on the head, shoulders, back, heels, elbows, and bony prominences (9)

ambulate   To walk or move about (6)

ambulation   To walk or move about in an upright position (6, 7)

anatomy   The study of the structure of an organism (14)

anemia   A shortage of red blood cells (18)

aneroid sphygmomanometer   Dial-type blood pressure equipment (19)

anesthesia   Loss of feeling or sensation in a part or all of the body (28)

anesthesiologist   The medical doctor who administers the anesthetic to the patient in the operating room (28)

anesthetic   A drug used to produce loss of feeling; can be given orally, rectally, by injection, or by inhalation; a person who has been given an anesthetic is anesthetized (28)

anesthetist   The registered nurse who assists the anesthesiologist (28)

anger   A strong emotional response of displeasure, irritation, and resentment (34)

anterior   Located in the front; opposite of posterior (14)

antiembolism stockings   Designed to promote blood to flow and to prevent the formation of blood clots in the bloodstream (29)

anuria   Inability to urinate, no urine output (22)

anus   Muscular opening that controls elimination of stool from the rectum (20)

apathy   A lack of feeling or interest in things (33)

aphasia   Loss of language or speech (26)

apical pulse   A measurement of the heartbeats at the apex of the heart, located just under the left breast (19)

apnea   Periods of not breathing (19)

appendicitis   Inflammation (swelling and irritation) and infection of the appendix, typically with pain in the right lower quadrant; surgery called appendectomy is usually performed to remove the appendix (20)

artery Blood vessel that carries oxygenated blood away from the heart (18)

arthritis Chronic condition of inflammation of the joints (16)

asepsis The absence of microorganisms (germs); free of disease-causing organisms (5, 23)

aseptic Germ free, without disease-producing organisms (5)

aspirate Material (vomitus, food, or liquids) inhaled into the lungs (28)

assessing Gathering facts to identify needs and problems (8)

atrophic skin Thin, fragile, less elastic skin frequently associated with aging (17)

atrophy Wasting away of muscles; decrease in muscle size (16)

autoclave Device used to achieve sterility of an item through heat, pressure, and steam (5)

autonomic nervous system The part of the nervous system that carries messages without conscious thought (26)

axillary The area under the arms; the armpits (19)

bacteria Unicellular microorganism (5)

bargaining Trying to make a deal to change the situation (34)

bed alarm A control unit that activates an audible alarm and the nurse call system when the patient's weight leaves the pressure-sensitive mat for a preselected amount of time (6)

bed cradle A frame shaped like a barrel cut in half lengthwise that is used to keep bed linens off a part of the patient's body (9)

bed-bound Unable to get out of bed (11)

bedpan A pan used by patients who must defecate or urinate while in bed (9, 12)

bedridden Unable to get out of bed (7)

benign tumor A tumor that stays at its site of origin and does not usually regrow once removed (30)

bile Substance manufactured by the liver that helps the food breakdown process (20)

binder A type of bandage applied to a large body area (abdomen or chest) to secure a dressing in place or to put pressure on or support a body part (29)

bioterrorism Terrorist attacks using chemical or biological materials (13)

bladder distention A stretching out of the bladder when urine produced is not excreted (22)

blood and lymph tissue Tissue composed of singular cells that move within a fluid to every part of the body, circulating nutrients, oxygen, and antibodies and removing waste products (14)

blood pressure The force of the blood pushing against the walls of the blood vessels; the force of the blood exerted on the inner walls of the arteries, veins, and chambers of the heart as blood flows or circulates through the structures (18, 19)

body alignment The correct, or anatomical, positioning of a patient's body; also the arrangement of the body in a straight line (7)

body language Communication through hand movements (gestures), facial expressions, body movements, and touch (3)

bony prominences Places where bones are close to the surface of the skin (17)

boot up To start up the computer (3)

brachycardia Heart rate below 60 (19)

calibrated Marked with lines and numbers for measuring (22)

calorie Unit for measuring the energy produced when food is digested in the body (21)

calorie count Counting or adding up a total of all calories consumed in a 24-hour period (21)

cancer Refers to malignant neoplasms, or tumors (30)

cannula A flexible tube that can be inserted into a body cavity and used to draw fluids out or give oxygen or fluids (6)

canthus The inner aspect of the eye closest to the nose (26)

carbohydrate Type of basic food element used by the body; composed of carbon, hydrogen, and oxygen; includes sugars and starches (24)

cardiac Pertaining to the heart (18)

cardiac arrest The unexpected stopping of the heartbeat and circulation (13)

cardiac muscle tissue Involuntary muscle tissue found only in the heart (14)

cardiopulmonary resuscitation (CPR) An emergency procedure used to reestablish effective circulation and respiration in order to prevent irreversible brain damage (13)

cardiovascular system Circulatory system which includes heart, arteries, veins, and capillaries (13)

caregiver The family member or significant other who is taking the major responsibility for care of a patient (11)

catheter A device for draining urine out of the body (22)

cell The basic unit of living matter (14)

centigrade A system for measurement of temperature using a scale divided into 100 units or degrees; in this system, the freezing temperature of water is 0°C and water boils at 100°C; often referred to as Celsius (19)

central processing unit (CPU) Central processing unit, the "computer brain" where information is stored or directed to appropriate pathways (3)

cerebral spinal fluid The fluid that circulates around and within the brain and spinal cord (26)

cerebrovascular accident (CVA) Stroke; blockage or bleeding of blood vessels in the brain, interrupting the blood supply to that part of the brain and damaging the surrounding area of the brain (26)

chair alarm A battery-operated control unit that activates an audible alarm immediately if the patient gets up and out of the chair (6)

chemotherapy Refers to the use of drugs to treat cancer (30)

Cheyne-Stokes respiration One kind of irregular breathing. At first the breathing is slow and shallow; then the respiration becomes faster and deeper until it reaches a peak. The respiration then slows down and becomes shallow again. The breathing may then stop completely for 10 seconds and then begin the pattern again; this type of respiration may be caused by certain cerebral (brain), cardiac (heart), or pulmonary (lung) diseases or conditions (19)

chronological age Actual age in years and months (15)

circulation The continuous movements of blood through the heart and blood vessels to all parts of the body (18)

circulatory system The heart, blood vessels, blood, and all organs that pump and carry blood and other fluids throughout the body (18)

circumcise Remove the foreskin of the penis by surgical procedure (31)

circumference The distance around an object or body part, such as the head (15)

clean catch Refers to the fact that the urine for this specimen is not contaminated by anything outside the patient's body (23)

client An individual cared for by a home health agency or provider (4)

closed bed Bed made with bedspread in place (10)

clove hitch A type of knot that can be easily released in case of emergency (6)

cognition Awareness; the mental processes by which knowledge is acquired (6)

cognitive Pertaining to the mental processes by which knowledge perception, memory, or judgment is acquired (15)

commode A movable chair enclosing a bedpan with an opening that can fit over a toilet (12)

communication The exchange of thoughts, messages, or ideas by speech, signals, gestures, or writing between two or more people (3)

competency A demonstrable skill or ability (2, 35)

complex partial seizure Seizure with motor and possible sensory symptoms (such as muscle twitching and smelling a foul odor) and a change in the level of consciousness (26)

complication An unexpected condition, such as the development of another illness in a patient who is already sick (28)

compress Folded piece of cloth used to apply pressure, moisture, heat, cold, or medication to a specific part of the body (27)

confusion Bewilderment; the state of being disoriented to person, place, or time (6)

connective tissue Tissue that connects, supports, covers, lines, pads, or protects other body structures (14)

constipation Difficult, infrequent defecation with passage of unduly hard and dry fecal material (20, 31)

constrict Get narrower (27)

continuing education Formal classes, courses, or training programs to develop new knowledge or qualify one for career advancement (35)

continuous Uninterrupted, without a stop (20)

contract Get smaller; shortening the length of muscle, thereby making the angle formed by bones and muscles smaller (16)

contracture An abnormal shortening of a muscle (16); drawing together, bunching up, or shortening of muscle tissue because of spasm or paralysis, either permanently or temporarily (26)

convalescence The period of recovery after an illness or surgery (8)

convert Change (22)

convulsive Involving convulsions—rhythmic, involuntary contraction of muscles (26)

cooperation Working or acting together; uniting to produce an effect or to share an activity for mutual benefit (2)

courtesy Being polite and considerate (3)

cubic centimeter Having a volume equal to a cube whose edges are 1 centimeter long (22)

culture The thoughts, beliefs, and values of a social group (4)

cursor Flashing bar, or symbol, that indicates where the next character is to be placed or location on the computer screen (3)

customer-focused care Care designed to meet the needs of patients, residents, and clients (customers) (4)

cyanosis When the skin looks blue or gray, especially on the lips, nailbeds, and under the fingernails; in a black patient, it may appear as a darkening of color. This occurs when there is not enough oxygen in the blood (3, 27)

cystitis   Inflammation of the urinary bladder (22)

dangling position   Sitting up on the edge of the bed with the feet hanging down loosely (32)

data   Information that a user enters into a computer (3)

decubitus ulcers   Tissue breakdown resulting from pressure or reduced blood flow (often called pressure sores or bed sores) (10)

deep   Distant from the surface of the body (14)

deficit   A temporary or permanent negative change in a patient's usual neurologic function (26)

dehydrate   Loss of body fluids (31)

dehydration   A decrease in the amount of water in the tissues occurring when fluid output exceeds input or intake (22)

delirium   A disordered mental state that develops over a short period or time (6)

dementia   A progressive mental condition characterized by personality change; decline in intellectual capacity, judgement and memory; and impairment of impulse control (6, 32)

denial   Refusal to admit the truth or face reality (34)

dentures   Artificial teeth. Dentures may replace some or all of a person's teeth; they are described as being partial or complete and upper or lower (12)

dependability   A quality shown by coming to work every day on time and doing what is asked at the proper time and in the proper way (2)

depression   A state of sadness, grief, or low spirits that may or may not cause change of activity (33, 34)

dermis   The inner layer of skin (17)

deteriorate   To make or grow worse; degenerate (32)

development   The motor, language, cognitive, and social skills changes that occur in a person over the course of the life span (15)

diabetes mellitus   Disorder of carbohydrate metabolism caused by inability to convert sugar into energy because of inadequate production or utilization of insulin (24)

diabetic coma   A coma (abnormal deep stupor) that can occur in a diabetic patient from lack of insulin (24)

diagnosis   Finding out what kind of disease or medical condition a patient has; a diagnosis is always made by a physician (1)

diagnosis-related groups (DRGs)   Diagnostically related groups of patients; a DRG includes patients whose diagnoses are related, usually by body system or broad disease type, such as heart disease (1)

diaper   Washable or disposable covering applied to the perineal area for the purpose of containing stool or urine (31)

diarrhea   Frequent, watery stools; some causes of this problem are infection, certain particular foods, or complication from tube feedings; abnormally frequent discharge of fluid fecal material from the bowel (20, 31)

diastolic blood pressure   In taking a patient's blood pressure, one records the bottom number as the reading for the diastolic pressure; this is the relaxing phase of the heartbeat (19)

digestion   Breaking down the food that is eaten into a form that can be used by the body cells; this process is both mechanical and chemical (20)

dilate   Get bigger; expand (27)

discharge   The official procedure for helping patients to leave the health care institution, including teaching them how to care for themselves at home (8); flowing out of material (secretion or excretion) from any part of the body such as pus, feces, urine, or drainage from a wound (22)

disinfection   The process of destroying as many harmful organisms as possible (5)

disoriented   Unaware of or unable to remember, recognize, or describe people, places, or times; confused perception of reality (32)

disposable equipment   Equipment that is used one time only or for one patient only and then thrown away (9)

dorsal   Refers to the back or to the back part of an organ (14)

dorsal flexion   Bending backward (33)

dorsal lithotomy position   The position in which a patient lies on the back, with legs spread apart and knees bent (7)

dorsal recumbent position   Lying down or reclining; refers to the back or the back part of an organ (7)

drape   A covering used to provide privacy during an examination or operation (7)

draping   Covering a patient or parts of a patient's body with a sheet, blanket, bath blanket, or other material during a physical examination or prior to surgery (7)

draw sheet   Small sheet made of plastic, rubber, or cotton placed across the middle of the bed to cover and protect the bottom sheet and assist in moving the patient (10)

dry application   A warm or cold application in which no water touches the skin (27)

duodenum   The first loop of the small intestine (20)

dysphagia   Difficulty in speaking usually requiring evaluation by speech therapist (32)

dyspnea   Insufficient oxygenation of the blood resulting in labored or difficult breathing (19)

dysuria   Painful voiding (22)

-ectomy   A suffix that means surgical removal (Appendix A)

edema   Abnormal swelling of a part of the body caused by fluid collecting in that area; usually the swelling is in the ankles, legs, hands, or abdomen (3, 22)

efficiency   Getting all of one's duties completed in an organized fashion within a designated work period (11)

elective surgery   Chosen and not vital for health (28)

eliminate (defecate)   To rid the body of waste products; to excrete, expel, remove, put out (to have a bowel movement; to excrete waste matter from the bowels) (12, 22)

embolus   Blood clot or mass of other undissolved matter that travels through the circulatory system from its place of formation to another site, lodges in a small blood vessel, and causes an obstruction (26)

emergency   Events that call for immediate action (13)

emergency surgery   Surgery performed to save life and limb (28)

emesis basin   A pan used for catching material that a patient spits out, vomits, or expectorates (9)

empathy   The ability to put yourself in another's place and to see things as they see them (3)

endocrine glands   Ductless glands that produce hormones and secrete them directly into the blood or lymph (24)

endocrine system   System composed of endocrine glands; regulates body function by secreting hormones (24)

enema   Procedure of evacuation or washing out of waste materials (feces or stool) from a person's lower bowel (20)

enterally   Delivery of a nutrition formula through a tube for patients with a functional GI tract who are unable to take in adequate calories or food by mouth (21)

environment   All the surrounding conditions and influences affecting the life and development of an organism (26)

epidermis   The outer layer or surface of the skin (17)

epithelial tissue   Tissue that lines, protects, secretes, absorbs, and receives sensations (14)

equipment   Materials, tools, devices, supplies, furnishings, necessary things used to perform a task (9)

essential nutrients   Nutrients needed for the human body to function; they must be consumed in the diet every day (21)

estrogen   A female hormone that causes a buildup of the lining of the uterus to prepare it for possible pregnancy; also responsible for the development of secondary sexual characteristics (25)

ethical behavior   To keep promises and do what you should do; to act in accordance with the rules or standards for right conduct or practice (2)

ethnic diversity   The variety of races, religions, and cultures in the world (4)

evacuation   Discharge of the contents of the lower bowel through the rectum and anus (20)

evaluating   Determining whether a plan (such as the patient care plan) has been effective (8)

evaluation   Assessment of one's ability or skill to perform a given task (35)

evaporate   To pass off as vapor, as water evaporating into the air (22)

exhaling   The process of breathing out air in respiration (19)

exocrine glands   Glands that produce hormones and secrete them either directly or through a duct to epithelial tissue, such as a body cavity or the skin surface (24)

expectorate   To cough up matter from the lungs, trachea, or bronchial tubes and spit it out (23)

expired   Deceased, dead (34)

extension   Straightening or lengthening a muscle, thereby making the angle formed by bones and muscles greater (16)

extra nourishment   Snacks (21)

Fahrenheit   A system for measuring temperature. In the Fahrenheit system, the temperature of water at boiling is 212°. At freezing, it is 32°. These temperatures are usually written 212°F and 32°F (19)

family unit   A group brought together by shared needs, interests, and mutual concern for the well-being of all its members (11)

fan-fold   Method of arranging bed linens so that the covers and bedspread are folded at the foot of the bed out of the way (10)

fatigue   A feeling of tiredness or weariness (33)

fecal impaction   Hard, putty-like fecal material resulting from long retention of stool in the rectum (20)

feces   Solid waste material discharged from the body through the rectum and anus; other names include excreta, excrement, bowel movement, stool, and fecal matter (23)

feedback   Response of the receiver to the sender's message; the response, or feedback, lets the sender know if the message is acknowledged and clearly understood (3)

fertile   Able to become pregnant; capable of reproduction (25)

fertilization   Joining of a sperm and ovum to form a new cell (25)

fine motor   Refers to the movement of small muscles, such as those in the hands and fingers (15)

first aid   The first action taken to help a person who is in crisis (13)

flammable   Capable of burning quickly and easily (9, 11, 32)

flatus   Intestinal gas (20)

flex   To bend; the act of bending a body part (16)

flexion   Bending of a joint (elbow, wrist, knee) (16)

flow sheet   A checklist or chart for recording the activities of daily living (12)

flowmeter   A device used to control and regulate the flow of oxygen (6)

fluid   Applies to liquid substances (22)

fluid balance   The same amount of fluid that is taken in by the body is given out by the body (22)

fluid imbalance   When too much fluid is kept in the body or when too much fluid is lost (22)

fluid intake   The fluid taken into the body, from whatever source (22)

fluid output   The fluid passed or excreted out of the body; for example urine, vomit, diarrhea (22)

force   Strength or power; used to describe the beat of the pulse (19)

force fluids (FF)   Extra fluids to be taken in by a patient according to the doctor's orders (22)

formula   A liquid food prescribed for an infant containing most required nutrients (11)

Fowler's position   The position in which the head of the patient's bed is at a 45° to 90° angle (7)

fracture   A break in a bone (16)

fracture pan   A bedpan with a flat end that goes under the patient (12)

friction   The process of rubbing two surfaces together, such as skin (5)

friction injuries   Injuries resulting from the patient sliding against hard surfaces (17)

functional nursing   A method of organizing the health care team in which the head nurse assigns and directs all patient care responsibilities for the nursing staff; this is sometimes called direct assignment (1)

gait training   Rehabilitative exercise to help the patient improve walking ability (6)

gastrointestinal (GI) system   The GI tract is about 30 feet long and consists primarily of the mouth, esophagus, stomach, small intestines, and large intestines (20)

gastrostomy   An opening made through the abdomen to the stomach for the purpose of feeding (20)

gastrostomy tube (GT)   Tube inserted into the abdomen for the introduction of fluids (20)

gavage   Feeding through a nasogastric tube (20)

general anesthetics   General anesthetics cause loss of sensation in the entire body (28)

generalized   Affecting, involving, or pertaining to the whole body (27)

generalized application   A warm or cold application applied to the entire body (27)

genital   The external reproductive organs (23)

geriatric person   Aging; elderly; over 65 years of age (32)

gland   An organ that is able to manufacture and discharge a chemical that will be used elsewhere in the body (24)

glucose   A sugar formed during metabolism of carbohydrates; blood sugar (24)

graduate   A measuring cup marked along its side to show various amounts so that the material placed in the cup can be measured accurately; the marks are called calibrations (22)

gross motor   Refers to the movement of large muscles, such as those used in walking or hitting a ball (15)

growth   The physical changes that take place in a person's body over the life span (15)

gynecological (GYN) patient   Patient being treated for diseases or conditions of the female reproductive organs, including the breasts (25)

hand hygiene   General term that applies to either handwashing, antiseptic handwash, antiseptic hand rub, or surgical hand antisepsis (5)

hardware   The actual physical equipment that is used by a computer to process data

hazard   A source of danger; a possible cause of an accident (2)

health care-associated infection (HAI)   An infection acquired in a health care setting (5)

health care institution (facility)   Hospital, hospice, nursing home, convalescent home, or clinic where health care services are provided both on an inpatient and outpatient basis (1)

Health Insurance Portability and Accountability Act (HIPAA)   Federal regulations governing the privacy of medical records and encouraging electronic transactions (1)

heart   A four-chambered, hollow, muscular organ that lies in the chest cavity and pumps the blood through the lungs and into all parts of the body (18)

heart attack   Interruption or damage to the blood supply to the heart muscle; myocardial infarction (13)

hemiplegia   Paralysis of one-half of the body (26)

hemisphere   Half of a sphere; in the nervous system, one-half of the brain (26)

hemorrhage   The extreme or unexpected loss of blood; heavy/excessive bleeding (13, 26)

hepatitis B   Blood-borne disease; affects the liver and is easily transmitted within the health care setting following parenteral exposure (5)

hepatitis C   Prior to 1988 known as non A-non B hepatitis. Transmitted best through needle sticks and may result in chronic liver disease (5)

HIV   Human immunodeficiency virus; the microorganism that causes AIDS (25)

holistic   An approach that reflects the four dimensions of a whole person: physiological, psychological, sociocultural, and spiritual (8); intended to meet the needs of the whole patient; based on the belief that human beings function as complete units and cannot be effectively treated part by part (33)

homeostasis   Stability of all body functions at normal levels (22)

hormones   Protein substances secreted by endocrine glands directly into the blood to stimulate increased activity (24)

hospice   An extended, or long-term, care facility that provides health care services to terminally ill patients and their families (1); program that allows a dying patient to remain at home or in a nonhospital environment and die there while receiving professionally supervised care (34)

hospice care   The care of patients with terminal conditions who choose to remain at home until their death (11)

hospital   A short-term, or emergency, care facility that provides health care services to patients (1)

hygiene   The science that deals with the preservation of health; when used to describe an object or a person, it means clean and sanitary (2)

hyperglycemia   Abnormally high blood sugar (24)

hypertension   High blood pressure (19)

hyperthermia   A higher than normal body temperature (27)

hypoglycemia   Abnormally low blood sugar (24)

hypotension   Low blood pressure (19)

hypothalamus   Area of the brain responsible for control of the pituitary gland (26)

hypothermia   A very low body temperature (27)

immediate supervisor   An individual responsible for providing direction, critiquing performance, and giving feedback related to that performance (1)

immunocompromised   Means that the immune system is not functioning normally; *immunocompromised* and *immunosuppressed* mean the same thing and are used interchangeably (30)

implementing   Carrying out or accomplishing a given plan (8)

impulse   An electrical or chemical charge transmitted through certain tissues, especially nerve fibers and muscles (26)

incident   An unforeseen event that occurs without intent (2)

incontinence   Inability to control the bowels or bladder; inability to control urination or defecation (12, 33)

incontinent   Unable to control the bowels or bladder; unable to control urine or feces (7, 17, 22)

indwelling urinary catheter   A bladder drainage tube that is allowed to remain in place within the bladder (22)

infant   A baby aged 1 month to 1 year (31)

infection   Due to a pathogen producing a reaction that may cause soreness, tenderness, redness, and/or pus, fever, change in drainage, and so on (5)

infection control   The effort to prevent the spread of pathogens; restraining or curbing the spread of microorganisms (5, 11)

inferior   The lower portion of the body (14)

infiltration   Occurs when an IV solution runs into nearby tissue instead of into a vein (29)

inflammation   A reaction of the tissues to disease or injury; there is usually pain, heat, redness, and swelling of the body part (27)

informed consent   A voluntary act by which a conscious and mentally competent person gives permission for someone else to do something for him (2)

inhaling   The process of breathing in air in respiration (19)

insensible fluid loss   Fluid that is lost from the body without being noticed, such as in perspiration or air breathed out (22)

insulin   A hormone produced by the pancreas to help the body change sugar into energy; can be produced from an animal pancreas for use in the treatment of diabetes; hormone that regulates the sugar content of the blood (24)

insulin shock   Serious complication related to diabetes; occurs when the diabetic receives too much insulin, misses a meal, or has too much physical activity (24)

integumentary system   The body system that includes the skin, hair, nails, and sweat and oil glands, that provides the first line of defense against infection, maintains body temperature, provides fluids, and eliminates wastes (17)

intermittent   Alternating; stopping and beginning again; procedure that is stopped from time to time (20, 27)

interpersonal skills   Skills used in interacting with other persons, such as courtesy; good interpersonal skills enable people to interact or work together in a productive and satisfying manner (2)

intervertebral discs   The material between the vertebral bodies that cushions the spinal column (26)

intravenous infusion   The injection of fluids, nutrients, or medication into a vein (29)

intravenous pole   A tall pole, also called IV pole, which attaches to a bed or is on rollers or casters; this pole is used to hold the containers or tubes needed, for example, during a blood transfusion (9)

involuntary   Without conscious will, control, or decision (26)

irregular respiration   The depth of breathing changes and the rate of the rise and fall of the chest is not steady (19)

isolation   To separate or set apart (5)

-itis   A suffix that means inflammation (Appendix A)

joint   A part of the body where two bones come together (16)

keyboard   An input device similar to a typewriter keyboard; has additional keys that allow the user to make selections to direct computer activity (3)

knee-chest position   A bent posture with the knees and chest touching the examining table, sometimes used for examining the rectum or for women who have recently given birth, to allow the uterus to fall forward into its natural position (7)

labored respiration   Working hard to breathe (19)

lamb's wool   A wide strip of lamb's hide with the fleece attached or an imitation material used to increase patient comfort (9)

large intestine   Distal colon that absorbs water from stool (20)

lavage   The washing out of the stomach through a nasogastric tube, usually with normal saline (20)

lesion   An abnormality, either benign or cancerous, of the tissues of the body, such as a wound, sore, rash, boil, tumors, or growths (17)

ligament   Tough, white fibrous cord that connects bone to bone (16)

light pen   A hand-held device shaped like a pen that has an electronic sensor for making selections on a computer screen (3)

liver   Responsible for manufacturing bile and is a storage area for glucose; the liver also is the place where toxins, or poisons, are removed from the blood (20)

local anesthetics   Local anesthetics cause numbness or a loss of sensation in only a part of the body (28)

localized   Limited to one place or part; affecting, involving, or pertaining to a definite area (27)

localized application   A warm or cold application applied to a specific area or small part of the body (27)

log on   To sign on to the computer using a password or personal identification number (3)

long-term supportive care   The care of chronically ill patients who are unable to care for themselves and live alone or have limited family support (11)

lumpectomy   Removal of a small part of the breast (30)

malignant (neoplasms)   New growths that spread, invade, and destroy organs (30)

malnutrition   Poor nutrition status (21)

malpractice   Negligence when applied to the performance of a professional (2)

mastectomy   Removal of the entire breast (30)

medical asepsis   Special practices and procedures for preventing the conditions that allow disease-producing bacteria to live, multiply, and spread (23)

medical terminology   The special vocabulary of words used in the health care professions (Appendix A)

memory   The capacity of the computer to store data (3)

meninges   The covering of the brain and spinal cord. There are three layers: the dura mater, the arachnoid, and the pia mater (26)

menopause   Time during which menstruation stops, resulting in decreased hormone production and an end of fertility (25)

menstruation   Periodic (monthly) loss of some blood and a small part of the lining of the uterus when a woman is not pregnant (25)

mental health   Describes the best adjustment an individual can make at a given time, based on internal and external resources (30)

mental illness   Describes a number of chemical imbalances in the brain or genetically based brain diseases that interfere significantly with people's abilities to live and work (30)

mercury sphygmomanometer   Blood pressure equipment containing a column of mercury (19)

metabolism   The total of all the physical and chemical changes that take place in living organisms and cells, including all the processes involved in the use of substances taken into the body; the process through which food elements are converted into energy for use in the human body (24)

metastasis   Refers to the spreading of cancer cells through the systems of the body (30)

microorganism   A living thing that is so small it cannot be seen with the naked eye but only through a microscope (5, 11)

midstream   Catching the urine specimen between the time the patient begins to void and the time he stops (23)

mobility   Ability to move (33)

mobilization   Making movable; putting into action (33)

moist application   A warm or cold application in which water touches the body (27)

monitor   A screen, similar to a television screen, that allows the user to see input and output (3)

morgue   A place for temporarily keeping dead bodies for identification, autopsy, retrieval by funeral home staff, and burial (34)

motivation   Reason, desire, need, or purpose that causes a person to do something (33)

mouse A pointing and selecting device to input data; a small tabletop electronic pointing device used to make selections on a computer screen (3)

multidisciplinary team A team of professionals and nonprofessionals from different disciplines that plans, makes decisions, and implements the delivery of patient care that is focused, or centered, on the patient's needs rather than any particular discipline's (department's) needs (1)

muscle tissue Tissue that ensures movement; it is capable of stretching and contracting (14)

myelin sheath Protective covering around most nerves (26)

nasal Pertaining to the nose and nasal cavity (6)

nasogastric tube A tube placed through one of the patient's nostrils (naso-), down the back of the throat, and through the esophagus into the patient's stomach (-gastric) (20)

need A requirement for survival (4)

negligence The commission of an act or failure to perform an act, where the respective performance or nonperformance deviates from the act that should have been done by a reasonably prudent person under the same or similar conditions (2)

neoplasm (tumor) New growth; the words *tumor* and *neoplasm* are interchangeable (30)

nerve tissue Tissue that carries nervous impulses between the brain, the spinal cord, and all parts of the body (14)

nervous system The group of body organs consisting of the brain, spinal cord, and nerves that controls and regulates the activities of the body and the functions of the other body systems (26)

network Several computers that are connected or wired together, having access to central computer programs; can interface to obtain information; located at different workstations (3)

neuron A type of nerve cell in the nervous system (26)

nonambulatory Unable to walk (7)

normal flora Microorganisms that are necessary for health and usually live and grow in specific locations; they are nonpathogenic when in or on a natural reservoir (5)

normal pressure hydrocephalus A disorder caused by enlargement of the ventricles, fluid-filled spaces in the brain (26)

nosocomial infection Hospital-acquired infection (5)

nothing by mouth (NPO) Cannot eat or drink anything at all, usually past midnight the night before surgery or a procedure (22, 28)

nurse A person educated and trained to provide health care for people and to help physicians and surgeons; nurses are licensed as registered nurses (RNs) and licensed practical nurses (LPNs) (1)

nurse manager The RN leader responsible for the care delivery, personnel supervision, and operating budget of a unit, area, or facility (1)

nursing assistant A person who helps the registered nurse to care for patients; nursing assistants work in hospitals, long-term care or other health care facilities, or in the patient's home (1)

nutrient Chemical substances found in foods (21)

nutrition status assessment Assessment by an RN or RD as to what a patient eats and how the body uses it; determination of any special nutritional needs (21)

obese Very overweight (17)

objective observations Signs that can be observed and reported exactly as they are seen (3)

objective reporting Reporting exactly what you observe (3)

OBRA regulations Federal rules and requirements established by the Omnibus Budget Reconciliation Act of 1987 (6)

observation Gathering information about the patient by noticing any change (3)

occupational therapist Person trained to assist the patient with performing activities of daily living (33)

occupied bed Bed with a patient in it (10)

omit Leave out (21)

open bed Bed made with top sheet folded so as to give patient easy entrance (10)

oral Anything to do with the mouth; examples are eating and speaking (19)

oral hygiene Cleanliness of the mouth (12)

organ A part of the body made of several types of tissue grouped together to perform a certain function; examples are the heart, stomach, and lungs (14)

orientation An individual's ability to identify who she is, where she is, and some information about time (month, year, time of day) (30)

orthopedics The medical specialty that covers the treatment of broken bones, deformities, or diseases that attack the bones, joints, and muscles (16)

orthotics The science concerned with making and fitting prosthetic devices (33)

osteoarthritis A degenerative, painful bone disease affecting the spine, hips, finger joints, or knees (16)

osteoporosis Condition in which bones become brittle or thin and break easily (26)

ostomy A surgical procedure (operation) in which a new opening, called a stoma, is created in the abdomen, usually for the discharge of wastes (urine or feces) from the body (20)

ostomy appliance Collecting pouch usually attached to the skin around the stoma with adhesive (20)

ova/ovum   The female reproductive cell produced in the ovaries which is capable of uniting with a sperm cell and developing into a new organism (25)

ovulation   Process whereby an ovum is released from one ovary into the opening of the fallopian tube and moves to the uterus (25)

oxygen   A colorless, odorless, tasteless gaseous element that is essential for respiration; air is 21 percent oxygen (6)

palliative care   Care designed to comfort, instead of cure, the patient (34)

pancreas   Produces digestive juices and enzymes responsible for food breakdown in the small intestines (20)

parenteral intake   Fluids taken in intravenously (22)

parenteral nutrition   Nutrition therapy delivered by an IV catheter for patients with a nonfunctioning GI tract (21)

passive motion   Not active, but acted upon; enduring with effort or resistance (33)

password   A word or phrase that identifies a person and allows access to or entry to a program or record (3)

pathogen   Disease-producing microorganism (5)

pathologic   Involved with or caused by a disease (32)

patient   An individual admitted to an inpatient or outpatient hospital, physician office, or clinic (4)

patient lift   A mechanical device with a sling seat used for lifting a patient into and out of such equipment as the hospital bed, bathtub, or wheelchair (9)

patient plan of care   A written plan stating the nursing diagnosis, the patient goals or expected outcomes, and the nursing orders, interventions, or actions to be taken (8)

patient unit   The space for one patient, including the hospital bed, bedside table, chair, and other equipment (9)

patient-focused care   A care delivery model in which multidisciplinary teams plan, make decisions, and deliver care with the patient's needs being the focus rather than the needs or convenience of various departments or caregivers (1)

pediatric patient   Any patient under the age of 16 years (3, 31)

pelvic inflammatory disease (PID)   Infection that spreads to all structures in the pelvic cavity (25)

perineal area   See *perineum* (25)

perineum (perineal area)   The area of the body between the thighs; includes the area of the anus and the external genital organs; area between and around the urinary opening and the rectum (12, 17, 25)

peristalsis   Rhythmic contractions of the muscle walls of the small and large intestines (20)

peristaltic waves   Waves of involuntary contractions (22)

personal identification number (PIN)   Password (3)

perspiration   Sweat (22)

phlebitis   Inflammation of a vein (29)

physical crisis management   Methods for dealing with a dangerous situation involving a patient, resident, or client (4)

physical therapist   Person trained to assist the patient with activities related to motion (33)

physiological   Referring to a person's biological response to alterations in the body's structures and functions (8)

physiology   The study of the functions of the body dealing with the physical and chemical processes of cells, tissues, and organs of living organisms (14)

planning   Deciding what to do and how to do it (8)

plaque   Fatty deposits within blood vessels attached to vessel walls (26)

plasma   The liquid portion of the blood (18)

poison   Any substance ingested, inhaled, injected, or absorbed into the body that will interfere with normal physiological functions (13)

posterior   Located in the back or toward the rear (14)

postmortem   After death (34)

postoperative   After surgery (28)

postoperative bed   Bed made with top sheet folded lengthwise and positioned to one side, allowing transfer of the patient from the surgical stretcher to the bed without unnecessary movement (10)

pouching   Also known as pocketing of food; the retaining or holding of food in the mouth between the cheek and teeth (32)

preferred provider organization (PPO)   Organization that contracts with an employer to provide health care and physician's services to employees at a discounted rate (1)

prefix   A word element added to the beginning of a root (Appendix A)

preoperative   Before surgery (28)

pressure-sensitive mat   A disposable mat that is connected to a bed or chair alarm (6)

pressure ulcers   Also called bedsores; areas of the skin that become broken and painful; caused by continuous pressure on a body part and usually occur when a patient is kept in one position for a long period of time (17)

primary nursing   A patient-oriented method of organizing the health care team in which the professional registered nurses are responsible for the total nursing care of the patient (1)

printer   An output device for creating a hard copy (3)

prompt   A reminder that the user must take some action so further processing of the data can continue (3)

prone position   Lying on one's stomach (7)

proper/protective body mechanics   Special ways of standing and moving one's body to make the best use of strength and to avoid fatigue (7)

prosthetics   Artificial limbs or substitutes for missing body parts (33)

protective devices   Measures taken to keep a patient safe or to prevent injury (6)

psychological   Referring to a person's cognitive and emotional responses to the self and the surrounding environment (8); involving aspects of the mind, such as feelings and thoughts (33)

psychosocial   Involving aspects of living together in a group of people (33)

pulmonary   Pertaining to the lungs (18)

pulse   The rhythmic expansion and contraction of the arteries caused by the beating of the heart; the expansion and contractions show how fast, how regular, and with what force the heart is beating (19)

pulse deficit   A difference between the apical heartbeat and the radial pulse rate (19)

punctuality   Arriving at one's planned destination on time (11)

radial pulse   This is the pulse felt at a person's wrist at the radial artery (19)

radiation therapy   The use of high doses of radiation, many times the dose used for x-ray exams, to treat the cancer (30)

range-of-motion exercises   Exercises that move each muscle and joint through its full range of motion and help a confined patient exercise the muscles and joints (33)

rate   Used to describe the number of pulse beats per minute (19)

rectal   Pertaining to the rectum (19)

rectal irrigation   Repeated washing out of the rectum; clean water runs into the rectum, gas (flatus) and water run out of the rectum, as in the Harris flush (20)

rectum   The lowest portion of the large intestine, which curves in an S-shape and stores fecal material (20)

registered dietitian (RD)   Person responsible for the preparation of well-balanced regular and therapeutic (special) diets to meet patients' nutritional needs (21)

regular diet   A basic, or well-balanced, diet containing appropriate amounts of foods from each of the food groups (21)

rehabilitation   The process by which people who have been disabled by injury or sickness are helped to recover as much as possible of their original abilities for the activities of daily living (33)

rehabilitation nurse   A nurse with special training in the causes and treatment of disabilities; may be certified in this specialty with the title certified rehabilitation registered nurse (CRRN) (33)

relax   To place in a resting position, in which muscle tension decreases and fibers lengthen (16)

reproductive system   The group of body organs that makes possible the creation of a new human life (25)

resident   An individual cared for in a nursing home or other long-term/extended care facility (4)

residual   Remaining or left over (22)

respiratory system   The group of body organs that carries on the body function of respiration; the system brings oxygen into the body and eliminates carbon dioxide (18)

respond   React; begin, end, or change activity in reaction to stimulation (26)

responsibility   A duty or obligation; that for which one is accountable (11)

restorative care   Care given to help patients attain or maintain their highest level of function and independence (32, 33)

restraint   A device that physically restricts a person's freedom of movement, physical activity, or normal access to his or her body. Restraints are used as part of an approved protocol or as a result of a physician's order (6)

restraint alternative   Protective measures such as a saddle or wedge cushion, self-releasing belt, or lap tray that are used to help prevent falls but do not physically restrain an individual (6)

restrict fluids   Fluids that are limited to certain amounts (22)

retain   To keep or hold in (22)

retention   The patient keeps the enema fluid (oil) in the rectum for 20 minutes (20)

retrieval   To recall data stored in computer memory (3)

rheumatoid arthritis   A chronic disease condition affecting the connective tissue of the body, especially the joints (16)

rhythm   Used to describe the regularity of the pulse beats (19)

Rickettsiae   An example of bacteria found in the tissues of fleas, lice, ticks, and other insects; Rickettsiae are transmitted to humans by insect bites (5)

rigor mortis   The natural stiffening of a body and limbs shortly after death (34)

Roman numerals   The letters used to represent numbers in the ancient Roman system (Appendix A)

root   The body or main part of the word (Appendix A)

rupture   Break open (26)

saliva   The secretion of the salivary glands into the mouth; saliva moistens food and helps in swallowing; substance containing chemicals that begin to digest the food being chewed (20, 23)

screen A portion of data that is displayed at one time within the confined area of the computer monitor (3)

scrotal prep The procedures for making the genital area of a male patient ready for surgery; the preparation includes thoroughly cleansing the skin and carefully shaving the hair in the area (28)

secrete Produce and release into the body; glands secrete hormones (24)

secretions The substances that flow out of or are produced by glandular organs; the process of producing this substance; for example: sweat, bile, lymph, saliva, or urine (3)

seizure An episode, either partial or generalized, which may include altered consciousness, motor activity, or sensory phenomena and convulsions (13, 26)

self-care Activities or care tasks performed by the patient (12)

semi-Fowler's position The position in which the head of the patient's bed is at a 30° to 45° angle (7)

service Factors such as attentiveness, quality of food, and cleanliness of environment that affect the care and comfort of the individual receiving health care (4)

severe acute respiratory syndrome (SARS) a viral respiratory illness spread by close person-to-person contact (5)

sexually transmitted diseases (STDs) Diseases acquired as a result of sexual intercourse with an infected person (25)

shallow respiration Breathing with only the upper part of the lungs (19)

shear injuries Result from the skin remaining in place on top of a surface while the underlying structures, such as the bone, slide downward (17)

shock The failure of the cardiovascular system to provide sufficient blood circulation to every part of the body (13)

short-term intermittent skilled nursing care The care provided to acutely ill patients or those with an exacerbated illness with the purpose of educating the patients to become independent in self-care and functional ability (11)

side-lying (lateral) positions positioning the body on the right or left side, often done for comfort, to relieve pressure points, or to prevent skin breakdown (7)

simple partial seizure A seizure when the patient is aware of his surroundings but experiences either motor (muscle twitching or movement) or sensory changes (see or hear things not present) (26)

Sims's position Position in which the patient lies on the left side with the right knee and thigh drawn up, often used for a rectal examination; often called the enema position (7, 20)

sitz bath A bath in which the patient sits in a specially designed chairtub or a regular bathtub with the hips and buttocks in water (27)

skin prep Shaving the area of the body where an operation is going to be performed in preparation for surgery (28)

small intestine The first, smaller portion of the bowel, including the duodenum, where most of digestion and food breakdown occurs; also known as the small bowel (20)

soak Immerse the body or body part completely in water (27)

sociocultural Referring to a person's interpersonal responses to socialization practices in the family and community (8)

software Set or sets of instructions that direct computer operations; computer programs (3)

spasm An involuntary sudden movement or convulsive muscular contraction (26)

special diet See *therapeutic diet* (21)

specialty bed A bed that constantly changes pressure under the patient. Used to minimize pressure points in the treatment or prevention of pressure ulcers (9)

specimen A sample of material taken from the patient's body; examples are urine specimens, feces specimens, and sputum specimens (23)

sperm The male reproductive cell produced in the testes, which is released from the male during intercourse (25)

sphincter Ring-shaped muscle that surrounds and controls a natural opening in the body, such as the anus (20)

sphygmomanometer An apparatus for measuring blood pressure (19)

spinal anesthetics Anesthetics that cause a loss of feeling in a large area of the body, usually from the umbilicus down to and including the legs and feet (28)

spiritual Referring to an individual's personal response to forces; inspirational (8)

spores Bacteria that have formed hard shells around themselves as a defense (5)

sputum Waste material coughed up from the lungs or trachea (23)

staff development On-the-job training or classes provided to enhance or expand an employee's skills or abilities (35)

sterile field An area created to work from when you are doing a sterile procedure (5)

sterilization The process of killing all microorganisms, including spores (5)

sterilize Destroying all microorganisms (11)

stertorous respiration The patient makes abnormal noises like snoring sounds when breathing (19)

stethoscope   An instrument that allows one to listen to various sounds in the patient's body, such as the heartbeat or breathing sounds (19)

stimuli   Changes in the external or internal environment strong enough to set up a nervous impulse or other responses in an organism (26)

stoma   A surgically made opening connecting the urinary or intestinal tract with the outside, such as in an urostomy or colostomy (20)

stool   Solid waste material discharged from the body through the rectum and anus; other names include feces, excreta, excrement, bowel movement, and fecal matter (23, 31)

stress   A physical, mental, or emotional tension or strain triggered by a stimulus that requires some response or type of adjustment (2)

stretcher   A narrow rolling table or cart with or without a mattress or simply a canvas stretched over a frame used to transport patients; the latter may also be called a litter or a gurney; a wheeled cart in which patients are moved from one place to another (7, 9)

stroke   Interruption or damage to the blood supply to the brain; a cerebrovascular accident (13)

subacute care   Ongoing medical, nursing, rehabilitative, or dietary care provided to patients who need a lower level of care than an acute care (i.e., hospital) setting provides; categories of subacute care are based on the patient's health status and the type of care and length of care needed (33)

subjective observations   Symptoms that can be felt and described only by the patient himself, such as pain, nausea, dizziness, ringing in the ears, and headaches (3)

subjective reporting   Giving your opinion about what you have observed; the nursing assistant should never use subjective reporting (3)

substance abuse   The excessive use of mood-altering drugs such as alcohol, cocaine, tobacco, or caffeine that results in negative changes to a person's life (30)

suction   Using negative pressure to remove material, usually fluid (20)

suffix   A word element used to change or add to the meaning of a root; it is always added to the end of a root (Appendix A)

sundowning syndrome   A state of increased confusion and disorientation that usually occurs in persons with cognitive dysfunction as evening approaches (32)

superficial   On or near the surface of the body (14)

superior   The upper portion of the body (14)

supine position   Lying on one's back (7)

suppository   A semisolid preparation, sometimes medicated, that is inserted into the vagina or rectum (33)

system   A group of organs acting together to carry out one or more body functions (14)

systolic blood pressure   The force with which blood is pumped when the heart muscle is contracting; when taking a patient's blood pressure, the systolic blood pressure is recorded as the top number (19)

tachycardia   Heart rate over 100 (19)

tact   Doing or saying the right things at the right time (3)

task oriented   Nursing care that is arranged according to what must be done (1)

team leader   The nurse responsible for one area of a nursing unit, including patient care assignments (1)

team nursing   A task-oriented method of organizing the health care team in which the team leader gives patient care assignments to each team member (1)

terminal   A computer monitor that allows the computer operator to see input and output on a screen (3)

terminally ill   Having an illness that can be expected to cause death, usually within a predictable time (34)

testosterone   The primary male sex hormone manufactured in the testes, which is essential for normal sexual behavior and the development of secondary sexual characteristics (25)

therapeutic diet   Any special diet (21)

thermometer   An instrument used for measuring temperature (19)

thrombophlebitis   Inflammation and blood clots in a vein (29)

thrombus   A blood clot that remains at its site of formation (26)

time/travel record   Record or log describing how time is spent in a patient's home and/or account of travel time to and from the patient's home or running errands (11)

tissue   A group of cells of the same type (14)

tissue fluid   A watery environment around each cell that acts as a place of exchange for gases, food, and waste products between the cells and the blood (22)

traction   Exertion of pull by means of weights or pulleys, often used for realignment of bones or other limb tissues (16)

transfer   Moving a hospital patient from one room, unit, or facility to another (8)

transmission   The spread of microorganisms (5)

transporting   Moving something or someone from one place to another (7)

trapeze   A triangle-shaped bar attached to the overbed frame of a traction setup which enables the patient to pull himself up in bed (16)

Trendelenburg's position   Position in which the bed or operating table on which a patient is lying is tilted so that the patient's head is about one foot below the level of his or her knees, to allow more blood flow to the head and prevent shock; also called shock position (7)

tuberculosis (TB)   A highly infectious disease that usually affects the lungs (18)

umbilical cord   Rather long, flexible, rough organ that carries nourishment from the mother to the baby; it connects the umbilicus of the unborn baby in the mother's uterus to the placenta (31)

unconscious   Unaware of the environment; occurs during sleep and in temporary episodes ranging from fainting or stupor or coma (28)

unilateral neglect   Failure of a patient disabled on one side of the body to dress, bathe, or otherwise care for that side because the patient forgets the side exists (33)

urethra   A small tube that serves to empty urine from the bladder to the external environment (22)

urinal   A portable container given to male patients in bed so they can urinate without getting out of bed (9,12)

urinary system (excretory system)   The group of body components including the kidneys, ureters, bladder, and urethra that removes wastes from the blood and produce and eliminates urine (22)

urinate   To discharge urine from the body; other words for this function are void, micturate, and pass water (12, 22)

urine   The fluid secreted by the kidneys, stored in the bladder, and excreted through the urethra (22)

vagina (vaginal canal)   The canal leading from the cervix to the outside of the female body; serves as the organ for intercourse and the birth canal (25)

vaginal irrigation (douche)   The introduction of a solution into the vagina with an immediate return of the solution by gravity; usually used for cleansing the vaginal canal or relieving inflammation of the vaginal tract (25)

vaginal prep   The procedures for making the genital area of a female patient ready for surgery; the preparation includes thoroughly cleansing the skin and carefully shaving the pubic hair; it may also include a cleansing douche (28)

validation therapy   A way of communicating with confused people (32)

vascular   Pertaining to blood vessels (26)

vein   Blood vessel that carries blood from parts of the body back to the heart (18)

ventilator   A machine that mechanically breathes for and provides oxygen to sustain a patient unable to inhale or exhale on his own (33)

ventral   On the abdominal, anterior, or front side of the body (14)

vertebral bodies   The bones around the spinal cord (26)

vertigo   Dizziness (32)

virus   A type of microorganism; much smaller than bacteria that can survive only in other living cells (5)

vital signs   Measurements reflecting the patient's physical well-being and condition (19)

void   To urinate, pass water (22, 28)

voluntary   Under control of the will; with conscious decision (26)

walker   A metal frame device with handgrips and four legs that is open on one side; provides stability and security for the patient who is weak on one side or restricted in the amount of weight he can put on one foot; a stable frame made of metal tubing used to support the unsteady patient while walking; the patient holds the walker while taking a step, moves it forward, and takes another step (9, 16)

wheelchair   A chair on wheels used to transport patients (9)

Index

S

PERSONAL CARE

What would you like to wear?	¿Qué se quiere poner?
Put on/Take off your...	Póngase / Quítese su/sus...
bathrobe	bata de baño
bra	sostén / sujetador
braces	frenillos
coat	abrigo
dentures	dentadura
glasses	anteojos / lentes
hearing aid	audífonos
make-up	maquillaje
pants	pantalones
shirt	camisa
shoes	zapatos
socks	medias / calcetines
underwear	ropa interior
Wash your...	Lave su/sus...
(Body parts are labeled on figures I and II)	
Brush your hair.	Cepille su pelo.

VITAL SIGNS

I'm going to take your temperature.	Voy a tomarle la temperatura.
I'm going to take your blood pressure.	Voy a tomarle la presíon arterial.
Give me your hand. I need to take your pulse.	Déme su mano. Necesito tomarle el pulso.
Get undressed, please, from the waist up.	Por favor, desvístase de la cintura para arriba.
Wait for the doctor here.	Espere al doctor aquí.
Put on this gown.	Póngase esta bata.

> ► The letter **v** is pronounced like a **b**.
> ► The letter **z** is pronounced like the **s** in *sock*.
> e.g., **zapatos** (shoes) *sah-pah-tos*

PAIN

Are you having any pain?	¿Tiene algún dolor?
Where does it hurt?	¿A dónde le duele?
How long have you had the pain?	¿Hace cuánto tiempo que tiene este dolor?
Is it constant?	¿Es un dolor constante?
Does it come and go?	¿El dolor viene y se va?
Is the pain..	¿Es el dolor.....
sharp?	agudo?
dull?	leve?
aching?	constante?
knifelike?	¿Como si le estuvieran acuchillando?
Have you had medicine for the pain?	¿Ha tomado medicina para el dolor?
Does the medicine relieve the pain?	¿La medicina alivia el dolor?

SYMPTOMS

Did you sleep well?	¿Duerme usted bien?
Are you nauseated?	¿Tiene usted náuseas?
Have you been vomiting?	¿Ha estado vomitando?
Do you have a fever?	¿Tiene fiebre?
Do you have chills?	¿Tiene escalofríos?
Do you feel dizzy?	¿Se marea usted?
Do you have a headache?	¿Tiene usted dolor de cabeza?
Do you feel short of breath?	¿Siente a veces problemas al respirar?
Do you cough a lot? Does anything come up? What color is it?	¿Tose mucho? ¿Vota algo al toser? ¿De qué color es?
green/yellow/clear/red	verde/amarillo/claro/rojo
Do you have..	¿Tiene..
double vision?	doble visión?
pain in your eyes?	dolor en los ojos?
Do you have spots before your eyes?	¿Ve chiribitas delante de sus ojos?

> ► The letter **j** is pronounced like an **h**. e.g., **rojo** (red) *ro-ho*
> ► The letter **r** is always rolled when it appears at the beginning of a word.

> ► When **c** appears before **a**, **o**, or **u**, it is pronounced as a **k**.
> e.g., **cara** (face) *ka-rah*

> ► When **c** appears before **e** or **i**, it is pronounced like an **s**.
> e.g., **cintura** (waist) *seen-too-rah*

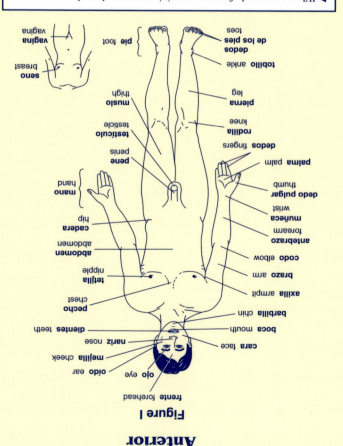

Figure I

Anterior

vagina — vagina
seno — breast
pie foot — pie
toes — dedos de los pies
tobillo — ankle
muslo — thigh
pierna — leg
testículo — testicle
rodilla — knee
pene — penis
dedos — fingers
palma — palm
mano — hand
pulgar — thumb
muñeca — wrist
cadera — hip
antebrazo — forearm
abdomen — abdomen
codo — elbow
tetilla — nipple
brazo — arm
pecho — chest
axila — armpit
barbilla — chin
dientes — teeth
boca — mouth
nariz — nose
mejilla — cheek
cara — face
oído — ear
ojo — eye
frente — forehead

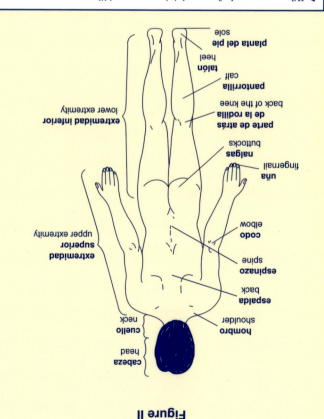

Figure II

Posterior

planta del pie — sole
talón — heel
pantorrilla — calf
parte de atrás de la rodilla — back of the knee
nalgas — buttocks
uña — fingernail
extremidad inferior — lower extremity
codo — elbow
espinazo — spine
espalda — back
extremidad superior — upper extremity
cuello — neck
hombro — shoulder
cabeza — head

CLINICAL POCKET TRANSLATOR

This handy reference is designed to help you provide the best care possible to your Spanish-speaking patients. English phrases and their Spanish translations are divided into ten practical topics for improved communication in the clinical setting.

Here are a few simple pronunciation tips to get you started...

❑ Knowing how to pronounce the Spanish vowels is key.

> **a** is pronounced like the a in *father*
> **e** is pronounced like the e in *bet*
> **i** is pronounced like the ee in *tree*
> **o** is pronounced like the o in *low*
> **u** is pronounced like the oo in *spoon*

❑ You will see that some words have an **a** or an **o** in parentheses. That means that you use an **a** or an **o** according to the gender of the person that you are speaking to. Usually, you use an **o** when speaking to a male and an **a** when speaking to a female. For example, if you wanted to say "welcome" to a new client you would say,

"Bienvenido" to a **male**   or   "Bienvenida" to a **female**

❑ To help you improve your pronunciation, additional tips appear at the bottom of each panel next to the ▶ icon.

PLEASE NOTE: THIS POCKET REFERENCE IS NOT A SUBSTITUTE FOR AN INTERPRETER. ALERT YOUR SUPERVISOR OR FOLLOW YOUR EMPLOYER'S POLICY TO ACCESS AN INTERPRETER'S SERVICE WHEN CIRCUMSTANCES REQUIRE MORE COMPLEX COMMUNICATION WITH A PATIENT.

GREETINGS AND INTRODUCTIONS

Hello/Hi	Hola
Welcome	Bienvenida(o)
Good morning; good afternoon;	Buenos días; buenas tardes;
good evening/goodnight	buenas noches
My name is _____.	Me llamo _____. Mi nombre _____.
What is your name?	¿Cómo se llama usted?
I only speak a little Spanish.	Sólo hablo un poco de español.
It is a pleasure to meet you.	Mucho gusto.
Is someone here with you today?	¿Ha venido con alguien?
Does he or she speak English?	¿Habla él o ella inglés?
I will call the interpreter.	Voy a llamar al intérprete.
The interpreter will be coming in a few minutes.	El intérprete vendrá en unos minutos.
How are you?	¿Cómo está usted?
How do you feel today?	¿Cómo se siente hoy?
well/so-so/not well	bien/regular/mal
Goodbye	Adiós
See you later.	Hasta luego.

ORIENTATION / MENTAL STATE

Can you tell me where you are?	¿Me puede decir a dónde está?
hospital / nursing home	hospital / casa de reposo
Can you tell me what day it is?	¿Me puede decir qué día es hoy?

Sunday	domingo
Monday	lunes
Tuesday	martes
Wednesday	miércoles
Thursday	jueves
Friday	viernes
Saturday	sábado

▶ The letter **h** is always silent, i.e. **hola** (hello) *oh-la*.

▶ The letter **ñ** has the nasal "ny" sound like the first **n** in the English word *union*. e.g., **español** (Spanish) *es-pahn-yol*

COURTESY AND ASSISTANCE

Please	Por favor
Thank you	Gracias
You're welcome.	De nada; No hay de qué.
Pardon me.	Perdón.
Excuse me.	Con permiso.
I'm sorry.	Lo siento.
Do you understand?	¿Entiende? / ¿Comprende?
I understand.	(Yo) entiendo. / (Yo) comprendo.
I don't understand.	No entiendo. / No comprendo.
I don't know.	No sé.
I'll be right back.	Regresaré enseguida.
I'm going to get someone who can help.	Voy a traer a alguien que le pueda ayudar.
Do you need the nurse?	¿Necesita a la enfermera?
If you need help, push this call button.	Si necesita ayuda, presione este botón.
I'll get the nurse.	Voy a traer a la enfermera.

DAILY ACTIVITIES

Would you like something to eat?	¿Le gustaría comer algo?
Would you like something to drink?	¿Le gustaría tomar / beber algo?
Do you need to go to the bathroom?	¿Necesita ir al baño?
I'm going to help you walk.	Le voy a ayudar a caminar.
I'm going to move you to the chair/bed/toilet.	Le voy a poner en la silla / la cama / el inodoro.
Sit down, please.	Por favor, siéntese.
I'm going to reposition you.	Le voy a cambiar de posición.
Do you feel hot/cold?	¿Siente calor / frío?
Are you comfortable?	¿Está comfortable?

▶ When **g** appears before **a**, **o** or **u**, it is pronounced as a **g**. e.g., **gracias** (thank you) *grah-see-ahs*

▶ Double **l** (**ll**) is pronounced like the **y** in *yes*. e.g. **silla** (chair) *see-yah*.

EATING AND ELIMINATION

How is your appetite?	¿Cómo está su apetito?
Do you like your diet?	¿Le gusta su dieta?
Are you hungry?	¿Tiene hambre?
Are you thirsty?	¿Tiene sed?
Do you have gas?	¿Tiene gases?
Do you suffer from indigestion?	¿Sufre usted de indigestión?
Urinary problems?	¿Problemas urinarios?
Are you constipated?	¿Está usted estreñida (o)?
When was your last bowel movement?	¿Cuándo fue la última vez que defecó?
Do you have diarrhea?	¿Tiene usted diarrea?
Do you urinate without difficulty?	¿Orína sin dificultad?
Do you have to get up at night to urinate?	¿Tiene que levantarse por las noches para orinar?
How many times?	¿Cuántas veces?

PEOPLE, PLACES AND THINGS

bath	tina/bañera	medicine	medicina
bathroom	cuarto de baño/ baño	nurse	enfermero(a)
bed	cama	oxygen	oxígeno
blanket	cobija	pillow	almohada
book	libro	shower	ducha
cane	bastón	staff	personal
chair	silla	telephone	teléfono
cup	taza	television	televisión
doctor	doctor(a)	tissue	pañuelo
door	puerta	toilet	inodoro / el water
food	comida/alimento	walker	andador
hydraulic lift	elevador mecánico	water	agua
juice	jugo/zumo	water pitcher	jarra de agua
light	luz	wheelchair	silla de ruedas
magazine	revista	window	ventana

▶ When **g** appears before **e** or **i**, it is pronounced as an **h**.
e.g., **oxígeno** (face) *ŏx-ee-hĕ-no*